Review for
NCLEX–PN

Fifth Edition

Sandra F. Smith, RN, MS

Los Altos, California

International Standard Book Number: 0-917010-57-4

In the writing of this text, the authors and publisher have made every attempt to follow current nursing practice and to ensure that suggested diets, drug selection and dosages, and nursing procedures are up to date and conform with current recommendations and practices at time of publication. However, in view of new research conclusions, technological advancements, and government regulations, it is the responsibility of the nurse to be aware of any changes that may alter suggested drug and diet therapies or nursing protocols. The authors recommend that nurses and nursing students be aware of hospital and school policies regarding their role and responsibilities in performing nursing actions. The authors and publisher disclaim any liability, loss or damage incurred as a result of direct or indirect use of this book.

Copies of this book may be obtained from:

National Nursing Review
342 State Street, Suite 6
Los Altos, CA 94022
1-800-950-4095

Contributing Authors

Chapter Contributors

Mary Bierly, RN, BSN
School of Practical Nursing
Columbus Public Schools, OH

Arlene Thorsness Kostoch, RN, PhD
Del Mar College, TX

Eva Nunn Gumke, RN, BSN
Hartnell College, CA

Patricia Ann Morrissey, RN, MS
Edna McConnell Clark School of Nursing, NY

Doris E. Nay, RN, MA
Boulder Valley Health Occupations, CO

Fay Alger O'Brien, RN, MA
De Anza College, CA

Section Contributors

Sharon Matusoff Bell, RN, BSN, MA
Health Occupations
Columbus Public Schools, OH

Barbara Enderle, RN, BSN
School of Practical Nursing
Columbus Public Schools, OH

Patricia Parr Graves, RN
School of Practical Nursing
Columbus Public Schools, OH

Judith Hankin, RN, BS, MS
Lively Area Vocational-Technical Center, FL

Sandra Harper, RN, BSN
Dallas Vocational Nursing Program, TX

Susan Tamburro Keiser, RN, BS, EdD
School of Practical Nursing
Columbus Public Schools, OH

PREFACE

During your practical nursing program, you have studied nursing theory and gained clinical experience. Now you face the important challenge of scoring sufficiently high in the National Council Licensure Examination to qualify for PN/VN licensure. The objective of this book is to provide you with a comprehensive, current and complete review of practical nursing content.

National Nursing Review is pleased to offer the fifth edition, totally revised and updated, of our PN/VN review book, written to assist you to prepare for your licensure exam. Most licensure candidates do not know how to review the vast amount of material to which they have been exposed during their nursing education. A key objective of this book is to help you prepare for NCLEX-PN in the easiest and most efficient manner.

An effective preparation method is to thoroughly review the material most likely to be covered on the exam and to take practice tests having similar questions. With this program in mind, **_Review for NCLEX-PN_** is organized into 14 chapters. The outline format is designed to help you review quickly, as well as to emphasize significant content. The selection and presentation of content in this book are directed toward minimizing your review time while maximizing your test results.

The question and answer sections, simulated NCLEX-PN CAT test, serve a dual purpose: (1) to acquaint you with the type of questions to expect on the examination, and (2) to give you an opportunity to test and improve your knowledge of nurse-patient situations. The answers and rationale sections are also intended to discourage rote memorization and reinforce learning by demonstrating the underlying principles which explain why the answers are right or wrong.

Acknowledgments

I wish to extend my thanks to all of the contributing authors and to the many other people who helped with the development of this book. Because of the invaluable assistance of the editors, graphic designers, typesetters, and book manufacturer, this review book is available to help students prepare for the current NCLEX.

Sandra F. Smith

CONTENTS

CHAPTER 7 MEDICAL-SURGICAL NURSING 119

CHAPTER 12 **PEDIATRIC NURSING   377**

1

PREPARING FOR NCLEX-PN

INTRODUCTION

Review for NCLEX-PN is designed to assist candidates for practical/vocational nurse licensure to prepare for the National Council Licensure Examination-PN. This text focuses on nursing skills, the practical nurse's responsibilities, major disease processes, and nursing care related to common health problems within the framework of the nursing process and client needs. The nursing content in this book is presented in outline format to help you focus your review on the most important information and utilize your review time most effectively.

A thorough review of the material in this book will enable you to recognize your areas of expertise. You can then concentrate on studying the less familiar content. The review questions at the end of the book will assist you to test your mastery of basic nursing principles and their application to clinical situations.

The following sections in this chapter provide general background information on PN licensure, the NCLEX Test Plan, and Computer Adaptive Testing, followed by helpful techniques for studying and achieving positive test results.

PN/VN LICENSURE PROCEDURES

The NCLEX-PN measures the licensure candidate's competence to perform safe and effective entry-level nursing practice. The boards of nursing of all 50 states, the District of Columbia, and the U.S. territories of Guam, the Virgin Islands, American Samoa, Puerto Rico, and the Northern Mariana Islands administer this screening test as developed by the National Council of State Boards of Nursing (NCSBN). This system of licensure provides protection for health care consumers and defines common entry-level standards throughout the U.S. In order to take the NCLEX, the candidate for licensure applies to the board of nursing in the state or jurisdiction in which the candidate plans to practice nursing. A complete list of the State Boards of Nursing is included as Appendix 1 to Chapter 14.

THE NCLEX-PN TEST PLAN FRAMEWORK

The NCSBN is responsible to provide its member boards of nursing with a psychometrically sound and legally defensible licensure examination. The purpose of the NCLEX-PN is to separate licensure candidates into two groups: those who can demonstrate minimal competence to perform safe and effective entry-level nursing care, and those who cannot. Although administration of the test via computerized adaptive testing (CAT) is a new procedure implemented in 1994, the basic test plan that provides the framework for presenting the questions has remained essentially unchanged since 1989. The NCSBN contracts with clinical nurses and nurse educators to write questions (referred to as test items) that test your ability to apply your knowledge of vocational/practical nursing. The test questions focus on job tasks normally performed by entry-level PNs during their first 6 to 12 months on the job. The NCSBN identifies these tasks by conducting extensive surveys, called job analyses, about every three years. It is entirely possible that your PN program may have included instruction on certain tasks that are not considered to be entry level by the NCSBN's job surveys. It is also possible that your PN program may not have provided you with instruction on some of the tasks about which questions have been included in the current test pool.

The job analysis studies are also used to help validate the test plan and to provide the basis for the proportional distribution of questions among the various subjects covered by the test. The test's two most significant conceptual areas are the Nursing Process and Client Needs. The following sections describe each phase of the Nursing Process, define the four broad categories of Client Needs, and list the 17 subcategories of Client Needs.

The Nursing Process

The phases of the Nursing Process that are measured by NCLEX-PN include Collecting Data, Planning, Implementing, and Evaluating. The accompanying chart shows the percentage of questions that are allocated to each phase.

The Nursing Process—Question Allocation	
Collecting Data	25–35%
Planning	15–25%
Implementing	25–35%
Evaluating	15–25%

Collecting Data for patient care contributes to the patient's data base by observing; collecting information from the patient, significant others, health team members, and the records; determining the need for additional information; communicating the findings; and using this data to participate in formulating a nursing diagnosis.

Planning patient care involves contributing to the development of a nursing care plan for patients with specific health needs; assisting in formulating goals; participating in identifying the patient's needs and nursing measures necessary to achieve goals; identifying needs; and communicating with the patient, significant others, and health team members in planning nursing care.

Implementing patient care includes performing basic therapeutic and preventive nursing measures; providing a safe and effective care environment; assisting the patient, significant others, and health care members to understand the care plan; and recording patient information and reporting it to the appropriate health team members.

Evaluating patient care involves assisting in evaluating the patient's response to nursing care and making appropriate alterations; evaluating the extent to which identified outcomes of the care plan are achieved; and recording and describing the patient's responses to the care.

Client Needs

The basic health needs of patients are grouped under 4 broad categories and 17 subcategories that are weighted according to the results of the job analysis studies conducted by the NCSBN. The emphasis on each category is summarized by the percentage breakdown of questions on NCLEX as noted in the accompanying chart.

Client Needs—Question Allocation	
Safe, Effective Care Environment	24–30%
Physiological Integrity	42–48%
Psychosocial Integrity	7–13%
Health Promotion and Maintenance	15–21%

Safe, Effective Care Environment

To assist in meeting the patient's needs in this area, the practical nurse must be able to provide the following:
• Coordinated Care
• Standards of Care
• Goal-oriented Care
• Environmental Safety
• Preparation for Treatments and Procedures
• Safe and Effective Treatments and Procedures†

Physiological Integrity

To assist in meeting the patient's needs for physiological integrity—this includes acute and/or chronically recurring physiological conditions, as well as potential complications—the practical nurse must be able to provide nursing care in the following areas:
• Physiological Adaptation
• Reduction of Risk Potential†
• Mobility
• Comfort
• Provisions of Basic Care†

† Indicates areas of greater job importance; therefore, more emphasis is given to presenting questions in these than other subcategories.

Psychosocial Integrity

To assist in meeting the patient's needs for psychosocial integrity during periods of illness and for common health problems that occur throughout the life cycle, the practical nurse must be able to provide nursing care in the following areas:
• Psychosocial Adaptation
• Coping/Adaptation†

Health Promotion and Maintenance

To assist in meeting the patient's needs for health promotion and maintenance throughout the life cycle, the practical nurse must be able to provide nursing care in the following areas:
• Continued Growth and Development
• Self-Care†
• Integrity of Support System
• Prevention and Early Treatment of Disease

Adapted from **NCLEX-PN Test Plan for the National Council Licensure Examination for Practical Nurses.** National Council of State Boards of Nursing, Chicago, 1989.

COMPUTERIZED ADAPTIVE TESTING

With the introduction of Computerized Adaptive Testing (CAT) in 1994, the procedures for taking the NCLEX changed radically from prior protocol. The major new elements include:
(1) Locating test sites throughout the U.S. where each candidate makes an appointment to take the test on an individual basis.
(2) Presenting the test on a computer screen rather than in a printed test booklet. Answer selections are made by pressing keys on a computer keyboard instead of marking an answer sheet with a pencil.
(3) Each candidate's test is unique because the computer selects each subsequent question based upon the candidate's prior answers.

The Advantages of CAT

CAT is described as providing a more comfortable and convenient way to take NCLEX. The testing environment at a Sylvan Technology Center will be similar to a small classroom or learning laboratory in contrast to a large hall or convention center with the distractions and tension associated with a large group of candidates taking the test simultaneously. From a procedural standpoint, the advantages of CAT are defined as:
(1) A more efficient way to test and measure competency than the prior pencil and paper test format.
(2) Reduction of testing time to a maximum of five hours in one test session.
(3) Greater security and the avoidance of inconvenience to candidates if security measures break down.
(4) Year-round testing schedules that provide applicants with greater flexibility and convenience than the prior twice-per-year system.
(5) Substantial reduction in the time required between applying to take NCLEX and receiving one's results.

NCLEX Administrative Organizations

Three organizations are involved with administering NCLEX: (1) boards of nursing from each state or jurisdiction, (2) the Educational Testing Service (ETS), and (3) Sylvan Learning Systems. As a candidate for licensure, it will help you to know the role of each organization.

As described earlier in this section, the NCSBN designs the test plan, conducts the job analysis, and sets the passing standard. The Educational Testing Service formulates the test questions to conform to the National Council's Test Plan. ETS maintains a test pool of several thousand questions written by specially selected item writers approved by the state boards of nursing. All NCLEX questions are drawn from this test pool. You will make an appointment with and physically take the NCLEX-PN at a Sylvan Technology Center.

Approximately 200 of these centers are available throughout the U.S. for NCLEX testing.

NCLEX-CAT Application Procedures

After the state (jurisdiction) in which you plan to practice accepts your application and verifies your eligibility to take the NCLEX, you will receive an Authorization to Test and other information that includes the locations and telephone numbers of the Sylvan Technology Centers. You will then contact a test center of your choice to make an appointment to take the test. The test center does not need to be located in the state to which you have applied for licensure. As a first time test taker, you should be able to schedule your appointment within 30 days of your call. Read all instructions carefully, especially noting the items that you must bring to the test center.

Taking the NCLEX-CAT

Upon arriving at the Sylvan Technology Center, you will present your Authorization to Test and two forms of identification, both signed and one with a photo. A driver's license, school or employee I.D., and passport are the most accepted forms. A social security card is an example of an unacceptable proof of identity. At check-in, you will be photographed and thumb printed. Before commencing the test questions, you will complete a brief computer tutorial to make certain that you are comfortable with the keyboard procedures. The National Council advises that no prior computer experience is necessary for CAT.

Two types of questions appear on NCLEX. The real questions test your competency and safety and provide the basis for your pass or fail score. The tryout questions are items being field tested for future NCLEX exams. You have no way of knowing the difference between real and tryout.

The minimum number of questions for each candidate will be 60 real and 15 to 25 tryout for a total of 75 to 85. The National Council maintains that the essential Test Plan categories can be covered by 60 carefully selected questions. The maximum number of real questions will be 180, so by adding the 15 to 25 tryouts, you could answer a total of 205 items.

Because the number of questions is flexible, from 75–85 to 195–205, there is no maximum time you should spend per question. However, because you won't know how long it will take you to reach the 95% confidence level, it is not wise to spend several minutes on many questions. If you don't know the answer, guess and move on, rather than spend five minutes and risk becoming immobilized.

CAT does not allow you to skip questions, change answers, or go back to look at questions already answered. Each question has an assigned degree of difficulty. Based on your prior answers—correct or incorrect—the computer selects the next question. Therefore, you must answer each question as it is presented. Because the computer draws from a large pool of questions, each candidate's test is unique. There is no absolute passing score in terms of the number or percent of questions that you must answer correctly in order to pass.

After you have answered the minimum number of questions, your test continues until the computer calculates with a 95% degree of confidence that you fall into the safe/competent group or that you do not. Although there is no minimum amount of time for your test, the maximum allowable test duration is five hours, including your computer tutorial and rest breaks. A mandatory rest break of 10 minutes is required after two hours of testing and an optional break is available after the next one and one-half hours.

The results of your test will be electronically transmitted from the Sylvan Technology Center where you take the test to Educational Testing Service in Princeton, New Jersey, for processing. Within 48 hours, ETS will forward your results to the board of nursing to which you applied for licensure. Your results—pass or fail—will be sent to you by the board of nursing. A failure report will be accompanied by a diagnostic analysis to help you identify your specific areas of weakness. The time required for the board of nursing to notify the candidate will vary from state to state.

NCLEX-PN/CAT Quick Reference

Test Location: Sylvan Technology Centers

Minimum Number of Questions: 75 to 85

Maximum Number of Questions: 195 to 205

Minimum Testing Time: None

Maximum Testing Time: 5 hours

GUIDELINES FOR NCLEX REVIEW

Familiarize Yourself with the Organization of Material in This Book

Review for NCLEX-PN summarizes extensive nursing content to which you have been introduced during your PN training. The material is organized into 14 chapters and presented in outline format for your review. Nursing theory and practical applications of this theory are included for each major subject area. Nursing theory includes pathophysiology, signs and symptoms of diseases, diagnosis and treatment of medical conditions, and the appropriate nursing care. The tables, appendices and glossaries are distributed throughout the book to assist you to efficiently review factual material. Familiarize yourself with how the contents are organized by chapter and how the Nursing Process is integrated throughout the book.

The multiple-choice questions that follow the content review are similar in format, subject matter, length, and degree of difficulty to those contained in the NCLEX-PN. The answer and rationale sections provide you with an added learning experience; if you understand the basic principles of nursing content, you can transfer that knowledge to the clinical situations and questions on the NCLEX.

Your Personal Review Program

Ideally, you will begin your review process several months prior to NCLEX; but if, like most students, you allocate only a few weeks to prepare for this exam, it is important that you conduct the review process in an efficient manner. The following recommendations are offered to help you achieve maximum results for the amount of time invested.

A. Schedule regular periods for your study and review.
   1. Arrange to study when mentally alert. Studying during periods of mental and physical fatigue reduces your efficiency.
   2. Allow short breaks at relatively frequent intervals. Breaks used as rewards for hard study serve as incentives for continued concentrated effort. A 10 to 15 minute break is recommended after each hour of concentrated study.

B. Analyze your strengths and weaknesses.
   1. Consider past performance on classroom tests and written clinical applications of factual material. Learn from your past errors on tests by looking up and studying the correct material in this book.
   2. Analyze your results on practice questions. Identify topics where your knowledge or understanding is weak. These areas will require a more thorough review.
   3. Allow sufficient time for repeated review in this book of subject areas that continue to be difficult for you.

C. Familiarize yourself with the examination format.
   1. Review the NCLEX Test Plan description so that you understand the Nursing Process and Client Needs categories. Notice which areas have the greater number of questions and allocate more of your review time to these topics.
   2. Study the format used for NCLEX-PN questions. You must know how to read, evaluate and respond to multiple-choice questions similar to the ones at the end of this book.

D. Systematically study the material contained in each chapter of this book.
1. First, gain a general impression of the content unit to be reviewed. Skim over the entire section and identify the main ideas.
2. Then, read and study the tables, glossaries, and appendices carefully.
3. Mark key material that is not thoroughly understood.
E. Follow up on your priority areas.
1. Set priorities on the material that is to be learned or reviewed. Identify the most crucial sections and underline the essential thoughts.
2. Review what you have read. Think of examples that illustrate the main points you have studied.
3. To be sure that you have learned the material, write down the main ideas or explain the major points to another person.
F. Test yourself by completing practice questions.
1. Complete the simulated NCLEX-PN CAT test of 180 practice questions included in this book. A computer disk, attached inside the back cover, contains the same questions that begin on page 467.
2. After completing the questions on the disk, you can obtain your Performance Summary which will help you identify your strengths and weaknesses in terms of Nursing Process, Client Needs and Clinical Area. You will also be able to obtain a list of the questions you answered incorrectly.
3. Refer to the rationales printed at the back of this book in order to understand the principles underlying the answers for all of the practice questions. By studying the rationales, you will learn new information and solidify material that you have mastered already.
4. If you do not have access to an IBM or IBM-compatible computer, you can complete the questions manually and check your results by referring to the answer and rationale section that follows the questions.
5. *NCLEX-PN Review Questions*, also by Sandra Smith, contains an additional 360 questions with answers and rationales.

Test-Taking Strategies

The following test-taking strategies can provide you with useful guidelines when answering questions. These strategies are neither absolute nor fool-proof; they are intended to guide you to choose the best response for each question.

A. Carefully read each question. Determine what the question is really asking. Some details may not be important. Mentally note important factors; pay attention to key terms and phrases. For example, do not misread grams as milligrams.

B. When answering multiple-choice questions, an effective strategy is to first eliminate the answers that you know are wrong, and then spend time deciding among the remaining answers. If you are not sure about any of the four possible answers, you will have to make an educated guess. Remember, you are not allowed to skip a question, nor will you be able to change any of the answers you have selected on earlier questions.

C. A first "hunch" is usually correct. Many candidates have a first impression, choose an answer, and, upon reflection, change their mind. Sensing that a particular alternative is correct has some basis. Your brain has made rapid connections. You came to an immediate conclusion based on your knowledge and experience. Because you did not go through the logical steps of arriving at the correct solution, it does not mean that your choice is incorrect.

D. Be alert for a question that requires you to identify which answer is not correct. Read the question as it is stated, not as you would like it to be stated.

E. The most comprehensive answer is often the best choice. For example, if two alternatives seem reasonable but one answer includes the other (i.e., it is more detailed, extends the first answer, or is more comprehensive), then this answer may be the best choice.

F. Eliminate answers that focus on medical knowledge or contain nursing actions that are performed by an RN. Remember, this is a

PN/VN test, and the questions are designed to test your competency and safety. It is unlikely that a question will require a medical or RN action for the correct answer; it may, however, offer these actions as distractors.

G. Evaluate the answers in relation to the stem (the question), not to other answers. Choose the answer that best fits the question rather than an answer that appears to be a correct statement but may not fit the question.

H. Eliminate answers that are obviously different from what is logically right, such as an answer given in grams when other choices are given in milligrams.

I. Do not look for a pattern to the answers. The questions are chosen at random, and the same number may possibly and correctly answer several consecutive questions.

J. Be on guard for answers that contain qualifiers such as always and never. They rarely fit within a logical framework. However, some situations may be true only when a qualifier is added.

K. If a clinical situation precedes a question, read the situation very carefully. Identify the essential ideas. Be careful of answer selections that divert your attention from key ideas.

L. Scratch paper will be available for you to use when making or checking calculations. This will assist you to determine the correct answer before entering your selection.

Final Preparation

A. The night before the test.
   1. Assemble the materials needed for the test as specified in your instructions from the Sylvan Technology Center.
   2. Get a good night's sleep. Do not stay up all night trying to learn new material.
   3. Avoid the use of stimulants or depressants, either of which may affect your ability to think clearly during the test.
   4. Approach the test with confidence and the determination to do your best. Think positively and concentrate on all that you do

know rather than on what you think you do not know.

B. The day of the test.
   1. Eat a good breakfast. Do not rush.
   2. Allow ample time to travel to your testing site, including time to park, and to present your Authorization to Test, two proofs of identity, and any other required documents.
   3. If possible, choose a station in the testing room where you are least likely to be distracted by other people taking tests.

THE IMPORTANCE OF A CONFIDENT ATTITUDE

Anxiety, a forceful deterrent to test-taking success, interferes with your ability to think clearly. Anxiety blocks the search and retrieval process so that you cannot access the knowledge held in your "memory bank." Fear of the unknown is a major source of anxiety. This fear can be overcome by diligent review. As you gain mastery over the nursing content, your self-confidence increases. It is also important to understand test construction and test-taking strategies. This introductory chapter is designed to reduce many of the unknowns associated with NCLEX-PN and to provide you with review guidelines and test-taking techniques.

These strategies are guidelines, not absolutes. Always use your own judgment, knowledge, and nursing experience. These personal assets will serve you well when taking the NCLEX-PN. Be confident that you will pass, and, in fact, you will.

Please Note: You will notice ❖ **PROCEDURE** ❖ appearing throughout this book. This symbol identifies a nursing skill. Because the current PN/VN test plan emphasizes performance of nursing skills, you can expect many NCLEX questions to focus on these procedures. Please review them thoroughly.

2

Nursing Through the Life Cycle

HOMEOSTASIS: STRESS AND ADAPTATION

Homeostasis

Definition: The maintenance of a constant state in the internal environment through self-regulatory techniques that preserve the organism's ability to adapt to stresses.

A. Dynamics of homeostasis.
   1. Danger or its symbols, whether internal or external, result in the activation of the sympathetic nervous system and the adrenal medulla.
   2. The organism prepares for flight or fight.
B. Adaptation factors.
   1. Age—adaptation is greatest in youth and young middle life, and least at the extremes of life.
   2. Environment—adequate supply of required materials is necessary.
   3. Adaptation involves the entire organism.
   4. The organism can more easily adapt to stress over a period of time than suddenly.
   5. Organism flexibility influences survival.
   6. The organism usually uses the adaptation mechanism that is most economical in terms of energy.
   7. Illness decreases the organism's capacity to adapt to stress.
   8. Adaptation responses may be adequate or deficient.
   9. Adaptation may cause stress and illness, i.e., ulcers, arthritis, allergy, asthma, and overwhelming infections.

Stress

A. Definitions of stress.
   1. A physical, a chemical, or an emotional factor that causes bodily or mental tension and that may be a factor in disease causation; a state resulting from factors that tend to alter an existing equilibrium.
   2. Selye's definition of stress.
      a. The state manifested by a specific syndrome that consists of all the nonspecifically induced changes within the biologic system.
      b. The body is the common denominator of all adaptive responses.
      c. Stress is manifested by the measurable changes in the body.
      d. Stress causes a multiplicity of changes in the body.
B. General aspects of stress.
   1. Body responses to stress are a self-preserving mechanism that automatically and immediately becomes activated in times of danger.
      a. Caused by physical or psychological stress: disease, injury, anger, or frustration.
      b. Caused by changes in internal and/or external environment.
   2. There are a limited number of ways an organism can respond to stress (for example, a cornered amoeba cannot fly).

Selye's Theory of Stress

A. General adaptive syndrome (GAS).
   1. Alarm stage (call to arms).
      a. Shock: the body translates as sudden injury, and the GAS becomes activated.
      b. Countershock: the organism restored to its preinjury condition.
   2. Stage of resistance: the organism is adapted to the injuring agent.
   3. State of exhaustion: if stress continues, the organism loses its adaptive capability and goes into exhaustion, which is comparable to shock.
B. Local adaptive syndrome (LAS).
   1. Selective changes within the organism.
   2. Local response elicits general response.
   3. Example of LAS: a cut, followed by bleeding, followed by coagulation of blood, etc.
   4. Ability of parts of the body to respond to a specific injury is impaired if the whole body is under stress.

C. Whether the organism goes through all the phases of adaptation depends both upon its capacity to adapt and the intensity and continuance of the injuring agent.
   1. Organism may return to normal.
   2. Organism may overreact; stress decreases.
   3. Organism may be unable to adapt or maintain adaptation, a condition that may lead to death.
D. Objective of stress response.
   1. To maintain stability of the organism during stress.
   2. To repair damage.
   3. To restore body to normal composition and activity.

Psychological Stress

Definition: All processes that impose a demand or requirement upon the organism, the resolution or accommodation of which necessitates work or activity of the mental apparatus.

Characteristics

A. May involve other structures or systems, but primarily affects mental apparatus.
   1. Anxiety is a primary result of psychological stress.
   2. Causes mental mechanisms to attempt to reduce or relieve psychological discomfort.
      a. Attack/fight.
      b. Withdrawal/flight.
      c. Play dead/immobility.
B. Causes of psychological stress.
   1. Loss of something of value.
   2. Injury/pain.
   3. Frustrations of needs and drives.
   4. Threats to self-concept.
   5. Many illnesses cause stress.
      a. Disfigurement.
      b. Sexually transmitted disease.
      c. Long-term or chronic diseases.
      d. Cancer.
      e. Heart disease.
   6. Conflicting cultural values, i.e., the American values of competition and assertive vs. the need to be dependent.
   7. Future shock: physiological and psychological stress resulting from an overload of the organism's adaptive systems and decision-making processes brought about by too rapidly changing values and technology.
   8. Cultural shock: stress developing in response to transition of the individual from a familiar environment to unfamiliar one.
      a. Involves unfamiliarity with communication, technology, customs, attitudes, and beliefs.
      b. Examples: individual moving to new area from foreign country or individual placed in hospital environment.

Assessment

   1. Assess increased anxiety, anger, helplessness, hopelessness, guilt, shame, disgust, fear, frustration, or depression.
   2. Evaluate behaviors resulting from stress.
      a. Apathy, regression, withdrawal.
      b. Crying, demanding.
      c. Physical illness.
      d. Hostility, manipulation.
      e. Senseless violence, acting out.

Implementation

A. Gather information about patient's internal and external environment.
B. Modify external environment so that adaptation responses are within the capacity of patient.
C. Support the efforts of patient to adapt or respond.
D. Provide patient with the materials required to maintain constancy of internal environment.
E. Understand body's mechanisms for accommodating stress.
F. Prevent additional stress.
G. Reduce external stimuli.
H. Reduce or increase physical activity depending on the cause of and response to stress.

GROWTH AND DEVELOPMENT MILESTONES

Children

One Month

A. Physical and motor development.
1. Follows with eyes to midline.
2. Follows bright, moving objects with eyes.
3. Lifts head slightly from prone.
4. Lies awake on back with head averted.
5. Keeps fists clenched.
6. Responds to sharp sounds, i.e., bell, etc.
7. Does not grasp objects.

B. Language and social development.
1. Regards face, may smile.
2. Responds to voice.
3. Makes throaty noises.
4. Is alert about one out of every ten hours.

C. Appropriate games and stimulation.
1. Smile and talk to infant.
2. Touch, stroke, cuddle.
3. Talk and sing to infant.
4. Play soft music.
5. Play with infant.
6. Hold infant while feeding.
7. Provide toys such as colorful, hanging mobiles.

Two Months

A. Physical and motor development.
1. Ceases activity to listen for a bell.
2. Follows better vertically and horizontally with jerky eye movements.
3. Moves arms and legs vigorously.
4. Lifts head to 45 degrees when prone on abdomen.
5. Turns from side to back.
6. Grasp becomes voluntary.
7. No longer exhibits crossed extensor reflex.

B. Language and social development.
1. Vocalizes and smiles responsively.
2. Visually follows moving person.
3. Makes single vowel sounds such as "ah," "eh," "uh."
4. Differentiates by crying.
5. Begins social smile.
6. Exhibits tactile and oral stimulation, not social.

C. Appropriate games and stimulation.
1. Smile and talk to infant.
2. Use cradle gym and infant seat.
3. Allow infant the freedom of kicking with clothes off.
4. Place infant in prone position on floor or in bed.
5. Expose infant to different textures.
6. Exercise infant's arms and legs.
7. Provide bright pictures and hanging objects that move.

Three Months

A. Physical and motor development.
1. Lifts head and chest when prone.
2. Brings objects to mouth.
3. Displays nimble and busy fingers.
4. Rotates head from side to side.
5. Improves convergence.
6. Discovers and stares at hands.
7. Briefly holds toy in hand.

B. Language and social development.
1. Babbles, pronounces initial vowels, and coos.
2. Smiles more readily.
3. Ceases to cry when mother enters room or caresses him or her.
4. Enjoys playing during feeding.
5. Stays awake longer without crying.
6. Turns head to follow familiar person.

C. Appropriate games and stimulation.
1. While infant prone on abdomen, move bright object upward to encourage head movement.
2. Bounce infant on bed.
3. Continue to introduce new sounds.
4. Provide social stimulation (important).
5. Play with infant during feeding.
6. Provide rattles, large soft animals.

Four Months

A. Physical and motor development.
1. Infant lifts head and shoulders to a 90-degree angle.
2. Looks ahead while in prone position on abdomen.
3. Can follow object 180 degrees.
4. Can move from side to side; tries to roll over.
5. Grasps for toy with whole hand.
6. Brings hands or toys to mouth.
7. Sucks thumb or fist.
8. Begins teething.
B. Language and social development.
1. Coos, gurgles, and laughs aloud.
2. Begins babbling.
3. Knows mother.
4. Imitates mother.
5. Demands attention by fussing.
6. Begins to respond to "no."
7. Enjoys being placed in sitting position with support.
8. Responds to and enjoys being handled.
C. Appropriate games and stimulation.
1. Show child his or her reflection in mirror.
2. Increase sensory stimulation.
3. Give frequent baths as infant enjoys splashing in tub.
4. Play music as child is quieted by it.
5. Move mobile out of reach; child may grab it and injure self.
6. Repeat child's sounds to him or her.
7. Provide soft, colorful squeeze toys; rattles, mirror; toys whose parts cannot be removed.

Five to Six Months

A. Physical and motor development.
1. Visually pursues lost object.
2. Holds block in each hand.
3. Exhibits hand-eye coordination.
4. Sits for short periods leaning forward on hands.
5. Creeps and rocks.
6. Reaches for objects beyond grasp.
7. Rolls from back to stomach and stomach to back.
8. Weighs twice as much as at birth.
B. Language and social development.
1. Begins to recognize strangers.
2. Shows fear and anger.
3. Vocalizes vowel sounds and well-defined syllables.
4. Shows anticipation; waves and raises arms to be picked up.
5. Expresses protest.
6. Understands name.
C. Appropriate games and stimulation.
1. Play sitting-up games.
2. Encourage reaching for objects.
3. Provide teething toys, soft blocks and squeeze toys, metal cup and wooden spoon for banging.

Seven to Nine Months

A. Physical and motor development.
1. Reaches for objects unilaterally.
2. Can transfer a toy.
3. Exhibits complete thumb opposition.
4. Sits alone steadily with good coordination.
5. Advances from creeping to crawling.
6. Can pull self to feet with assistance.
7. Feeds self a cracker.
8. Develops eye-to-eye contact while talking.
9. Engages in social games.
B. Language and social development.
1. Begins imitative expressions.
2. Shows fear of strangers.
3. Makes polysyllable vowel sounds.
4. Play is self-contained.
5. Laughs out loud.
6. Listens to conversations.
C. Appropriate games and stimulation.
1. Play social games such as peek-a-boo and pat-a-cake.
2. Allow child to drop and retrieve toys.
3. Allow child to play with spoon at feeding.
4. Give child soft finger-foods.
5. Take safety precautions as child puts everything into mouth.
6. Show excitement at child's achievements.

7. Provide squeeze toys in bath, toys that make noise, large nesting toys, crumpled paper.

Ten to Eleven Months

A. Physical and motor development.
   1. Sits without support indefinitely.
   2. Pulls self to feet.
   3. Stands on toes with support.
   4. Creeps and cruises very well.
   5. Can pick up objects fairly well.
   6. Uses index finger and thumb to grasp.
   7. Can hold own bottle or cup.
   8. Shows interest in tiny objects.
B. Language and social development.
   1. Has vocabulary of one to two words ("Mama," "Dada").
   2. Recognizes meaning of "no."
   3. Shows moods; looks hurt, sad.
   4. Is very aware of environment.
   5. Responds to own name.
   6. Imitates gestures, facial expressions, sounds.
   7. Begins to test parental reaction during feeding and at bedtime.
   8. Entertains self for long periods of time.
C. Appropriate games and stimulation.
   1. Use plastic bottle.
   2. Protect child from dangerous objects.
   3. Have child with family at mealtime.
   4. Allow exploration outdoors.
   5. Provide new objects (blocks); toys that stimulate; containers (milk cartons); toys that can be filled, emptied, knocked down, and stacked up; fabric books.

Twelve to Eighteen Months

A. Physical and motor development.
   1. Stands and walks alone.
   2. Puts objects in and out of containers; can release objects at will.
   3. Points to indicate wants.
   4. Holds a cup with both hands.
   5. Throws a ball.
   6. Looks at pictures with interest.

7. Triples birth weight at 12 months; has closed anterior fontanel.
   8. Begins to develop fine muscle coordination.
   9. Has protruding abdomen.
B. Language and social development.
   1. Is aware of expressive function of language; uses jargon, imitates sounds.
   2. Cooperates in dressing; removes socks.
   3. Likes an audience and will repeat performance.
   4. Shows anxiety about strangers.
   5. Distinguishes self from others.
   6. Has a vocabulary of ten meaningful words.
   7. Finds security in a blanket, favorite toy, or thumb sucking.
   8. Plays alone but near others (parallel play).
   9. Is dependent upon parents but shows first signs of desire for autonomy.
C. Appropriate games and stimulation.
   1. Make no attempt to change from use of left to right hand.
   2. Provide frequent changes of environment.
   3. Allow self-directed play rather than adult-directed play.
   4. Continue to expose child to different foods.
   5. Show affection and encourage child to reciprocate.
   6. Create safe environment (medications locked up and harmful items out of reach).
   7. Provide pull and push toys, Teddy bears, pots and pans, musical toys, telephone, sand box and fill toys, cloth picture books with colorful, large pictures.

Eighteen Months to Two Years

A. Physical and motor development.
   1. Exhibits well developed eye accommodation.
   2. Walks up and down stairs one at a time with pauses.
   3. Turns door knobs; climbs on furniture.
   4. Chews more effectively.
   5. Walks and runs with a stiff gait and wide stance.

6. Uses a spoon without spilling.
7. Builds tower of six cubes.
8. Kicks a ball in front of him or her without support.
9. Has daytime bladder and bowel control; occasional accidents; nighttime control not complete.

B. Language and social development.
1. Displays receptive vocabulary of 200 to 300 words; speaks vowels correctly.
2. Begins to use short sentences.
3. Has fear of parents leaving.
4. Helps to undress; tries to button.
5. Wants to hoard and not share: "snatch and grab stage."
6. Violently resists having toys taken away.
7. Begins to have feelings of autonomy.
8. Begins process of identification; uses "no" as assertion of self.
9. Begins cooperation in toilet training.

C. Appropriate games and stimulation.
1. In toilet training, allow child to follow own pattern.
2. Provide peer companionship.
3. Allow child to eat with family.
4. Provide role-modeling for positive behavior (important for child).
5. Provide building blocks, wagons, pull toys, pounding toys like a drum, books with pictures.

Two and One-Half Years

A. Physical and motor development.
1. Pushes and pulls large toys.
2. Jumps; squats to play.
3. Builds tower of eight blocks.
4. Copies horizontal and vertical strokes.
5. Feeds self, uses fork.
6. Pours from pitcher.
7. Can undress.
8. Begins to use scissors.
9. Has full set (20) of baby teeth.

B. Language and social development.
1. Knows full name.
2. Refers to self by pronoun "I."

3. Shows negativism, has temper tantrums, and is ritualistic.
4. Learns power of "yes" and "no."
5. Shows poorly developed judgment.
6. Can tolerate short periods of separation from parents.
7. Begins to identify sex (gender) roles.
8. Explores environment outside the home.
9. Engages in associative play.

C. Appropriate games and stimulation.
1. Allow child his or her preferences.
2. Control temper tantrums.
3. Allow ritualism, especially at night.
4. Be aware that negativism and ritualism is normal behavior at this age.
5. Provide discipline as a way of socializing and educating child. Discipline simply for the sake of establishing authority is counterproductive.
6. Use firmness and consistency.
7. Read simple book to child to help develop language and memory skills.
8. Provide manipulative toys for muscle coordination, crayons and paper, simple games.

Three Years

A. Physical and motor development.
1. Goes up and down stairs, alternating feet.
2. Rides tricycle.
3. Stands momentarily on one foot.
4. Swings, climbs.
5. While running, can stop suddenly or turn corners.

B. Language and social development.
1. Begins to cooperate but is still self-centered.
2. Begins imaginative and make-believe play.
3. Wants to please.
4. Knows own age and sex, and the concept of *one*.
5. Verbalizes toilet needs and goes to toilet by self (needs help wiping).
6. Uses "I," "me," "you" speech.
7. Has vocabulary of 900 words.

8. Begins to understand what it means to take turns.
9. Can remember and repeat three numbers.
C. Appropriate games and stimulation.
1. Encourage and promote social contacts and imaginative outlets.
2. Alternate group activity with solitary play.
3. Listen to child's conversations and narratives.
4. Base expectations within child's limitations.
5. Provide climbing apparatus, keys, tricycle, wagons, dump trucks, simple puzzles, music, record player.

Three to Four Years

A. Physical and motor development.
1. Has 20/20 vision.
2. Races up and down steps.
3. Skips, hops, performs stunts; has good balance.
4. Draws man with two to four parts besides the head.
5. Cuts on line with scissors.
6. Feeds self.
7. Dresses self; laces shoes but cannot tie; buttons.
8. Brushes teeth.
B. Language and social development.
1. Asks abundant questions: What? Why? How?
2. Recites nursery rhyme or poem, or sings a song.
3. Gives full name.
4. Shows interest in world: nurses, firemen, police, doctors.
5. Begins to share; seeks peer relationships.
6. Exhibits excessive imaginative and make-believe play.
7. Displays less negative behavior.
8. Can tolerate separation from mother longer.
C. Appropriate games and stimulation.
1. Encourage widening horizon and exploration of environment, imagination, peer relationships.

2. Encourage pretending, story telling, expressing.
3. Give simple explanation as to cause and effect.
4. Provide alternate periods of active and quiet play.
5. Provide books, puzzles, drawing materials, puppets.

Four to Five Years

A. Physical and motor development.
1. Exhibits improved muscle coordination; is more agile and graceful; jumps, hops, skips on alternate feet.
2. Draws recognizable pictures.
3. Is quieter and less restless; has greater concentration.
4. Draws triangle and square from copy.
5. Names four colors, the heavier of two weights, and the longer of two lines.
6. Builds steps.
7. Exhibits good posture; carries arms near body; narrows stance.
8. Transports objects in trucks and cars.
9. Dresses and undresses with skill but still needs some supervision.
B. Language and social development.
1. Exhibits improved concept and language development.
2. Asks questions about the meaning of words.
3. Prints simple words.
4. Is cooperative, has poise, and controls behavior.
5. Is creative.
6. Is capable of longer attention span; completes activities; shows imaginative, dramatic play.
7. Displays planning, space, depth, expression, and creativity in drawing.
8. Begins to develop an elementary conscience.
9. Displays high energy during play.
C. Appropriate games and stimulation.
1. Give kind but unmistakable discipline.
2. Build self-confidence.

3. Provide consistent control.
4. Encourage responsibility for putting things away.
5. Widen and vary experiences in reading and music.
6. Enroll child in kindergarten.
7. Encourage group play and cooperation and sharing in projects.

Five to Six Years

A. Physical and motor development.
   1. Improves balance.
   2. Begins to ride two-wheel bicycle.
   3. Runs skillfully and plays games at the same time.
   4. Is able to wash without wetting clothing.
   5. Begins to lose baby teeth.
   6. Exhibits good control with small motor movements.
   7. Catches a ball.
   8. Shows little awareness of dangers, but has good motor development.
   9. Uses hands as manipulative tools in cutting, pasting, hammering.
B. Language and social development.
   1. Has well-developed vocabulary.
   2. Repeats sentence of 10 syllables or more.
   3. Talks constantly.
   4. Is cooperative.
   5. Does simple chores at home.
   6. Begins to take responsibility for actions.
   7. Understands units such as a week or month.
   8. Knows right and left hand.
   9. Still requires parental support but pulls away from overt signs of affection.
C. Appropriate games and stimulation.
   1. Provide family atmosphere conducive to child's emotional development.
   2. Give guidance and limits, but avoid humiliating punishment.
   3. Provide sufficient exercise to stimulate motor and psychosocial development.
   4. Include other children for stimulation during play.
   5. Provide books, games, bicycle.

Six to Seven Years

A. Physical and motor development.
   1. Begins growth spurt.
   2. Is very active, impulsive.
   3. Dresses self.
B. Language and social development.
   1. Defines words by use.
   2. Shows more independence in play.
   3. Enjoys group play in small groups.
   4. Begins to accept authority outside home.
   5. Considers ideas of teachers important.
   6. Learns to read.
   7. Knows number combinations to ten.
C. Appropriate games and stimulation.
   1. Provide opportunity for collecting various items.
   2. Provide imaginary dramatic play: "dress up," school, firemen, soldiers; table games (tiddlywinks, marbles); dolls.

Seven to Eight Years

A. Physical and motor development.
   1. Has fully developed eyes.
   2. Is less impulsive and boisterous in activities.
   3. Frequently develops nervous habits such as nail-biting.
   4. Is more coordinated.
   5. Is capable of fine hand movements.
B. Language and social development.
   1. Is more competitive.
   2. Recognizes differences between his or her home and others.
   3. Wishes to be like his or her friends.
   4. Tells time; knows days of the week.
   5. Shows curiosity about sex differences.
   6. May have periods of shyness.
C. Appropriate games and stimulation.
   1. Recognize child's periods of shyness as normal behavior.
   2. Give reassurance and understanding if and when nightmares occur.
   3. Provide table games and card games; magic tricks; games that develop physical and mental skill.

Eight to Nine Years

A. Physical and motor development.
   1. Exhibits long arms in proportion to body.
   2. Shows good coordination of fine muscles.
   3. Engages in active play.
   4. May begin secondary sex characteristics (females).
   5. Learns to use script.

B. Language and social development.
   1. Is more self-assured in environment.
   2. Likes group projects, clubs.
   3. Has increased modesty.
   4. Recognizes property rights.
   5. Needs help accepting defeat in games.
   6. Begins to have sense of humor.
   7. Through play, learns new ideas and independence: competition, compromise, cooperation, and beginning collaboration.

C. Appropriate games and stimulation.
   1. Give child opportunity to obtain adult approval.
   2. Give small household responsibilities.
   3. Answer child's questions regarding sex in simple, honest words.
   4. Do not become overly concerned with common problems such as teasing and quarreling, as they are usually temporary.
   5. Provide sports, books (geography and adventure), erector sets, comics and funny papers.

Nine to Ten Years

A. Physical and motor development.
   1. Shows skill in manual activities because hand-eye coordination is developed.
   2. Exhibits decreased growth in height.
   3. Is very active physically.
   4. Cares completely for own physical needs.

B. Language and social development.
   1. Shows sex differences in play.
   2. Likes to have secrets.
   3. Displays antagonism between the sexes.
   4. Grasps easy multiplication and division.
   5. Has special friend to confide in.

C. Appropriate games and stimulation.

   1. Determine cause if lying and stealing occur.
   2. Provide parental understanding.
   3. Provide opportunity to enroll in clubs and organizations.
   4. Provide books, musical instruments, TV, records, practical projects.

Ten to Eleven Years

A. Physical and motor development.
   1. Shows onset of major secondary sex characteristics (males).
   2. Attempts perfection of physical skills.

B. Language and social development.
   1. Enjoys companionship more than play.
   2. Needs privacy occasionally.
   3. Exhibits increased ability to discuss problems.
   4. Has growing capacity for thought and conceptual organization.
   5. Sees physical qualities as constant despite changes in size, shape, weight, volume.
   6. Shows group conformity.

C. Appropriate games and stimulation.
   1. Continue sex education and preparation for adolescent body changes.
   2. Encourage participation in organized clubs, youth groups.

Eleven to Twelve Years

A. Physical and motor development.
   1. Begins puberty; physical changes appear in both males and females.
   2. Begins menstruation (females).
   3. May require more sleep due to body changes.

B. Social development.
   1. Participates in community and school affairs.
   2. Tends toward segregation of the sexes.
   3. Likes to be alone occasionally.
   4. Exhibits interest in world affairs.
   5. Comprehends world of possibility and abstraction.
   6. Begins to question parental values.

C. Appropriate games and stimulation.
1. Provide help in school and sports to channel energy in proper direction.
2. Provide guidance during dependence/independence conflict.
3. Set realistic limits.
4. Give adequate explanation of body changes.
5. Provide special consideration for child who lags behind in physical development.

Early Adolescence

A. Physical development.
1. Exhibits further development of secondary sex characteristics.
2. Shows poor posture.
3. Exhibits rapid growth and becomes awkward and uncoordinated.
4. Shows changes in body size and development.
B. Social development.
1. Needs social approval of peer group.
2. Strives for independence from family.
3. Has one or two very close friends in peer group.
4. Becomes more interested in opposite sex.
5. Period of upheaval: displays confusion about body image.
6. Must again learn to control strong feelings (love, aggression).
C. Counseling guidelines.
1. Provide adult understanding when adolescent deals with social, intellectual, and moral issues.
2. Allow some financial independence.
3. Provide limits to ensure security.
4. Provide necessary assurance to help adolescent accept changing body image.
5. Show flexibility in adjusting to emotional and erratic mood swings.
6. Be calm and consistent when dealing with an adolescent.
D. Developmental tasks.
1. Finds identity; moves out of role diffusion.

a. Integrates childhood identifications with basic drives.
b. Expands concept of social roles.
2. Moves toward heterosexuality.
3. Begins separation from family.
4. Integrates personality.

Adolescence to Young Adulthood

Developmental Milestones

A. Physical development.
1. Completes sexual development.
2. Exhibits signs of slowing down of body growth.
3. Is capable of reproduction.
4. Shows more energy after growth spurt tapers off.
5. Exhibits increased muscular ability and coordination.
6. Menarche—onset of menstruation—usually occurs between the ages of 11 and 14.
B. Social development.
1. Is less attached to peers.
2. Shows increased maturity.
3. Exhibits more interdependence with family members.
4. Begins romantic love affairs.
5. Increases mastery over biologic drives.
6. Develops more mature relationship with parents.
7. Values fidelity, friendship, cooperation.
8. Begins vocational development.
C. Counseling guidelines.
1. Assist adolescent in vocational choice.
2. Provide safety education, especially regarding driving.
3. Encourage good attitudes toward health in issues of nutrition, drugs, smoking, and drinking.
4. Attempt to understand own (parental) difficulties in accepting transition of adolescent to independence and adulthood.
D. Developmental tasks.
1. Intimacy and solidarity versus isolation.

a. Moves from security of self involvement to insecurity of building intimate relationships with others.
b. Becomes less dependent and more self-sufficient.
2. Able to form lasting relationships with others.
3. Learns to be productive and creative.
4. Handles hormonal changes of developmental period.

Adulthood

Developmental Tasks

A. Achieves goal of generativity versus stagnation or self-absorption.
1. Shows concern for establishing and guiding next generation.
2. Exhibits productiveness, creativity, and an attitude of looking forward to the future.
3. Stagnation results from the refusal to assume power and responsibility of the goals of middle age.
a. Suffers pervading sense of boredom and impoverishment.
b. Undergoes but does not resolve midlife crisis.
B. Has relaxed sense of competitiveness.
C. Opens up new interests.
D. Shifts values from physical attractiveness and strength to intellectual abilities.
E. Shows productivity (may be most productive years of one's life).
F. Has more varied and satisfying relationships.
G. Exhibits no significant decline in learning abilities or sexual interests.
H. Shifts sexual interests from physical performance to the individual's total sexuality and need to be loved and touched.
I. Assists next generation to become happy, responsible adults.
J. Achieves mature social and civic responsibility.
K. Accepts and adjusts to physiological changes of middle life.

L. Uses leisure time satisfactorily.
M. Failure to complete developmental tasks may cause the individual to approach old age with resentment and fear.
1. Neurotic symptoms may appear.
2. Increased psychosomatic disorders may develop.

Values of Adulthood

A. Becomes more introspective.
B. Shows less concern as to what others think.
C. Identifies self as successful even though all life goals may not be achieved.
D. Shows less concern for outward manifestations of success.
E. Lives more day-to-day and values life more deeply.
F. Has faced one's finiteness and eventual death.

Parenting in Adulthood

A. Characteristics.
1. Tendency toward smaller families.
2. Career-oriented women who limit family size or who do not want children.
3. Early sexual experimentation, necessitating sexual education, contraceptive information.
4. Tendency toward postponement of children.
a. To complete education.
b. Economic factors.
5. High divorce rates.
6. Alternate family designs.
a. Single parenthood.
b. Communal family.
B. Family planning.
1. General concepts.
a. Dealing with individuals with particular ideas regarding contraception.
b. No perfect method of birth control.
c. Method must be suited to individual.
d. Individuals involved must be thoroughly counseled on all available methods and how they work—including advan-

tages and disadvantages. This includes not only female but also sexual partner (if available).
  e. Once a method is chosen both parties should be thoroughly instructed in its use.
  f. Individuals involved must be motivated to succeed.
2. Effectiveness depends upon:
  a. Method chosen.
  b. Degree to which couple follows prescribed regimen.
  c. Thorough understanding of method.
  d. Motivation on part of individuals concerned.

Psychosocial Changes

Midlife Crisis

A. A normal stage in the ongoing life cycle in which the middle-aged person reevaluates his or her total life situation in relation to youthful achievements and actual accomplishments.
  1. Struggles to maintain physical attractiveness in relation to younger people.
  2. Partner or lover critical self-definition.
  3. Feels he or she has peaked in ability.
  4. Blames environment or others for failure to succeed.
  5. Displays increased interest in sexuality.
  6. Exhibits competitiveness in career plans.
B. Unresolved crisis.
  1. May result in stagnation, boredom, and decreased self-esteem and depression.
  2. Age for crisis varies.
    a. Women pass through it between 35 to 40 years old.
    b. Men experience the crisis between 40 to 45 years old.

Major Causes of Psychological Problems

A. Fears losing job.
B. Competition with younger generation.

C. Loss of job.
D. Loss of nurturing functions.
E. Loss of spouse, particularly females. (Forty-five percent of women over 65 are widowed.)
F. Realization that person is not going to accomplish some of the things that he or she wanted to do.
G. Changes in body image.
H. Illness.
I. Role change within and outside of family.
J. Fear of approaching old age.
K. Physiological changes.

The Aged

Developmental Tasks

A. Maintains ego integrity versus despair.
  1. Integrity results when an individual is satisfied with his or her own actions and lifestyle, feels life is meaningful, remains optimistic, and continues to grow.
  2. Despair results from the feeling that he or she has failed and that it is too late to change.
B. Continues a meaningful life after retirement.
C. Adjusts to income level.
D. Makes satisfactory living arrangements with spouse.
E. Adjusts to loss of spouse.
F. Maintains social contact and responsibilities.
G. Faces death realistically.
H. Provides knowledge and wisdom to assist those at other developmental levels to grow and learn.
I. Societal concerns.
  1. There are approximately 20 million people over the age of 65 in the United States today.
  2. Five percent of the aged are currently institutionalized.

Physiological, Psychological and Socioeconomic Implications

A. Physical changes.
   1. Decrease in physical strength and endurance.
   2. Decrease in muscular coordination.
   3. Tendency to gain weight.
   4. Loss of pigment in hair and skin.
   5. Increased brittleness of the bones.
   6. Greater sensitivity to temperature changes with low tolerance to cold.
   7. Degenerative changes in the cardiovascular system.
   8. Diminution of sensory faculties.
   9. Decreased resistance to infection, disease and accidents.
B. Developmental process retrogresses.
   1. Increasing dependency.
   2. Concerns focus increasingly on self.
   3. Interests may narrow.

4. Needs tangible evidence of affection.
C. Major fears of the aged.
   1. Physical and economic dependency.
   2. Chronic illness.
   3. Loneliness.
   4. Boredom resulting from not being needed.
D. Major problems of the aged.
   1. Economic deprivation.
      a. Increased cost of living on a fixed income.
      b. Increased need for costly medical care.
   2. Chronic disease and disability.
   3. Social isolation.
   4. Blindness.
   5. Organic brain changes.
      a. Not all persons become senile.
      b. Most people have memory impairment.
      c. The change is gradual.
   6. Nutritional deprivation.
E. Death in the life cycle.

Table 1. Erikson's Stages of Personality Development

Stage	Approx. Age	Psychological Crises	Significant Persons	Accomplishments
Infant	0–1	Basic trust vs. mistrust	Mother or maternal figure	Tolerates frustration in small doses Recognizes mother as separate from others and self
Toddler	1–3	Autonomy vs. shame and doubt	Parents	Begins verbal skills Begins acceptance of reality vs. pleasure principle
Preschool	3–6	Initiative vs. guilt	Basic family	Asks many questions Explores own body and environment Differentiates between sexes
School	6–12	Industry vs. inferiority	Neighborhood school	Gains attention by accomplishments Explores things Learns to relate to own sex
Puberty and adolescence	12–?	Identity vs. role diffusion	Peer groups External groups	Moves toward heterosexuality Begins separation from family Integrates personality (altruism, etc.)
Adolescence and young adult	—	Intimacy and solidarity vs. isolation	Partners in friendship, sex	Is able to form lasting relationships with others Learns to be creative and productive

Based on Erikson: *Childhood and Society*

1. In American culture death is very distasteful.
2. The elderly may see death as an end to suffering and loneliness.
3. Death is not feared if the person has lived a long and fulfilled life, having completed all developmental tasks.
4. Religious beliefs and/or philosophy of life important.

F. The elderly may provide knowledge and wisdom from their vast experiences, which can assist those at other developmental levels to grow and learn.

G. There will be approximately 33 million people over the age of 65 in the United States by the year 2000.

DEATH, DYING, AND GRIEF PROCESS

The Grief Process

Definition: A process that an individual goes through in response to the loss of a significant or loved person. The grieving process follows certain predictable phases—classic description originally done by Dr. Eric Lindeman. The normal grieving process is described by George Engle, M.D., in "Grief and Grieving," *American Journal of Nursing*, September 1964.

A. First response is shock and refusal to believe that the loved one is dead.
1. Displays inability to comprehend the meaning of loss.
2. Attempts to protect self against painful feelings.

B. As awareness increases, the bereaved experiences severe anguish.
1. Crying is common in this stage.
2. Anger directed toward those people or circumstances thought to be responsible.

C. Mourning is the next stage where the work of restitution takes place.

1. Rituals of the funeral help the bereaved accept reality.
2. Support from friends and spiritual guidance comfort the bereaved.

D. Resolution of the loss occurs as the mourner begins to deal with the void.

E. Idealization of the deceased occurs next where only the pleasant memories are remembered.
1. Characterized by the mourner's taking on certain qualities of the deceased.
2. This process takes many months as preoccupation with the deceased diminishes.

F. Outcome of the grief process takes a year or more.
1. Indications of successful outcome are when the mourner remembers both the pleasant and unpleasant memories.
2. Eventual outcome influenced by:
   a. Importance of the deceased in the life of mourner.
   b. The degree of dependence in the relationship.
   c. The amount of ambivalence toward the deceased.
   d. The more hostile the feelings that exist, the more guilt that interferes with the grieving process.
   e. Age of both mourner and deceased.
   f. Death of a child is more difficult to resolve than that of an aged loved one.
   g. Number and nature of previous grief experiences.
   h. Degree of preparation for the loss.

Counseling Guidelines

A. Recognize that grief is a syndrome with somatic and psychological symptomatology.
1. Weeping, complaints of fatigue, digestive disturbance, and insomnia.
2. Guilt, anger, and irritability.
3. Restless, but unable to initiate meaningful activity.
4. Depression and agitation.

B. Be prepared to support the family as they learn of the death.

1. Know the general response to death by recognizing the stages of the grief process.
2. Understand that the behavior of the mourner may be unstable and disturbed.

C. Use therapeutic communication techniques.
1. Encourage the mourner to express feelings, especially tears.
2. Attempt to meet the needs of the mourner for privacy, information, and support.
3. Show respect for the religious and social customs of the family.

Death and Dying

Impact of Dying Process for Adults

A. Physical symptoms of dying.
1. Cardiovascular collapse.
2. Renal failure.
3. Decreased physical and mental capacity.
4. Gradual loss of consciousness.

B. Stages of dying.
1. The dying process is ably portrayed in *Death and Dying*, by Elisabeth Kübler-Ross, New York, Macmillan Publishing Company, Inc., 1970.
2. Individual is stunned at the knowledge he or she is dying and denies it.
3. Anger and resentment usually follow as the individual questions, "Why me?"
4. With the beginning of acceptance of impending death comes the bargaining stage, that is, bargaining for time to complete some situation in his or her life.
5. Full acknowledgment usually brings depression; individual begins to work through feelings and to withdraw from life and relationships.
6. Final stage is full acceptance and preparation for death.
7. Throughout the dying process, hope is an important element that should be supported but not reinforced unrealistically.

C. Psychosocial clinical manifestations.
1. Depression and withdrawal.
2. Fear and anxiety.

3. Focus is internal.
4. Agitation and restlessness.

The Concept of Death in the Aging Population

A. In American culture, death is very distasteful.
B. The elderly may see death as an end to suffering and loneliness.
C. Death is not feared if the person has lived a long and fulfilled life, having completed all developmental tasks.
D. Religious beliefs and/or philosophy of life important.

Death and Children

A. Understanding of death for the young child.
1. Death is viewed as a temporary separation from parents, sometimes viewed synonymously with sleep.
2. Child may express fear of pain and wish to avoid it.
3. Child's awareness is lessened by physical symptoms if death occurs suddenly.
4. Gradual terminal illness may simulate the adult process: depression, withdrawal, fearfulness, and anxiety.

B. Older children's concerns.
1. Death is identified as a "person" to be avoided.
2. Child may ask directly if he or she is going to die.
3. Concerns center around fear of pain, fear of being left alone, and fear of leaving parents and friends.

C. Adolescent concerns.
1. Death is recognized as irreversible and inevitable.
2. Adolescent often avoids talking about impending death, and staff may enter into this "conspiracy of silence."
3. Adolescents have more understanding of death than adults tend to realize.

Nursing Management for Dying Patient

A. Nursing management of the adult.

1. Minimize physical discomfort.
   a. Attend to all physical needs.
   b. Make patient as comfortable as possible.
2. Recognize crisis situation.
   a. Observe for changes in patient's condition.
   b. Support patient.
3. Be prepared to give the dying patient the emotional support needed.
4. Encourage communication.
   a. Allow patient to express feelings, to talk, or to cry.
   b. Pick up cues that patient wants to talk, especially about fears.
   c. Be available to form a relationship with patient.
   d. Communicate honestly.
5. Prepare and support the family for their impending loss.
6. Understand the grieving process of patient and family.

B. Nursing management for the dying child.
1. Always elicit the child's understanding of death before discussing it.
2. Before discussing death with child, discuss it with parents.
3. Parental reactions include the continuum of grief process and stages of dying.
   a. Reactions depend on previous experience with loss.
   b. Reactions also depend on relationship with the child and circumstances of illness or injury.
   c. Reactions depend on degree of guilt felt by parents.
4. Assist parents in expressing their fears, concerns, and grief so that they may be more supportive to the child.
5. Assist parents in understanding siblings' possible reactions to a terminally ill child.
   a. Guilt: belief that they caused the problem or illness.
   b. Jealousy: demand for equal attention from the parents.
   c. Anger: feelings of being left behind.

HUMAN SEXUALITY

Overview

A. Biological sexuality is determined at conception.
   1. Male sperm contributes an X or a Y chromosome.
   2. Female ovum has an X chromosome.
   3. Fertilization results in either an XX (female) or an XY (male).
B. Preparation for adult sexuality originates in the sexual role development of the child.
   1. Significant differences between male and female infants are observable even at birth.
   2. Biological changes are minimal during childhood, but parenting strongly influences a child's behavior and sexual role development.
   3. Anatomical and physiological changes occur during adolescence which establish biological sexual maturation.
C. Human sexuality pervades the whole of an individual's life.
   1. More than a sum of isolated physical acts.
   2. Functions as a purposeful influence in human nature and behavior.
   3. Observable in everyday life in endless variations.
D. Each society develops a set of normative behaviors, attitudes, and values in respect to sexuality which are considered "right" and "wrong" by individuals.
E. Freud described the bisexual (androgynous) nature of the person.
   1. Each person has components of maleness-femaleness, masculinity-femininity, and heterosexuality-homosexuality.
   2. These components are physiological and psychological in nature.
   3. All components influence an individual's sexuality and sexual behavior.
F. Gender identity (identified at birth) refers to whether a person is male or female.

1. Cases of "ambiguous genitalia" are rare (1:3000 births), and require special care for the infant and parents.
2. Ambiguous genitalia is a clinical label similar to slang term "morphodite," or biological term "hermaphrodite."

G. Sexual object choice is the selection of a mode of outlet for sexual desire, usually with another person.
   1. Generally occurs during adolescence and beyond.
   2. Includes heterosexuality, homosexuality, bisexuality, celibacy, and narcissism/ onanism.

H. Sexual object choice has strong influence on person's lifestyle.
   1. Individual must establish patterns of intimacy and sexual behavior that are acceptable to self, to significant others, and to society to a certain extent.
   2. Psychological demands and expectations throughout life influence an individual's sexual interest, activity, and functional capacity.
   3. Sexual object choice can affect a person's choices in life such as whether to be a parent, where to live, and what career to maintain.

Sexual Behavior

A. Sexual behavior is a composite of developed patterns of intimacy, psychological demands and expectations, and sexual object choice.
   1. Can be genital (sexual intercourse), intimate (holding, hugging), or social (dating, choice of clothing).
   2. Beyond the obvious examples, one never stops "behaving sexually."
   3. Dress, communication, and activity are all expressions of sexuality.
   4. Every person exhibits sexual behavior continually; no one is sexless.

B. "Transvestite" and "transsexual" are two terms that often cause confusion and need definition and differentiation.
   1. Transvestite refers to one who enjoys wearing clothing of the opposite sex; may or may not be homosexual.
   2. Transsexual is a person who chooses sexual reassignment: a complex physical (surgical), psychological, and social process of taking on the gender identity, sex role, sexual object choice, and sexual behavior of the opposite sex.

C. Sexuality, although difficult to define, is pervasive from birth to death, and nurses need to look beyond the framework of reproduction and procreation to understand the influence of sexuality on patients' health and illness.

D. Characteristics.
   1. Difficult to define precisely, human sexuality is considered to be a pervasive life force and includes a person's total feelings, attitudes, and behavior.
   2. It is related to gender identity, sex-role identity, and sexual motivation.
   3. Touching, intimacy, and companionship are factors that have unique meaning for each person's sexuality.
   4. Sex role describes whether a person assumes masculine or feminine behaviors, usually a combination of both.
      a. This role generally considered to be fairly established by age five.
      b. Usually referred to by the concepts boy/girl and man/woman.

Nursing Care Related to Sexual Behavior

A. Assist in providing sex education and counseling.
   1. Patients consider nurses to be experts in sexuality.
   2. Intervention requires knowledge and skill.
   3. Nurses need to know referral sources for interventions beyond their ability.

B. Give patients "permission" or acceptance to maintain sexuality and sexual behavior.

C. Be aware of the effect of medications on patients' sexuality and sexual functioning.
   1. Oral contraceptives are considered by some to have played a major role in creat-

ing a sense of sexual freedom in contemporary society.

2. Drugs that decrease sexual drive or potency may act directly on the physiological mechanisms or may decrease interest through a depressant effect on the central nervous system.

3. Drugs with an adverse effect on sexual activity include antihypertensive drugs, antidepressants, antihistamines, antispasmodics, sedatives and tranquilizers, ethyl alcohol, and some hormone preparations and steroids.

4. There are no known drugs that specifically increase libido or sexual performance; those that seem to enhance sexual behavior do so indirectly through transient relaxation of tensions, alleviation of discomfort, or release of inhibitions.

5. Long-term use of any drug or medicine will likely have a negative effect on sexual interest and capability.

D. Be aware of the problems to which nursing personnel should direct themselves in relation to the area of human sexuality.

1. Attitudes.
   a. Nurses should increase their self-awareness of their own attitudes and the effect of these attitudes on the sexual health care of their patients.
   b. Nurses should suppress negative biases and prejudices and/or make appropriate referrals when they cannot give effective sexual health care.

2. Knowledge.
   a. May have to be actively sought although nursing programs are increasing the sexuality content in their curricula.
   b. Also available through books, journal articles, classes and workshops, and preparation for sexuality therapy on the graduate level.

3. Skills.
   a. Primary skills needed are interpersonal techniques such as therapeutic communication, interviewing, and teaching.

   b. As with any skill, practice is needed for proficiency in sexual-history taking, education, and counseling.

Common Problems and Implications for Nursing

A. Masturbation.
   1. A common sexual outlet for many people.
   2. For patients requiring long-term care, masturbation may be only means for gratifying sexual needs.
   3. Nurses frequently react negatively to any type of masturbatory activity, especially by male patients.
   4. Patients should be allowed privacy; if nurse walks in on a patient masturbating, he or she should leave with an apology for having intruded on the patient's privacy.
   5. Frequent or inappropriate masturbation may be harmful to the patient's health. Limits need to be set to protect patient and other patients if behavior is inappropriate.

B. Homosexuality.
   1. Homosexuality is accepted by many as a viable life style.
   2. Nurses have tended to have negative attitudes and incorrect knowledge about homosexuality.
   3. A patient's homosexual (gay) life style should be accepted and respected.
   4. As with any patient, visitors should be encouraged as appropriate for the health/illness status, and these people should not be embarrassed or ridiculed.
   5. For chronically ill patients, such as in a nursing home, it is essential that sexuality needs be considered in the total care plan and special efforts be made to have these needs met.

C. Inappropriate sexual behavior.
   1. Difficult to precisely define "inappropriate" sexual behavior.
   2. Sometimes sexual behavior is in reaction to unintentional "seductive" behavior of the nurses.

3. Specific nursing interventions.
   a. Set limits to unacceptable behavior immediately.
   b. Interact without rejecting patient.
   c. Help patient express feelings in an appropriate manner.
   d. Teach alternative behaviors that are acceptable.
   e. Provide acceptable outlets to sexual feelings.
D. Rape.
   1. Rape is basically an act of violence and is only secondarily a sex act.
   2. Treatment should consist of both medical and psychological intervention.
   3. Sexual assault can have a long-term impact on the victim.
   4. Victims may need encouragement and support to report rape occurrences to authorities.
   5. Female nurses especially can play a valuable role in giving assistance and support to female rape victims.
   6. Many communities have "hot-lines" that offer telephone information and crisis counseling to victims of sexual assault and to professionals.
E. Child sexual abuse.
   1. There is only a beginning awareness of this problem area.
   2. Most child sexual abuse involves a male adult and female child, but male children can also be victims of female or male sexual abusers.
   3. The child may need special protection or temporary placement outside the home, but often the family unit can be maintained.
   4. Child sexual abuse is a form of child abuse, and nurses should know local regulations and procedures for case finding and reporting.
F. Sexuality and disability.
   1. Physically and developmentally disabled persons are sexual beings also.
   2. Developmentally disabled persons should be given sexuality education and counsel-

ing in preparation for responsible sexual expression and behavior.
   3. After spinal cord injury, the level of the lesion and degree of interruption of nerve impulses influence sexual functioning; adaptation of previous sexual practices may be needed after the injury.
   4. Fertility and the ability to bear children are usually not compromised in women with spinal cord injury.
   5. Nurses working with disabled patients must make special effort to include sexuality in total health care and services.
G. Contraception.
   1. Nurses are considered experts on forms of birth control.
   2. Nurses should be familiar with different methods and relative effectiveness of each one.
   3. Patients should be assisted to make their own choices as to whether to use contraception and what method is best for them.
   4. More detailed outline of contraception appears in maternity chapter.
H. Therapeutic abortion.
   1. Patients need information about resources for and procedures of therapeutic abortions.
   2. Patients should be given nonjudgmental assistance and support in decision-making process.
   3. If nurse cannot in good conscience assist the patient, referral should be made to someone who can.
   4. More detailed outline of abortion appears in maternity chapter.

SEXUALLY TRANSMITTED DISEASES (STDs)

Chlamydia

Characteristics

A. Most common sexually transmitted disease (STD) in the U.S.
B. 4 to 5 million people contract disease each year.
C. High risk women: young, nonwhites with multiple sex partners and woman not using barrier contraceptives.
D. Chlamydia is not a reportable disease in 50 percent of states.
E. Statistics:
   1. 20 percent men and 40–50 percent women with gonorrhea also are infected with chlamydia.
   2. 25–50 percent of pelvic inflammatory diseases (PID) are caused by chlamydia.
   3. 155,000 infants born to mothers with chlamydia are at risk for pneumonia and inclusion conjunctivitis.
   4. Each year 1 billion dollars spent on infection.
F. Chlamydiae are bacteria microorganisms, but have characteristics of both viruses and bacteria.
G. Sensitive to antibiotics.
H. Spread through sexual contact. Incubation period 5–10 days or longer (28 days) gonorrhea is only 2–10 days).
I. Tests for chlamydia include Chlamydiazyme—enzyme immuno assay test and Microtak—direct fluorescent antibody test.

Assessment

A. Observe for a discharge—vaginal or urethral.
B. Assess for burning.
C. Check for lower abdominal pain or testicular pain.
D. Assess for bleeding or pain with coitus.
E. Assess for rectal pain or discharge.
F. 33 percent women report no symptoms.

Implementation

A. Administer antibiotics as ordered.
   1. Tetracycline 500 mg 4x/day for seven days or Doxycycline 100 mg 2x/day for seven days.
      a. Take on an empty stomach.
      b. May cause sensitivity to the sun.
      c. Avoid becoming pregnant.
   2. Erythromycin 500 mg 4x/day for seven days as second choice (take with meals).
   3. Penicillin does not cure chlamydia.
B. Educate men and women about transmission, symptoms and prevention.
   1. Frequent examinations if people are not monogamous.
   2. If symptoms/signs occur, seek help immediately—teach importance of taking medication as prescribed.
   3. Suggest sexually active people use barrier methods of contraception.
   4. Avoidance of sex until completion of treatment.
C. Provide accurate information about disease, health care and prevention.

Syphilis

Definition: A chronic infectious disease caused by *Treponema pallidum.*

Characteristics

A. Transmission is by intimate physical contact with syphilitic lesions, which are usually found on the skin or the mucous membranes of the mouth and the genitals.
B. Incubation period is two to six weeks following exposure.
C. Primary stage.

1. Most infectious stage.
2. Appearance of chancres, ulcerative lesions.
3. Usually painless, produced by spirochetes at the point of entry into the body.

D. Secondary stage.
   1. Lesions appear about three weeks after the primary stage and may occur anywhere on the skin and the mucous membranes.
   2. Highly infectious.
   3. Generalized lymphadenopathy.

E. Tertiary stage.
   1. The spirochetes enter the internal organs and cause permanent damage.
   2. Symptoms may occur 10 to 30 years following the occurrence of an untreated primary lesion.
   3. Invasion of the central nervous system.
      a. Meningitis.
      b. Locomotor ataxia: foot slapping and broad-based gait.
      c. General paresis.
      d. Progressive mental deterioration leading to insanity.
   4. Cardiovascular: most common site of damage is at the aortic valve and the aorta itself.

F. Characteristics relating to pregnancy.
   1. May cause abortion or premature labor.
   2. Infection is passed to the fetus after the fourth month of pregnancy as congenital syphilis.

Assessment

A. Evaluate serum test (STS) for syphilis on first prenatal visit.
B. May repeat just before fourth month, as disease may be acquired after initial visit.

Implementation

A. Educate women to recognize signs of syphilis.
B. Educate women to seek immediate treatment if known exposure occurs.
C. Educate women as to the need for simultaneous treatment of partner as reinfection may occur.

D. Monitor treatment: during pregnancy, 4.8 million units of procaine penicillin G with 2% aluminum monostearate, IM normally in divided doses.
E. Report all cases of syphilis to health authorities for treatment of contacts.

Gonorrhea

Definition: An infection caused by *Neisseria gonorrhoeae*, which causes inflammation of the mucous membrane of the genitourinary tract.

Characteristics

A. Transmission is almost completely by sexual intercourse.
B. Incidence is of epidemic proportions in the United States.
C. Signs and symptoms.
   1. Male.
      a. Painful urination.
      b. Pelvic pain and fever.
      c. Epididymitis with pain, tenderness, and swelling.
   2. Female (usually asymptomatic).
      a. Vaginal discharge.
      b. Urinary frequency and pain.
D. Complications.
   1. Female: pelvic inflammatory disease (PID) with abdominal pain, fever, nausea, and vomiting.
   2. Male: postgonococcal urethritis and spread of infection to posterior urethra, prostate, and seminal vesicles.
   3. PID can lead to sterility.
   4. A secondary infection can develop in any organ.
E. Infection may be transmitted to baby's eyes during delivery, causing blindness.

Assessment

A. Obtain culture for gonorrhea (usually done on first prenatal visit).

B. Repeat later as infection may occur during pregnancy.

Implementation

A. Educate women to recognize signs of gonorrhea and to seek immediate treatment.

B. Administer prophylactic medication of 1% silver nitrate to newborn.

C. Monitor treatment: same as for syphilis. Other antibiotics may be used for sensitivity to penicillin.

D. Important to treat sexual partner, as patient may become reinfected.

Herpes Simplex Type 2 (Genital Herpes)

Characteristics

A. Involves external genitalia, vagina, and cervix.

B. Development and draining of painful vesicles.

C. Virus may be lethal to fetus if inoculated during vaginal delivery. Delivery usually by C-section.

D. Safe use of Acyclovir has not been established for pregnant women.

Assessment

A. Evaluate for presence of painful, draining vesicles on external genitals, vagina, and cervix.

B. Check for increased temperature and vital signs.

Implementation

A. Educate patient as to dangers to fetus.

B. Encourage patient to report symptoms.

C. Explain to patient as to the possibility of a cesarean section should an outbreak occur around the time of delivery. Policy regarding time limit of outbreak in relation to time of delivery varies, but usual policy is an outbreak within two weeks.

D. Maintain precautions during vaginal examinations of patient.

E. Maintain isolation precautions during hospitalization if disease is active.

F. Encourage careful handwashing by patient.

G. Infant and mother may be separated during active period depending upon hospital policy or other special precautionary measures may be used to avoid transmission of disease to neonate. Encourage mother to express her feelings regarding separation and to talk about baby.

Genital Warts

Characteristics

A. Almost one million Americans develop this condition—major STD of 1990s. Caused by the human papilloma virus (HPV).

B. The virus affects cervix, urethra, penis, scrotum, and anus.

C. Warts appear one or two months after exposure, transmitted through intimate sexual contact.

Assessment

A. Assess for small to large wartlike growths on genitals (no symptoms other than lesions).

B. Assess for cervical cell changes—HPV associated with up to 90 percent of cervical malignancies.

Implementation

A. There is no cure for HPV—treatment is cryotherapy, liquid nitrogen, or electrocautery to remove lesions.

B. Key is prevention—similar to any other STD: limit sexual contacts and use condoms.

C. Suggest Pap test every year (cancer risk).

See also AIDS, page 175.

3

GENERAL NURSING CONCEPTS

FUNDAMENTAL CONCEPTS

Environment of the Patient

Safety and Comfort

A. Adequate space.
B. Privacy.
C. Comfortable room temperature.
   1. 66 to 76°F is normal.
   2. Warmer temperature for very young, old, sedentary, or ill patients.
D. Room humidity 30 to 60 percent.
E. Adequate lighting.
   1. Natural light if available; avoid glare.
   2. Use of night lights especially with elderly, very young, very ill.
F. Adequate ventilation.
G. Comfortable sound levels.
H. Pleasing, easy-to-clean decor/furniture.
I. Protection from hazards.
   1. Use of handrails, side rails.
   2. Items placed within reach at the bedside.
J. Identification bands/bracelets.
K. Functional call system within patient's reach.

Assessment

Purpose of Assessment

A. Determine person's current health status.
B. Provide baseline for nursing diagnosis and care planning.
   1. First step in the nursing process.
   2. May not be duty of LVN/LPN but importance should be understood.

Assessment Procedure

A. Collect data by reading chart/care plan.
B. Interview to obtain subjective information/symptoms.

C. Collect cardinal or vital signs.
   1. Temperature.
      a. Oral—inappropriate for use with infants, after oral surgery, or with patients who are unconscious or receiving oxygen by mask.
      b. Rectal—inappropriate for use with patients who have a rectal disorder or following rectal surgery.
   2. Pulse.
      a. Usually palpated over radial artery.
      b. Apical—used with babies and irregular heart rates.
      c. Pulse deficit—apical rate minus radial rate.
   3. Blood pressure—arterial.
      a. Systolic—the pressure in vessel when heart is contracting.
      b. Diastolic—the pressure in vessel when heart is at rest.
      c. Pulse pressure—the difference between systolic and diastolic.
D. Measure weight and height.
E. Perform a detailed assessment.
   1. May be done from the patient's head-to-toes.
   2. May be done on a system basis.
   3. May be used to determine patient's strengths and/weaknesses. (See specific chapters for outlines.)
   4. Phases.
      a. Inspection—overview of patient.
      b. Auscultation—use of stethoscope to listen to heart.
      c. Palpation—use of entire surface of all five fingers.
      d. Percussion—use of middle finger for "tapping."
F. Use data to plan patient care or report the care plan to responsible nurse/team leader for validation, interpretation, or use in planning care.
G. Assist RN to formulate nursing diagnoses.
H. Follow steps of the Nursing Process.

Recording/Charting

Purpose of Written Records

A. Method of precise communication between staff members.

B. Legal documentation.

C. Provides for continuity of care and documents progress.

D. Research, statistics, and education.

Types of Charting

A. Computer-assisted.

B. Source-oriented.
1. Most common.
2. Organized by sources of information.
3. Types of forms.
   a. Order sheets.
   b. X-ray reports.
   c. Graphs—vital signs.
   d. Flow sheets—intake and output.
   e. Narrative nurses' notes.
      (1) Objective, not interpretive.
      (2) Brief and concise.
      (3) Use of approved symbols and abbreviations.
      (4) Accurate spelling.
      (5) Prepared legibly in ink.
      (6) Signed with name and status.

C. SOAP charting (also called SOAPIER notes).
1. *Subjective:* patient's symptoms and own description of problem.
2. *Objective:* factual data, e.g., intake and output, vital signs, drainage, etc.
3. *Assessment:* your conclusions about the problem.
4. *Plan:* what you decide to do about the problem.
5. *Implementation:* your nursing interventions.
6. *Evaluation:* how the implementation worked.
7. *Revision:* how you plan to change the PCP if improvement is needed.
8. A separate SOAP note is needed for each problem. Do not combine problems.

9. It is not always necessary to include the I, E, and R portions of the note; always include the S, 0, A, and P parts, even if the patient does not supply subjective statements.

Nursing Diagnosis

A. A statement of an actual health problem or a potential one.
1. Derived from the assessment phase of the nursing process.
2. Based on both objective and subjective data.
3. As data base is collected, deviations from normal health patterns are identified.

B. Specific problem identified is related to a nursing intervention—not a medical one.

C. There are three major categories.
1. Diagnosis or condition—either potential or actual.
2. Etiology to which condition is related.
3. Defining characteristics that support the etiology.
4. State: Impairment of: *related to*, followed by etiology, if known and the defining characteristics.

Patient Care Plans

A. The two accepted types are: individualized care plan and standard care plan.
1. Individualized care plans have mutually agreed-upon goals set by the patient, family, and health team members.
2. Specific directions are written to define how these goals can be achieved.
3. The usual care plan format contains a problem list, a health team action section, and expected outcomes with deadline dates.
4. Standard care plans provide a guide for patient care.
   a. Identify problem relating to all patients having a specific medical condition.
   b. Health team actions include routine preventive nursing interventions.

B. The information contained in the care plan must be specific.
C. Care plans become a permanent part of the patient's chart.
   1. They must be written in ink.
   2. Resolved problems should be crossed out using a colored felt tip pen.
D. Care plans must be updated on a routine basis (generally every 24 to 48 hours or as the patient's condition changes).

The Nurse-Patient Relationship

Definition: The nurse-patient relationship is a therapeutic, professional relationship in which interaction occurs between two individuals—the vocational nurse, who possesses the skills, abilities, and resources to relieve another's discomfort; and the patient, who is seeking assistance for alleviation of some existing problem.

Characteristics

A. Give the patient the feeling of being accepted.
   1. Accept the patient as having value and worth as an individual.
   2. Empathize (feel with the patient) but do not sympathize or use platitudes.
   3. Offer emotional involvement but maintain objectivity.
   4. Protect and promote patient's self-esteem.
B. Indicate desire to develop mutual trust.
   1. Exhibit verbal and nonverbal behavior that is consistent and congruent.
   2. Encourage reality orientation.
   3. Interact at patient's level of understanding.
   4. Understand your own motives and needs.
   5. Provide open and honest communication.
   6. Communicate with the patient using therapeutic communication techniques.
C. Provide a reality-oriented supportive environment.
   1. Focus on the total patient so as to include all physical needs.
   2. Set appropriate behavioral limits.

3. Assist patient to identify and cope with feelings.
4. Encourage expression of feelings within a safe limit.
5. Recognize signs of a high anxiety level and seek appropriate help.

Phases of the Relationship

A. Initiating phase.
   1. Identify problems.
   2. Get to know each other.
   3. Test each other's attitudes.
   4. Identify expectations.
   5. Plan for the conclusion at the beginning of the relationship.
B. Continuing phase.
   1. Accept each other.
   2. Use specific therapeutic problem-solving techniques.
   3. Work actively on problems.
   4. Assess and evaluate problem continually.
   5. Encourage patient to become more independent and to rely less on the nurse.
C. Terminating phase.
   1. Evaluate the initial plan for conclusion.
   2. Anticipate problems of termination.
      a. Excessive dependence of patient on nurse, who must encourage independence.
      b. Patient may have feelings of abandonment, rejection, and/or depression about termination.
      c. Discuss patient's feelings about termination.

Communication Techniques

Definition: Communication is the process of sending and receiving messages by means of symbols, words, signs, gestures, or other actions. It is a multi-level process consisting of the content or information of the message, as well as the part that defines the meaning of the message. Messages sent and received define the relationship between individuals.

EFFECTIVE COMMUNICATION TECHNIQUES

Listen
: The act of consciously receiving another person's message. Listen eagerly, actively, responsively, and seriously.

Acknowledge
: Recognize the person without inserting your own values or judgments. Acknowledgment may be simple and with or without understanding. Example, in the response "I hear what you're saying," the person acknowledges a statement without agreeing with it. Acknowledgment may be verbal or nonverbal.

Give Feedback
: The process of the receiver relaying to the sender the effect the message has had. Helps keep the sender on course or alter his course. Involves acknowledging, validating, clarifying, extending, and altering. *Nurse to patient:* "You did that well."

Be Congruent (Mutual Fit)
: Verbal and nonverbal messages coincide. Example, a patient is crying, and the nurse says, "I want to help," and places her hand on the patient's shoulder.

Clarify
: Checking out or making clear either the intent or hidden meaning of message or determining if the message sent was the message received. *Nurse:* "You said that you felt warm. Would you like to open the window?"

Focus or Refocus
: Pick up on central topic or cue given by the patient. *Nurse:* "You were telling me how hard it was to talk to your mother."

Validate
: The process of verifying the accuracy of the sender's message by paraphrasing thought. *Nurse:* "Yes, it is confusing with so many people around."

Reflect
: Identify sender's message and return a message that expresses sender's implied feeling rather than overt idea (conveys acceptance and great understanding). *Nurse:* "You distrust your doctor?"

Ask Open-Ended Questions
: Ask questions that cannot be answered "Yes" or "No" or "Maybe" and generally require an answer or several words in order to broaden conversational opportunities and help the patient to communicate. *Nurse:* "What kind of job would you like to do?"

Encourage Nonverbally
: Use body language to indicate interest, understanding, support, caring, and/or listening to extract further information. *Nurse:* Nodding appropriately as patient talks.

Restate
: Echo last few words. This encourages patient to elaborate thought. *Nurse:* "You hear voices."

Paraphrase
: Reword. This enables sender to hear message meaning in another form. *Nurse:* "You mean you're unhappy."

Respond Neutrally
: Show interest and involvement without indicating assent or dissent. Nurse: "Yes . . . ." "Uh hm . . . ."

Use Incomplete Sentences
: Encourage patient to continue. *Nurse:* "Then your life is . . ."

EFFECTIVE COMMUNICATION TECHNIQUES (*Continued*)

Minimize Verbalization	Keep your own verbalization at a minimum, and let the patient the conversation. *Nurse:* "You feel . . . ?"
Initiate Broad Statements	Open the communication by allowing the patient freedom to talk and focus on himself. *Nurse:* "How have you been feeling?"

BLOCKS TO EFFECTIVE COMMUNICATION

Make Assumptions	(Jumping to conclusions.) Suppose or guess meaning of sender's behavior when not validated by sender. The nurse finds the suicidal patient smiling and joking, and tells the staff he's in a cheerful mood.
Give Advice	Tell the patient what to do, give an opinion, or make a decision that implies sender cannot cope with own self-determination and that receiver will accept responsibility for sender. *Nurse:* "If I were you . . . .
Change the Subject	Introduce new topics inappropriately, a pattern that may indicate anxiety. The patient is crying and discussing her fear of surgery, when the nurse asks, "How many children do you have?"
Use Social Response	Focus attention on receiver of message rather than sender. *Nurse:* "This sunshine is good for my roses. I have a beautiful rose garden."
Invalidate Patient	Ignore or deny another's presence, thoughts, or feelings. *Patient:* "Hi, how are you?" *Nurse:* "I can't talk now. I'm on my way to lunch."
Use False Reassurance	Use cliches, pat answers, cheery words, advice, and comforting statements as an attempt to reassure the patient. Most of what is called "reassurance" is really false reassurance. *Nurse:* "It's going to be all right."
Overload Conversation	Speak rapidly, change subjects, and give receiver more information than can be absorbed at one time. *Nurse:* "What's your name? I see you are 48 years old and that you like sports. Where do you come from?"
Underload Conversation	Remain silent and unresponsive, fail to pick up cues, and fail to give feedback. *Patient:* "What's your name?" *Nurse:* Smiles and walks away.
Use Incongruent Messages	Send verbal and nonverbal messages that contradict one another; two or more messages, sent via different levels, seriously do contradict one another. The contradiction may be between the content, verbal, nonverbal, and/or content (time, space). This contradiction is a double message. *Patient:* "I like your dress." *Nurse:* Annoyed, frowns and looks disgusted.
Make Value Judgments	Give one's own opinion, moralize or imply one's own values by using words such as "nice," "good," "bad," "right," "wrong," "should," and ought." *Nurse:* "I think he's a very good doctor."

Characteristics

A. An individual cannot *not* communicate.

B. Communication is a basic human need.

C. It is both verbal and nonverbal expression (also tone, pace, and manner of dress).

D. Effective communication includes:
    1. Feedback.
    2. Appropriateness.
    3. Efficiency.
    4. Flexibility.

E. Communication skills are learned as the individual grows and develops.

F. The foundation of the individual's perception of self and the world is based on communicated messages received from significant others.

G. Factors that affect communication.
    1. Intrapersonal framework of the individual.
    2. Relationship between the participants.
    3. Purpose of the sender.
    4. Content.
    5. Context.
    6. Manner in which the message is sent.
    7. Effect on the receiver.

Interviewing Skills

A. Help the patient feel comfortable so that there is no need to be defensive.

B. Use "I" messages, not "you" messages (e.g., "I feel angry," not "you make me angry").

C. Observe carefully and be alert to cues given by the patient.

D. Participate in planning a goal- and direction-oriented approach.

Implementation

A. Encourage the patient to verbalize his or her thoughts and feelings.

B. Assist the patient to clarify or make clear what he or she is saying.

C. Focus on the patient, not on yourself or others.

D. Help the patient understand how he or she affects others.

E. Communicate at the patient's level of understanding.

F. Use "how" questions rather than "why" questions.

G. Focus on the present "here and now" rather than on the past "there and then."

H. Help the patient learn new ways of problem solving.

I. Give constructive feedback so that the patient can self-correct unclear statements.

J. Use nonverbal communication to convey empathy, interest, and encouragement.

K. Send verbal messages that are congruent with your nonverbal messages.

L. Be honest in your answers or statements; say what you mean and mean what you say.

M. Use effective communication techniques (see page 37).

N. Recognize blocks to effective communication (see page 38).

O. Make a sustained effort to give and receive a message.

PAIN MANAGEMENT

Characteristics

A. Classification of pain fibers.
    1. Class A—large myelinated (fast pain).
    2. Class B—smaller unmyelinated.
    3. Class C—unmyelinated (slow pain).

B. The experience of pain.
    1. Pain source—direct causative factor.
    2. Stimulation of pain receptor—mechanical, chemical, thermal, electrical, ischemic.
    3. Pain pathway.
        a. Sensory pathways through dorsal root, ending on second order neuron in posterior horn.
        b. Afferent fibers cross over to anterolateral pathway, ascend in lateral spinothalamic tract to thalamus.

    c. Fibers then travel to postcentral gyrus in parietal lobe.

C. Types of pain.
1. Superficial—localized, shorter duration, sharp sensation.
2. Deep pain—long duration, diffuse, dull aching quality; associated autonomic responses, musculoskeletal tension, nausea.
    a. Visceral—internal organs.
    b. Somatic—neuromuscular, segmental distribution.
    c. Preferred—area stimulated (deep) and area pain referred to (superficial) are innervated by nerve fibers arising from same segment of spinal cord.
    d. Secondary to skeletal muscle.
3. Central pain—autonomic reflex pain syndrome.
    a. Causalgia—lesion peripheral nerve.
    b. Phantom—after amputation.
    c. Central—lesion in CNS, affecting pain pathway.
4. Psychogenic—due to emotional factors without anatomic or physiological explanation.

D. Gate control theory.
1. Pain impulses can be modulated by a transmission blocking action within CNS.
2. Large diameter cutaneous pain fibers can be stimulated (rubbing, scratching) and may inhibit smaller diameter excitatory fibers and prevent transmission of that impulse.
3. Cerebral cortical mechanisms that influence perception and interpretation may also inhibit transmission.

E. Pain perception—thalamus/awareness and parietal/integration.

F. Pain interpretation—cerebral cortex; delayed response influenced by previous experiences, culture, existing physical/psychological state.

G. Reactions—psychic and/or physiologic.

Assessment

A. Assess type of pain.
1. Acute pain: short duration of a few seconds to six months.
2. Chronic pain: longer duration of six months to years.
3. Intractable pain: severe and constant and resistant to relief measures.

B. Assess location.
1. Ask patient to identify area of the body affected.
2. Superficial or deep.
3. Diffuse or localized.
4. Radiates and where it goes.

C. Assess quality.
1. Stabbing, knifelike.
2. Throbbing.
3. Cramping.
4. Viselike, suffocating.
5. Searing, burning.
6. Other.

D. Assess intensity.
1. Ask patient to indicate intensity of pain on a scale of zero to ten, zero being no pain and ten being the most pain ever experienced.
2. Use this scale to assess relief of pain after intervention.

E. Assess onset and precipitating factors.
1. How movement affects pain.
2. If coughing affects pain.
3. Impact of emotion on pain, e.g., arguing with spouse or receiving disturbing news.

F. Assess aggravating factors.
1. How position affects pain.
2. Environmental stressors.
3. Fatigue.

G. Assess associated factors.
1. Nausea.
2. Vomiting.
3. Bradycardia/tachycardia.
4. Hypotension/hypertension.
5. Profuse perspiration.
6. Apprehension or anxiety.

H. Assess alleviating factors.
1. Position.
2. Elevation of inflamed extremity.
3. Techniques used at home for pain relief.

I. Assess patient's behavioral responses to pain.
   1. Depression, withdrawal, or crying.
   2. Stoicism or expressive.

Implementation

A. Assess pain before treating.
B. Give reassurance, reduce anxiety and fears.
C. Offer distraction.
D. Give comfort measures as ordered: positioning rest, elevation, heat/cold applications; protect from painful stimuli.
E. Massage—but never massage calf due to danger of emboli.
F. Administer pain medication as ordered: monitor therapeutic, toxic dose, and side effects.
   1. Check physician's orders.
   2. Use a preventive approach to pain management. Give medication before pain becomes severe.
   3. Follow steps outlined in assessment to determine the nature, quality, and extent of pain.
   4. Start with PO medications. If ineffective or only mildly effective, give IM medications, or combine PO and IM medications.
   5. Evaluate result of pain medication. Was it effective? How long did the effect last? What was the extent of relief?
   6. Evaluate patient for possible side effects of the medication.
   7. Discuss with charge nurse the effects of medication and whether a change of prescription is needed.
G. Monitor alternative methods to control pain.
   1. Dorsal column stimulator: stimulation of electrodes at dorsal column of spinal cord by patient-controlled device to inhibit pain.
   2. Analgesics: alter perception, threshold, and reaction to pain.
   3. Anesthesia: block pain pathway.
   4. Local nerve block.
   5. Neurosurgical procedures: interrupt sensory pathways; usually also affect pressure and temperature pathways.
      a. Neurectomy: interrupt cranial or peripheral nerves.
      b. Sympathectomy: interrupt afferent pathways (ganglia).
H. Nurse's role in pain relief.
   1. Prevent pain from retarding recovery.
   2. Prevent pain from causing nausea and vomiting which could result in fluid and electrolyte imbalance.
   3. Prevent pain from causing undue fatigue.
   4. Prevent pain from inhibiting moving, ambulating, turning and coughing, and thereby increasing possibilities of secondary problems from inactivity (pneumonia, emboli).
   5. Relieve pain or prevent pain from escalating by relaxing muscles (muscle tension increases with pain).
   6. Decrease anxiety that present and future pain relief will not be achieved.
   7. Bring pain relief to a level acceptable to the patient.

DISEASE PROCESS

Definition: A definite morbid process that affects the body or any of its parts. Symptoms accompany the process; the etiology, course, extent, and prognosis vary.

Etiology

A. Mechanical.
   1. Trauma—accidental injury.
   2. Extremes of heat or cold.
   3. Radioactive elements.
   4. Obstaction of normal body passage.
B. Chemical agents.
   1. Caustic substances.
   2. Drugs.
   3. Insect bites.
   4. GI secretions, or blood that is not in GI tract or in vascular system, etc.
   5. Hormones/electrolytes.
C. Genetic/hereditary factors.
D. Infectious agents.
   1. Bacteria.

a. Cocci—round.
b. Bacilli—rod-shaped.
c. Spirochetes—spiral.
2. Virus—very small, must grow on living cells.
3. Rickettsias—small, round or rod-shaped microorganisms, transmitted by bites of fleas, lice, ticks.
4. Fungi—yeasts or molds that thrive in a warm, moist place and feed on living plants or animals and decaying organic material.
5. Protozoa—one-celled microscopic organism that belongs to the animal family.

Inflammation

A. Normal body response/homeostatic mechanism.
B. Common local signs/symptoms.
1. Heat.
2. Redness.
3. Swelling.
4. Pain.
5. Loss of motion.

Immunity

A. The body's ability to resist infectious disease.
B. Types.
1. Natural immunity—"born with"; inborn body characteristic.
2. Acquired or adaptive immunity.
a. Develops after exposure to infectious disease or to some form of a particular pathogen or its toxins.
b. Active—attack of the disease, vaccination, injection of toxoids.
c. Passive—receive antibodies or antitoxins from mother to unborn fetus or injections of immune serum, gamma globulin, antivenin.
C. Antigens.
1. Substance that causes an immune response.
2. Examples: pathogen, toxin, foreign protein.
D. Antibodies—substance that protects the body from antigen.

FLUID AND ELECTROLYTES

Fluid Composition of the Body

Body Water

Definition: Total body water represents the largest constituent (45 to 80 percent) of total body weight, depending on the amount of fat present.

A. Intracellular—represents three-fourths of total body water fluid; contained inside the cell; includes the red blood cells.
B. Extracellular—represents one-fourth of total body water; includes remaining fluid not contained within the cell.
1. Intravascular (plasma)—liquid in which the blood cells are suspended.
2. Interstitial—liquid surrounding tissue cells.

Electrolytes

Definition: Electrolytes are compounds that dissolve in a solution to form ions. Each ion carries either a positive or negative electrical charge.

A. Types.
1. Cations—positive charge (Na^+, K^+, Ca^{++}, Mg^{++})
2. Anions—negative charge (Cl^-, HCO_3^-, HPO_4^-, SO_4^-)
3. Equal number of cations and anions (154 each).
B. Concentration in solution is expressed in mEq/L. Total number of cations (mEq) plus total number of anions (mEq) will be the same in both the intracellular fluid and extracellular fluid, thereby rendering the body's fluid composition electrically neutral.
C. Compartment composition.
1. Extracellular—large quantities of sodium, chloride, and bicarbonate ions.
2. Intracellular—large quantities of potassium, phosphate, and proteins.

Table A. Major Electrolytes

Cations$^+$		Anions$^-$	
Na$^+$	Sodium	Cl$^-$	Chloride
K$^+$	Potassium	HCO$_3^-$	Bicarbonate
Ca^{++}	Calcium	HPO$_4^-$	Phosphate
Mg^{++}	Magnesium		

Dynamics of Intercompartmental Fluid Transfer

A. Osmosis—the movement of water molecules across a semipermeable membrane in a direction that equalizes the concentration of water. The flow of water is into a solution that has a high solute concentration.

B. Diffusion—movement of a substance from an area of high concentration to an area of low concentration.

C. Active transport—transport of substances across a membrane from an area of low concentration to an area of high concentration.

D. Filtration—passage of fluids through a semipermeable membrane as a result of a difference in hydrostatic pressures (pressure exerted by a fluid within a closed system).

Balance of Body Fluid

A. Intake.
   1. Ingestion of foodstuff and water.
   2. Oxidation of foodstuff.
B. Output.
   1. Skin and lungs.
      a. Water is lost through vaporization from the skin surface and through expired air from the lungs.
      b. The amount lost increases as metabolism increases.
   2. Gastrointestinal tract.
      a. Routes include saliva, gastric secretions, bile, pancreatic juices, and intestinal mucosa.
      b. A volume in excess of seven liters is transferred from the extracellular fluid (ECF) into the gastrointestinal tract, only to be reabsorbed, excepting some 200 ml which is passed with feces.
   3. Kidneys.
      a. Carry the heaviest load.
      b. Through glomerular filtration and tubular reabsorption, the kidneys maintain homeostasis.

Fluid Imbalance

Dehydration

A. Loss of skin turgor (after being pinched and lightly pulled upward, skin very slowly returns to normal).
B. Thirst.
C. Skin dry and warm.
D. Febrile (usually means there is fluid loss through perspiration).
E. Cracked lips.
F. Decreased urinary output (normal output is 30 ml/hr).
G. Concentrated urine—dark amber color and odorous.
H. Weight loss.
I. Low central venous pressure (CVP).

Circulatory Overload

A. Headache.
B. Flushed skin.
C. Tachycardia.
D. Venous distention, particularly neck veins.
E. Increased blood pressure and CVP.
F. Tachypnea (an increase in respiratory rate), coughing, dyspnea (shortness of breath), cyanosis, and pulmonary edema.

Implementation

A. Take central venous pressure to determine fluid balance if CVP catheter is in place. CVP reflects competency of the heart (particularly the right side) to handle the volume of blood returning to it.

1. CVP indicates the comparison of the pumping capacity of the heart and the volume of the circulating blood.
2. Normal CVP reading: 5 to 10 cm H_2O.
3. Increased CVP (above 15 cm H_2O) can be indicative of congestive heart failure or circulatory overload.
4. Decreased CVP (below 5 cm H_2O) is indicative of hypovolemia (decreased fluid volume) whether from blood loss or other fluid losses.

B. Monitor patient's condition every two hours.
1. Check condition of skin.
2. Check body temperature—fever suggests loss of body fluids.
3. Check for venous distention.
4. Ask patient about unusual related symptoms: headache, shortness of breath.

Electrolyte Imbalance

Potassium Imbalance

Definition: Normal serum or plasma level is 3.5 to 5.5 mEq/L. Deficiency or excess of potassium in the blood varies from these levels.

Hyperkalemia (Potassium Excess)

A. Signs and symptoms.
1. Weakness, flaccid paralysis.
2. Hyperreflexia proceeding to paralysis.
3. Bradycardia.
4. Ventricular fibrillation.
5. ECG changes.
6. Nausea.
7. Dizziness.
8. Oliguria.
9. Apprehension.
10. Cardiac arrest.

B. Causes of excess potassium levels.
1. Usually renal disease (cannot excrete potassium).

2. Burns (due to cellular destruction releasing potassium).
3. Crushing injuries (due to cellular breakage releasing potassium from cells).
4. Adrenal insufficiency.
5. Respiratory or metabolic acidosis.

C. Treatment of hyperkalemia.
1. Decrease potassium intake.
2. IV infusion of sodium chloride, providing kidney function is normal.
3. Kayexalate enemas.
4. Dialysis.
5. Observe ECG tracings.
6. Measure intake and output.

Hypokalemia (Potassium Deficiency)

A. Signs and symptoms.
1. Muscle weakness, muscle pain and hyporeflexia.
2. Hypotension.
3. Arrhythmias—PVCs particularly.
4. Anorexia advancing to nausea, vomiting.
5. Apathy, drowsiness leading to coma.
6. ECG changes.
7. Fatigue.
8. Weak pulse.
9. Shortness of breath.
10. Shallow respirations.

B. Causes of hypokalemia.
1. Renal loss most common (usually caused by use of diuretics).
2. Insufficient potassium intake.
3. Loss from vomiting and diarrhea or from gastrointestinal tract via NG tube placement without replacement of electrolyte solution.

C. Treatment of hypokalemia—replacement of potassium, orally or parenterally.

Sodium Imbalance

Definition: Normal serum or plasma level is 135 to 145 Eq/L. Deficiency or excess of sodium varies from these levels.

Hypernatremia (Sodium Excess)

A. Signs and symptoms.
  1. The same as for extracellular fluid excesses.
    a. Pitting edema.
    b. Excessive weight gain.
    c. Increased blood pressure.
    d. Dyspnea.
  2. If hypernatremia is due to dehydration, in which there is a loss of fluid thereby increasing the number of ions, the signs and symptoms include:
    a. Concentrated urine and oliguria.
    b. Dry mucous membranes.
    c. Thirst.
    d. Flushed skin.
    e. Increased temperature.
    f. Tachycardia.
B. Causes of hypernatremia.
  1. Usually from administration of excessive amount of sodium chloride.
  2. Dehydration from excessive loss of fluids.
C. Nursing care.
  1. Record intake and output.
  2. Restrict sodium in diet.
  3. Weigh daily.
  4. Observe vital signs.

Hyponatremia (Sodium Deficiency)

A. Signs and symptoms.
  1. The same as those for extracellular fluid deficiency.
    a. Weakness.
    b. Restlessness.
    c. Delirium.
    d. Hyperpnea.
    e. Oliguria.
    f. Increased temperature.
    g. Flushed skin.
    h. Abdominal cramps.
    i. Convulsions.
  2. If sodium is lost but fluid is not, the following signs and symptoms will be present (similar to those of water excess).
    a. Mental confusion.
    b. Headache.
    c. Muscle twitching and weakness.
    d. Coma.
    e. Convulsions.
    f. Oliguria.
B. Causes of hyponatremia.
  1. Excessive perspiration.
  2. Use of diuretics.
  3. Gastrointestinal losses.
  4. Lack of sodium in diet.
  5. Renal disease.
  6. Burns.
C. Nursing care.
  1. Monitor IV fluids with sodium.
  2. Maintain accurate intake and output.

Calcium Imbalance

Definition: Normal serum level is 4.5 to 6.0 mEqL. Imbalances vary from these levels. Ninety-nine percent of all calcium is found in bones and teeth.

Hypocalcemia (Calcium Deficiency)

A. Signs and symptoms.
  1. Abdominal cramps, muscle cramps.
  2. Tetany, carpopedal spasms.
  3. Circumoral tingling, tingling in fingers.
  4. Convulsions.
B. Causes of hypocalcemia.
  1. Acute pancreatitis.
  2. Burns.
  3. Removal of parathyroid glands.
C. Treatment—reestablish normal plasma level and/or treat underlying cause.

Hypercalcemia (Calcium Excess)

A. Signs and symptoms.
  1. Anorexia, nausea.
  2. Lethargy.
  3. Weight loss.
  4. Polydipsia, polyuria.
  5. Flank pain, bone pain.
  6. Decreased muscle tone.
B. Causes of hypercalcemia.
  1. Excessive intake of vitamin D (milk).
  2. Hyperparathyroidism, neoplasm of parathyroids.

3. Thyrotoxicosis.
4. Immobilization.
5. Paget's disease.
C. Treatment—treat the underlying cause and/or reestablish normal plasma level of calcium.

Intravenous Regulation ❖ PROCEDURE ❖

A. Calculation of drip factor.
1. Microdrop—60 gtt/ml fluid.
2. Adult drop factor usually depends on administration set 10–20 gtt/ml fluid.
B. General formula.

$$\frac{\text{Drops/}}{\text{min}} = \frac{\text{Total volume infused} \times \text{drops/ml}}{\text{Total time for infusing in minutes}}$$

Example: Ordered 1000 ml D_5W administered over eight-hour period of time.

1. With microdrip, it is easy to remember that the number of drops per minute equals the number of ml's or ml's to be administered per hour.

Example: $\dfrac{1000}{8} = 125$ ml/hour

Using formula:

$$(8 \times 60) \frac{1000 \times 60}{480} = \frac{60,000}{480} = \frac{125}{\text{gtt/min}}$$

2. With administration set that delivers 10 gtt/cc

$$\frac{1000 \times 10}{480} = \frac{10,000}{480} = 20.8 \text{ or } 21 \text{ gtt/min}$$

3. With administration set that delivers 15 gtt/cc

$$\frac{1000 \times 15}{480} = \frac{15,000}{480} = 31 \text{ gtt/min}$$

C. Nursing care with IV therapy.
1. Before infusion, ensure patient is in comfortable position.
2. Carefully check label against physician's orders.
3. Check circulation in the immobilized extremity.

4. Frequently check rate of infusion.
5. Observe for signs of swelling at infusion site.
6. Take vital signs at least every 15 minutes for replacement fluid administration.

ACID-BASE BALANCE

Normal Acid-Base Balance

Principles

A. Acid-base balance is the ratio of acids and bases in the body that are necessary to maintain a chemical balance conducive to life.
B. Acid-base ratio is 20 base to 1 acid.
C. Acid-base balance is measured by arterial blood samples and recorded as blood pH. Range is 7.35 to 7.45.
D. Acids are hydrogen ion donors. They release hydrogen ions to neutralize or decrease the strength of the base.
E. Bases are hydrogen ion acceptors. They accept hydrogen ions to convert strong acids to weak acids (for example, hydrochloric acid is converted to carbonic acid.)

Regulatory Mechanisms

A. The body controls the pH balance by use of:
1. Chemical buffers.
2. Lungs.
3. Cells.
4. Kidneys.
B. The chemical buffer system works fastest, but other regulatory mechanisms provide more reliable protection against acid-base imbalance. The three primary buffer systems are:
1. Bicarbonate—maintains blood pH at 7.4 with ratio of 20 parts bicarbonate to 1 part carbonic acid.
2. Plasma proteins (along with the liver)—vary the amounts of hydrogen ions in the

chemical structure of the protein. They can both attract and release hydrogen ions.

3. Hemoglobin—maintains balance by chloride shift. Chloride shifts in and out of red blood cells according to the level of oxygen in blood plasma. Each chloride ion that leaves the cell is replaced by a bicarbonate ion.

C. Lungs.
1. Next to react are the lungs.
2. It takes 10 to 30 minutes for lungs to inactivate hydrogen molecules by converting them to water molecules.
3. Lungs can only inactivate the hydrogen ions carried by carbonic acid. The other ions must be excreted by the kidneys.

D. Cells.
1. Cells absorb or release extra hydrogen ions.
2. Cells react in two to four hours.

E. Kidneys.
1. Kidneys are the mainstay of regulatory mechanisms.
2. Excretion of excessive acid or base is slow. Compensation takes a few hours to several days, but it is the most effective process.
3. Primary function of kidneys is bicarbonate regulation. Kidneys restore bicarbonate by releasing hydrogen ions and holding bicarbonate ions.

Acid-Base Imbalances

Metabolic Acidosis

Definition: Metabolic acidosis occurs when there is a deficit of bases or an accumulation of fixed acids.

A. Changes in pH and serum carbon dioxide.
1. The pH will become acidic (fall below 7.35).
2. The serum CO_2 level will be below 22 mEq/L (normal range of CO_2 is 26–28 mEq/L).

B. Compensatory mechanisms.
1. When compensating for metabolic acidosis, the one clinical manifestation usually observed is the "blowing ￼ acids. This is manifeste ￼ rate increase.
2. The lungs are the faste ￼ to compensate for meta ￼

C. Causes of metabolic acido ￼ in the surgical patient).
1. Diabetes—diabetic ketoacidosis.
2. Renal insufficiency—kidneys retain the products of protein metabolism, thereby decreasing the bicarbonate that is available to maintain an acid-base balance.
3. Diarrhea—excessive amounts of base are lost from the intestines and pancreas, resulting in acidosis.

D. Signs and symptoms.
1. Headache.
2. Drowsiness.
3. Nausea, vomiting, diarrhea.
4. Stupor, coma.
5. Twitching, convulsions.
6. Kussmaul's respiration (increased respiratory rate).
7. Fruity breath (as evidenced in diabetic ketoacidosis as a result of improper fat metabolism).

E. Treatment and nursing care.
1. These drugs may be given intravenously:
   a. Sodium bicarbonate.
   b. Sodium lactate.
   c. Insulin (in ketoacidosis).
2. Watch laboratory values closely while treating metabolic acidosis.
3. Watch for signs of hyperkalemia and dehydration in the patient (oliguria, vital sign changes, etc.).
4. Record intake and output.

Metabolic Alkalosis

Definition: Metabolic alkalosis is a malfunction of metabolism that causes an increase in blood base or a reduction of available acids in the serum.

A. Changes in pH and serum carbon dioxide.
1. The pH will become more alkaline (above 7.45).

CO_2 will increase above 35 mEq/L. ote that this measures the amount of circulating bicarbonate or the base portion of the plasma. (A good way to remember these acid-base values is to recall that as the pH increases, so does the CO_2. The reverse is true for acidosis.)

B. Compensatory mechanisms.
1. The lungs will attempt to hold on to the carbonic acid in an effort to neutralize the base state.
2. As a result, the rate of respiration will decrease.

C. Causes of metabolic alkalosis.
1. Ingestion of excessive soda bicarbonate (used by individuals for acid indigestion).
2. Excessive vomiting, which results in the loss of hydrochloric acid and potassium.
3. Placement of NG tube which causes a depletion of both hydrochloric acid and potassium.
4. Use of potent diuretics, particularly by cardiac patients. Not only potassium but also hydrogen and chloride ions are lost, causing an increase in the bicarbonate level of the serum.

D. Signs and symptoms.
1. Nausea, vomiting.
2. Diarrhea.
3. Irritability, agitation.
4. Coma, convulsions.
5. Restlessness.
6. Twitching of extremities.
7. ECG changes.

E. Treatment and nursing care.
1. Maintain diet of foods high in potassium and chloride (bananas, apricots, dried peaches, Brazil nuts, dried figs, oranges).
2. Monitor IV solution of added electrolytes.
3. Give Diamox to promote kidney excretion of bicarbonate.
4. Administer potassium chloride maintenance doses to patients on long-term diuretics.
5. Give ammonium chloride to increase the amount of available hydrogen ions, thereby increasing the availability of acids in the blood.
6. Check laboratory values frequently to watch for electrolyte imbalance.
7. Watch patient for physical signs indicative of hypokalemia or metabolic alkalosis.
8. Keep accurate records of intake and output and vital signs.

Respiratory Acidosis

Definition: Respiratory acidosis refers to increased carbonic acid concentration (accumulated CO_2, which has combined with water) caused by retention of carbon dioxide through hypoventilation. Differs from metabolic acidosis in that it is caused by defective functioning of the lungs.

A. Changes in pH, pCO_2 and pO_2.
1. With an increased acidic state, the pH will fall below 7.35.
2. The pCO_2 will be increased above 50 mmHg.
3. The pO_2 is normal (90–100 mmHg) or it can be decreased as hypoxia increases.
4. The HCO_3 will be normal if respiratory acidosis is uncompensated.

B. Compensatory mechanisms.
1. Because the basic problem in respiratory acidosis is a defect in the lungs, the kidneys must be the major compensatory mechanism.
   a. The kidneys work much slower than the lungs.
   b. As a result, compensation may take from hours to days.
2. The kidneys will retain and return bicarbonate to the extracellular fluid compartment.

C. Causes of respiratory acidosis.
1. Sedatives.
2. Over-sedation with narcotics in postoperative period.
3. A chronic pulmonary disorder, such as emphysema, asthma, bronchitis or pneumonia, leading to
   a. Inability of the lungs to expand and contract adequately.

b. Difficulty in the expiratory phase of respiration, which causes retention of carbon dioxide.
4. Poor gaseous exchange during surgery.

D. Signs and symptoms.
1. Dyspnea after exertion.
2. Hyperventilation when at rest.
3. Cyanosis.
4. Sensorium changes (drowsiness leading to coma).
5. Carbon dioxide narcosis.
   a. When body has adjusted to higher carbon dioxide levels, the respiratory center loses its sensitivity to elevated carbon dioxide.
   b. Medulla fails to respond to high levels of carbon dioxide.
   c. Patient is forced to depend on anoxia for respiratory stimulus.
   d. If a high level of oxygen is administered, patient will cease breathing.

E. Treatment and nursing care.
1. Turn, cough, and hyperventilate patients at least every two to four hours postoperatively. Use oropharyngeal suction if necessary.
2. When pulmonary complications present a threat, do postural drainage, percussion, and vibration, followed by suctioning.
3. Keep patient well hydrated to facilitate removal of secretions. If patient is dehydrated, secretions become thick and more difficult to expectorate.
4. Watch vital signs carefully, particularly rate and depth of respirations.
5. Teach pursed-lip breathing to chronic respiratory patients.
6. If oxygen is administered, watch carefully for signs of carbon dioxide narcosis.
7. Place patient on mechanical ventilation if necessary.
8. Administer aerosol medications through IPPB.
   a. Bronchodilators (aminophylline)—relieve bronchospasms.
   b. Detergents (Tergemist)—liquefy tenacious mucus.
   c. Antibiotics specific to causative agent.
9. Drugs that may be given intravenously:

a. Sodium bicarbonate.
b. Sodium lactate.
c. Ringer's lactate—to replace electrolyte loss.

Respiratory Alkalosis

Definition: Respiratory alkalosis occurs when an excessive amount of carbon dioxide is exhaled, usually caused by hyperventilation. The loss of carbon dioxide results in a decrease in H^+ concentration along with a decrease in pCO_2 and an increase in the ratio of bicarbonate to carbonic acid. The result is an increase in the pH level.

A. Changes in pH, pCO_2 and pO_2.
1. With an increased alkalotic state, the pH will increase above 7.45, indicating there is a decreased amount of carbonic acid in the serum.
2. The pCO_2 will be normal-to-low, as this measures the acid portion of the acid-base system (30 to 45 mmHg).
3. The pO_2 should be unchanged.
4. The bicarbonate level (HCO_3 or CO_2 content) should be normal unless the patient is compensating.

B. Compensatory mechanisms.
1. Since the basic problem is related to the respiratory system, the kidneys will compensate by excreting more bicarbonate ions and retaining H^+.
2. This process will return the acid-base balance to a normal ratio.

C. Causes of respiratory alkalosis.
1. Hysteria—patient hyperventilates and exhales excessive amounts of carbon dioxide.
2. Hypoxia—stimulates patient to breathe more vigorously.
3. Following head injuries or intracranial surgery.
4. Increased temperature.
5. Salicylate poisoning.
   a. Stimulation of respiration causes alkalosis through hyperventilation.
   b. Acidosis may occur from excessive salicylates in the blood.

D. Signs and symptoms.
  1. Hyperreflexia.
  2. Muscular twitching.
  3. Convulsions.
  4. Gasping for breath.
E. Treatment and nursing care.
  1. Eliminate cause of hyperventilation.
  2. Remain with patient and be supportive to reduce anxiety.
  3. Use rebreathing bag to return patient's carbon dioxide to self (paper bag works just as well).

BLOOD AND BLOOD FACTORS

Blood Grouping

Major Blood Groups

A. ABO blood group.
  1. A.
  2. AB.
  3. B.
  4. O.
B. Rh blood group.
  1. Positive (85 percent of the population).
  2. Negative (15 percent of the population).

Antigens and Antibodies

A. Blood type based on type of antigens present in red blood cells as well as type of antibodies in the serum.

B. A and B antigens.
  1. Persons with type A blood have antigen A present; persons with type B blood have antigen B present.
  2. Persons with type AB blood have both A and B antigens present.
  3. Persons with type 0 blood have no antigens present.
C. Anti-A and Anti-B antibodies.
  1. Antibodies develop as a response to exposure. Persons with type A blood have anti-B antibodies. They do not have anti-A antibodies because the blood cells would be destroyed by agglutination.
  2. Persons with type B blood have anti-A antibodies.
  3. Persons with type AB blood have no antibodies.
     a. Considered *universal recipients*.
     b. Cannot destroy donor's red blood cells.
  4. Persons with type 0 blood have both anti-A and anti-B antibodies.
     a. Considered *universal donors*.
     b. Red blood cells do not contain antigens that could be destroyed by antibodies in recipients' blood.

Transfusion Administration ❖ PROCEDURE ❖

Procedure

A. Check carefully for correct name and ID number. Double check blood group donor number (have two persons check information).
B. Do not warm blood, as bacteria thrives in this medium.

Table B. Summary of ABO Blood Grouping

Blood Type	Antigen in RBCs	Antibodies in Plasma	Incompatible Donor Blood	Compatible Blood Donor
A	A	Anti-B	AB and B	A and O
B	B	Anti-A	A and AB	B and O
AB	A and B	None	None	All blood groups
O	None	Anti-A and Anti-B	All blood groups	O

C. Do not allow blood to be unrefrigerated for more than 30 minutes before administration.
D. Use blood filter to prevent fibrin and other materials from entering the bloodstream.
E. Transfusion will be started with normal saline or another electrolyte solution; blood will agglutinate without the presence of electrolytes.

Implementation

A. Transfusion usually started at 20 to 40 drops per minute. Closely observe transfusion as reaction usually occur during the first 15 minutes.
B. Take base line vital signs at beginning and five minutes after beginning transfusion.
C. Transfusion is usually completed in no less than two hours and in no more than five hours.
   1. Usually administered at a rate of 60 to 80 drops per minute.
   2. If patient is hypovolemic, blood can be administered at the rate of 500 ml in 10 minutes by use of a blood pump. Observe for pulmonary edema and hypervolemia.

Transfusion Reactions

A. Hemolytic or incompatibility reaction.
   1. Most severe complication.
   2. Caused by mismatched blood.
   3. Clinical manifestations.
      a. Increased temperature.
      b. Decreased blood pressure.
      c. Pain across the chest and at the site of needle insertion.
      d. Chills.
      e. Hematuria.
      f. Backache in the kidney region.
      g. Dyspnea and cyanosis.
      h. Jaundice can occur in severe cases.
   4. The reaction is caused by agglutination of the donor's red cells.
      a. The antibodies in the recipient's plasma react with the antigens in the donor's red cells.

b. The clumping blocks off capillaries and therefore obstructs the flow of blood and oxygen to cells.
   5. Nursing care.
      a. Stop transfusion immediately upon appearance of symptoms.
      b. Return remaining blood and the patient's blood sample to the laboratory for type and cross match.
      c. Keep IV patent after changing blood tubing with either normal saline or preferably D_5W.
      d. Take vital signs every 15 minutes.
      e. Insert Foley catheter for a urine sample for red blood cells and an accurate output record.
      f. Check for oliguria.
      g. Administer medications such as vasopressors if indicated.
      h. Administer oxygen as necessary.
B. Bacterial contamination.
   1. Check blood for discoloration, cloudiness, and bubbles, which are indicative of contamination.
   2. Signs and symptoms.
      a. Sudden increase in temperature.
      b. Sudden chill.
      c. Headache.
      d. Peripheral vasodilation.
      e. Malaise.
      f. Lumbar pain.
   3. Nursing care.
      a. Do not use blood that is cloudy or discolored or appears to have bubbles present.
      b. If transfusion has been started, discontinue immediately.
      c. Send remaining blood to laboratory for culture and sensitivity. If transfusion has been started, send patient's blood sample as well.
      d. Change IV tubing and keep it patent.
      e. Check vital signs, including temperature, every 15 minutes.
      f. Insert Foley catheter for accurate output and urine specimen as ordered.

g. Control hyperthermia, if present, with antipyretics, cooling blankets, or with sponge baths.

C. Allergic reactions.
  1. Allergic response to any type of allergen in the donor's blood.
  2. Common reaction, usually mild in nature.
  3. Signs and symptoms.
     a. Hives.
     b. Urticaria.
     c. Wheezing.
     d. Laryngeal edema.
  4. Nursing care.
     a. Administer an antihistamine such as Benadryl to control itching and to relieve edema.
     b. If reaction is severe, discontinue the transfusion; otherwise, decrease the flow rate.

COMMON PROCEDURES

General Principles

Nursing Actions Prior to Procedures

A. Most procedures require a physician's order.
B. Review written procedure in your hospital's/agency's procedure book; seek help from team leader/head nurse if you do not know method.
C. Explain all procedures to patient; ask patient's cooperation.
D. Wash hands before beginning procedure and maintain medical or surgical asepsis.
E. Provide privacy for patient.

Restraints

A. Uses.
  1. Immobilize a part.
  2. Provide support to a part.
  3. Prevent patient from injuring self or another.
  4. Promote safety while sitting in chair or in bed.
B. Application. ❖ **PROCEDURE** ❖
  1. Check for physician's order.
  2. Explain purpose of restraint to patient and his/her family.
  3. Apply restraint.
  4. Check circulation of extremities distal to restraint.
  5. Chart application and reason.
  6. Intervene every two hours.
     a. Remove restraint.
     b. Observe condition of skin.
     c. Check circulation.
     d. Reapply restraint.

Infection Control

A. Methods of microorganism transmission.
  1. Direct contact.
  2. Air, droplet.
  3. Fomite (toys, books, etc.).
  4. Food, water.
  5. Animals, insects.
B. Medical asepsis—"clean."
  1. Limits spread of microorganisms.
  2. Handwashing best single technique.
  3. First rinse washable articles in cold water to remove protein; then wash in hot, soapy water.
C. Surgical asepsis—"sterile."
  1. Absence of all forms of microorganisms, including spores.
  2. Method used in surgical procedures/operations.
D. Isolation technique.
  1. Used to confine pathogens (disease-producing microorganisms).
     a. General principles.
        (1) Floors are contaminated.
        (2) Keep doors closed.
        (3) Double bag all items to be removed from room.
        (4) Wash hands immediately after leaving room.

b. Types of restriction.
   (1) Respiratory.
   (2) Wound and skin.
   (3) Enteric (GI tract).
   (4) Strict—prevents transmission by all methods.
2. Protective or reverse barrier—used to keep potential pathogens from patient.
   a. Used for patients with increased susceptibility to disease.
   b. All equipment sterile when brought into room; no special care necessary to remove equipment from room.
   c. Staff wears "space suits."

Catheterization ❖ PROCEDURE ❖

A. Procedure involves putting plastic or rubber tube/catheter in bladder via urethra in order to empty bladder or obtain specimen.

B. It is a sterile procedure—use surgical aseptic technique and avoid contaminating equipment.

C. Position for female patient.
   1. Dorsal recumbent most common.
   2. Sims' or lateral.

D. Make provisions for privacy.

E. Procedure protocol.
   1. Screen, position, and drape patient.
   2. Place catheter tray for convenience and open it.
   3. Put on sterile gloves and arrange equipment.
   4. Place sterile drapes.
   5. Lubricate catheter.
   6. Expose urinary meatus (this gloved hand now considered contaminated). Leave hand in position until procedure completed.
   7. Cleanse urinary meatus with provided equipment.
   8. Pick up lubricated catheter (do not contaminate it). Insert catheter into urethra until urine flows.
   9. When urine stops flowing, pinch and withdraw catheter. (If more than 1000 ml obtained, some facilities suggest clamping catheter for 20 minutes before removing more urine to prevent bladder spasm).
   10. Remove gloves.
   11. Clean patient and position for comfort.
   12. Clean all equipment or discard disposable equipment.
   13. Chart time procedure done and amount and character of urine.

F. Retention or Foley catheter (R/C) is inserted in the same manner.
   1. When in place, sterile water or sterile air is instilled into a balloonlike structure near the catheter tip. This "balloon" keeps the catheter in the bladder.
   2. The catheter is usually attached to a drainage tube and bag.

R/C or Bladder Irrigation ❖ PROCEDURE ❖

A. Surgical aseptic technique used.

B. Check amount and type of solution ordered.

C. Open method.
   1. Cleanse catheter at connection with drainage tube and separate. Protect drainage tube from contamination.
   2. Fill sterile irrigating syringe with sterile solution and gently put into catheter.
   3. Remove syringe and allow solution to drain into emesis basin—do not contaminate end of catheter.
   4. Repeat as necessary until ordered amount is used or desired returns are obtained.
   5. Connect catheter to drainage tube.

D. Closed method—most common.
   1. Place clamp on catheter immediately above drainage tube connector.
   2. Place 22- or 24-gauge sterile needle on sterile syringe. Fill syringe with ordered sterile solution.
   3. Cleanse catheter between side arm and clamp with an alcohol swab, and insert needle.
   4. Gently inject solution. When ordered amount injected, withdraw needle and remove clamp.

E. Chart method used, amount and type of solution, description of returns, and patient's reaction.

PREOPERATIVE AND POSTOPERATIVE CARE

Routine Preoperative Care

Psychological Support

A. Reinforce the physician's teaching regarding the surgical procedure.
B. Identify patient's anxieties; notify physician of extreme anxiety.
C. Listen to patient's verbalization of fears.
D. Provide support to the patient's family (where family can wait during surgery, approximately how long surgery will take, etc.).

Preoperative Teaching

A. Postoperative exercises: leg, coughing, deep breathing, etc.
B. Equipment which will be used during postoperative period: intermittent positive pressure breathing machine (IPPB), NG tube to suction, etc.
C. Pain medication and when to ask for it.
D. Explanation of NPO.

Physical Care

A. Observation and recording of patient's overall condition.
    1. Nutritional status.
    2. Physical defects, such as loss of limb function, skin breakdown.
    3. Hearing or sight difficulties.
B. Chest x-ray, ECG, and blood and urine samples as ordered.

C. Preoperative history and present physical condition.
D. Determination of any drug allergies.
E. Skin prep and shave when necessary; shower with antibacterial soap if ordered.
F. Retention or indwelling catheter, NG tube, or enema if ordered.
G. Have patient void immediately before medicating.
H. Preoperative medications administered.
I. Following preoperative medication, quiet rest with siderails up and curtains drawn.

Nurse's Responsibility

A. Check and report abnormal lab values and vital signs.
B. Complete preoperative check list.
    1. Remove dentures, nail polish, hairpins, artificial eyes, contact lenses, glasses.
    2. Give preoperative medicines.
C. Complete ordered preoperative nursing interventions.
D. See that consent form is signed.
E. Check ID band.
F. Perform or check skin prep/shave.

Anesthesia

Preoperative Medications

A. Purpose.
    1. Decrease secretions of the mouth and respiratory tract.
    2. Depress vagal reflexes.
    3. Produce drowsiness and relieve anxiety.
    4. Allow anesthesia to be induced more smoothly and in smaller amounts.
B. Types of drugs administered.
    1. Barbiturates.
        a. Intermediate-acting barbiturate at bedtime.
        b. Short-acting barbiturate one hour preoperatively.
    2. Belladonna alkaloids.

a. Decrease salivary and bronchial secretions; allow inhalation anesthetics to be administered more easily and prevent postoperative complications.

b. Scopolamine is used in conjunction with morphine or Demerol to produce amnesic block.

c. Atropine blocks the vagus nerve response of decreased heart rate which can occur as a reaction to some inhalation anesthetics.

3. Central nervous system depressants.

General Anesthesia

A. General anesthesia produces a depression of the CNS, amnesia, loss of reflexes, and unconsciousness.

1. Inhalation agents.
   a. Halothane.
   b. Ether.
   c. Chloroform.

2. Intravenous anesthesia—thiopental (Pentothal).

3. Dissociative anesthesia (ketamine HCL and Innovar). Used with nitrous oxide and oxygen for short anesthesia.

B. Stages and planes of general anesthesia.

1. Stage one: early induction—from beginning of inhalation to loss of consciousness.

2. Stage two: delirium or excitement.
   a. No surgery is performed at this point—very dangerous stage.
   b. Breathing is irregular.

3. Stage three: surgical anesthesia.
   a. Begins when patient stops fighting and is breathing regularly.
   b. Four planes, based on respiration, pupillary and eyeball movement, and reflex muscular responses.

4. Stage four: medullary paralysis—respiratory arrest.

C. Anesthetic Agents.

1. Anesthesia produces insensitivity to pain or sensation.

2. Dangers associated with anesthesia depend on overall condition of patient.

a. High risk if associated cardiovascular, renal, or respiratory conditions.

b. High risk for unborn fetus and mother.

c. High risk if stomach full (chance of vomiting and aspiration).

3. Types of anesthesia.

a. General—administered IV or by inhalation. Produces loss of consciousness and decreases reflex movement.

b. Local—applied topically or injected regionally. Patient is alert, but pain and sensation are decreased in surgical area.

Routine Postoperative Care

Recovery Room ❖ PROCEDURE ❖

A. Immediate postoperative care.

1. Maintain patent airway.

2. Administer oxygen by mask or nasal cannula.

3. Check gag reflex.

4. Position patient for adequate ventilation.

5. Observe for adverse signs of general anesthesia or spinal anesthesia.
   a. Level of consciousness.
   b. Movement of limbs.

6. Monitor vital signs.
   a. Check every 10 to 15 minutes.
      (1) Pulse—check rate, quality, and rhythm.
      (2) Blood pressure—check pulse pressure and quality as well as systolic and diastolic pressure.
      (3) Respiration—check rate, rhythm, depth, and type of respiration (abdominal breathing, nasal flaring).
   b. Vital signs are sometimes difficult to obtain due to hypothermia.
   c. Movement from operating room table to gurney can alter vital signs significantly, especially with cardiovascular patients.
   d. Maintain temperature (operating room is usually cold)—apply warm blankets.

7. Check patency of IV; check IV insertion site.
8. Observe dressings and surgical drains.
   a. Mark any drainage on dressings, and note time by drawing a line around the drainage.
   b. Note color and amount of drainage on dressings and in drainage tubes.
   c. Ensure that dressing is secure.
   d. Reinforce dressings as needed.
B. Overall observations of condition.
   1. Check skin for warmth, color, and moisture.
   2. Check nailbeds and mucous membranes for color (report if cyanotic) and blanching.
   3. Observe for return of reflexes.
C. Medications—begin routine drugs and administer all STAT drugs.
D. Assessment for return to room.
   1. Be sure vital signs are stable and within normal limits.
   2. See if patient is awake and reflexes are present (gag and cough reflex).
   3. Take oral airway out (if not out already).
   4. Check for movement and sensation in limbs (particularly legs, with spinal anesthesia).
   5. Watch for cyanosis.
   6. Be sure dressings are intact and there is no excessive drainage.

Surgical Floor

A. Assessment.
   1. Maintain patent airway; administer oxygen as necessary.
   2. Take vital signs—usual orders are VS q 15 minutes until stable; then q ½ hour x 2, q hour x 4; then q 4 hours for 24–48 hours.
   3. Check IV site and patency frequently.
   4. Observe and record urine output.
   5. Keep accurate records of intake and output.
B. Nursing care.
   1. Position patient for comfort and maximum airway ventilation.
   2. Turn q 2 hours and prn.
3. Give back care at least every four hours.
4. Encourage coughing and deep breathing every two hours (may use IPPB or blow bottles).
5. Keep patient comfortable with medications.
6. Check dressings and drainage tubes q 2–4 hours unless abnormal amount of drainage; then, more frequently.
7. Give oral hygiene at least q 4 hours; q 2 hours if NG tube, nasal oxygen, or endotracheal tube inserted.
8. Bathe patient when temperature can be maintained—bathing removes the antiseptic solution and stimulates circulation.
9. Keep patient warm and avoid chilling, but do not increase temperature above normal.
   a. Increased temperature increases metabolic rate and need for oxygen.
   b. Excessive perspiration causes fluid and electrolyte loss.
10. Irrigate NG tube q 2 hours and prn with normal saline to keep patent.
11. Maintain dietary intake—type of diet depends on type and extent of surgical procedure.
    a. Minor surgical conditions—the patient may drink or eat as soon as he or she is awake and desires food or drink.
    b. Major surgical conditions.
       (1) NPO until bowel sounds return.
       (2) Clear liquid advanced to full liquid as tolerated.
       (3) Soft diet advanced to full diet within three to five days (depending on type of surgery and physician's preference).
12. Place on bedpan two to four hours postoperatively if catheter not inserted.

Postoperative Medications

Narcotic Analgesics

A. Pharmacological action—reduces pain and restlessness.

B. General side effects.
1. Drowsiness.
2. Euphoria.
3. Sleep.
4. Respiratory depression.
5. Nausea and vomiting.
C. Types of analgesics.
1. Opiates.
a. Morphine sulfate—potent analgesic.
(1) Specific side effects: miosis (pin-point pupils); bradycardia.
(2) Usual dosage: ¼ to ⅙ gr IM q 3–4 hours prn.
b. Codeine sulfate—mild analgesic.
(1) Specific side effects: constipation.
(2) Usual dosage: 30 mg to 60 mg q 3–4 hours IM
c. Dilaudid—potent analgesic.
(1) Specific side effects: hypotension, constipation, euphoria.
(2) Usual dosage: 2 to 4 mg PO, IM or IV q 4–6 hours.
d. Numorphan—potent analgesic.
(1) Specific side effects: urinary retention, ileus, euphoria.
(2) Usual dosage: 1–1.5 mg sub q. or IM q 4–6 hours; 0.5 mg IV q 4–6 hours.
2. Synthetic opiatelike drugs.
a. Demerol (meperidine)—potent analgesic.
(1) Specific side effects: miosis or mydriasis (dilation of pupils); hypotension; tachycardia.
(2) Usual dosage: 25 mg to 100 mg q 3–4 hours IM.
b. Talwin (pentazocine)—potent analgesic.
(1) Specific side effects: gastrointestinal disturbances, vertigo, headache, and euphoria.
(2) Usual dosage: 50 mg oral tablets q 3–4 hours; 30 mg IM q 3–4 hours prn.

Antiemetics

A. Pharmacological action.

1. Reduces the hyperactive reflex of the stomach.
2. Makes the chemoreceptor trigger zone of medulla less sensitive to nerve impulses passing through this center to the vomiting center.
B. General side effects.
1. Drowsiness.
2. Dry mouth.
3. Nervous system effects.
C. Common drugs.
1. Phenothiazines.
a. Compazine (prochlorperazine).
(1) Specific side effects: amenorrhea, hypotension, and vertigo.
(2) Normal dosage: 5–10 mg q 3–4 hours IM.
b. Phenergan (promethazine).
(1) Specific side effects.
(a) Dryness of mouth.
(b) Blurred vision.
(2) Normal dosage: 12.5–50 mg q 4 hours prn.
2. Nonphenothiazines.
a. Dramamine (dimenhydrinate).
(1) Specific side effects: drowsiness.
(2) Normal dosage: 50 mg IM q 3–4 hours.
b. Tigan (trimethobenzamide).
(1) Specific side effects (rare).
(a) Hypotension.
(b) Skin rashes.
(2) Normal dosage: 200 mg (2 ml) tid or qid IM.

COMMON POSTOPERATIVE COMPLICATIONS

Respiratory Complications

Prevention

A. Turn, cough, hyperventilate.

B. Mechanical interventions (provide a means of forced-expiration exercise).
   1. Spirometers.
   2. Blow bottles.
   3. IPPB.
C. Pharmacological therapy (through nebulization or oral route).
   1. Antibiotics—to fight infection by causative organism.
   2. Bronchodilators—to act on smooth muscle to reduce bronchial spasm.
      a. Sympathomimetics (beta$_2$ agonists preferred).
      b. Theophylline (aminophylline).
      c. Anticholinergics (atropine sulfate inhalant).
   3. Adrenocorticosteroids—to reduce inflammation (Prednisone).
   4. Enzymes—to liquefy thick, purulent secretions through digestion.
      a. Dornavac.
      b. Varidase.
   5. Expectorants—to aid in expectoration of secretions.
      a. Mucolytic agents reduce viscosity of secretion (Mucomyst).
      b. Detergents liquefy tenacious mucus (Tergemist, Alevaire).

General Signs and Symptoms

A. Complaint of tightness or fullness in chest.
B. Cough, dyspnea, or shortness of breath.
C. Increased vital signs, particularly temperature and respiratory rate.
D. Restlessness.

Common Respiratory Conditions

A. Pneumonia (see section on respiratory system.)
B. Atelectasis, collapse of pulmonary alveoli, caused by mucous plug or by inadequate ventilation.
C. Signs and symptoms.
   1. Asymmetrical chest movement.
   2. Decreased or absent breath sounds over affected area.
   3. Shortness of breath leading to cyanosis.
   4. Painful respirations.
   5. Increased vital signs: temperature, respiration, pulse.
   6. Anxiety and restlessness.

Implementation

A. Encourage coughing and deep breathing exercises; splint incision.
B. Turn frequently and position to facilitate expectoration.
C. Suction as necessary.
D. Instruct in proper use of mechanical measures (blow bottles, etc.).
E. Do clapping, percussion, vibration, postural drainage every four hours.
F. Encourage oral fluid intake to reduce tenacious sputum and to facilitate expectoration.
G. Administer expectorants and other medications as ordered.
H. Place patient in cool room with mist mask or vaporized steam.
I. Administer oxygen if necessary.
J. Mobilize patient as soon as possible.
K. Auscultate breath sounds every two to four hours and report unusual occurrences.

Thrombophlebitis

Definition: Thrombophlebitis is the formation of a clot in a vein. It occurs most often in the femoral vein.

Etiology

A. Dehydration leading to increased cellular components in vessel.
B. Decreased blood flow due to hypothermia and/or decreased metabolic rate during surgery.
C. Injury to vessel during surgery.

D. Incidence most common following abdominal or circulatory surgery.

A. Red, tender, painful calf.
B. Edema of affected leg.
C. Increased temperature in affected area as well as generalized elevation of temperature.
D. Positive Homan's sign.

Implementation

A. Maintain strict bed rest.
B. Do not use knee gatch or pillows under knees.
C. Elevate lower extremities slightly; if ordered, raise entire foot of bed.
D. Administer anticoagulants only after checking lab values.
E. Check for extension of clot.
   1. Check breath sounds for possible emboli.
   2. Check extremity involved for extension of signs (tenderness further up leg, etc.), especially in groin.
   3. Check for circulatory difficulties.
F. Position patient to avoid venous stasis, and turn every two hours.
G. Take vital signs at least every four hours.
H. Apply hot packs if ordered.
I. Use range-of-motion exercises on unaffected limbs only.
J. Do not massage or exercise affected leg unless specified by physician.
K. Apply antiembolic stockings to unaffected leg.
L. Begin exercise gradually with leg-raises to standing briefly every hour, then ambulation.

Patient Instruction

A. Avoid standing in one position for any length of time (when exercise program instituted, patients are told to either walk or to lie flat).
B. Avoid wearing constrictive clothing or garments.
C. Keep extremities at consistent, moderate temperature.

D. Wear support hose consistently.
E. Understand correct use of anticoagulants and the necessity for lab tests.

Wound infections

Etiology

A. Usual causative agents.
   1. Staphylococcus.
   2. Pseudomonas aeruginosa.
   3. Proteus vulgaris.
   4. Escherichia coli.
B. Usually occur within five to seven days of surgery.

Assessment

A. Slowly increasing temperature and tachycardia.
B. Pain and tenderness surrounding surgical site.
C. Edema and erythema surrounding suture site.
D. Increased warmth around suture site.
E. Purulent drainage.
   1. Yellow if staphylococcus.
   2. Green if Pseudomonas.

Implementation

A. Administer specific antibiotics for causative agent.
B. Irrigate wound with solution as ordered (usually hydrogen peroxide and normal saline).
C. Keep dressing and skin area dry to prevent skin excoriation and spread of bacteria.
D. Use sterile technique in changing dressings.
E. If excoriation occurs, use karaya powder and drainage bags around area of wound.
F. Changing wet to dry dressings.
   1. Wet-to-damp—*Purpose*: To prevent damage to granulating tissue.
      a. Cover wound with second moist dressing.
      b. Remove dressing while still damp.

2. Wet-to-dry—*Purpose*: To assist in debriding wounds.
   a. Cover wound with second moist dressing.
   b. Remove dressing after it dries.
3. Wet-to-wet—*Purpose*: To dilute thick exudate for easier removal.
   a. Cover wound with second saturated dressing.
   b. Keep entire dressing moist with periodic application of irrigating solution.

Wound Dehiscence and Evisceration

Definition: Dehiscence is the splitting open of wound edges. Evisceration is the extensive loss of pinkish fluid (purulent if infection is present) through a wound and the protrusion of a loop of bowel through an open wound. Patient feels as though "everything is pulling apart."

Etiology

A. Usual causes.
   1. General debilitation.
      a. Poor nutrition.
      b. Chronic illness.
      c. Obesity.
   2. Inadequate wound closure.
   3. Wound infection.
   4. Severe abdominal stretching (by coughing or vomiting).
B. Occurs about seventh postoperative day.

Implementation

A. Lay patient in supine position.
B. Cover protruding intestine with moist, sterile, normal saline packs; change packs frequently to keep moist.
C. Notify physician.
D. Take vital signs for baseline data and detection of shock.
E. Apply scultetus binder following dehiscence (preventative measure in obese or debilitated patients).

Shock

Definition: Shock is an abnormal physiological state in which there is insufficient circulating blood volume for the size of the vascular bed, thereby resulting in circulatory failure and tissue anoxia.

Classification of Shock

A. Hematogenic.
   1. Reduced circulating blood volume.
      a. Hemorrhage.
      b. Burns.
      c. Diabetes.
   2. Can be termed hypovolemic shock, referring to decreased fluid volume and other fluid losses from wounds or GI tract.
B. Neurogenic—decreased vasoconstriction leading to vasodilatation.
   1. Insulin shock.
   2. Spinal anesthesia.
C. Vasogenic (septic shock)—vasodilatation and loss of vasomotor stimulation caused by toxic substances (toxic or septic shock, such as gram negative sepsis).
D. Cardiogenic—cardiac pump failure.
   1. Congestive heart failure.
   2. Following left ventriculotomy.

Assessment of Early Shock

A. Early stages, regardless of the cause.
   1. Decreased tissue perfusion.
   2. Cellular hypoxia.
   3. Increased sympathetic nervous system activity.
B. Oliguria—usually the first sign of shock.
   1. Decreased blood volume through kidneys.
   2. Decreased urine output; hyperkalemia can be a problem.
C. Hypotension.
   1. Due to compensatory peripheral vasoconstriction (not evident initially, but it does appear in early shock).
   2. Narrowing pulse pressure, due to systolic pressure falling and diastolic pressure being maintained.

D. Tachycardia—due to heart's responding to increased sympathetic activity.

E. Tachypnea.
   1. Medulla is stimulated by buildup in lactic acid through anaerobic metabolism.
   2. As blood pH is lowered, the respiratory rate increases in an effort to blow off excess carbon dioxide and return body to acid-base balance.

F. Cool, dry, or moist skin.
   1. Caused by peripheral vasoconstriction.
   2. Blood is supplied to vital organs rather than to skin.

G. Sensorium changes—due to brain cell hypoxia.
   1. Restlessness.
   2. Apprehension and anxiety.
   3. Lethargy.
   4. Confusion.
   5. Semiconsciousness to coma.

H. Excessive thirst—due to loss of fluids or blood volume as well as peripheral vasoconstriction which decreases salivary secretions.

I. Fatigue and muscle weakness—result of shift from aerobic to anaerobic metabolism leading to lactic acid buildup.

Assessment of Severe Shock

A. Blood pressure below 70 mmHg and narrowing of pulse pressure (body loses ability to compensate and blood pressure drops rapidly).

B. Respirations become shallow and irregular.

C. Tachycardia continues.

D. Unconsciousness to coma occurs as blood supply to brain cells is decreased.

E. Pupils become dilated and fixed, due to decreased oxygen to brain.

F. Anuria is present as blood supply to kidneys is sharply decreased.

G. Skin becomes cyanotic, along with mucous membranes and nailbeds.

Implementation

A. Monitor plasma expanders, IV fluids, or blood replacement.

B. Place patient in supine position with feet and/or head slightly elevated (Trendelenburg's position compromises venous return as well as respirations).

C. Insert Foley catheter for hourly urine volumes, if ordered.
   1. Record intake and output.
   2. Notify physician if urine output is below 30 ml/hour.

D. Take vital signs every 15 minutes.

E. Place light covering over patient to prevent chilling, but not enough to cause vasodilatation.

F. Provide oxygen via nasal catheter, mask, or cannula.

G. Treat the cause of the shock (stop bleeding, prepare for surgery, etc.).

Pulmonary Embolism

Definition: A type of embolism usually caused by clot lodging in pulmonary artery.

Assessment

A. Sudden sharp pain in chest.

B. Shortness of breath.

C. Cyanosis.

D. Increased pulse and respirations.

E. Hypotension—symptoms of shock.

F. Distended neck veins caused by congestive heart failure.

G. Decreased breath sounds.

H. Arrhythmias.

I. Anxiety.

Implementation

A. Provide patent airway.
   1. Position in semi- to high-Fowler's position if vital signs allow.
   2. Administer oxygen as needed.
   3. Assist with intubation as needed.
   4. Auscultate breath sounds every one to two hours.

5. Obtain arterial blood gases to ascertain acid-base imbalance.
6. Check sputum for presence of blood or blood-tinged mucus.
7. May administer diuretics or cardiotonics.

B. Administer anticoagulants following initial anticoagulation (check lab values each day before administering medication).

C. Take vital signs every two to four hours.

D. Turn as directed by physician; do not do percussion or clapping or administer back rubs.

E. Encourage patient to cough and deep breathe every one to two hours.

F. Give emotional support.

G. Observe for possible extension of emboli or occurrence of other emboli.
1. Check urine for hematuria or oliguria.
2. Check legs, especially calf.

Fat Embolism

Definition: A type of embolism caused by fat droplets released into the blood stream.

Etiology

A. Embolism occurs after long bone fractures (particularly from mishandling or incorrect splinting of fractures).

B. Fat droplets are released from the marrow and enter circulation. They usually lodge in the lungs. If they lodge in the brain the embolism is severe and sometimes fatal.

C. Fat emboli usually occur within the first 24 hours following an injury.

Assessment

A. Classical sign: petechiae across chest, shoulders, and axilla; can also involve conjuctiva.

B. Related pulmonary signs: shortness of breath leading to pallor, cyanosis, and hypoxemia.

C. Diaphoresis.

D. Tachycardia without apparent cause.

E. Change in level of consciousness.

F. Shock.

Implementation

A. Position patient in high-Fowler's position to allow for respiratory exchange.

B. Administer oxygen to decrease anoxia and to reduce surface tension of fat globules.

C. Obtain arterial blood gases to maintain sufficient pO_2 levels.

D. Intubate and place on respirator if respirations are severely compromised.

E. Institute preventative treatment to avoid further complications such as shock and heart failure.

F. Monitor administration of medications.
1. Alcohol drip.
2. Cortisone therapy to reduce inflammation.
3. Decholin to emulsify fat.
4. Antihyperlipemic drugs.

REHABILITATIVE NURSING

Definition: The process of restoring a person's ability to live and work in as normal a manner as possible after a disabling injury.

General Principles

Goals

A. Strive for optimal function.

B. Prevent further injury or complications.

C. Restore normal function.

D. Accept philosophy underlying rehabilitative nursing.
1. Rehabilitation begins with initial contact.
2. Every illness has intrinsic threat of disability.
3. Principles of rehabilitation are basic to care of all patients.

Effects of Disability

A. Impact upon the individual's body image.
   1. Physical appearance.
   2. Bodily sensations.
B. Behavior during reaction period.
   1. Appears confused and disorganized.
   2. Denies disability exists.
   3. Overreacts to situations and physical condition.
   4. Assumes false positive attitude.
   5. Becomes self-centered.
   6. Becomes depressed.
   7. Mourns loss of function or body part.
C. Adaptation and adjustment.
   1. Revises body image by modifying former picture of self.
   2. Reorganizes values.
   3. Accepts degree of dependency.
   4. Accepts limitations imposed by disability.
   5. Begins to develop realistic goals.

Duties of the Rehabilitative Nurse

General Duties

A. Assist in developing nursing care plan to meet patient's needs.
B. Provide direct nursing care.
C. Establish supportive relationship.
D. Teach activities of daily living.
   1. Activities which must be accomplished each day in order for the individual to care for his or her own needs.
   2. Assist in patient evaluation.
      a. Medical condition.
      b. Functional capacity.
      c. Therapeutic goal.
      d. Family background.
      e. Educational background.
   3. Assist in ascertaining best method for patient.
   4. Demonstrate and encourage individual to practice.
   5. Increase activities as individual progresses and is able to assume activity.
   6. Give positive reinforcement for all effort expended.
E. Record and report nursing observations.
F. Evaluate nursing care plan and alter as necessary.
G. Assist in developing discharge plan.

Prevention of Deformities and Complications

A. Specific nursing actions.
   1. Turn and position in good alignment.
      a. Prevent contractures.
      b. Stimulate circulation.
      c. Prevent thrombophlebitis.
      d. Prevent decubiti.
   2. Prevent edema of extremities.
   3. Promote lung expansion.
B. Types of Exercises. ❖ PROCEDURE ❖
   1. Passive.
      a. Carried out by the therapist or nurse without assistance from patient.
      b. Purpose—retain as much joint range of motion as possible, and maintain circulation.
   2. Active assistive.
      a. Carried out by the patient with assistance of therapist or nurse.
      b. Purpose—encourage normal muscle function.
   3. Active.
      a. Accomplished by the individual without assistance.
      b. Purpose—increase muscle strength.
   4. Resistive.
      a. Active exercise carried out by the individual working against resistance produced by manual or mechanical means.
      b. Purpose—provide resistance in order to increase muscle power.
   5. Isometric or muscle setting.
      a. Performed by the individual without assistance.
      b. Purpose—maintain strength in a muscle when a joint is immobilized.
   6. Range of Motion (ROM).
      a. Movement of a joint through its full range in all appropriate planes.

b. Purpose—maintain joint mobility and increase maximal motion of a joint.
c. Nursing care.
  (1) Assess general condition of patient.
  (2) Establish extent of ROM before present condition.
  (3) Ensure comfortable position.
  (4) Discontinue ROM at point of pain.
d. Deterrents to ROM exercises: fear and pain.

Proper Use of Aids/Devices

A. Cane ❖ **PROCEDURE** ❖
  1. Purpose.
    a. Provide greater stability and speed when walking.
    b. Relieve pressure on weight-bearing joints.
    c. Provide force to push or pull body forward.
  2. Safety factors.
    a. Handle at level of greater trochanter.
    b. Elbow flexed at 25 to 30 degree angle.
    c. Light-weight material.
    d. Rubber suction tip.
  3. Techniques for walking with cane.
    a. Hold cane close to body.
    b. Hold in hand on unaffected side.
    c. Move cane at same time as affected leg.

B. Crutches. ❖ **PROCEDURE** ❖
  1. Purpose—provide support during ambulating when lower extremities unable to support body weight.
  2. Safety factors.
    a. Measure 1½ to 2 inches from axillary fold to floor (4 inches in front and 6 inches to side of toes).
    b. Hand piece adjusted to allow 30 degree elbow flexion.
    c. Rubber suction tips on crutches.
    d. Wear well-fitting shoes with nonslip soles.
  3. Techniques for teaching crutch walking.
    a. Four-point gait: move right crutch, left foot, left crutch, right foot.

b. Three-point gait: move crutches and affected leg forward, move unaffected leg forward.
c. Upstairs: crutches and unaffected leg on same level; put weight on crutch handles and lift unaffected leg to first step; put weight on unaffected leg and lift other leg and crutches to step.
d. Downstairs: uninjured leg and crutches on same step; put crutches on first step; put weight on crutch handles and transfer unaffected leg to first step.

C. Tilt table.
  1. Board or table that can be tilted gradually from a horizontal to a vertical position.
  2. Purpose.
    a. Assist individual in gradually adjusting to upright position.
    b. Start weight-bearing activities.
    c. Increase standing tolerance.
    d. Prevent disuse syndrome.
    e. Prevent demineralization of bones.

D. Prosthesis—artificial replacement for a missing body part.

E. Brace—support that protects or supports weakened muscles.

Common Problems from Immobility

Pressure Ulcers

A. Localized areas of necrosis of skin and subcutaneous tissue due to pressure.

B. Cause—pressure exerted on skin and subcutaneous tissue by bony prominences and the object on which the body rests.

C. Predisposing factors.
  1. Malnutrition.
  2. Anemia.
  3. Hypoproteinemia.
  4. Vitamin deficiency.
  5. Edema.

D. Common sites: bony prominences of body such as sacrum, greater trochanter, heels, elbows, etc.

E. Prevention.
1. Purpose.
   a. Relieve or remove pressure.
   b. Stimulate circulation.
   c. Keep skin dry.
2. Nursing care.
   a. Encourage patient to keep active.
   b. Change position frequently.
   c. Maintain good skin hygiene.
   d. Provide for active and/or passive exercises.
   e. Ambulate.
   f. Use alternating air pressure mattress, etc.
   g. Use sheepskin padding.
   h. Inspect skin frequently.
   j. Provide for adequate nutritional intake.
F. Treatment protocol.
1. Stage 1—transparent dressing (Op-Site or Tegaderm).
2. Stage 2—transparent dressing—if wound is draining, irrigate with normal saline and apply hydrocolloid dressing (DuoDERM).
3. Stage 3—debride area (check orders with RN), then irrigate with normal saline and cover with hydrocolloid dressing.
4. Stage 4—debride by dressing changes (physician will do surgery or chemical debridement). Wet-to-damp dressing used.

External Rotation of Hip

A. Outward rotation of the hip joint.
B. Cause—lying for long periods of time on back without support to hips or incorrect positioning in bed.
C. Prevention.
1. Trochanter roll extending from crest of ilium to midthigh when positioned on back.
2. Frequent change of position.
3. Proper positioning.

Footdrop

A. Tendency for the foot to plantar flex.
B. Causes.
1. Prolonged bed rest.
2. Lack of exercise.
3. Weight of bed clothing forcing toes into plantar flexion.
C. Complications.
1. Individual will walk on his toes without touching heel on ground.
2. Unable to walk.
D. Prevention.
1. Position feet against footboard.
2. Use footcradle to keep weight of top linen off toes.
3. Provide range of motion exercises.

Contractures

A. Abnormal shortening of muscle, tendon, or ligament so joint cannot function properly.
B. Cause—improper alignment, lack of movement.
C. Prevention.
1. Properly align at all times.
   a. Use pillows.
   b. Provide supportive splints.
2. Provide for range of motion exercises.

Bladder Dysfunction

A. Cause.
1. Disease process.
2. Lack of innervation.
3. Lack of motivation.
B. Bladder training.
1. Purpose.
   a. Prevent urinary tract infection and preserve renal function.
   b. Keep individual dry and odor free.
   c. Help individual maintain social acceptance.
2. Nursing care. ❖ PROCEDURE ❖
   a. Set up specific time to empty bladder.
   b. Give measured amounts of fluids.
   c. Position in normal voiding position.
   d. Instruct to Crede bladder.
   e. Keep record of amount and time of intake and output.
   f. Encourage patient to wear own clothing, particularly underwear.

Bowel Dysfunction

A. Cause.
1. Disease process.
2. Inadequate intake.
3. Poor prior habits.
B. Bowel training.
1. Purpose.
   a. Develop regular bowel habits.
   b. Prevent fecal incontinence, impaction, and/or irregularity.
2. Nursing care. ❖ **PROCEDURE** ❖
   a. Establish specific time.
   b. Provide for adequate roughage and fluid intake.
   c. Use normal posture.
   d. Instruct to bear down and contract abdominal muscles.
   e. Provide privacy and time.
   f. Provide exercise.

Hypostatic Pneumonia

A. Incidence.
1. Very young, very old.
2. Debilitated.
3. Immobile.
B. Cause—stasis of secretions in lungs.
C. Prevention.
1. Assess lung function.
2. Encourage deep breathing, coughing.
3. Turn every two hours.
4. Provide for postural drainage, if indicated.
5. Ensure adequate hydration.

Other Common Problems

A. Muscle atrophy.
B. Venous thrombosis.
C. Psychological deterioration.

4

PHARMACOLOGY

PHARMACOLOGICAL CONCEPTS

Drug Metabolism

Stages of Metabolism

Definition: Drug metabolism in the human body is accomplished in four basic stages—absorption, transportation, biotransformation, and excretion. In order for a drug to be completely metabolized, it must first be given in sufficient concentration to produce the desired effect on body tissues. When this critical drug concentration level is achieved, body tissues change.

A. Absorption.
1. The first stage of metabolism refers to the route a drug takes from the time it enters the body until it is absorbed in the circulating fluids.
2. Drugs are absorbed by the mucous membranes, the gastrointestinal tract, the respiratory tract, and the skin.
   a. The mucous membranes are one of the most rapid and effective routes of absorption because they are highly vascular.
   b. Drugs are absorbed through these membranes.
3. Drugs given by mouth are absorbed in the gastrointestinal tract.
   a. Portions of these drugs dissolve and absorb in the stomach.
   b. Drugs are enteric coated to prevent absorption in the stomach.
   c. The rate of absorption depends on the pH of the stomach's contents, the food content in the stomach at the time of ingestion, and the presence of disease conditions.
   d. Most of the drug concentrate dissolves in the small intestine where the large vascular surface and moderate pH level enhance the process of dissolution.
4. Methods of administration include intradermal, subcutaneous, intravenous, and intraarterial injections.
   a. Parenteral methods are the most direct, reliable, and rapid route of absorption.
   b. The actual administration site will depend on type of drug, its action, and the patient.
5. Another route of administration is inhalation or nebulization through the respiratory system.
   a. This method is not as rapid as parenteral injections but faster than the gastrointestinal tract.
   b. Drugs administered through the respiratory tract must be made up of small particles that can pass through to the alveoli in the lungs.
6. The final mode of absorption is the skin.
   a. Most drugs, when applied to the skin, produce a local rather than a systemic effect.
   b. The degree of absorption will depend on the strength of the drug as well as where it is applied on the body surface.

B. Transportation.
1. The second stage of metabolism refers to the way in which a drug is transported from the site of introduction to the site of action.
2. First, a drug enters or is absorbed by the body.
   a. Drug is transported through circulation to all parts of the body.
   b. If drug binds to plasma protein, it is not effective.
3. As a drug moves from the circulatory system, it crosses cell membranes and enters the body tissues.
   a. Some of the drug is distributed to and stored in fat and muscle.
   b. Greater masses of tissue (such as fat and muscle) attract the drug.
4. The amount of drug that is distributed to body tissues depends on the permeability of the membranes and the blood supply to the absorption area.
5. A drug that first accumulates in the brain may move into fat and muscle tissue and then back to the brain because the drug is still chemically active.

a. The drug is released in small quantities from the tissues and travels back to the brain.
b. Equal drug and blood concentration levels in the body are maintained.

C. Biotransformation.
   1. The third stage of metabolism takes place as the drug, a foreign substance in the body, is converted by enzymes into a less active and harmless agent that can be easily excreted.
   2. Most of this conversion occurs in the liver.
      a. Both synthetic and biochemical reactions take place.
      b. Some conversion does take place in the kidney, plasma, and intestinal mucosa.
   3. Synthetic reactions: liver enzymes conjugate the drug with other substances to make it less harmful for the body.
   4. Biochemical reactions: drugs are oxidized, reduced, hydrolyzed, and synthesized so they become less active and more easily eliminated from the body.

D. Excretion.
   1. The final stage in metabolism takes place when the drug is changed into an inactive form or excreted from the body.
   2. The kidneys are the most important route of excretion.
   3. The kidneys eliminate both the pure drug and the metabolites of the parent drug.
      a. During excretion these two substances are filtered through the glomeruli.
      b. They are then secreted by the tubules.
      c. Finally, they are reabsorbed through the tubules or directly excreted.
   4. Other routes of excretion include the lungs (which exhale gaseous drugs), feces, saliva, tears, and mother's milk.

Factors That Affect Drug Metabolism

A. Personal attributes.
   1. Body weight.
   2. Age.
   3. Sex.
B. Physiological factors.
   1. State of health.
   2. Disease processes.
C. Acid-base and fluid and electrolyte balance.
D. Permeability.
E. Diurnal rhythm.
F. Circulatory capability.
G. Genetic and immunologic factors.
H. Drug tolerance.
I. Cumulation effect of drugs.
J. Other factors.
   1. Psychological.
   2. Emotional.
   3. Environmental
K. Responses to drugs vary.
   1. Responses depend on the speed with which the drug is absorbed into the blood or tissues.
   2. Responses depend on the effectiveness of the body's circulatory system.

Origin and Naming of Drugs

Common Sources

A. Plant sources.
   1. Roots, bark, sap, leaves, flowers, and seeds from medicinal plants can be used as drug components.
   2. Component substances.
      a. Alkaloid.
         (1) Alkaline (base) in reaction.
         (2) Bitter in taste.
         (3) Physiologically powerful in activity.
      b. Glycoside: a compound containing a carbohydrate molecule.
      c. Resin: soluble in alcohol; insoluble in water.
      d. Gum.
         (1) Mucilaginous (gelatinlike) excretion.
         (2) Used in bulk laxatives; may absorb water.
         (3) Used in skin preparations as a soothing effect, e.g., Karaya gum.
      e. Oil.

(1) Fixed oil: does not evaporate on warming; occurs as a solid, semi-solid, or liquid, e.g., castor oil.

(2) Volatile oil: evaporates readily; occurs in aromatic plants, e.g., peppermint.

B. Animal sources.
1. Processed from an organ, from organ secretion, or from organ cells.
2. Insulin, as an example, is a derivative from the pancreas of sheep, cattle, or hogs.

C. Mineral sources.
1. Inorganic elements occurring in nature, but not of plant or animal origin; may be metallic or nonmetallic.
2. Usually form a base or acid salt in food.
3. Dilute hydrochloric acid (HCl), as an example, is diluted in water and then taken through a straw to prevent damage to teeth by acid.

D. Synthetic sources.
1. A pure drug made in a laboratory from chemical, not natural, substances.
2. Many drugs, sulfonamides for example, are synthetics.

Methods of Naming Drugs

A. Chemical name.
1. Precise description of chemical constituents with the exact placement of atom groupings.
2. "N-Methyl-4-carbethoxypiperidine hydrochloride" is an example of a chemical name.

B. Generic name.
1. Reflects chemical name to which drug belongs, but is simpler.
2. It is never changed and used commonly in medical terminology.
3. The synthetic narcotic meperidine is an example of a generic name.

C. Trademark name (brand name, proprietary name).
1. Appears in literature with the sign ®, e.g., Demerol®.

2. The sign indicates the name is registered; use of the name is restricted to the manufacturer who is the legal owner.
3. Trademark name is capitalized or shown in parentheses if generic name stated.

Drug Classification

Classification by Action

A. Anti-infectives.
1. Antiseptics.
   a. Action—inhibit growth of microorganisms (bacteriostatic).
   b. Purpose—application to wounds and skin infections, sterilization of equipment, and hygienic purposes.
2. Disinfectants.
   a. Action—destroy microorganisms (bactericidal).
   b. Purpose—destroy bacteria on inanimate objects (not appropriate for living tissue).

B. Antimicrobials.
1. Sulfonamides.
   a. Action—inhibit the growth of microorganisms.
   b. Reduce or prevent infectious process especially for urinary tract infections.
2. Antibiotics (e.g., penicillin).
   a. Action—interfere with microorganism metabolism.
   b. Usage—reduce or prevent infectious process.
   c. Specific drug and dosage based on culture and sensitivity of organism.

C. Metabolic drugs.
1. Hormones obtained from animal sources, found naturally in foods and plants.
2. Synthetic hormones.

D. Diagnostic materials.
1. Action—dyes and opaque materials ingested or injected to allow visualization of internal organs.
2. Purpose—to analyze organ status and function.

E. Vitamins and minerals.
   1. Action—necessary to obtain healthy body function.
   2. Found naturally in food or through synthetic food supplements.
F. Vaccines and serums.
   1. Action—prevent disease or detect presence of disease.
   2. Types.
      a. Antigenics produce active immunity.
         (1) Vaccines—attenuated suspensions of microorganisms.
         (2) Toxoids—products of microorganisms.
      b. Antibodies—stimulated by microorganisms or their products.
         (1) Antitoxins.
         (2) Immune serum globulin.
      c. Allergens—agents for skin immunity tests.
         (1) Extracts of materials known to be allergenic.
         (2) Can be used to relieve allergies.
      d. Antivenins—substances which neutralize venom of certain snakes and spiders.
G. Antifungals—check growth of fungi.
H. Antihistaminics.
   1. Action—prevent histamine action.
   2. Purpose—relieve symptoms of allergic reaction.
I. Antineoplastics—prevent growth and spread of malignant cells.

Classification by Body Systems

CENTRAL NERVOUS SYSTEM

A. Drugs affect CNS by either inhibiting or promoting the actions of neural pathways centers.
   1. Action promoting drug groups (stimulants).
      a. Antidepressants—psychic energizers used to treat depression.
      b. Caffeine—increases mental activity and lessens drowsiness.
      c. Ammonia—used as revival from fainting spell (patient smells cap, not contents of bottle).

   2. Action inhibiting drug groups (depressants).
      a. Analgesics—reduce pain by interfering with conduction of nerve impulses.
         (1) Narcotic analgesics—opium derivatives may depress respiratory centers; must be used with caution and respiratory rate above 12.
            (a) A narcotic antagonist drug counteracts depressant drugs.
            (b) Such antagonist drugs are Lorfan, Narcan, and Nalline.
         (2) Nonnarcotic antipyretics—reduce fever and relieve pain.
         (3) Antirheumatics—analgesics given to relieve arthritis pain; may reduce joint inflammation.
      b. Alcohol—stimulates appetite when given in small doses but classified as a depressant.
      c. Hypnotics—sedatives that induce sleep; common form is the barbiturates.
      d. Antispasmodics—relieve skeletal muscle spasms; anticonvulsants prevent muscle spasms or convulsions.
      e. Tranquilizers.
         (1) Relieve tension and anxiety, preoperative and postoperative apprehension, headaches, menstrual tension, chronic alcoholism, skeletal muscle spasticity, and other neuromuscular disorders.
         (2) Tranquilizers and analgesics frequently given together (in reduced dosage); the one drug enhances the action of the other (synergy).
      f. Anesthetics—produce the state of unconsciousness painlessly.
B. Precautions to be taken with CNS drugs.
   1. Drugs which act on CNS may potentiate other CNS drugs.
   2. Patient may be receiving other medications; find out drug name and dosage.
   3. Dependence on CNS drugs may occur.

Autonomic Nervous System

A. This system governs several body functions so that drugs that affect the ANS will at the same time affect other system functions.

B. The ANS is made up of two nerve systems—the sympathetic and parasympathetic.
   1. Parasympathetic is the stabilizing system.
   2 Sympathetic is the protective emergency system.

C. Each system has a separate basic drug group acting on it.
   1. Adrenergics—mimic the actions of sympathetic system.
      a. Vasoconstrictors—stimulants such as Adrenalin.
         (1) Action is to constrict peripheral blood vessels, thereby increasing blood pressure.
         (2) Dilate bronchial passages.
         (3) Relax gastrointestinal tract.
      b. Vasodilators—depressants such as nicotinic acid.
         (1) Antagonists of epinephrine and similar drugs.
         (2) Vasodilate blood vessels.
         (3) Increase tone of GI tract.
         (4) Reduce blood pressure.
         (5) Relax smooth muscles.
         (6) *Caution:* If drug is to be stopped, reduce dosage gradually over a period of a week; do not stop it suddenly.
   2. Cholinergics—mimic actions of parasympathetic system.
      a. Cholinergic stimulants (e.g., Prostigmin or neostigmine).
         (1) Decrease heart rate.
         (2) Contract smooth muscle.
         (3) Contract pupil in eye.
         (4) Increase peristalsis.
         (5) Increase gland secretions.
      b. Cholinergic inhibitors (anticholinergics).
         (1) Decrease gland secretion.
         (2) Relax smooth muscle.
         (3) Dilate pupil in eye.
         (4) Increase heart action.

Gastrointestinal System

A. Drugs affecting GI system act upon muscular and glandular tissues.

B. Drug groups and actions.
   1. Antacids—counteract excess acidity.
      a. Have alkaline base.
      b. Used in the treatment of ulcers.
      c. Neutralize hydrochloric acid in the stomach.
      d. Given frequently (two hour intervals or more often).
      e. May cause constipation, depending on type of medication.
      f. Baking soda is a systemic antacid which disturbs the pH balance in the body. Most other antacids coat the mucous membrane and neutralize hydrochloric acid.
   2. Emetics—produce vomiting (emesis).
   3. Antiemetics—prevent vomiting or nausea but may cause drowsiness.
   4. Digestants—relieve enzyme deficiency by replacing secretions in digestive tract.
   5. Antidiarrheics—prevent diarrhea.
   6. Cathartics—affect intestine and produce defecation.
      a. Provide temporary relief for constipation.
      b. Rid bowel of contents before surgery, and prepare viscera for diagnostic studies.
      c. Counteract edema.
      d. Treat diseases of GI tract.
      e. Contraindicated when abdominal pain is present.
      f. Classifications.
         (1) By degree of action.
            (a) Laxative—mild action.
            (b) Cathartic—moderate action.
            (c) Purgative—severe action.
         (2) By method of action.
            (a) Increase bulk.
            (b) Lubricate mechanically.
            (c) Irritate chemically.
            (d) Increase or decrease water content with saline.
            (e) Disperse detergent or wetting agent.

RESPIRATORY SYSTEM

A. Drugs act on respiratory tract, tissues, and cough center.
B. Action is to suppress, relax, liquefy, and stimulate.
   1. Respiratory stimulants stimulate depth and rate of respiration.
   2. Bronchodilators relax smooth muscle of trachea.
   3. Drug groups that provide cough relief:
      a. Antitussive agents (narcotic, non-narcotic).
         (1) Sedatives prevent cough.
         (2) Not to be accompanied by water.
      b. Demulcents soothe respiratory tract.
      c. Expectorants liquefy bronchial secretions and increase amount of excretions in respiratory tract.

URINARY SYSTEM

A. Drugs that act on kidneys and urinary tract.
B. Action is to increase urine flow, destroy bacteria, and perform other important body functions.
   1. Diuretics.
      a. Rid body of excess fluid and relieve edema.
      b. Some drugs that act on the GI tract and circulatory system also are diuretic in action.
   2. Urinary antiseptics.
   3. Acidifiers and alkalinizers—certain foods also increase body acids or alkalies.

CIRCULATORY SYSTEM

A. Drugs that act on heart, blood, and blood vessels.
B. Action is to change heart rhythm, rate, and force and to dilate or constrict vessels.
   1. Cardiotonics used for heart-strengthening.
      a. Direct heart stimulants that speed heart rate, e.g., caffeine, Adrenalin.
      b. Indirect heart stimulants, e.g., digitalis.
         (1) Stimulate vagus nerve.
         (2) Slow heart rate and strengthen it.
         (3) Improve heart action, thereby improving circulation.

         (4) Do not administer if apical pulse below 60.
   2. Antiarrhythmic drugs used clinically to convert irregularities to a normal sinus rhythm.
      a. Monitor constantly with ECG when administering these drugs.
      b. Quinidine used for its vasodepressor action.
         (1) Slows impulse of sinoauricular node.
         (2) Slows heart rate.
         (3) Side effects include ringing in ears.
   3. Drugs that alter blood flow.
      a. Anticoagulants—inhibit blood clotting action.
      b. Coagulants—maintain blood fluidity.
   4. Blood replacement.

Dosage and Preparation Forms

Solids

A. Extract—obtained by dissolving drug in water or alcohol and allowing solution to evaporate; residue is the extract.
B. Powder—finely ground drugs.
C. Pills—common term for tablet; made by rolling drug and binder into a sphere.
D. Suppository.
   1. Contains drugs mixed with a firm base.
   2. Liquefies at body temperature when inserted into orifice.
   3. Releases drug to produce a local or systemic effect.
E. Ointment—semisolid mixture of drugs with a fatty base.
F. Lozenge—flavored flat tablet that releases drug slowly when held in mouth.
G. Capsule.
   1. Drugs in small, cylindrical gelatin containers that disguise the taste of the drug.
   2. Capsule can be opened and drug mixed with food or jam to mask taste.
H. Tablets.

1. Dried, powdered drugs that are compressed into a small disk which easily disintegrates in water.
2. Enteric coated—tablet does not dissolve until reaching intestines, where release of drug occurs.

Liquids

A. Fluid extract.
   1. Concentrated fluid preparation of drugs produced by dissolving crude plant drug in a solvent.
   2. Strength of extract is such that 1 ml (about ¼ teaspoon or 15 to 16 gtt) represents 1 gram of the drug at 100 percent strength.
B. Tincture.
   1. Diluted alcoholic extract of a drug.
   2. Varies in strength from 10 to 20 percent.
C. Spirit—preparation of volatile (easily vaporized) substances dissolved in alcohol.
D. Syrup—drug contained in a concentrated sugar solution.
E. Elixir—solution of drug made with alcohol, sugar, and some aromatic or pleasant-smelling substance.
F. Suspension.
   1. Undissolved, finely divided particles of drug dispersed in a liquid.
   2. Gels and magma are other forms of suspensions.
   3. Shake all bottles of suspension well before giving.
H. Emulsion—suspension of unmixed oils, fats, or petrolatum in water.
I. Liniment and lotion—liquid suspension of medication applied to the skin.

Packaging Methods and Dispensing

A. Unit dosage package method.
   1. Package contains premeasured amount of drug in proper form for administering.
   2. Pharmacy may deliver the daily needs for each patient to the floor.
   3. Procedures for delivery and storage vary from hospital to hospital.

4. Nurse administers the medication to the patient.
B. Traditional method.
   1. Nurse prepares medication on the unit.
   2. Supplies come from stock or bulk on the ward or from a multiple dose bottle of patient's.
C. The nurse is responsible for accuracy of the medication given, regardless of the packaging or dispensing method used.

Routes of Administration

Oral Route

A. Ingested (swallowed).
B. Sublingual (under tongue).
C. Buccal (on mucous membrane of cheek or tongue).

Rectal Route

A. Suppository.
B. Liquid (retention enema).

Parenteral Route

A. Intravenous.
   1. The response is fast and immediate.
   2. Over 5 ml medication can be given.
   3. Drug *must* be given slowly and usually in diluted form.
   4. Check medication leaflets to determine if medication route is IM or IV.
B. Intradermal.
   1. Injected into skin; usual site is inner aspect of forearm or scapular area of back.
   2. A short bevel 26-gauge, 1-cm needle is used.
   3. Needle should be inserted with bevel up.
   4. This route is usually used to inject antigens for skin or tuberculin tests.
   5. Amount injected ranges from 0.01 to 0.1 ml.
C. Subcutaneous.

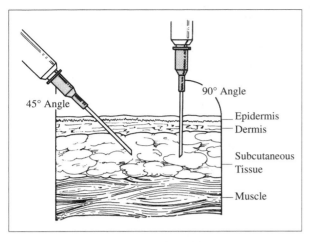

Insert needle at 45- or 90-degree angle for subcutaneous injection.

Insert needle at 15-degree angle under the epidermis for intradermal injection.

1. A 25-gauge, 1.3- to 1.6-cm needle is used.
2. Injection site is the fatty layer under skin.
   a. Abdomen at navel.
   b. Lateral upper arm or thigh.
3. This route usually used for injecting medication that is to be absorbed slowly with a sustained effect.
4. Amount injected ranges from 0.5 to 1.5 ml.
5. If repeated doses are necessary, as with insulin for a diabetic person, rotate the injection sites.

D. Intramuscular.
   1. Needle gauge and length will vary with site.
      a. Deltoid—located by having patient raise arm.
         (1) A 23- to 25-gauge, 1.6- to 2.5-cm needle is used.
         (2) Administer no more than 2 ml.
      b. Thigh and buttock.
         (1) Needle must be long enough to reach muscle; may vary from 2 to 8 cm.
         (2) Needle gauge depends upon substance of medication.
         (3) Oil bases require 20 gauge; water bases require 22 gauge.

2. Absorption rate of IM medication dependent upon circulation of person injected.
3. This route usually used for systemic effect of an irritating drug.
4. Amount of medication must not be over 5 cc's, as absorption would be difficult and painful.
5. Techniques for lessening pain for the patient receiving an IM medication:
   a. Encourage relaxation of area to be injected; request patient to lie on side with flexed knee or out flat on abdomen, if giving injection in buttock.
   b. Reduce puncture pain by "darting" needle.
   c. Prevent antiseptic from clinging to needle during insertion by waiting until skin antiseptic is dry.
   d. If medication must be drawn through a rubber stopper, use a new needle for injection.
   e. Avoid sensitive or hardened body areas.
   f. After needle is under skin, aspirate to be certain that needle is not in a blood vessel.
   g. Inject slowly.
   h. Maintain grasp of syringe.

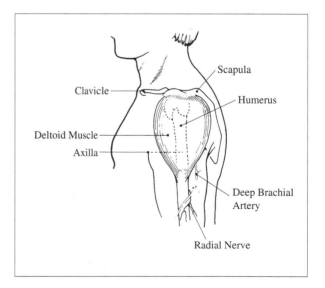

Inject no more than 2 ml IM into deltoid muscle.

i. Withdraw needle quickly after injection.

j. Massage relaxed muscle gently to increase circulation and to distribute medication.

6. Observe for side effects of medication following injection.

Administration of Medications

Basic Guidelines for Medication Administration

A. Determine the correct dosage, actions, side effects, and contraindications of any medication before administration.

B. Check with head nurse if medications ordered by the physician do not seem appropriate for patient's condition. This is part of the nurse's professional responsibility.

C. Question the physician about any medication orders that are incomplete, illegible, or inappropriate for the patient's condition.
   1. Remember, the nurse may be liable if a medication error is made.
   2. Report every medication error to the head nurse and/or physician.
   3. Complete a medication incident report.

D. Check to determine if the medication ordered is compatible with the patient's condition and with other medications prescribed.

E. Check on what the patient has been eating or drinking before administering a medication.
   1. Determine what effect the patient's diet has on the medication.
   2. Do not administer medication if contraindicated by diet. For example, do not give an MAO inhibitor to a patient who has just ingested cheddar cheese or wine.

F. Check that calculated drug dosage is accurate for young children, elderly people, or for very thin or obese patients. These age and weight groups require smaller or larger dosages.

Anatomical view of thigh and buttock for intramuscular injection.

Safety Rules

A. The five rights.
   1. Right medication.
      a. Compare drug card with drug label three times.
      b. Know general purpose, dosage, method of administration.
      c. Know side effects of drug.
   2. Right patient: check ID band and door number.
   3. Right time.
   4. Right method of administration.
   5. Right amount.

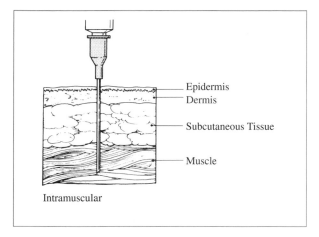

Epidermis
Dermis

Subcutaneous Tissue

Muscle

Intramuscular

Insert needle at 90-degree angle and deep into muscle tissue for intramuscular injection.

a. Check all calculations of divided dosages with another nurse.
b. Check heparin and insulin doses with another nurse.

B. The five rights should be practiced each and every time a medication is given.

Documentation of Medications

Medication Orders

A. Medication administered to patient must have a physician's order or prescription before it can be legally administered.

B. Physician's order is a verbal or written order, recorded in a book or file or in patient's chart.

C. If order is given verbally over the telephone, nurse must write a verbal order in patient's chart for the physician to sign at a later date.

D. Written orders are safer—they leave less room for potential misunderstanding or error.

E. Drug order should consist of seven parts:
1. Name of the patient.
2. Date the drug was ordered.
3. Name of the drug.
4. Dosage.
5. Route of administration and any special rules of administration.

6. Time and frequency the drug should be given.
7. Signature of the individual who ordered the drug.

Types of Medication Schedules

A. Routine orders.
1. Administered according to instructions until it is canceled by another order.
2. Can also be used for p.r.n. drugs.
    a. Administered when patient needs the medication.
    b. Not given on a routine time schedule.
3. Continued validity of any routine order should be assessed—physicians occasionally forget to cancel an order when it is no longer appropriate for patient's condition.

B. One-time orders.
1. Administered as stated, only one time.
2. Given at a specified time or "stat," which means immediately.

Medication Errors

A. Nurse who prepares a medication must also give it to patient and chart it.
1. If patient refuses drug, chart that medication was refused—report this information to the physician.
2. When charting medications, use the correct abbreviations and symbols.

B. If error in a drug order is found, it is nurse's responsibility to question the order.
1. If order cannot be understood or read, verify with the physician.
2. Do not guess at the order as this constitutes gross negligence.
3. In many hospitals it is the pharmacist's responsibility to contact physicians when medication orders are unclear.

C. Always report medication errors to the head nurse and/or physician immediately.
1. This action minimizes potential danger to the patient.
2. Measures can be taken immediately to assess and evaluate the patient's status.

3. A plan of action can be implemented to reverse the effects of the medication.

D. Errors in medication are documented in a medication incident report and on the patient's record.
   1. This action is necessary for both legal reasons and nursing audits.
   2. Nursing audits are conducted to determine problems in medication administration:
      a. A particular source of problems.
      b. A range of problems that seem to have no connection.

Legal Issues in Drug Administration

A. Nurse must not administer a specific drug unless allowed to do so by the particular state's Nurse Practice Act.

B. Nurse is to take every safety precaution in whatever he or she is doing.

C. Nurse is to be certain that employer's policy allows him or her to administer a specific drug.

D. A drug may not lawfully be administered unless all the above items are in effect.

E. General rules.
   1. Never leave tray with prepared medicines unattended.
   2. Always report errors immediately.
   3. Send labeled bottles that are unintelligible back to pharmacist for relabeling.
   4. Store internal and external medicines separately if possible.

ADMINISTERING MEDICATIONS

Administering Oral Medications

Preparation ❖ PROCEDURE ❖

A. Check medication orders for their completeness and accuracy.

B. Assess patient's physical ability to take medication as ordered.

1. Swallow reflex present.
2. State of consciousness.
3. Signs of nausea and vomiting.
4. Uncooperative behavior.

C. Check to make sure you have the correct medication for the patient.

D. Assess correct dosage when calculation is needed.

E. Preparing the oral medication.
   1. Obtain patient's medication record. Medication record may be a drug card, medication sheet, or drug Kardex.
   2. Compare the medication record with the most *recent* physician's order.
   3. Wash your hands.
   4. Gather necessary equipment.
   5. Remove the medication from the drug box or tray on medication cart.
   6. Compare the label on the bottle or drug package to the medication record.
   7. Correctly calculate dosage if necessary and check the dosage to be administered.
   8. Pour the medication from the bottle into the lid of the container and then into the medicine cup. With unit dosage, take drug package from medication cart and place in medication cup. Do not remove drug from drug package.
   9. Check medication label again to ensure correct drug and dosages if drug is not prepackaged.
   10. Place medication cup on a tray, if not using medication cart.
   11. Return the multidose vial bottle to the storage area. If medication to be given is a narcotic, sign out the narcotic record sheet with your name.
   12. Check medication label for third time before returning bottle to storage.

Implementation

A. Procedure for administering oral medications to adults. ❖ PROCEDURE ❖
   1. Take medication tray or cart to patient's room; check room number against medication card or sheet.

2. Place patient in sitting position, if not contraindicated by his or her condition.
3. Tell the patient what type of medication you are going to give and explain the actions this medication will produce.
4. Check the patient's Identaband and ask patient to state name so that you are sure you have correctly identified him or her.
5. If prepackaged medication is used, read label, take medication out of package, and put into medication cup.
6. Give the medication cup to the patient.
7. Offer a fresh glass of water or other liquid to aid swallowing, and give assistance with taking medications.
8. Make sure the patient swallows the medication.
9. Discard used medicine cup.
10. Position patient for comfort.
11. Record the medication on the appropriate forms.

B. Procedure for administering oral medications to children. ❖ **PROCEDURE** ❖
1. Follow the procedures for the previous intervention, keeping the following guidelines in mind:
   a. Play techniques may help to elicit a young child's cooperation.
   b. Remember, the smaller the quantity of diluent (food or liquid), the greater the ease in eliciting the child's cooperation.
   c. Never use a child's favorite food or drink as an enticement when administering medication because the result may be the child's refusal to eat or drink anything.
   d. Be honest and tell the child that you have medicine, not candy.
2. Assess child for drug action and possible side effects.
3. Explain medication action and side effects to parents.

Administering Parenteral Medications

Preparation ❖ **PROCEDURE** ❖

A. Check appropriate method for administration of drug:
1. Intradermal (intracutaneous): injection is made below surface of the skin.
2. Subcutaneous: small amount of fluid is injected beneath the skin in the loose connective tissues.
3. Intramuscular: larger amount of fluid is injected into large muscle masses in the body.
4. Intravenous: medication is injected or infused directly into a vein—route used when immediate drug effect is desired.

B. Evaluate condition of administration site for presence of lesions, rash, inflammation, lipid dystrophy, ecchymosis, etc.

C. Assess for tissue damage from previous injections.

D. Assess patient's level of consciousness.
1. For patient in shock: certain methods (subcutaneous) will not be used.
2. For presence of anxiety: make sure patient is allowed to express his or her fear of injections and offer explanations of ways in which injections will be less frightening.

E. Check patient's written and verbal history for past allergic reactions. Do *not* rely solely on patient's chart.

F. Review patient's chart noting previous injection sites, especially insulin and heparin administration sites.

G. Check label on medication bottle to determine if medication can be administered via route ordered.

H. Preparing the medication.
1. Wash your hands and don gloves.
2. Obtain equipment for injection: needle and syringe, alcohol wipes, medication tray (medication container if needed).
3. Assemble the needle and syringe. Select the appropriate size needle, considering the size of the patient's muscle mass and the viscosity of the medication.

4. Open the alcohol wipe and cleanse the top of the vial or break top of ampule.

5. Remove the needle guard and place on alcohol wipe or medication tray.

6. Pull back on barrel of syringe to markings where medication will be inserted.

7. Pick up vial, insert needle into vial, and inject air in an amount equal to the solution to be withdrawn by pushing barrel of syringe down. If using an ampule, break off top at colored line, insert syringe, but do not inject air into ampule as it causes a break in the vacuum and possible loss of medication through leakage.

8. Extract the desired amount of fluid. Remove needle from container and cover needle with guard. Needle should be changed to prevent tracking medication on skin and subcutaneous tissue.

9. Double-check drug and dosage against drug card or medication sheet and vial or ampule.

10. Place syringe on tray if tray available.

11. Check label and drug card or medication sheet for accuracy before returning multidose vial to correct storage area.

12. Return multidose vial to correct storage area or discard used vial or ampule.

Implementation

A. Administering intradermal injections.
   ❖ **PROCEDURE** ❖
   1. Take medication to patient's room.
   2. Explain the medication's action and the procedure for administration to patient.
   3. Check patient's Identaband and ask patient to state name.
   4. Wash your hands and don gloves.
   5. Select the site of injection.
   6. Cleanse the area with an alcohol wipe, wiping in circular area from inside to outside.
   7. Take off needle guard and place on tray.
   8. Grasp patient's forearm from underneath and gently pull the skin taut.
   9. Insert the needle at 10- to 15-degree angle with the bevel of needle facing up.

10. Inject medication slowly. Observe for wheals and blanching at the site.

11. Withdraw the needle, wiping the area gently with a dry 2 × 2 bandage to prevent dispersing medication into the subcutaneous tissue.

12. Return the patient to a comfortable position.

13. Discard supplies in appropriate area.

14. Chart the medication and site used.

B. Administering subcutaneous (sub q) injections.
   ❖ **PROCEDURE** ❖
   1. Take medication to patient's room.
   2. Set tray on a clean surface, not the bed.
   3. Check patient's Identaband and ask patient to state name.
   4. Explain action of medication and procedure of administration.
   5. Provide privacy when injection site is other than on the arm.
   6. Wash your hands and don gloves.
   7. Select site for injection by identifying anatomical landmarks. Remember to alternate sites each time injections are given.

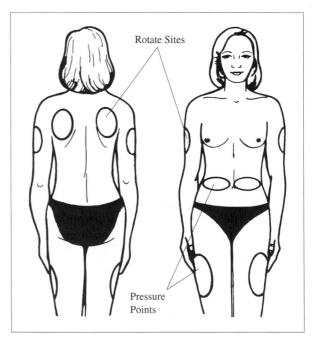

Rotate sites for subcutaneous injections given on a continuing basis.

8. Cleanse area with alcohol wipe. Using a circular motion cleanse from inside outward.
9. Take off needle guard.
10. Express any air bubbles from syringe.
11. Insert the needle at a 45-degree angle.
12. Pull back on the plunger.
13. Inject the medication slowly.
14. Withdraw needle quickly and massage area with alcohol wipe to aid absorption and lessen bleeding. Put on Bandaid if needed.
15. Return patient to a position of comfort.
16. Discard used supplies in proper areas.
17. Chart the medication and site used.

C. Administering insulin injections.
   ❖ **PROCEDURE** ❖
   1. Gather equipment and check medication orders, injection site, and rotation chart. Insulin does not need to be refrigerated.
   2. Wash your hands and don gloves.
   3. Obtain specific insulin syringe for strength of insulin being administered (U100).
   4. Rotate insulin bottle between hands to bring solution into suspension.
   5. Wipe top of insulin bottle with alcohol.
   6. Take off needle guard.
   7. Pull plunger of syringe down to desired amount of medication and inject that amount of air into the insulin bottle.
   8. Draw up ordered amount of insulin into syringe.
   9. Expel air from syringe.
   10. Replace needle guard.
   11. Check medication card, bottle, and syringe with another RN for accuracy.
   12. Take medications to patient's room.
   13. Double-check site of last injection with patient.
   14. Provide privacy.
   15. Wash your hands.
   16. Follow protocol for administration of medications by subcutaneous injections.

D. Administering two insulin solutions.
   ❖ **PROCEDURE** ❖
   1. Follow steps 1 to 6 above.
   2. Inject prescribed amount of air into intermediate acting (NPH, Lente) or long acting (PZI, Ultralente) bottle.

INSULIN TYPES AND ACTION

Types	Onset	Peak	Duration
Rapid Acting			
Regular	½ to 1	2 to 4	5 to 10
Semilente	½ to 1	5 to 7	12 to 16
Humulin R	½ to 1	2 to 3	5 to 7
Intermediate			
Humulin N	1½ to 3½	8 to 12	18 to 24
NPH	1 to 1½	8 to 12	24
Lente	1 to 1½	8 to 12	24
Long Acting			
Protamine zinc (PZI)	4 to 8	14 to 20	24 to 36
Ultralente	4 to 8	16 to 24	36

3. Pull needle out of insulin bottle and withdraw plunger to prescribed regular insulin dosage.
4. Inject air into regular bottle and withdraw medication.
5. Expel all air bubbles.
6. Insert needle into second insulin bottle taking care not to push any regular insulin into bottle. This can be avoided by putting pressure on plunger with your small finger when inserting into bottle.
7. Invert bottle and pull back on plunger to obtain prescribed amount of insulin. Remember the total insulin dose will include the amount of regular insulin already drawn up into syringe.
8. Follow steps 9 to 16 above to complete procedure.

E. Administering intramuscular (IM) injections.
   ❖ **PROCEDURE** ❖
   1. Take medication to patient's room. Check room number against medication card or sheet.
   2. Set tray on a clean surface, not the bed.
   3. Explain the procedure to patient.
   4. Check patient's Identaband and have patient state name.
   5. Provide privacy for patient.
   6. Wash your hands and don gloves.

7. Select the site of injection by identifying anatomical landmarks. Remember to alternate sites each time injections are given.
8. Cleanse the area with alcohol wipe. Using a circular motion, cleanse from inside outward.
9. Hold the syringe; take off needle cover.
10. Express air bubbles from syringe. Some clinicians suggest leaving a small air bubble at the tip so that all medicine will be expelled.
11. Insert the needle at 90-degree angle.
12. Pull back on plunger. If blood returns, you know you have entered a blood vessel and need to reposition the needle and aspirate again.
13. Inject the medication slowly.
14. Withdraw the needle and massage the area with an alcohol wipe. Put on a Bandaid, if needed.
15. Return patient to a comfortable position.
16. Discard supplies in appropriate area.
17. Chart the medication and site used.
F. Administering IM injections using Z-track method. ❖ **Procedure** ❖
    1. Used for iron injections.

Z-Track Injection

Medication

Z-track is used to prevent tracking of medications on the skin.

2. Draw up prescribed medication into syringe.
3. Draw up 0.3 to 0.5 ml of air into syringe.
4. Replace needle with 3-inch needle to penetrate deep into muscle.
5. Pull skin laterally away from injection site.
6. Cleanse site with alcohol.
7. Insert needle.
8. Inject medication slowly—and wait ten seconds keeping skin taut.
9. Withdraw needle and then release skin.
10. Discard supplies in appropriate area.
11. Chart medication and site used.

Administering Medications to the Skin

Preparation

A. Observe skin for open lesions, rashes, or areas of erythema.
B. Check for allergies.

Implementation

A. Obtain patient's medication record.
    ❖ **Procedure** ❖
B. Compare the medication record with the most recent physician's order. Medication record may be a drug card, medication sheet, or drug Kardex, depending on the method of dispensing medications in your facility.
C. Wash your hands.
D. Gather necessary equipment including gloves or tongue blade as needed.
E. Remove the medication from the drug box or tray on medication cart.
F. Compare the label on the medication tube or jar to the medication record.
G. Place medication tube or jar (include a tongue blade with jar) on a tray if not using medication cart.
H. Take medication to patient's room.
I. Wash your hands.
J. Provide patient privacy.

K. Squeeze medication from a tube or, using a tongue blade, take ointment out of jar.

L. Spread a small, smooth, thin quantity of medication evenly over patient's skin surface using your fingers or a tongue blade.

M. Protect skin surface with a dressing, if needed, so that medication cannot rub off.

N. Cleanse skin surface with soap and water between medication applications, unless contraindicated by patient's condition.

O. Return medication to appropriate storage area.

P. Check to see that patient is comfortable before leaving room.

Q. Wash hands.

R. Chart administration.

Administering a Topical Vasodilator

Implementation

A. Take medication to patient's room.
   ❖ PROCEDURE ❖

B. Wash your hands.

C. Provide patient privacy.

D. Put on gloves to prevent absorbing any medication yourself.

E. Obtain premeasured paper, which accompanies medication tube.

F. Place prescribed medication directly on paper (usually one-half to one-inch strip).

G. Apply medicated paper to anterior surface of chest.

H. You may apply medicated paper to any area of the body; however, most patients feel the medication works better if applied to the chest surface.

I. Alternate areas of the chest with each dose of medication.

J. Return medication to appropriate storage area.

K. Check to see that patient is comfortable before leaving room.

L. Wash hands.

M. Chart administration.

Mathematic Conversions

Approximate Equivalents

A. The metric system is the universal system of weights and measures.

B. Apothecary and metric do not use same size units; denominations of one system not compatible with the other.

C. Equivalency tables established to list measurement denominations of one system in terms of another. (See Appendix 1.)
   1. Conversion from one system to another can be computed, but is not equivalent in absolute terms.
   2. If there is occasion to compute, have computations checked by another licensed nurse.
      a. Do not compute unless allowed to do so by your state's Nurse Practice Act.
      b. Check hospital policy for further guidelines.

Computation

A. Drugs are not always labeled clearly as to number of tablets to administer so computation may be necessary. Always have your computation checked by another licensed nurse.

B. Method.
   1. Both desired (ordered) dose and dose on hand must be in same unit of measurement, e.g., grains, grams, milligrams.
   2. If not same, convert so that unit of measure is the same.
      a. Refer to conversion table. (Appendix 1.)
      b. To convert one measure unit to another, basic equivalencies must be memorized.
   3. After converting, divide desired dose by dose on hand to find amount to administer.

Calculation of Dosages

A. Using equivalent tables to calculate drug dosages.

1. To convert milligrams to grains, use the following formula:

Example: Convert 180 milligrams to grains.

$$\frac{1 \text{ gr}}{\text{mg in gr}} = \frac{\text{dose desired}}{\text{dose on hand}}$$

$$\frac{1}{60} = \frac{x}{180}$$

$$60x = 180$$

$$x = 3 \text{ grains}$$

2. You may also make this conversion as a ratio:

1 gr : 60 mg : :x gr : 180 mg
60x = 180   x = 3 grains

3. Check equivalency tables in the drug supplement.

B. Calculating oral dosages of drugs.

❖ **PROCEDURE** ❖

1. To calculate oral dosages, use the following formula:

$$\frac{D}{H} = X$$

where D = dose desired
        H = dose on hand
        X = dose to be administered

Example: Give 500 mg of ampicillin when the dose on hand is in capsules containing 250 mg.

$$\frac{500 \text{ mg}}{250 \text{ mg}} = 2 \text{ capsules}$$

2. To calculate oral dosages of liquids, use the following formula:

$$\frac{D}{H} \times Q = X$$

where Q = quantity

Example: Give 375 mg of ampicillin when it is supplied as 250 mg/5 ml.

$$\frac{375 \text{ mg}}{250 \text{ mg}} \times 5$$

$$1.5 \times 5 = 7.5 \text{ ml}$$

You can also set up a direct proportion and following the algebraic principle, cross multiply:

$$\frac{375 \text{ mg}}{x} = \frac{250 \text{ mg}}{5 \text{ ml}}$$

$$250x = 1875$$

$$x = 7.5 \text{ ml (of strength 250 mg/5 ml)}$$

C. Calculating parenteral dosages of drugs.

1. To calculate parenteral dosages, use the following formula:

$$\frac{D}{H} \times Q = X$$

Example: Give patient 40 mg gentamicin. On hand is a multidose vial with a strength of 80 mg/2 ml.

$$\frac{40}{80} \times 2 = 1 \text{ ml}$$

2. Check your calculations before drawing up medication.

GOVERNING LAWS

Federal Food, Drug, and Cosmetic Act of 1938

A. The act is an update of the Food and Drug Act first passed in 1906.

B. It designates *United States Pharmacopeia and National Formulary* as official standards.

C. The federal government has the power to enforce standards.

D. Provisions of the act.
   1. Drug manufacturer must provide adequate evidence of drug's safety.
   2. Correct labeling and packaging of drugs.

E. Amended in 1952 to include control of barbiturates by restricting prescription refills.

F. Amended in 1962 to require substantial investigation of drug and evidence that drug is effective in terms of labeling claims.

Harrison Narcotic Act of 1914

A. Provisions of the act.
   1. Regulates manufacture, importation, and sale of opium, cocaine, and their derivatives.
   2. Amendments have added addictive synthetic drugs to the regulated drug listing.
B. Applications of the act.
   1. Individuals who produce, sell, dispense (pharmacists), and prescribe (dentists, physicians) these drugs must be licensed and registered; prescriptions must be in triplicate.
   2. Hospitals order drugs on special blanks that bear hospital registry number. The following information is recorded for each dose:
      a. Name of drug.
      b. Amount of drug.
      c. Date and time drug obtained.
      d. Name of physician prescribing drug.
      e. Name of patient receiving drug.
      f. Nurse's signature and type of license (RN, LVN, or LPN).

The Controlled Substance Act of 1970

A. Provisions of the act.
   1. Regulates potentially addictive drugs as to prescription, use, and possession.
      a. Regulations refer to use in hospital, office, research, and emergency situations.
      b. Regulations cover narcotics, cocaine, amphetamines, hallucinogens, barbiturates, and other sedatives.
   2. Controlled drugs are placed in five different schedules or categorical listings, each governed by different regulations.
      a. The regulations govern manufacture, transport, and storage of the controlled drugs.

b. The use of the drugs is controlled as to prescription, authorization, mode of dispensation, and administration.
B. Application of the act for use of controlled drugs in hospital.
   1. The nurse is to keep the stock supply of controlled drugs under lock and key.
      a. Nurse must sign for each dose (tablet, cc) of drug.
      b. Key is held by the nurse responsible for administration of medication.
      c. At the end of each shift, nurse must account for all controlled drugs in the stock supply.
   2. Violations of the Controlled Substance Act.
      a. Violations are punishable by fine, imprisonment, or both.
      b. Nurses, upon conviction of violation, are subject to losing their licenses to practice nursing.

Prescription and Medication Orders

A. Prescription is a written order for dispensation of drugs that can be used only under physician's supervision.
B. Prescriptions outside the hospital.
   1. Formula to pharmacist for dispensing drugs to patient.
   2. Consists of four parts.
      a. Superscription (symbolized by Rx, meaning "take").
         (1) Patient's name.
         (2) Patient's address (required only for controlled drugs).
         (3) Age (required only if age is factor in dose preparation).
         (4) Date (must always be included).
      b. Inscription.
         (1) Specifies ingredients and their quantities.
         (2) May specify other ingredients necessary to specific drug form.
      c. Subscription—directions to pharmacist as to method of preparation.
      d. Signature—consists of two parts.
         (1) Accurate instructions to patient as to when, how, and in what quanti-

ties to take medication; typed on label.

    (2) Physician's signature and refill instructions.

C. Orders inside the hospital.

  1. Physician writes medication order in book, file, or patient's chart; if given over phone, nurse writes verbal order which physician later signs.

  2. Order consists of six parts.

    a. Name of drug.

    b. Dosage.

    c. Route of administration with time drug was given.

    d. Reason drug required (not always included).

    e. Length of time patient is to receive drug (not always included).

    f. Signature of individual who ordered drug.

      Example: Aspirin gr x PO q3h for pain for three days.

                  D. Smith, M.D.

Informational Resources

Official Publications

A. A drug listed in the following publications is designated as official by the Federal Food, Drug and Cosmetic Act (FDC).

  1. *The United States Pharmacopeia* (USP).

  2. *National Formulary* (NF).

  3. *Homeopathic Pharmacopeia of the United States.*

B. These publications establish standards of purity and other criteria for product acceptability; these standards are binding according to law.

C. Publications contain information on each drug entry.

  1. Source.

  2. Chemical and physical composition.

  3. Method of storage.

  4. General type or category.

  5. Range of dosage and usual therapeutic dosage.

Other Publications

A. *American Hospital Formulary* is a publication indexed by generic and proprietary names.

B. *Physicians' Desk Reference* (PDR).

  1. Annual publication with quarterly supplements.

  2. Handy source of information about dosage and drug precautions.

Miscellaneous Resources

A. Package inserts from manufacturers that accompany the product.

B. Pharmacist.

C. Physician.

D. Nursing journals.

E. Pharmaceutical and medical treatment texts.

APPENDIX 1. CONVERSION TABLES

Table A. Household Equivalents (Volume)

Metric	Apothecary	Household
0.06 ml	1 minim	1 drop
5(4) ml	1 fluidram	1 teaspoonful
15 ml	4 fluidrams	1 tablespoonful
30 ml	1 fluidounce	2 tablespoonfuls
180 ml	6 fluidounces	1 teacupful
240 ml	8 fluidounces	1 glassful

Table B. Apothecary Equivalents (Volume)

Metric		Apothecary
1	ml	= 15 minims
1	cc	= 15 minims
0.06	ml	= 1 minim
4	ml	= 1 fluidram
30	ml	= 1 fluidounce
500	ml	= 1 pint
1000	ml (1 L)	= 1 quart

Table C. Apothecary Equivalents (Weight)

Metric			Apothecary
1.0	Gm or	1000 mg	= gr xv
0.6	Gm or	600 mg	= gr x
0.5	Gm or	500 mg	= gr viiss
0.3	Gm or	300 mg	= gr v
0.2	Gm or	200 mg	= gr iii
0.1	Gm or	100 mg	= gr 1 1/2
0.06	Gm or	670 mg	= gr 1
0.05	Gm or	50 mg	= gr 3/4
0.03	Gm or	30 mg	= gr 1/2
0.015	Gm or	15 mg	= gr 1/4
0.010	Gm or	10 mg	= gr 1/6
0.008	Gm or	8 mg	= gr 1/8
		4 gm	= 1 dr
		30 gm	= 1 oz
		1 kg	= 2.2 lbs

APPENDIX 2. ABBREVIATIONS AND SYMBOLS FOR ORDERS, PRESCRIPTIONS, AND LABELS

$\overline{aa}$	of each
ac	before meals
ad lib	freely, as desired
Ba	barium
bid	twice each day
$\overline{c}$	with
C	carbon
Ca	calcium
Cl	chlorine
dr or ʒ	dram
et	and
GI	gastrointestinal
gt or gtt	drop(s)
H_2O	water
H_2O_2	hydrogen peroxide
IM	intramuscular
in	inch
K	potassium
lb or #	pound
m	minimum (a minim)
Mg	magnesium
N	nitrogen, normal
Na	sodium
NPO	nothing by mouth
od	everyday
oob	out of bed
os	mouth
oz or ʒ	ounce
pc	after meals
per	by, through
prn	whenever necessary
qh	every hour
qid	four times each day
qs	as much as required
q2h	every two hours
q3h	every three hours
q4h	every four hours
R_x	treatment, "take thou"
$\overline{s}$	without
$\overline{ss}$	one-half (½)
stat	immediately
tid	three times a day
tsp	teaspoon
WBC	white blood cell
°	degree
−	minus, negative, alkaline reaction
+	plus, positive, acid reaction
%	percent
v	roman numeral five
vii	roman numeral seven
ix	roman numeral nine
xiii	roman numeral thirteen

5

NUTRITION

ESSENTIAL BODY NUTRIENTS

Carbohydrates

A. Chief source of energy.
B. Monosaccharides.
   1. Glucose, fructose, galactose.
   2. Easily digested.
C. Disaccharides: sucrose, lactose, maltose.
D. Polysaccharides.
   1. Starch, dextrin, glycogen, cellulose, hemi-cellulose.
   2. More complex and harder to digest.
E. Convert to glucose.
   1. Appears in body as blood sugar.
   2. Metabolizes in cells.
   3. Converted in liver to glycogen for storage.

Fats

A. Provide energy.
B. Act as barriers for fat-soluble vitamins.
C. Fatty acids are the basic components of fat and comprise two main groups.
   1. Saturated fatty acids usually come from animal sources.
   2. Unsaturated fatty acids primarily come from vegetables, nuts, or seed sources.
      a. This group contains three essential fatty acids.
      b. These acids are called "essential" because they are necessary to prevent a specific deficiency disease.
      c. The body cannot manufacture these acids. They are obtained only from the diet.
      d. These acids are called linoleic acid, arachidonic acid, and linolenic acid.

Proteins

A. Complex organic compounds that contain amino acids.
B. Critical to all aspects of growth and development of body tissues; necessary for the building of muscles, blood, skin, internal organs, hormones, and enzymes.
C. Source of energy.
   1. When there is insufficient carbohydrate or fat in the diet, protein is burned.
   2. When protein is spared, it is either used for tissue repair and maintenance or converted by the liver and stored as fat.
D. When digested and broken down, proteins form 22 amino acids.
   1. Amino acids are absorbed from the intestine into the bloodstream.
   2. They are carried to the liver for synthesis into the tissues and organs of the body.
E. Amino acids are the chemical basis for life, and if just one is missing, protein synthesis will decrease or even stop.
   1. *All* but eight can be produced by the body; these eight must be obtained from the diet.
   2. If all eight are present in a particular food, the food is a "complete protein"; foods that lack one or more are called "incomplete proteins."
   3. Most meat and dairy products are complete proteins; most vegetables and fruits are incomplete proteins.
   4. When animal protein is restricted, complementing or combining proteins from plant foods will assure adequate nutrition. For example, the combination of beans and rice is a complete protein food.
F. The National Research Council recommends that 0.42 grams of protein be consumed per 0.4 kg of body weight.

Water

A. While not specifically a nutrient, water is essential for survival.
   1. Water is involved in every body process from digestion and absorption to excretion.
   2. It is a major portion of circulation and is the transporter of nutrients throughout the body.
B. Body water performs three major functions.
   1. Water gives form to the body, comprising from 50 to 75 percent of the body mass.
   2. It provides the necessary environment for cell metabolism.
   3. It maintains a stable body temperature.

C. Almost all foods contain water that is absorbed by the body.

D. The average adult body contains 59 liters of water and loses about three liters a day.
1. If a person suffers severe water depletion, dehydration and salt depletion can result and can eventually lead to death.
2. A person can survive longer without food than without water.

Vitamins

A. Vitamins are organic food substances and are essential in small amounts for growth, maintenance, and the functioning of body processes.

B. Vitamins are found only in living things—plants and animals—and usually cannot be synthesized by the human body.

C. Vitamins can be grouped according to the substance in which they are soluble.

D. The fat-soluble group includes vitamins A, D, E, and K.

E. The water-soluble vitamins include B_1, B_2, B_6, B_{12}, niacin, pantothenic acid, folacin, viotin, choline, mesoinositol, para-aminobenzoic acid, and ascorbic acid (vitamin C).

F. Vitamins have no caloric value, but they are as necessary to the body as any other basic nutrient.
1. Currently, there are about 20 substances identified as vitamins.
2. Recent research is concerned with identifying even more of these substances since they are so essential to survival.

G. The most commonly used are the listings of the Recommended Dietary Allowances (RDA), based on standards established by the National Academy of Sciences.

Minerals

A. Minerals are inorganic substances, widely prevalent in nature, and essential for metabolic processes.

B. Minerals are grouped according to the amount found in the body.

C. Major minerals include calcium, magnesium, sodium, potassium, phosphorus, sulfur, and chlorine, all of which have a known function in the body.

D. Trace minerals are iron, copper, iodine, manganese, cobalt, zinc, and molybdenum and their function in the body remains unclear.

E. There remains another group of trace minerals found in scanty amounts in the body and whose function is also unclear.

F. Minerals form 60 to 90 percent of all inorganic material in the body, and are found in bones, teeth, soft tissue, muscle, blood, and nerve cells.

G. Minerals act on organs and in metabolic processes.
1. They serve as catalysts for many reactions such as controlling muscle responses, maintaining the nervous system, and regulating acid-base balance.
2. They assist in transmitting messages, maintaining cardiac stability, and regulating the metabolism and absorption of other nutrients.

H. Even though they are considered separately, all minerals work synergistically with other minerals, and their actions are interrelated.
1. A deficiency in one mineral will affect the action of others in the body.
2. Adequate minerals must be ingested because a mineral deficiency can result in severe illness.
3. Excessive amounts of minerals can throw the body out of balance.
4. Additional information can be found in section on Fluid and Electrolyte Balance.

Assimilation of Nutrients

Gastrointestinal Tract

A. The main functions of the gastrointestinal system consist of the following.
1. Secretion of enzymes and electrolytes to break down raw materials that are ingested.

Essential Body Nutrients

Carbohydrates

Monosaccharides
Glucose, fructose, galactose
Disaccharides
Sucrose, lactose, maltose
Polysaccharides
Starch, dextrin, glycogen, cellulose, hemicellulose

Fats

Linoleic acid, linolenic acid, arachidonic acid

Proteins

Amino acids
Phenylalanine, lysine, isoleucine, leucine, methionine, valine, tryptophan, threonine

Vitamins

Fat-soluble
Vitamins A, D, E, and K
Water-soluble
Vitamins B_1, B_2, B_6, B_{12}, niacin, pantothenic acid, folacin, biotin, choline, mesoinositol, para-aminobenzoic acid, and vitamin C

Minerals

Major elements
Calcium, chlorine, iron, magnesium, phosphorus, potassium, sodium, sulfur
Trace elements

Water

Foods Rich in Fat- and Water-Soluble Vitamins

Foods Rich in Fat-Soluble Vitamins

Vitamin A—liver, egg yolk, whole milk, butter, fortified margarine, green and yellow vegetables, fruits

Vitamin D—fortified milk and margarine, fish oils

Vitamin K—egg yolk, leafy green vegetables, liver, cheese

Foods Rich in Water-Soluble Vitamins

Vitamin C—citrus fruits, tomatoes, broccoli, cabbage

Thiamine (B_1)—lean meat such as beef, pork, liver; whole grain cereals and legumes

Riboflavin (B_2)—milk, organ meats, enriched grains

Niacin—meat, beans, peas, peanuts, enriched grains

Pyridoxine (B_6)—yeast, wheat, corn, meats, liver, and kidney

Cobalamin (B_{12})—lean meat, liver, kidney

Folic acid—leafy green vegetables, eggs, liver

2. Movement of ingested products through the system.
3. Complete digestion of nutrients.
4. Absorption of nutrients into the blood.
5. Storage of nutrients.
6. Excretion of the end products of digestion.

B. Mechanical digestion.
 1. Begins in the mouth with chewing and swallowing.
 2. Nutrients are churned, and peristaltic waves move the material through the stomach.
 3. At intervals, with relaxation of the pyloric sphincter, they move into the duodenum.
 4. Peristaltic waves move the mass through the small intestines where some absorption occurs.
 5. The large intestine provides for the absorption of nutrients and the elimination of waste products.
  a. Vitamins K and B_{12}, riboflavin, and thiamin are formed.
  b. Water is absorbed from the fecal mass.

C. Chemical digestion relies on the action of digestive enzymes and other substances.
 1. See table of Major Enzymes of Digestion.
 2. Hydrochloric acid is secreted by the stomach. Aids pepsin in its action on protein.

Accessory Organs

A. The accessory organs of the gastrointestinal tract play an important role in the utilization of nutrients.

B. The liver plays a major role in the metabolism of carbohydrates, fats, and proteins.
 1. Liver converts glucose to glycogen and stores it. It reconverts glycogen to glucose when the body requires higher blood sugar. The process of releasing carbohydrates (end products) into the bloodstream is called glycogenolysis.
 2. Fats are metabolized through the process of oxidation of fatty acids and the formation of acetoacetic acid.
 3. Lipoproteins, cholesterol, and phospholipids are formed, and carbohydrates and protein are converted to fats.

Major Enzymes of Digestion

Enzyme	Source/ Secretion	Substance Acted On
Ptyalin	Oral/Saliva	Starch
Maltose	Oral/Saliva	Maltose
Pepsin	Gastric	Protein
Lipase	Gastric	Fat
Rennin	Gastric	Casein (protein in milk)
Trypsin	Pancreatic	Protein
Steapsin	Pancreatic	Fats
Amylopsin	Pancreatic	Starch
Amylase	Intestinal	Starch
Maltase	Intestinal	Maltose
Lactase	Intestinal	Lactose
Sucrase	Intestinal	Sucrose
Erepsin	Intestinal	Proteins
Enterokinase	Intestinal	Proteins

4. Proteins are metabolized.
5. The formation of urea and plasma proteins is completed.
6. Bile is secreted.

C. The gallbladder's primary function is to act as a reservoir for bile.
   1. Bile emulsifies fats through constant secretion.
   2. Secretion rate is 500 to 1000 ml every 24 hours.

D. The pancreas secretes pancreatic juices that contain enzymes for the digestion of carbohydrates, fats, and proteins. These enzymes are activated in the small intestine.

Nutritional Concepts

Normal and Therapeutic Nutrition

A. Normal nutrition.
   1. A guide for determining adequate nutrition is the U.S. Department of Agriculture recommended daily dietary allowances.
      a. The guide is scientifically designed for the maintenance of healthy people in the United States.
      b. The values of the caloric and nutrient requirements given in the guide are used in assessing nutritional states.
      c. Stress periods in the life cycle, which require alterations in the allowances, should be considered during the planning of menus.
   2. The basic four food groups are described in *A Daily Food Guide: the Basic Four* (see Appendix 2).
      a. Choices in four food groups are offered to meet the nutrient recommendations during the life cycle. (Caloric requirement is not included.)
      b. Basic nutrients in each food group should be related to dietary needs during the life cycle when menus are planned for each age group.

B. Therapeutic nutrition.
   1. The therapeutic or prescription diet is a modification of the nutritional needs based on the disease condition and/or the excess or deficit nutrition state.
   2. Combination diets, which include alterations in minerals, vitamins, proteins, carbohydrates, and fats, as well as fluid and texture, are prescribed in therapeutic nutrition.
   3. Although not all such diets will be included in this review, study of the selected diet concepts will enable you to combine two or more diets when necessary.

C. Normal and therapeutic nutrition considerations.
   1. Cultural, socioeconomic, and psychological influences, as well as physiological requirements, must be considered for effective nutrition.
   2. In any given situation, the nutrition requirements must be considered within the context of the bio-psycho-social needs of an individual.

Nutritional Problems in the Hospital

A. Nutrition is frequently neglected as an important part of patient care.
B. The nurse must consistently assess the patient (see Appendix 1) to assist in determining needed diet alterations.
   1. Inability to feed self or absence of dentures.
   2. Feelings of depression or fear.
   3. Unpleasant environmental factors prior to meals.
   4. Pain or nausea.

Providing Appropriate Nutrition

   1. Verify dietary order.
   2. Notify charge nurse and/or physician if patients' needs are not being met.
   3. Determine patients' food preferences.
   4. Check all diet trays before serving to ensure the diet provided is the one ordered.
   5. Ensure that hot food is hot and cold food is cold.
   6. Keep food trays attractive. Avoid spilling liquids on tray.
   7. Position the patient in a chair or up in bed (unless otherwise ordered) to assist in feeding.
   8. Assist the patient with cutting meat and opening milk cartons as needed.
   9. Feed the patient if necessary.

Malnutrition Disorders

A. Kwashiorkor—caused by a lack of protein; frequently seen in ages one to three, when high-protein intake is necessary.
B. Nutritional marasmus—a disease caused by a deficiency of food intake. It is a form of starvation.
C. Vitamin A deficiency—night blindness may progress to xerophthalmia and, finally, keratomalacia.
D. Vitamin C deficiency: scurvy—symptoms begin with muscle tenderness as walls of capillaries become fragile. Hemorrhage of vessels results.
E. Vitamin D deficiency: rickets—caused because vitamin D is necessary for adequate calcium absorption by the bones.
F. Thiamine deficiency: beriberi—primarily a disease of rice-eating people; symptoms include numbness in extremities and exhaustion.
G. Niacin deficiency: pellagra—symptoms include dermatitis, diarrhea, dementia, and, finally, death.
H. Iodine deficiency—leads to hyperplasia of the thyroid gland, or goiter.

Nutrients via Tube Feeding

Characteristics

A. Purpose is to maintain adequate food-fluid intake.
B. Reasons for procedure
   1. Patient is unconscious.
   2. Refusal to take in fluids or solid foods (anorexic).
   3. Trauma to upper GI tract.
   4. Patient is unable to chew or swallow.

Nasogastric Tube Insertion ❖ PROCEDURE ❖

A. Check order for tube feeding.
B. Warm feeding to room temperature.
C. Discuss procedure with the patient.
D. Demonstrate and display items to be used in order to allay the patient's fear and to gain cooperation.
E. Wash your hands and don gloves.
F. Position the patient at 45-degree angle or higher.
G. Examine nostrils and select the most patent nostril by having the patient breathe through each one.
H. Measure from tip of nose to earlobe to xiphoid process of sternum to determine appropriate length for tube insertion. If tube is to go below stomach, add additional 15 to 25 cm. Mark point on tube with tape.

Recommended Nutrient Requirements

Total Calories

2800 for tissue repair; 6000 for extensive repair

Protein

50 to 75 g/day early in postoperative period; 100 to 200 g/day if needed for new tissue synthesis

CHO—sufficient in quantity to meet calorie needs and allow protein to be used for tissue repair

Fat—not excessive as it leads to poor tissue healing and susceptibility to infection

Vitamins

Vitamin C—up to 1 g/day

Vitamin B—increased above normal

Vitamin K—normal amounts

I. Lubricate first 10 cm of tube with water-soluble lubricant.

J. Insert tube through nostril to back of throat and ask the patient to swallow. (Do not have patient hyperextend neck.) Sips of water may aid in advancing tubing past oropharynx.

K. Continue advancing tube until taped mark is reached.

L. Check position of tube.
   1. It is no longer considered safe to place end of NG tube in glass of water and observe for bubbling.
   2. Inject 10 ml of air through nasogastric tube and listen with the stethoscope over stomach for a rush of air. (Not method of choice.)
   3. Aspirate gastric contents and check pH (sometimes difficult with small-bore tubes). If pH is acidic—below 3 with litmus paper red— tube is in stomach.
   4. X-ray confirmation. If nasoduodenal or nasojejunal feedings required, patient should have x-ray to confirm correct placement.
   5. Tape tube securely to nose and to cheek.

M. Remain with and talk with the patient until the anxiety level is decreased (tube insertion often raises anxiety).

Diabetic Exchange Diets

Food Group	Unit of Exchange	Calories	Foods Allowed
Milk			
whole	1 cup	170	1 cup whole milk = 1 cup
skim	1 cup	80	skim milk and 2 fat exchanges
Fruit	Varies according to calories allotted	40	Fresh or canned without sugar or syrup
Vegetables			
A	1 cup	Vary	Green leafy vegetables; tomatoes
B	½ cup	35	Vegetables other than green, leafy
Bread	1 slice	70	Can exchange cereals, starch items, some vegetables
Meat	1 ounce	75	Lean meats, egg, cheese, seafood
Fat	1 teaspoon	45	1 teaspoon butter or mayonnaise = bacon, oil, olives, avocado
Unlimited foods			Coffee, tea, bouillon, spices, flavorings

Tube Feeding Administration ❖ Procedure ❖

1. Obtain order from the physician for appropriate formula (calories and/or amount).
2. Send requisition for formula to diet kitchen.
3. Check early in shift to ensure adequate formula is available.
4. Warm formula to room temperature using a microwave or set formula in basin of hot water.

5. Assemble feeding equipment. If using bag, fill with ordered amount of formula.
6. Explain procedure to the patient and assure privacy.
7. Place the patient on right side in high-Fowler's position.
8. Aspirate stomach contents to determine amount of residual. Return aspirated contents to stomach to prevent electrolyte imbalance.
9. Check position of tube by injecting 10 ml of air, if gastric contents not available.
10. Pinch the tubing to prevent air from entering stomach.
11. Attach barrel of syringe to nasogastric tube.
12. Fill syringe with formula. (If using feeding bag, adjust drip rate to infuse over 30 minutes.)
13. Hold syringe no more than 39 cm above patient.
14. Allow formula to infuse slowly (between 20 to 35 minutes) through the tubing.
15. Follow tube feeding with water in amount ordered.
16. Clamp end of the tube.
17. Wash tray and return it to patient's bedside.
18. Give water in between feedings if tube feeding is the sole source of nutrition.

Nasogastric Tube Irrigation ❖ PROCEDURE ❖

1. Obtain a disposable irrigation set or emesis basin for irrigation solution, a 20-ml syringe, and a normal saline irrigation solution.
2. Wash your hands and don gloves.
3. Place patient in a semi-Fowler's position.
4. Check for nasogastric tube placement by instilling air and listening for "woosh" sound.
5. Draw up 20 ml normal saline into the irrigating syringe.
6. Gently instill the normal saline into the nasogastric tube. Do not force the solution.
7. Withdraw the 20 ml irrigation solution and empty into basin.
8. Repeat the procedure twice.

9. Record on I&O sheet the irrigation solution that has not been returned.

Continuous Tube Feedings (Dobhoff, Keofeed Tubes) ❖ PROCEDURE ❖

1. Insert tube (tubes are weighted at the distal end with mercury or tungsten) or check patency of existing tube.
2. Irrigate feeding tube with sterile water or saline at least every eight hours.
3. Administer formula at prescribed infusion rate. Infusion pumps are used to maintain continuous flow.
4. Avoid keeping formula at room temperature for longer than four hours to prevent spoilage and bacterial contamination.
5. Routinely assess the abdomen for abdominal distention and bowel sounds.
6. Keep patient in semi-Fowler's position.
7. Turn off flow when placing patient supine.

Gastrostomy Feeding ❖ PROCEDURE ❖

1. Assess gastric contents to determine amount per intermittent feeding. Hold feeding if more than 50–100 ml.
2. Feed slowly for intermittent feeding or keep at prescribed rate for continuous feeding.
3. Observe gastrostomy tube insertion site for signs of dislodging, infection, or skin breakdown.
4. Provide site care; wash area with warm water and soap.
5. Apply skin protective barrier. Cover area with sterile dressing.

Therapeutic/Prescription Diets

Diets Associated with Carbohydrate Control

A. The source of glucose from food: carbohydrate—100 percent; protein—58 percent; fat—10 percent. The control of glucose in diets is based on these three nutrients.
B. Hypoglycemic diet.

1. A hypoglycemic diet is utilized to reduce stimulation of excessive insulin by avoiding highly concentrated carbohydrate foods.
   a. Foods prescribed are high protein, high fat, and low carbohydrate.
   b. Foods not allowed are high carbohydrate, for example, sugar, syrup, candy.
2. A diabetic diet modifies the insulin disorder and controls sugar intake.
   a. Foods prescribed usually use food exchange method.
   b. Foods not allowed are refined sugars.

Diets Associated with Protein Control

A. Low protein diet.
   1. Utilized for renal impairments (uremia), hepatic coma, and cirrhosis (according to individual requirements).
   2. Purpose of diet: to control by limiting protein intake the end (breakdown) products of protein metabolism which are disturbing the fluid and electrolytes and/or acid-base balances.
   3. Diet allowances/requirements.
      a. The number of grams of protein allowed is stated for each diet.
      b. Examples of high protein foods to be avoided: eggs, meat, milk and milk products.
B. High protein diet.
   1. Utilized for tissue building conditions, correction of protein deficiencies, burns, liver diseases, malabsorption syndromes, undernutrition, and maternity.
   2. Purpose of diet: to correct protein loss, and/or maintain and rebuild tissues by increasing intake of high quality protein food sources.
   3. Protein supplements are ordered by physician for individual needs. Examples of protein supplements: Sustagen, Meritene, Proteinum.
C. Amino acid metabolism abnormalities diet.
   1. Utilized for phenylketonuria (PKU), galactosemia, and lactose intolerance.
   2. Purpose of diet: to reduce and/or eliminate the offending enzyme in the food intake of protein and utilize substitute nutrient foods.
   3. The main source of enzymes for the three diseases is milk. Milk and milk products must be avoided and substitutes used to meet daily allowances.

Diets Associated with Fat Control

A. Restricted cholesterol diet.
   1. Utilized for cardiovascular diseases, diabetes mellitus, high serum cholesterol levels.
   2. Purpose of diet: to decrease the blood cholesterol level and/or maintain blood cholesterol at a normal level by restricting foods high in cholesterol.
   3. High cholesterol foods to be restricted or avoided (primarily originating from animal sources).
      a. Saturated fats.
      b. Examples: egg yolk, shell fish, organ meats, bacon, pork.
   4. Low cholesterol foods allowed (primarily originating from plant sources).
      a. Polyunsaturated fats.
      b. Examples: vegetable oils, raw or cooked vegetables, fruits, lean meats, fowl.
B. Modified fat diet.
   1. Utilized according to individual tolerance in malabsorption syndromes, cystic fibrosis, gall bladder disease, obstructive jaundice, and liver diseases.
   2. Purpose of diet: to lower fat content in diet to stop contractions of diseased organs; to reduce fat content where there is inadequate absorption of fat.
   3. Diet allowances/requirements.
      a. Moderate fat diet.
         (1) Foods to be avoided: gravies, fat meat and fish, cream, fried foods, rich pastries.
         (2) Foods allowed: eggs, lean meat, butter/margarine, cheese.
      b. Low fat diet.
         (1) Foods to be avoided: gravies, fat meat and fish, cream, fried foods, rich pastries, whole milk products,

cream soups, salad and cooking oils, nuts, chocolate, avocado.
      (2) Foods allowed: eggs (two to three per week), lean meat, butter/margarine.
   c. Fat free diet.
      (1) No fat is allowed in diet; fatty meats are omitted from diet.
      (2) Foods to be avoided: eggs, butter/margarine.
      (3) Foods allowed: vegetables, fruits, lean meats, fowl, fish, bread, cereal.

Diets Associated with Renal Disease

A. Low protein, essential amino acid diet (modified Giovannetti diet: 20 gm. protein, 1500 mg. potassium).
   1. Utilized for renal failure.
   2. Purpose of diet: to prevent electrolytes and by-products of metabolism from accumulating to a fatal level between artificial kidney treatments.
   3. Foods allowed:
      a. Eggs (one daily).
      b. Milk (6 ounces).
      c. Low protein bread.
      d. Fruit (two to four servings): apples, peaches, pears, cherries, pineapple, strawberries, grapefruit, grapes.
      e. Vegetables (two to four servings): usually any vegetable.
      f. Free list: for calories—butter, oil, jelly, candy with chocolate; tea, coffee.
   4. Foods restricted or not allowed:
      a. Meat: chicken, roast beef, fish, lamb, veal.
      b. Peanuts; bread other than low protein bread.
B. Low calcium diet.
   1. Utilized to prevent formation of renal calculi (96 percent calculi are calcium compounds).
   2. Purpose of diet: to decrease the total daily intake of calcium to prevent further stone formation. Total 400 mg. calcium instead of normal 800 mg. calcium per day.
   3. Foods allowed:
      a. Milk (one cup daily).
      b. Fruit juices, tea, coffee.
      c. Eggs (one daily); fats.
      d. Fresh fruits; vegetables (except dried).
   4. Foods restricted:
      a. Rye and whole grain breads and cereals.
      b. Dried fruits and vegetables (peas and beans).
      c. Fish, shellfish, dried and cured meats.
      d. Cheese, chocolate, nuts.
C. Acid ash diet.
   1. Utilized to prevent precipitation of stone elements.
   2. Purpose of diet: to establish well-balanced diet with total acid ash greater than total alkaline ash daily.
   3. Foods allowed:
      a. Breads and cereals of any type.
      b. Fats.
      c. Fruits (one serving), except those restricted.
      d. Vegetables; potatoes, noodles, rice.
      e. Meat, eggs, cheese, fish, fowl (two servings).
      f. Spices.
   4. Foods restricted:
      a. Carbonated beverages.
      b. Foods containing baking powder or soda.
      c. Dried fruits, bananas, figs, raisins.
      d. Dried beans; carrots.
      e. Chocolate candy.
      f. Nuts, olives, pickles.
D. Low purine diet.
   1. Utilized to prevent uric acid stones; also utilized for gout patients.
   2. Purpose of diet: to restrict purine, which is the precursor of uric acid; 4 percent of urinary stones are composed of uric acid.
   3. Foods allowed:
      a. Carbonated beverages, milk, tea, fruit juices.
      b. Breads, cereals.
      c. Cheese, eggs, fat.
      d. Most vegetables.
   4. Foods restricted:
      a. Glandular meats, gravies.

b. Fowl, fish, meat (restricted in amount).

Diets Associated with Vitamin Control

A. Diets adequate in caloric and nutrient requirements usually contain adequate amounts of vitamins.
B. Increased vitamin diet.
   1. Utilized for treatment based on specific deficiencies of vitamins.
      a. Dietary increases are needed for patients with burns, healing wounds, raised temperatures, infections, pregnancy.
      b. Water-soluble vitamins may be prescribed for certain diseases such as cystic fibrosis and liver disease.
C. There are no specific diets associated with low vitamin control.

Selected Diets Associated with Mineral Control

A. Restricted sodium diet.
   1. Utilized for hypertension, hepatitis, congestive heart failure, renal deficiencies, cirrhosis of liver, adrenal corticoid treatment.
   2. Purpose of diet: to correct and/or control the retention of sodium and water in the body by limiting sodium intake. May be done strictly by food restriction or in combination with medications.
   3. Restriction varies from eliminating salt in cooking or at the table to strict food restrictions of any product containing sodium, such as soda bicarbonate.
B. Increased or high potassium diet.
   1. Utilized for diabetic acidosis, extended use of certain diuretic drugs, burns (after first 48 hours), vomiting and fevers.
   2. Purpose of diet: to replace potassium loss from the body. (Severe potassium loss is managed with intravenous therapy.)
C. High iron diet.
   1. Utilized for anemias (hemorrhagic, nutritional, pernicious), postgastrectomy syndrome, malabsorption syndrome.

Definitions of Sodium Restrictions

Categories

- Mild: 2 to 3 g sodium
- Moderate: 1000 mg sodium
- Strict: 500 mg sodium
- Severe: 250 mg sodium

Foods High in Sodium

Table salt and all prepared salts, such as celery salt

Smoked meats and salted meats

Most frozen or canned vegetables with added salt

Butter, margarines, and cheese

Quick-cooking cereals

Shellfish and frozen or salted fish

Seasonings and sauces

Canned soups

Chocolates and cocoa

Beets, celery, and selected greens (spinach)

Foods with salt added, such as potato chips, popcorn

Foods High in Potassium

Fruit juices such as orange, grapefruit, banana, apple

Instant, dry coffee powder

Egg, legumes, whole grains

Fish, especially fresh halibut and codfish

Pork, beef, lamb, veal, chicken

Milk, skim and whole

Dried dates, prunes

Bouillon and meat broths

   2. Purpose of diet: to replace a deficit of iron due to either inadequate intake or chronic blood loss.
   3. Foods high in iron content: organ meats (especially liver), meats, egg yolks, whole wheat, seafood, leafy green vegetables, nuts, dried fruit, legumes.

Diet Associated with Fiber Control

A. High residue (roughage) diets.
   1. Prescribed for constipation and diverticulosis (prescription varies with physician).

2. Purpose of diet: to mechanically stimulate the gastrointestinal tract.
3. Diet allowances/requirements.
   a. Foods high in residue.
      (1) Any meat or fish—fried, canned, or smoked; any poultry with skin.
      (2) Cheese.
      (3) Fat in any form.
      (4) Milk and fruit juices.
      (5) Whole wheat breads, unrefined bran, cereals, shredded wheat.
   b. Foods low in carbohydrates are usually high in residue.

B. Low residue (roughage) diets.
   1. Utilized for ulcerative colitis, postoperative colon and rectal surgery, diverticulitis (when inflammation decreases diet may revert to high residue), rheumatic fever, diarrhea and enteritis.
   2. Purpose of diet: to soothe and be nonirritating residue in the large intestine.
   3. Diet allowances/requirements.
      a. Foods low in residue.
         (1) Ground, tender meat; fresh fish; any boiled, roasted, or broiled poultry without skin or fat.
         (2) Hard-boiled egg.
         (3) Creamed cottage cheese and mild cheeses.
         (4) Limited fat, crisp bacon, plain gravies.
         (5) Warm drinks (not iced); no milk.
         (6) Refined, strained, precooked cereals like pablum; enriched white bread; crackers; toast.
      b. Foods low in carbohydrates usually add high residue.

Bland Food Diets

A. These diets are presented in stages, with gradual addition of specific foods.
B. Frequent, small feedings during active stress periods; then regular meals and patterns should be established.
C. Utilized for duodenal ulcer, gastric ulcers, postoperative stomach surgery.

D. Purpose of diet: to promote the healing of the gastric mucosa by eliminating food sources that are chemically and mechanically irritating.
E. Diet allowances/requirements.
   1. Foods allowed.
      a. Milk, butter, eggs (not fried), custard, vanilla ice cream, cottage cheese.
      b. Cooked refined or strained cereal, enriched white bread.
      c. Jello; homemade creamed, pureed soups.
      d. Baked or broiled potatoes.
   2. Examples of foods that are eliminated.
      a. Spicy and highly seasoned foods.
      b. Raw foods.
      c. Very hot and very cold foods.
      d. Gas-forming foods (varies with individuals).
      e. Coffee, alcoholic beverages, carbonated drinks.
      f. High fat contents (some butter and margarine allowed).

Diets Associated with Calorie Control

A. Restricted calorie diet.
   1. Utilized in obesity, overnutrition in the aged, and specific conditions requiring weight reduction.
   2. Purpose of diet: to reduce the caloric intake of food below the energy demands of the body so weight loss will occur. Psychological support and exercise are important components of therapy along with diet.
   3. Individual diet plan is based on nutritional requirements for age group. Low caloric intakes may require nutrient supplements.
      a. Food exchange patterns are widely used for weight control diets.
      b. Aging adult requires less calories to maintain normal weight.
   4. Foods restricted.
      a. CHO.
      b. Fat.
B. Increased calorie diet.
   1. Utilized in burns, pregnancy, aging, childhood, surgery, undernutrition.

2. Purpose of diet: to meet the increased metabolic needs of the body. There is usually an increase in protein and vitamins when increased calories are ordered.
3. Foods allowed:
   a. Any food group.
   b. CHO, particularly high calorie.

Diets Associated with Surgery

A. Preoperative diet.
   1. Purpose of diet.
      a. Maintenance of normal serum protein levels.
      b. Provide adequate carbohydrate to maintain liver glycogen.
      c. Provide adequate amino acids to promote wound healing.
      d. Restore nitrogen balance if protein-depleted (burn, elderly, severely debilitated patient).
   2. Recommended nutrient requirements.
      a. 0.8 to 1.5 gm of protein/kg body weight/day.
      b. 25 to 50 Kcal/kg/day.
         (1) A calorie is a unit of heat measurement defined as the amount of heat required to raise 1 kg of water to 1°C.
         (2) One gram of protein equals 4 kilogram calories (Kcal).
   3. Recommended diet.
      a. 2500 Kcal.
      b. A high energy, moderate protein diet.
      c. High protein supplements.
   4. Elemental diet.
      a. Low residue diet.
      b. Contains synthetic mixture of CHO, amino acids, essential fatty acids with added minerals and vitamins.
      c. Bulk free, easily assimilated and absorbed.
      d. Replace clear liquid diet for patients with colon surgery.
      e. Diet products: Vivonex and Precision.
B. Postoperative surgical diets.
   1. Purpose of diet.
      a. Promote wound healing by adequate protein intake.
      b. Avoid shock from decreased plasma proteins and circulating red blood cells by increasing protein intake.
      c. Prevent edema by adequate protein intake (maintains colloidal osmotic pressure).
      d. Promote bone healing in orthopedic surgery by adequate protein and mineral replacement.
      e. Prevent infection by adequate amino acid replacement (amino acids are involved in body defense mechanisms).
   2. Recommended nutrient requirements.
      a. Total calories: 2800 for tissue repair; 6000 for extensive repair.
      b. Fluid intake.
         (1) Uncomplicated surgery: 2000 to 3000/day.
         (2) Complicated surgery (sepsis, renal damage): 3000 to 4000/day.
         (3) Seriously ill with drainage: 7000/day.
   3. Diet progresses from nothing by mouth (NPO) the day of surgery to a general diet. Phases/steps include:
      a. A clear-liquid diet is 1000 to 1500 ml/day and is comprised of water, tea, broth, jello, and juices (avoid juices with pulp).
      b. A full-liquid diet is clear liquids, milk and milk products, custard, puddings, creamed soups, sherbet, ice cream, and any fruit juice.
      c. A soft diet is full liquid and, in addition, pureed vegetables, eggs (not fried), milk, cheese, fish, fowl, tender beef, veal, potatoes, and cooked fruit.
      d. General diet, taking into consideration specific alterations necessary for patient's health status.

APPENDIX 1. BASIC NUTRITIONAL ASSESSMENT

Assessment	Normal	Abnormal
Appetite	Remains unchanged	Recently increased or decreased Particular cravings
Weight	Previous weight maintained Normal for patient Appropriate for age and body build	Changed—recently increased or decreased Rapid or slow changes
Nutritional Intake	Adequate foods and fluids to supply body nutrients Nonallergic response to major food groups No pattern of fad diets Absence of drugs, chemicals, or other substances that influence appetite or metabolism	Elimination of certain food categories that results in limited nutrients Emphasis on some food groups (sugar) to the exclusion of others (vegetables) Allergic response to certain foods Constant use of fad diets to lose weight Use of drugs or chemicals that interferes with appetite nutrient assimilation Presence of emotional disorder (depression, anorexia, manic response) that interferes with food ingestion
Meal Patterns	Three to six home-prepared meals per day Adequate time and calm atmosphere for meals	Fast-food or packaged foods Missed meals, constant snacking, or over-eating Eating "on the run" or hurried
Physical Factors	Adequate chewing and swallowing capability Mouth and gums healthy so food can be ingested Physical exercise adequate for calorie intake	Teeth and/or gums in poor condition or ill-fitting dentures Swallowing impairs ingestion Inadequate physical exercise to burn calories
Presence of Disease	No disease process that interferes with nutrient assimilation No congenital condition or postsurgery condition that interferes with nutrient assimilation	Disease present that interferes with ingestion, digestion, assimilation, or excretion Congenital condition, rehabilitation phase, or postsurgery that interferes with food assimilation
Sociocultural—Religious Factors	Ability to afford adequate foods in all food categories Cultural beliefs that do not eliminate whole food groups Religious beliefs that do not eliminate whole food groups Food does not lose all nutrient value in preparation	Economic position that precludes purchase of adequate foods Religious or cultural beliefs that interfere with receiving balanced diet (macrobiotic diets) Inadequate knowledge, experience, or intelligence to prepare healthy meals
Elimination Schedule	Regular, adequate elimination of foods Absence of constant flatus, discharge, or mucus	Irregular and/or painful elimination Presence of constant flatus Presence of discharge, blood, or mucus

APPENDIX 2. THE BASIC FOUR FOOD GROUPS

Dairy Products

Foods Included

- Milk: whole, evaporated, skim, dry, buttermilk
- Cheese: cottage, cream, cheddar, natural or processed
- Ice cream

Contribution to Diet   Milk is a leading source of calcium, which is needed for bones and teeth. It also provides a high-quality protein, riboflavin, vitamin A (if milk is whole or fortified), and other nutrients.

Amounts Recommended   Two servings for adults. Recommended amounts are given below in terms of whole fluid milk for other groups.

	237 ml (8-ounce) cups
Children under 9	2 to 3
Children 9 to 12	3 or more
Teenagers	4 or more
Adults	2 or more
Pregnant women	3 or more
Nursing mothers	4 or more

Part or all of the milk may be fluid skim milk, buttermilk, evaporated milk, or dry milk.

Cheese and ice cream may replace part of the milk. To substitute, figure the amount on the basis of calcium content. Common portions of various kinds of cheese and ice cream and their milk equivalents in calcium are:

16 ml (1-inch cube) cheddar-type cheese	= ½ cup milk
½ cup cottage cheese	= ⅓ cup milk
2 tablespoons cream cheese	= 1 tablespoon milk
½ cup ice cream or ice milk	= ⅓ cup milk

Protein

Foods Included

- Beef; veal; lamb; pork; variety meats, such as liver, heart, kidney
- Poultry and eggs
- Fish and shellfish
- Alternates: dry beans, dry peas, lentils, nuts, peanuts, peanut butter

Contribution to Diet   Foods in this group are valued for their protein, which is needed for growth and repair of body tissues, muscle, organs, blood, skin, and hair. These foods also provide iron, thiamin, riboflavin, and niacin.

Amounts Recommended   Choose two servings every day.

Count as a serving: 57 to 85 G (not including bone weight) cooked lean meat, poultry or fish. Count as alternates for ½ serving meat or fish: 1 egg, ½ cup cooked dry beans, dry peas, or lentils, or 2 tablespoons peanut butter.

Vegetable-Fruit Group

Foods Included

All vegetables and fruit. This guide emphasizes those that are valuable as sources of vitamin C and vitamin A.

Sources of Vitamin C

Good Sources: Grapefruit or grapefruit juice, orange or orange juice, cantaloupe, guava, mango, papaya, raw strawberries, broccoli, brussels sprouts, green pepper, sweet red pepper.

Fair Sources: Honeydew melon, lemon, tangerine or tangerine juice, watermelon, asparagus tips, raw cabbage, cauliflower, collards, garden cress, kale, kohlrabi, mustard greens, potatoes and sweet potatoes cooked in the jacket, rutabagas, spinach, tomatoes or tomato juice, turnip greens.

Sources of Vitamin A

Dark-green and deep-yellow vegetables and a few fruits, namely, apricots, broccoli, cantaloupe, carrots, chard, collards, cress, kale, mango, persimmon, pumpkin, spinach, sweet potatoes, turnip greens and other dark-green leaves, winter squash.

Contribution to Diet   Fruits and vegetables are valuable chiefly because of the vitamins and minerals they contain. In this plan, this group is counted on to supply nearly all the vitamin C needed and over half the vitamin A.

Vitamin C is needed for healthy gums and body tissues. Vitamin A is needed for growth, normal vision, and healthy condition of skin and other body surfaces.

Amounts Recommended   Choose five or more servings every day, including:

- One serving of a good source of vitamin C or two servings of a fair source.
- One serving, at least every other day, of a good source of vitamin A. If the food chosen for vitamin C is also a good source of vitamin A, the additional serving of a vitamin A food may be omitted.
- The remaining three or more servings may be of any vegetable or fruit, including those that are valuable for vitamin C and vitamin A.

Count as one serving: ½ cup of vegetable or fruit; or one medium apple, banana, orange, or potato, half a medium grapefruit, a slice of cantaloupe, or the juice of one lemon.

APPENDIX 2. THE BASIC FOUR FOOD GROUPS (*Continued*)

Complex Carbohydrates

Foods Included

All breads and cereals that are whole grain, enriched, or restored; *check labels to be sure*.

Grains (wheat, corn, rice, millet, oats), cornmeal, crackers, flour, grits, pasta, potatoes, beans, and nuts.

Amounts Recommended   Choose six or more servings every day.

Other Foods

To round out meals and meet energy needs, almost everyone will use some foods not specified in the four food groups. Such foods include unenriched, refined bread, cereal, flour; sugar; butter, margarine, other fats. Often these are ingredients in a recipe, or are added to other foods during preparation or at the table. Include some vegetable oil among the fats used.

6

LABORATORY TESTS

ROUTINE BLOOD CHEMISTRY TESTS

Test	Purpose	Normal Values
Erythrocytes		
Red Blood Cell Count	Determines actual number of formed blood elements in relation to volume. Identifies abnormalities.	Males: 4.5–6.2 million/cu mm Females: 4.0–5.5 million/cu mm Children: 3.2–5.2 million/cu mm
Hematocrit (HCT)	Measures percentage of red blood cells per fluid volume of whole blood.	Males: 40–54/100 ml Females: 37–47/100 ml Children: 29–54/100 ml
Hemoglobin (Hgb)	Measures amount of hemoglobin/100 ml blood to determine oxygen-carrying capacity.	Males: above 13–18 g/100 ml Females: above 12–16 g/100 ml
Platelet Count	Determines number of platelets.	Adults: 100,000–400,000/cu mm
Prothrombin Time (PT)	Evaluates thrombin generation. Detects deficiencies in extrinsic clotting mechanism.	11–15 seconds
Partial Thromboplastin Time (PTT)	Evaluates adequacy of plasma-clotting factors—intrinsic clotting mechanism.	30–45 seconds Prolonged values indicate coagulation factor deficiency
Thrombin Time	Screening test to detect abnormalities in thrombin fibrinogen reaction. (Conversion to fibrin in stage 3 of clotting sequence.)	10–15 seconds
Leukocytes		
White Blood Cell Count (WBC)	Establishes quantity and maturity of white blood cell elements.	Adults: 4500–11,000/cu mm Children: 5000–13,000/cu mm Neutrophils: 3000–7500/cu mm Band Neutrophils: 150–700/cu mm Basophils: 25–100/cu mm Eosinophils: 50–400/cu mm Lymphocytes: 1500–4500 cu/mm Monocytes: 100–500/cu mm
Erythrocyte Sedimentation Rate (ESR)	Measures rate of red blood cells settling from plasma—reflects infections.	<u>Wintrobe Method</u> Males: 9 mm/hr Females: 0–15 mm/hr Children: 0–13 mm/hr <u>Westergren Method</u> Males: 0–15 mm/hr Females: 0–20 mm/hr Children: 0–20 mm/hr
Schilling Test	Determines absorption of vitamin B_{12} necessary for erythropoiesis. Definitive test for pernicious anemia.	7% of radioactive B_{12} excreted in urine in first 24 hours Diagnosis is made when less than 3% excreted

Serum Electrolyte Levels

Potassium (K⁺)

A. Normal serum level 3.5 to 5.0 mEq/L.

B. Purpose—test for electrolyte imbalance.

C. Indications.
1. Increased K^+—acute renal disease, burns, crushing injuries, adrenal insufficiency, dehydration, anorexia nervosa, excessive intake caused by specific drugs (potassium penicillin), salt substitute, or the most common, too rapid infusion of IV solution containing potassium.
2. Decreased K^+—renal loss (due to diuretics), loss from the GI tract via NG tube, vomiting or diarrhea, and reduced potassium intake.

D. Nursing considerations.
1. Critical values may lead to fatal cardiac arrhythmias.
2. Assess for signs and symptoms of potassium excess or loss (see page 44).
3. Hyperkalemia—remove excess potassium.
   a. Administer diuretics (as ordered) if kidney function adequate.
   b. Administer exchange resins through NG tube or via Kexalate enema.
   c. Administer hypertonic IV glucose with insulin as ordered—moves potassium back into cells.
   d. Administer sodium bicarbonate—shifts potassium back into cells.
   e. Hemo- or peritoneal dialysis.
4. Hypokalemia—replace lost potassium.
   a. Administer oral potassium, monitor IV infusion of potassium.
   b. Replace no more than 20 mEq of KCL in one hour.
   d. Observe ECG monitor if possible to observe for cardiac effect of KCL.
   e. Give foods rich in potassium—bananas, molasses, oranges, raisins, seafood.

Sodium (Na⁺)

A. Normal serum level 135 to 145 mEq/L.

B. Purpose—test for deficiency or excess of electrolyte.

C. Indications.
1. Increased level is a very high concentration of sodium in the extracellular fluid—dehydration, severe diarrhea, decreased water intake, fever, renal failure, and ingestion of sodium chloride.
2. Decreased level is a very low concentration of sodium in the extracellular fluid—diuretics, excessive perspiration, GI loss (vomiting, diarrhea), lack of sodium in diet, adrenal insufficiency, burns, excessive IV solutions without NaCl replacement.

D. Nursing considerations.
1. Assess for signs and symptoms of sodium excess or loss (see page 45).
2. Assess for critical levels (below 120 or above 155).
3. Hypernatremia.
   a. Administer salt-free IV solutions (dextrose), monitor for hyponatremia, and administer 0.45% NaCl to prevent hyponatremia.
   b. Restrict sodium in diet.
   c. Discontinue drugs that cause sodium retention.
   d. Weigh daily and record intake and output.
4. Hyponatremia—replace lost sodium.
   a. Administer IV fluids with sodium (3% or 5% saline)—monitor venous pressure to prevent circulatory overload.
   b. Restrict water intake—monitor intake and output.

Calcium (Ca⁺⁺)

A. Normal serum level is 8.4 to 10.5 mg/100 ml.

B. Purpose—test for deficit or excess of calcium electrolyte.

C. Indications.
1. Increased level—excess of calcium in the extracellular fluid. Excess of vitamin D (from milk), hyperparathyroidism, cancer (neoplasm of parathyroid, multiple myeloma), immobilization, Paget's disease, thyro-

toxicosis, acromegaly, specific drugs (thiazide diuretics), and calcium supplements with inadequate assimilation.
2. Decreased level—deficit of calcium in the extracellular fluid. Vitamin D deficiency, magnesium deficiency, excessive laxatives, malabsorption syndrome, hypothyroidism, chronic renal insufficiency, burns, acute pancreatitis, removal of the parathyroid glands, blood transfusions (over 2000 ml) without calcium supplements, and specific drugs (anticonvulsant therapy).

D. Nursing considerations.
  1. Assess for signs and symptoms of excessive calcium or loss (see page 45).
  2. Assess for critical levels of calcium (below 7.0 or above 13.5 mg/100 ml). Notify head nurse or physician immediately.
    a. Assess for tetany and convulsions indicating hypocalcemia.
    b. Excess calcium may lead to coma.
  3. Hypercalcemia.
    a. Treat underlying cause of high serum calcium level.
    b. Force fluids.
    c. Limit dietary intake of calcium.
    d. Promote calcium excretion (sodium salts IV and diuretics).
  4. Hypocalcemia—replace low levels of calcium.
    a. Monitor by checking for positive Trousseau's test or Chvostek's sign.
    b. Administer calcium gluconate IV or serum albumin if low levels are due to low serum albumin concentration.
    c. Administer oral calcium supplements and a diet high in calcium (dairy products, bone meal, molasses, yogurt).

Magnesium (Mg⁺⁺)

A. Normal serum level is 1.5 to 2.5 mEq/L.

B. Purpose—test for excess or deficit serum levels of magnesium to evaluate kidney function and metabolic disorders.

C. Indications.

1. Increased Magnesium—renal insufficiency, severe dehydration, adrenal insufficiency, hypothyroidism, leukemia, overuse of antacids with magnesium (Gelusil), specific drugs.
2. Decreased Magnesium—acute pancreatitis, chronic nephritis, diuretic phase of renal failure, gastric drainage, abnormal loss due to diarrhea, impaired absorption, specific drugs (diuretics), hypercalcemia, acute alcoholism and cirrhosis, prolonged IV (three weeks) without magnesium.

D. Nursing consideration.
  1. Assess for signs and symptoms of magnesium excess or loss.
  2. Assess for critical values indicating immediate interventions.
    a. Increased level—above 2.5 mEq/L. The higher the level of magnesium, the more sedative the effect.
    b. Assess for loss of deep tendon reflexes, respiratory decrease, and cardiac arrest.
  3. Hypermagnesemia.
    a. Increased fluid intake—for magnesium intoxication give IV calcium gluconate slowly in peripheral veins (do not use a CVP line) to promote excretion of excess Mg.
    b. Administer diuretics with possible renal dialysis if renal function is impaired.
    c. Increased levels potentiate cardiac effect of increased potassium.
  4. Hypomagnesemia.
    a. Assess for severe deficiency—muscle twitching indicates neurological signs; nausea and vomiting indicate GI signs.
    b. Administer magnesium sulfate IV (10 to 40 mEq/L in IV fluid) or IM slowly. Observe for urine output and keep antidote (calcium gluconate) available.
    c. Monitor daily ingestion of magnesium PO and promote diet high in Mg—nuts, green vegetables, seafood.

Chloride (Cl⁻)

A. Normal serum value is 100 to 106 mEq/L.

B. Purpose—test for excess or deficit levels.

C. Indications.
1. Increased Chloride—prolonged diarrhea leading to metabolic acidosis, acute renal failure, respiratory alkalosis (hyperventilation, CNS damage), diabetes insipidus, dehydration, specific drugs (salicylate intoxication, steroids).
2. Decreased Chloride—prolonged vomiting or NG suction, loss of HCl, diarrhea, metabolic acidosis, adrenocortical insufficiency, renal disease that loses salt, specific drugs.
D. Nursing considerations.
1. Assess for signs and symptoms of chloride excess and loss.
2. Assess for critical values, below 70 or above 120 mEq/L.
3. Excess chloride—conditions that cause increased sodium levels may also cause increased chloride.
4. Record intake and output and daily weights to monitor electrolyte imbalances.

Phosphorus (Ph)

A. Normal serum value is 2.3 to 4.7 mg/dl.
B. Purpose—test for excess or deficit levels.
C. Indications.
1. Increased phosphorus—hypocalcemia, tetany, hypoparathyroidism, headaches, GI irritation, kidney disease, specific drugs, and vitamin D excess.
2. Decreased phosphorus—hypocalcemia, hypomagnesemia, hyperparathyroidism, vitamin D deficiency, alcohol intoxication, malabsorption.
D. Nursing considerations.
1. Assess for signs and symptoms of phosphorus excess and loss.
2. Assess for critical values—hyperphosphatemia may occur with hypocalcemia and cardiac complications (arrhythmias).
3. Hyperphosphatemia.
a. May require dialysis to lower serum phosphorus.
b. Gastric lavage with potassium may lower level of phosphorus.
c. Blood transfusions may be necessary.

4. Hypophosphatemia.
a. Administer phosphate salt tablets or foods high in phosphorus (eggs, fish, meat, poultry, grains, peas, peanuts, walnuts, whole wheat, rye, and chocolate).
b. Administer IV potassium phosphate.

Cardiac Function Tests

A. Enzyme activity evaluation denotes heart muscle damage.
1. When the heart muscle is without oxygen for 30–60 minutes, intracelluar enzymes are released.
2. Specific enzymes are released into the bloodstream at varying intervals.
a. CPK-isoenzymes (CPK-MB)—most valuable measurement; level rises within six hours.
b. LDH, LDH_2-isoenzymes—level rises in 6–8 hours; persists longer.
c. SGOT+—not specific to heart disease alone; serial tests helpful.
d. Alpha hydroxybutyric dehydrogenase.
B. The greater the peak in enzymes and the longer the level remains, the more serious the heart damage.

Lipoprotein and Lipid Tests

A. Normal values.
1. Cholesterol—below 200 mg/100 ml (teenager's level should be below 180 mg/100 ml).
2. Triglycerides—40 to 150 mg/100 ml.
3. Low-density lipoproteins (LDLs)—60 to 180 mg/100 ml.
4. Very low-density lipoproteins (VLDLs)—25 to 50% of total cholesterol.
5. High-density lipoproteins (HDLs)—male level, 30 to 70 mg/100 ml; female level, 30 to 80 mg/100 ml.
B. Purpose—total cholesterol, lipoproteins and triglycerides are screening tests to determine risk of atherosclerosis and heart disease.

1. High cholesterol—increased risk of heart disease.
2. High-density lipoprotein—lower risk of heart disease.
3. Low-density lipoprotein—higher risk of heart disease.
4. High triglycerides—higher risk of acute myocardial infarction.

C. Variations.
1. Serum cholesterol increased in: biliary obstruction (cirrhosis), hypothyroidism, pancreatic disease, uncontrolled diabetes, and pregnancy.
2. Serum cholesterol decreased in: liver disease, hyperthyroidism, malnutrition, anemias, malabsorption of cholesterol.
3. Triglycerides increased in: hepatitis, pancreatitis, cirrhosis due to alcoholism, renal failure, acute myocardial infarction.
4. Triglycerides decreased in: hyperparathyroidism, pulmonary disease, malnutrition.

Arterial Blood Studies

A. Arterial blood gases.
1. Indicate respiratory function by measuring:
   a. Oxygen (pO_2).
   b. Carbon dioxide (pCO_2).
   c. pH.
   d. Oxygen saturation and bicarbonate (HCO_3).
2. Determine state of acid-base balance.
3. Reveal the adequacy of the lungs to provide oxygen and to remove carbon dioxide.
4. Assess degree to which kidneys can maintain a normal pH.

B. Normal arterial values.
1. Oxygen saturation—93 to 98 percent.
2. PaO_2—95 mm Hg.
3. Arterial pH—7.35 to 7.45 (7.4).
4. pCO_2—35 to 45 mm Hg (40).
5. HCO_3 content—23 to 27 mEq (25).
6. Base excess— -3 to +3 (0).

C. Acid-base imbalances.
1. Respiratory acidosis.
   a. pH—7.32.
   b. pCO_2—52 mmHg.
   c. pO_2—90 mmHg.
   d. HCO_3—24 mEq/L.
2. Respiratory alkalosis.
   a. pH—7.51.
   b. pCO_2—32 mm pressure.
   c. pO_2—95 mmHg.
   d. HCO_3—24 mEq/L.
3. Metabolic acidosis.
   a. pH—7.30.
   b. HCO_3—16 mEq/L.
   c. pCO_2—38 mm.
   d. pO_2—95 mm.
   e. Cl—120 mEq/L.
   f. K—5.5 mEq/L.
4. Metabolic alkalosis.
   a. pH—7.50.
   b. HCO_3—38 mEq/L.
   c. pCO_2—38 mm pressure.
   d. pO_2—95 mm pressure.
   e. K—3.0 mEq/L.
   f. Cl—88 mEq/L.

Hematological Tests

Blood Grouping

A. Normal values summary of ABO blood grouping.
B. Purpose—test correctly matches donated blood with recipients.
C. Rh blood group.
1. Positive (85 percent of the population).
2. Negative (15 percent of the population).

Antigens and Antibodies

A. Based on type of antigens present in red blood cells as well as type of antibodies in the serum.
B. A and B antigens.
1. Patients with type A blood have antigen A present; patients with type B blood have antigen B present.
2. Patients with type AB blood have both A and B antigens present.
3. Patients with type O blood have no antigens present.

Normal Values Summary of ABO blood grouping

Blood Type	Antigen in RBCs	Antibodies in Plasma	Incompatible Donor Blood	Compatible Blood Donor
A	A	Anti-B	AB and B	A and O
B	B	Anti-A	A and AB	B and O
AB	A and B	None	None	All blood groups
0	None	Anti-A and Anti-B	All blood groups	O

C. Anti-A and anti-B antibodies present.
1. Patients with type A blood do not have anti-A antibodies because the blood cells would be destroyed by agglutination.
2. They have anti-B antibodies.
3. Type B blood has anti-A antibodies.

Blood Coagulation

A. Clotting takes place in three phases.
1. Phase I—prothrombin activator formed in response to ruptured vessel or damage to blood.
2. Phase II—prothrombin activator catalyzes conversion of prothrombin into thrombin.
3. Phase III—thrombin acts as an enzyme to convert fibrinogen into fibrin thread.
B. Types of clotting factors.
1. Calcium ions.
   a. Cofactor in coagulation.
   b. Does not enter into reaction.
   c. If absent, neither extrinsic or intrinsic system will operate.
2. Phospholipids.
   a. Necessary for formation of final pro-thrombin activator.
   b. Thromboplastin is phospholipid in extrinsic system.
   c. Platelet factor III is phospholipid for intrinsic system.
3. Plasma protein—all clotting factors from V to XIII.
C. Coagulation mechanisms.
1. Extrinsic mechanisms.
   a. Extract from damaged tissue is mixed with blood.

b. Trauma occurs to tissue or endothelial surface of vascular wall, releasing thromboplastin.
2. Intrinsic mechanisms.
   a. Blood itself comes into contact with roughened blood vessel wall.
   b. Platelets adhere to vessel and disintegrate, which releases blood factor III containing thromboplastin.
D. Fibrinolytic system.
1. Adequate function is necessary to maintain hemostasis.
2. Dissolves clots through formation of plasmin.

Prothrombin Time (PT)

A. Normal values—10 to 15 seconds (some labs use 11 to 16 seconds).
B. Purpose—prothrombin time provides data on thrombin generation.
1. It is a screening test to detect deficiencies in the extrinsic clotting mechanism.
2. Useful for control of long-term anticoagulant therapy.
C. Critical values.
1. If value is above 30 seconds, hemorrhage may occur—observe for bleeding.
2. Administer vitamin K as ordered.
D. Prolonged clotting time.
1. Inadequate vitamin K in premature and newborn infants or in diet.
2. Poor fat absorption (obstructive jaundice).
3. Liver damage.
4. Specific drugs (heparin, Coumadin, salicylates).

Partial Thromboplastin Time (PTT)

A. Normal values—30 to 45 seconds.

B. Purpose—best single screening test for coagulation disorders.
1. Test evaluates adequacy of plasma clotting factors—intrinsic clotting mechanism.
2. Monitors heparin therapy.
3. Used for patient with hemophilia.

C. Arterial values—if PTT is very prolonged (100 seconds), assess for spontaneous bleeding.

D. Prolonged clotting time.
1. Vitamin K deficiency.
2. Liver disease.
3. Hemophilia.
4. Specific drugs (heparin, warfarin, Coumadin, salicylates).

Renal Function Tests

A. Phenolsulfonphthalein (PSP) test indicates the functional ability of the kidney to:
1. Excrete waste products.
2. Concentrate and dilute urine.
3. Carry on absorption and excretion activities.
4. Maintain body fluids and electrolytes.

B. Renal concentration tests.
1. Evaluate the ability of the kidney to concentrate urine.
2. As kidney disease progresses, renal function decreases. Concentration tests evaluate this process.
3. Renal concentration is measured by specific gravity readings.

C. Specific gravity.
1. Normal value—1.003 to 1.035, usually 1.010 to 1.025.
2. If specific gravity is 1.018 or greater, it may be assumed that the kidney is functioning within normal limits.
3. Specific gravity that stabilizes at 1.010 indicates kidney has lost ability to concentrate or dilute.

D. Blood urea nitrogen (BUN).
1. Normal value—7 to 18 mg/100 ml.
2. Purpose—tests for impaired kidney function by testing the body's urea production and urine flow.
3. BUN level affected by protein intake and tissue breakdown.

E. Serum creatinine.
1. Normal value—male: 0.8 to 1.2 mg/dl; female: 0.6 to 0.9 mg/dl.
2. Purpose—tests renal function by evaluating the balance between production and filtration of glomeruli.
3. This is the most sensitive of renal function tests.

F. Concentration and dilution tests.
1. Fishberg concentration test—high protein dinner with 200 ml fluid is ordered. Next A.M. on arising, client voids q 1/hr. One specimen should have specific gravity more than 1.025.
2. Dilution test—NPO after dinner. Morning voiding discarded. Client drinks 1000 ml in 30 to 45 minutes. Four specimens at one hour intervals are collected. One specimen will fall below 1.003.
3. Specific gravity—urine 1.003 to 1.030. Increased solutes cause increased specific gravity.

G. Glomerular filtration test (endogenous creatinine clearance).
1. Normal value—125 ml/minute (male) and 110 ml/minute (female).
2. Purpose—kidney function is assessed by clearing a substance from the blood (filtration in the glomerulus).
3. Common test is the amount of blood cleared of urea per minute.
4. Test done on 12-hour or 24-hour urine specimen.

H. Electrolyte tests.
1. Kidney function is essential to maintain fluid and electrolyte balance.
2. Tests for electrolytes (sodium, potassium, chloride, and bicarbonate) measure the ability of the kidney to filter, reabsorb, or excrete these substances.

3. Impaired filtration leads to retention, and impaired reabsorption leads to loss of electrolytes.
4. Tests are performed on blood serum, so venous blood is required.

Urine Analysis

A. Normal values.
   1. Specific gravity—1.005 to 1.020.
   2. Urine pH—4.5 to 8.0.
   3. Color—straw.
   4. Odor—aromatic.
   5. Appearance—clear.
   6. Protein—negative or zero.
   7. Glucose—negative or zero.
   8. Ketones—negative or zero.
   9. Red blood cells—0 to 3.
   10. White blood cells—0 to 4.
   11. Casts—none; occasional.
   12. Crystals—negative.
   13. Yeast cells—none.
   14. Parasites—none.
B. Urinalysis is a critical test for total evaluation of the renal system and for indication of renal disease.
C. Specific gravity shows the degree of concentration in urine.
   1. Normal value—1.005 to 1.020.
   2. Indicates the ability of the kidney to concentrate or dilute urine.
   3. Change from normal range indicates diabetes mellitus (greater than 1.030) or kidney damage (less than 1.010).
   4. Renal failure—specific gravity constant at 1.010.
D. Analysis of the pH of urine.
   1. pH is the symbol for the logarithm of the reciprocal of the hydrogen ion concentration.
   2. A measurement of hydrogen ion concentration is taken—the lower the number, the higher the acidity of urine.
      a. Normal value—4.5 to 8.0 (normal pH is 6 to 7).

      b. Lower than 6 is acidic urine, and higher than 7 is alkaline urine.
   3. Regulation of urine pH is important for treatment of certain conditions.
      a. Above pH 6.
         (1) Treatment of hypertension with mecamylamine hydrochloride (Inversine).
         (2) Management of blood transfusions.
         (3) Streptomycin and sulfonamide therapy.
         (4) Management of renal calculi.
      b. Below pH 6—treatment of urinary tract infections.
E. Chemical analysis of urine.
   1. Protein or albumin—zero is normal for a 24-hour specimen.
      a. Presence may indicate renal disease, such as nephritis or nephrosis.
      b. Inflammatory processes any place in the body may result in proteinuria.
      c. Toxemia of pregnancy yields a finding of proteinuria.
      d. Renal calculi indicate positive test results.
      e. Appearance in urine may be due to dehydration, strenuous exercise, high protein diet.
   2. Glucose—normal range is zero.
      a. Presence of glucose may indicate head injury or diabetes.
      b. Test is usually done by test strips or tablets; change in color indicates presence of glucose.
   3. Ketone bodies—normal range is zero.
      a. Ketonuria primarily indicates diabetic acidosis but is also present with starvation and pernicious vomiting.
      b. Test is usually done by strip or powder mixed with urine; purple color indicates positive test.
   4. Bilirubin—normal range is zero.
      a. Presence in urine may indicate liver disease and may appear before the clinical symptom of jaundice.
      b. Detected in the urine by qualitative methods, such as inspection of color.
   5. Blood—normal range is zero.

a. If red blood cells present, may indicate disease of kidney or urinary tract, and the source of hemorrhage must be determined.

b. Specific diagnosis is made by complete urine analysis for casts and epithelial cells.

F. Microscopic examination of urine.
   1. Evaluation of urinary sediment is important for diagnostic purposes.
   2. Test for cellular elements (epithelial cells, white and red blood cells).
   3. Test for casts, fat bodies, and crystals.

G. Levels of albuminuria.
   30 mg/100 ml = 1 +
   100 mg/100 ml = 2 +
   300 mg/100 ml = 3 +
   1000 mg/100 ml = 4 +

Analysis of GI Secretions

A. Contents of the GI tract may be examined for the presence or absence of digestive juices, bacteria, parasites, and malignant cells.

B. Stomach contents may be aspirated and analyzed for volume and free and total acid.

Gastric Analysis

A. Performed by means of a nasogastric tube.
   1. Maintain NPO six to eight hours prior to the test.
   2. Pass nasogastric tube; verify its presence in the stomach; tape to patient's nose.

B. Collect fasting specimens.
   1. Administer agents, such as alcohol, caffeine, histamine (0.2 mg subcutaneous), as ordered, to stimulate the flow of gastric acid.
      a. Watch for side effects of histamine, including flushing, headache, and hypotension.
      b. Do not give drug to patients with a history of asthma or other allergic conditions.
   2. Collect specimens as ordered, usually at 10 to 20 minute intervals.

3. Label specimens and send to laboratory.
4. Withdraw nasogastric tube; offer oral hygiene; make patient comfortable.
5. Gastric acid is high in the presence of duodenal ulcers, and is low in pernicious anemia.

C. Tubeless gastric analysis.
   1. Enables the determination of acidity or its absence.
   2. Have patient fast for six to eight hours prior to the examination.
   3. Administer gastric stimulant followed by Azuresin or Diagnex Blue, as ordered.
   4. Acid in the stomach displaces the dye, which is then released, absorbed by the bowel mucosa, and excreted in the urine.
   5. The bladder is emptied; the specimen saved. One hour after taking dye resin, patient is instructed to void again. Urine is analyzed, and an estimation is made of the amount of free acid in the stomach.

D. Gastric washings for acid-fast bacilli.
   1. Have client fast six to eight hours prior to the procedure.
   2. Insert nasogastric tube and secure gastric washings.
   3. Send specimens to the laboratory to determine the presence of acid-fast bacilli.
   4. Wash your hands carefully and protect yourself from direct contact with specimens.
   5. This procedure is performed on suspected cases of active pulmonary tuberculosis when it is difficult to secure sputum for analysis.

Stool Analysis

A. Stool specimens are examined for amount, consistency, color, shape, blood, fecal urobilinogen, fat, nitrogen, parasites, food residue, and other substances.
   1. Stool cultures are also done for bacteria and viruses.
   2. Some foods and medicines can affect stool color—spinach, green; cocoa, dark red; senna, yellow; iron, black; upper GI bleed-

ing, tarry black; lower GI bleeding, bright red.

B. Stool abnormalities.
   1. Steatorrhea—bulky, greasy and foamy, foul odor.
   2. Biliary obstruction—light gray or clay-colored.
   3. Ulcerative colitis—loose stools, with copious amounts of mucus or pus.
   4. Constipation or obstruction—small, hard masses.

C. Specimen collection.
   1. Specimens for detection of parasites should be sent to the laboratory while the stool is still warm and fresh.
   2. Examinations for blood are performed on small samples. A tongue blade may be used to place a small amount of stool in a disposable waxed container.
   3. Stools for chemical analysis are usually examined for the total quantity expelled, so the complete stool is sent to the laboratory.

Liver Function Tests

Biliary Excretion

A. Serum bilirubin—abnormal in biliary and liver disease causing jaundice.
   1. Direct (conjugated)—normal: 0.2 mg/100 ml, soluble in H_2O.
   2. Indirect (unconjugated)—normal: 0.8 mg/100 ml, insoluble in H_2O.
   3. Total serum bilirubin—normal: 1.0 mg/100 ml.

B. Urine bilirubin—normally none is found.

C. Urine urobilinogen—0 to 4 mg/24 hours.

D. Fecal urobilinogen—40 to 280 mg/24 hours.

E. Serum cholesterol—150 to 250 mg/100 ml.

Protein Studies

A. Total protein—6 to 8 g/100 ml.

B. Serum albumin—3.5 to 5.0 mg/100 ml.

C. Serum globulin—1.5 to 3.0 mg/100 ml.

D. Prothrombin time—11 to 16 sec.

E. Cephalin—0 to 1+.

F. In liver damage, fewer plasma proteins are synthesized; thus, albumin synthesis is reduced.
   1. Serum globulins produced by the plasma cells are increased.
   2. PT is reduced in liver cell damage.

Fat and Carbohydrate Metabolism

A. Fat metabolism—serum lipase 1.5 units.

B. Carbohydrate metabolism—glucose tolerance levels should return to normal in one to two hours.

Liver Detoxification

A. Bromsulphalein excretion (BSP).

B. Less than 5 percent dye retention after one hour.
   1. Dye is injected intravenously and removed by the liver cells, conjugated, and excreted.
   2. Blood specimen is obtained at 30-minute and one-hour intervals after injection.
   3. Increased retention occurs in hepatic disorders.

Enzyme Production

A. Elevations reflect organ damage.

B. Levels.
   1. SGOT—10 to 40 units/ml.
   2. SGPT—5 to 35 units/ml.
   3. LDH—120 to 340 units/ml.

Alkaline Phosphatase

A. 2 to 5 units.

B. Elevated in obstructive jaundice and in liver metastasis.

Blood Ammonia

A. 30–70 µ/100 ml.

B. Ammonia level rises in liver failure since liver converts ammonia to urea.

C. Metabolic alkalosis increases the toxicity of NH_3.

Thyroid Function Tests

Radioactive Iodine (RAI) Uptake (Radioiodine ^{131}I)

A. Normal values—5 to 35 percent in 24 hours (recently lowered values in United States due to increased ingestion of iodine).
   1. Elevated values indicate—hyperthyroidism, thyrotoxicosis, hypofunctioning goiter, iodine lack, excessive hormonal losses.
   2. Depressed values indicate—low T_4, antithyroid drugs, thyroiditis, myxedema, or hypothyroidism.

B. Purpose—measures the absorption of the iodine isotope to determine how the thyroid gland is functioning.

C. Principles.
   1. The use of ^{123}I rather than ^{131}I is now preferred because of its lower radiation hazard. (^{123}I can be used on pregnant women while ^{131}I is contraindicated.)
   2. The amount of radioactivity is measured 2, 6, and 24 hours after ingestion of the capsule.
   3. ^{131}I (as does ^{123}I) evaluates the storage of iodine and gives a distribution pattern.

T_3 and T_4 Resin Uptake Tests

A. Normal values.
   1. T_4—3.8 to 11.4%.
   2. T_3—25 to 35%.
   3. T_4.
      a. Elevated—hyperthyroidism, early hepatitis, exogenous T_4.
      b. Decreased—hypothyroidism, abnormal binding, exogenous T_4.
   4. T_3.
      a. Elevated—hyperthyroidism, T_3 toxicosis.

   b. Decreased—advancing age.

B. Purpose—both of these in vitro tests are used as screening tests for diagnosis in thyroid disorders. T_4 is 90 percent accurate in diagnosing hyperthyroidism and hypothyroidism.

C. Principles.
   1. Levels of T_3 and T_4 in the blood regulate thyroid stimulating hormone (TSH).
   2. These levels alter according to a balancing system of negative feedback.
   3. Venous blood sample is obtained to directly measure concentration of unsaturated thyroxine-binding globulin in the serum.
   4. Thyroid function tests should be interpreted according to the clinical situation.

Thyroid Stimulation Test

A. Normal values less than $10\mu U/ml$ (may vary with laboratory).
   1. Increased values indicate primary hypothyroidism.
   2. Decreased values indicate hyperthyroidism, large doses of glucocorticoids, secondary hypothyroidism.

B. Purpose—differentiates primary from secondary hypothyroidism and assesses level of thyroid gland activity.

C. Principles.
   1. Administration of IM TSH (thyrotropin) measures the responsiveness of the thyroid gland.
   2. Blood samples are obtained at intervals.

Glucose Tolerance Test

A. Normal values are between 60 to 125 mg fasting and no sugar in the urine.
   1. Increased values indicate hyperinsulinism, Addison's disease, hypothyroidism, or celiac disease.
   2. Decreased values indicate diabetes, hyperthyroidism, hyperplasia, anemia, or certain central nervous system disorders.

B. Purpose—primary aim is to diagnose or rule out diabetes, but also important for unexplained hypoglycemia and malabsorption syndrome.

C. Principles.
1. This test determines rate of removal of a concentrated dose of glucose from the bloodstream.
2. Test is indicated when there is sugar in the urine or when fasting blood sugar is elevated.
3. This is a timed test done in the morning after fasting for at least 12 hours. Blood and urine samples are taken at intervals up to three hours.
4. This test is contraindicated for recent surgical patients or patients with history of myocardial infarctions.

Immunodiagnostic Tests

HIV-1 Antibody Test

A. The ELISA (enzyme-linked immunosorbent assay) test was developed to screen national donor blood.
1. This test does not test for AIDS, but the antibodies to the HIV virus.
2. Once exposed to a virus, it takes the body time to produce antibodies. A person may already be infected and if the body has not yet produced antibodies, the ELISA test will be negative.
3. Test is also imperfect in that it may produce a false positive or false negative.

B. All positive results must be retested via ELISA.

C. If second test is positive, the Western blot test is given for final confirmation.

Coombs' Test

A. Normal values—negative.

B. Purpose—test to discover presence of antibodies present in Rh negative mother's blood.
1. Test also will confirm diagnosis of hemolytic disease in the newborn.

2. Titration determines extent to which antibodies are present.

C. Types of test for Rh incompatibility.
1. Indirect Coombs'—mother's blood reveals antibodies as result of previous transfusion or pregnancy.
2. Direct Coombs'—tests newborn's cord blood—determines presence of maternal antibodies attached to baby's cells.

Venereal Disease Research Laboratory Test (VDRL)

A. Normal values—serum is nonreactive.

B. Purpose—to screen for primary or secondary syphilis.

C. Differential diagnosis.
1. Biological false positive tests may occur with: hepatitis, mononucleosis, leprosy, malaria, rheumatoid arthritis, lupus erythematosus.
2. A nonreactive result does not rule out syphilis, as it takes 14–21 days after infection to cause an immunologic response.

Epstein-Barr Virus Antibodies (EBV)

A. Normal values—negative (antibodies appear within first three weeks, then decline rapidly).

B. Purpose—to diagnose infectious mononucleosis or to determine the antibody status of EBV infected people.

C. Test—serum is tested for heterophile antibodies (Monospot test).

D. Differential diagnosis.
1. Positive results may occur with: infectious mononucleosis, hepatitis A and B, cancer of the pancreas.
2. A negative Monospot does not always rule out acute or past EBV.

Serologic Tests for Hepatitis A, B

A. Normal values—negative for hepatitis A, B, non-A, non-B, and D.

B. Purpose—serologic tests diagnose and differentiate different forms of hepatitis.

C. Test variations.
   1. Hepatitis A (HAV).
      a. Anti-HAV IgM presence confirms recent infection of hepatitis A—detectable for 3–12 weeks.
      b. Anti-HAV IgG indicates previous exposure to HAV, recovery and immunity. Appears after acute infection and is detectable for life.
   2. Hepatitis B (HBV).
      a. Hepatitis B Surface Antigen—appears in 27–41 days and is the earliest indicator of HBV.
      b. Antibody to hepatitis B Surface Antigen indicates clinical recovery with subsequent immunity.
   3. Hepatitis Non-A, Non-B has no serologic or laboratory test to establish diagnosis—usually made by excluding other causes of hepatitis. Now, this form is labeled hepatitis C.
   4. Hepatitis D or Delta is associated with hepatitis B and depends on HBV for replication. It is found in the serum 7–14 days during acute infection.

Rubella Viral Serologic Test

A. Normal values.
   1. Negative titer of less than 1.8 or 1.10 (depending on test)—no antibody detected, therefore, not immune.
   2. Positive titer of more than 1.10—antibody detected, therefore immune.
B. Purpose—exposure to rubella is important to detect because exposure to this virus—if a woman is in the first trimester of pregnancy—may result in congenital abnormalities, abortion or stillbirth.

Papanicolaou Smear

A. Diagnosis for cervical cancer.
B. Vaginal secretions and secretions from posterior fornix are swabbed and smeared on a glass slide.
C. Pathological classifications.
   1. Class I—no abnormal or atypical cells present.
   2. Class II—atypical or abnormal cells present but no malignancy found; repeat pap smear and follow-up if necessary.
   3. Class III—cytology, suggestive of malignancy; additional procedures indicated (biopsy, D and C).
   4. Class IV—cytology, strongly suggestive of malignancy; additional procedures indicated (biopsy, D and C).
   5. Class V—cytology results conclusive of malignancy.

7

MEDICAL-SURGICAL NURSING

NEUROLOGIC SYSTEM

The nervous system (together with the endocrine system) provides the control functions for the body. It handles thousands of bits of information and stimuli from the sensory organs. This system of nerves and nerve centers coordinates and regulates all of this data and determines the responses of the body.

ANATOMY AND PHYSIOLOGY OF THE NERVOUS SYSTEM

Structure and Function

Neuron

A. Structure.
  1. Cell body (gray matter).
  2. Processes—dendrites (to cell body) and axon (from cell body).
  3. Synapse—chemical transmission of impulses from axon to dendrites.
  4. Nerve fiber—axon and its myelin sheath (white matter).
    a. Myelin sheath insulates; correlates with function and speed of conduction.
    b. Produced by neurolemma cells in peripheral nerve fibers and neuroglia cells in CNS fibers.
B. Classification by function.
  1. Sensory (afferent)—conduct impulses from end organ to CNS.
  2. Motor (efferent)—conduct impulses from CNS to muscles, glands.
  3. Internuncial (connector)—conducts impulses from sensory to motor neurons.
  4. Somatic—innervate body wall.
  5. Visceral—innervate the viscera.
C. Regeneration of destroyed nerve fibers.
  1. Peripheral nerve—can regenerate, possibly due to neurolemma.

2. CNS—cannot regenerate as it lacks neurolemma.
D. Reflex arc—basic unit of function.
  1. Involuntary stereotyped response to stimulus.
  2. Components—sensory receptor, sensory neuron, internuncial neuron, motor neuron, and effector.
  3. Classification of reflexes—three types: superficial (cutaneous), deep (tendon), pathological.

Central Nervous System—Brain and Spinal Cord

A. Forebrain.
  1. Cerebrum—highest level of functioning.
    a. Governs all sensory and motor activity, thought, and learning.
    b. Analyzes, associates, integrates, and stores information.
    c. Cerebral cortex (outer gray layer) divided into four major lobes.
      (1) Frontal.
        (a) Motor function.
        (b) Motor speech area.
        (c) Prefrontal lobe—controls morals, values, emotions, judgment.
      (2) Parietal.
        (a) Integrates general sensation.
        (b) Interprets pain, touch, temperature, and pressure.
        (c) Governs discrimination.
      (3) Temporal.
        (a) Auditory center.
        (b) Sensory speech center.
      (4) Occipital—visual area.
  2. Basal ganglia.
    a. Part of extrapyramidal tract.
    b. Controls associated motor movements.
  3. Internal capsule—contains projection fibers connecting cortical areas with other parts of the CNS.
B. Brainstem.
  1. Diencephalon.
    a. Thalamus.

(1) Screens and relays sensory impulses to cortex.

(2) Lowest level of crude conscious awareness.

    b. Hypothalamus—regulates autonomic nervous system, stress response, sleep, appetite, body temperature, water balance, emotion.

2. Midbrain—motor coordination, conjugate eye movements.

3. Pons.

    a. Contains projection tracts between spinal cord, medulla, and brain.

    b. Controls the involuntary respiratory reflexes.

4. Medulla oblongata.

    a. Contains all afferent and efferent tracts.

    b. Contains cardiac, respiratory, vomiting, and vasomotor centers.

C. Cerebellum.

1. Connected by afferent/efferent pathways to all other parts of CNS.

2. Coordinates muscle movement, posture, equilibrium, and muscle tone.

D. Pyramidal tract.

1. Initiates skilled voluntary movements.

2. Originates with cell bodies in motor cortex; fibers form projection tracts which pass through internal capsule and medulla where most decussate; fibers from corticospinal tracts which terminate at anterior horn.

E. Extrapyramidal (outside of pyramidal tract).

1. Inhibitory or facilitory effect on motor function.

2. Includes basal ganglia, cerebellum, reticular formation, cortex, and spinal cord.

F. Spinal cord—conveys messages between brain and periphery.

1. Structure.

    a. Extends from foramen magnum to second lumbar vertebra.

    b. Inner column of H-shaped gray matter which contains the two anterior and two posterior horns.

    c. Posterior horns—contain cell bodies which connect with afferent (sensory) nerve fibers from posterior root ganglia.

    d. Anterior horns—contain cell bodies giving rise to efferent (motor) nerve fibers.

    e. Lateral horns—present in thoracic segments; origin of autonomic fibers of sympathetic nervous system.

2. Ascending tracts (sensory pathways).

3. Descending tracts (motor pathways).

G. Protection for CNS.

1. Skull—rigid chamber with opening at the base (foramen magnum).

2. Meninges.

    a. Dura mater—tough, outermost, fibrous membrane.

    b. Arachnoid membrane—delicate membrane that contains subarachnoid fluid.

    c. Pia mater—vascular membrane.

3. Cerebral spinal fluid.

    a. Protective cushion; aids exchange of nutrients, wastes.

    b. Secreted from choroid plexuses in the four ventricles.

    c. Circulates within interconnecting ventricles and subarachnoid space.

4. Blood-brain barrier.

    a. Prevents damaging substances from entering CSF.

    b. Brain parenchyma.

5. Blood supply—conductor of oxygen vitally needed by nervous system.

    a. Internal carotids.

    b. Vertebral arteries.

    c. Circle of Willis.

Peripheral Nervous System

A. Carries voluntary and involuntary impulses.

B. Cranial nerves (12 pairs).

1. Motor, sensory, or mixed nerve fibers.

2. Names: olfactory, optic, oculomotor, trochlear, trigeminal, abducens, facial, acoustic, glossopharyngeal, vagus, accessory, hypoglossal.

C. Spinal nerves (31 pairs).

1. All mixed nerve fibers formed by joining of anterior motor and posterior sensory roots.
2. Anterior root—efferent nerve fibers to glands and voluntary and involuntary muscles.
3. Posterior root—afferent nerve fibers from sensory receptors. Contains posterior ganglion (cell body of sensory neuron).

Autonomic Nervous System

A. Structure and function.
1. Part of peripheral nervous system controlling smooth muscle, cardiac muscle, and glands.
2. Two divisions make involuntary adjustments for integrated balance (homeostasis).
B. Sympathetic nervous system—thoracolumbar division.
1. Fight, flight, or freeze; diffuse response.
2. Increases heart rate, blood pressure.
3. Dilates pupils, bronchi.
C. Parasympathetic nervous system—craniosacral division.
1. Repair, repose; discrete response.
2. Decreases heart rate, blood pressure.
3. Constricts pupils, bronchi.

Basic Neurological Assessment

Signs and Symptoms

A. Numbness, weakness.
B. Dizziness, fainting, loss of consciousness.
C. Headache, pain.
D. Speech disturbances.
E. Visual disturbances.
F. Disturbances in memory, thinking, personality.
G. Nausea, vomiting.

Level of Consciousness

A. Most sensitive, reliable index of cerebral function.

B. Assessment of consciousness.
1. Orientation of patient as to place, purpose, time.
2. Response to verbal and tactile stimuli or simple commands.
3. Response to painful stimuli.
C. Describe behaviors indicating levels of consciousness: clouding, confusion, delirium, stupor, coma.

Pupillary Signs

A. Light reflex—most important sign differentiating structural from metabolic coma.
B. Pupil assessment.
1. Size—measure in millimeters.
2. Equality—equal, unequal, fluctuations.
3. Reactions to light—brisk, slow, fixed.
4. Unusual eye movements or deviations from midline.
C. Pupillary abnormalities.
1. Unilateral dilation.
2. Mid-position, fixed (often unequal).
3. Pinpoint, fixed.

Motor Function

A. Pattern of motor dysfunction gives information about anatomic location of lesions, independent of level of consciousness.
B. Assessment of face, upper and lower extremities.
1. Muscle tone, strength, equality.
2. Voluntary movement.
3. Involuntary movements.
4. Reflexes:
   a. Babinski—dorsiflexion ankle and great toe with fanning of other toes.
   b. Corneal—blink reflex.
   c. Gag—gag and vomiting reflex.
C. Patterns of motor function.
1. Appropriate—spontaneous movement to stimulus or command.
2. Absent: hemiplegia, paraplegia, quadriplegia.
3. Inappropriate (nonpurposeful).
   a. Posturing in response to stimuli.

b. Involuntary: choreiform (jerky, quick); athetoid (twisting, slow); tremors; spasms; or convulsions.

Sensory Function

A. Assess general sensory function in all extremities: touch, pressure, pain.
B. If no motor response to command, may elicit response by sensory stimuli such as supraorbital pressure.
C. Use minimal amount of stimulus necessary to evoke a response.

Vital Signs

A. Monitor for trends—changes often unreliable and occur late with increasing intracranial pressure.
B. Blood pressure and pulse—changes may indicate increasing intracranial pressure.
C. Respiration.
   1. Rate, depth, and rhythm more sensitive indication of intracranial pressure than blood pressure and pulse.
   2. Cheyne-Stokes—respiratory increase and decrease in rate and depth, rhythmically alternating with periods of apnea.
   3. Neurogenic hyperventilation—sustained regular, rapid, and deep.
   4. Ataxic—totally irregular, random rhythm and depth.
D. Temperature (rectal).
   1. Early rise may indicate damage to hypothalamus or brainstem.
   2. Slow rise may indicate infection.
   3. Elevated temperature increases brain's metabolic rate.

Signs of Meningeal Irritation

A. Brudzinski's sign—flexion of head causes flexion of both thighs at the hips and flexion of the knees.
B. Kernig's sign—in supine position, thigh and knee flexed to right angles; extension of leg causes spasm of hamstring, resistance, and pain.

Diagnostic Procedures

Radiologic Procedures

A. Skull series.
   1. Procedure—x-rays of head from different angles.
   2. Purpose—to visualize configuration, density, and vascular markings.
   3. Tomograms—layered vertical or horizontal x-ray exposures.
B. Ventriculography.
   1. Procedure—injection of air directly into lateral ventricles followed by x-rays.
   2. Purpose—to visualize ventricles, localize tumors. May be used if increased intracranial pressure contraindicates pneumoencephalography.
   3. Potential complications—headache, nausea and vomiting, meningitis, increasing intracranial pressure.
   4. Nursing care.
      a. Monitor vital signs.
      b. Check neurological status.
      c. Elevate head.
      d. Administer ice bag and analgesics for headache.
C. Myelography.
   1. Procedure—injection of dye or air into lumbar or cisternal subarachnoid space followed by x-rays of the spinal column.
   2. Purpose—to visualize spinal subarachnoid space for distortions caused by lesions.
   3. Potential complications.
      a. Same as for lumbar puncture.
      b. Cerebral meningeal irritation from dye.
   4. Nursing care.
      a. Same as for lumbar puncture.
      b. If dye is used, elevate head and observe for meningeal irritation.
      c. If air is used, keep head lower than trunk.
D. Cerebral angiography.

1. Procedure—injection of radiopaque dye into carotid and/or vertebral arteries followed by serial x-rays.
2. Purpose—to visualize cerebral vessels and localize lesions such as aneurysms, occlusions, angiomas, tumors, or abscesses.
3. Potential complications.
   a. Anaphylactic reaction to dye.
   b. Local hemorrhage.
   c. Vasospasm.
   d. Adverse intracranial pressure.
4. Nursing care.
   a. Prior to procedure.
      (1) Check allergies.
      (2) Take baseline assessment.
      (3) Measure neck circumference.
   b. During and after procedure.
      (1) Have emergency equipment available.
      (2) Monitor neurological and vital signs for shock, level of consciousness, hemiparesis, hemiplegia, and aphasia.
      (3) Monitor for swelling of neck, difficulty in swallowing or breathing.
      (4) Administer ice collar.

Magnetic Resonance Imaging (MRI)

A. Procedure—visualization of distribution of hydrogen molecules in the body in three dimensions.
B. Technique has revolutionized diagnostic medicine and is surpassing more conventional methods.
   1. Procedure is noninvasive.
   2. Does not use harmful ionizing radiation.
   3. Superior imaging of body's soft tissue.
C. Purpose—to differentiate types of tissues, including those in normal and abnormal states. Includes brain, both tumors and vascular abnormalities; cardiac and respiratory conditions; blood vessels; liver disease, renal abnormalities, gallbladder, and tumors.
D. Safety measures.
   1. Patients with pacemakers are excluded from MRI.

2. Metal objects must be removed from patients.
3. Patients with metal implants (hip prostheses, vascular clips, artificial valves, etc.) are prohibited from MRI imaging.
4. Closely monitor patients with potential respiratory or cardiac collapse.
E. Nursing implementation.
   1. Maintain safety measures with MRI use.
   2. Explain procedure and machine to allay anxiety.
   3. Provide patient and family teaching.

Brain Scan

A. Procedure—intravenous injection of radioactive isotope substance followed by anterior-posterior and lateral scanning. Concentration of substance is greatest in pathological areas.
B. Purpose—to localize tumors with high degree of accuracy. Accuracy is increased if scanning is combined with arteriography or encephalography.
C. Tomography—type of brain scan that relies on tissue density—EMI or CAT.

Electroencephalography (EEG)

A. Procedure—graphic recording of brain's electrical activity by electrodes placed on the scalp.
B. Purpose—to detect intracranial lesion and abnormal electrical activity (epilepsy); now used to detect and indicate "brain death."
C. Nursing care.
   1. Wash hair.
   2. Withhold sedatives or stimulants.
   3. Administer fluids as ordered.

Echoencephalogram

A. Procedure—recording of reflected ultrasonic waves from brain structures.
B. Purpose.
   1. To measure position and shifting of midline structures.
   2. To detect subdural hematoma or tumors.

Electromyography (EMG)

A. Procedure—recording of muscle action potential by surface or needle of needle electrodes.

B. Purpose—to diagnose or localize neuromuscular disease.

Lumbar Puncture (LP)

A. Procedure—insertion of spinal needle through L_3-L_4 or L_4-L_5 interspace into lumbar subarachnoid space.

B. Purpose.
   1. To obtain cerebral spinal fluid (CSF).
   2. To measure intracranial pressure.
   3. To instill air, dye, or medications.

C. Potential complications—headache, backache, and herniation with brainstem compression (especially if intracranial pressure is high).

D. Nursing care.
   1. Have patient empty bowel and bladder.
   2. Assist with specimens and pressure measurement.
   3. Maintain strict asepsis.
   4. Monitor vital signs.
   5. Maintain patient in horizontal position.
   6. Encourage fluids if not contraindicated.
   7. Inspect puncture site.

E. Queckenstedt-Stookey test.
   1. Normal if pressure increases with jugular compression and drops to normal 10 to 30 seconds after release of compression.
   2. Partial block if slow rise and return to normal.
   3. Complete block if no rise.

Cisternal Puncture

A. Procedure—needle puncture into cisterna magna just below the occipital bone.

B. Purpose—same as for lumbar puncture. May be used if intracranial pressure is high or for infants.

C. Potential complications—respiratory distress.

D. Nursing care.
   1. Same as for lumbar puncture.
   2. Observe for cyanosis, dyspnea, and apnea.

CONDITIONS OF THE NEUROLOGIC SYSTEM

The Unconscious or Immobilized Patient

Definition: Unconsciousness is the state of depressed cerebral function with altered sensory and motor function. Immobilization is the loss of normal sensory/motor function without loss of consciousness.

Treatment and Implementation

A. Maintain open airway and adequate ventilation.
   1. Airway obstruction.
   2. Breath sounds.
   3. Positioning.
      a. Semiprone (to prevent tongue from occluding airway and secretions from pooling in pharynx).
      b. Frequent change of position.
   4. Bronchial hygiene.
      a. Include deep breathing and coughing when possible.
      b. Suctioning.
   5. Assisted ventilation.

B. Maintain adequate circulation.
   1. Positioning.
      a. Avoid Trendelenburg's position with head or neck injuries.
      b. Change position frequently, from horizontal to sitting or standing, as soon as possible.
      c. Passive, active ROM.
      d. Encourage self-help.
   2. Caution against Valsalva's maneuver (technique of clearing or testing patency of the eustachian tubes).

C. Observe signs and symptoms for potential complications.
   1. Neurological (see Basic Neurological Assessment, p. 122).
   2. Respiratory function.
      a. Color, chest expansion, deformities.

b. Rate, depth, and rhythm of respirations.
c. Movement of air at nose/mouth or intratracheal tube.
d. Breath sounds.
e. Accumulation of secretions or blood in the mouth.
f. Signs of respiratory distress, failure, hypoxemia, hypercapnia, infection, atelectasis.

3. Cardiovascular function.
   a. Blood pressure, pulses.
   b. Skin color, temperature, edema, leg pain.
   c. Heart sounds, arrhythmias.
   d. Signs of shock, hypertension, orthostatic hypotension.

4. Condition of skin.
   a. Inspect entire body, especially susceptible pressure points (heels, malleoli, trochanteric areas, ischium, sacrum).
   b. Note redness, pallor, edema, excoriation, or skin breakdown.

5. Bladder/bowel function.
   a. Bladder distention—urinary stasis, incontinence.
   b. Urinary tract infection.
   c. Urinary calculi—stasis, infection, alkalinity, decreased volume of urine and citric acid.
   d. Abdominal distention—paralytic ileus, constipation, impaction, diarrhea, trauma.

6. Nutrition, fluid, and electrolyte balance.
   a. Intake—NPO, oral, tube feedings, IV.
   b. Output—urinary, feces; unconsciousness, check emesis, nasogastric.
   c. Electrolytes, acid-base.
   d. Dehydration, fluid overload.
   e. Thirst, loss of sensation of thirst.
   f. Swallowing, gag reflex.

7. Musculoskeletal function.
   a. Muscle strength—weakness, paralysis.
   b. Muscle tone or resistance to passive movement—flaccid, atrophied, spastic.
   c. Limitation of function—deformities, contractures.
   d. Osteoporosis.

8. Process of psychological adaptation—patient/family.
   a. Changes in body image; social and family roles.
   b. Sensory deprivation.
   c. Emotional/physiological stress.
   d. Adaptation to loss—anxiety, fear, denial, depression, dependency.

D. Maintain optimal positioning and movement.
   1. Prevent further trauma.
      a. Maintain body alignment, support head and limbs when turning, logroll.
      b. Do not flex or twist spine or hyperextend neck if spinal cord injury suspected.
   2. Positioning.
      a. Maintain and support joints and limbs in most functional anatomic position.
      b. Avoid improper use of knee gatch or pillows under knee.
   3. Avoid complete immobility.
      a. Perform ROM (against resistance if able), weight bearing; provide tilt table.
      b. Encourage self-help.

E. Maintain integrity of the skin.
   1. High risk of decubitus ulcers.
      a. Loss of vasomotor tone.
      b. Impaired peripheral circulation.
      c. Paralysis, immobility, and loss of muscle assistance to blood flow.
      d. Hypoproteinemia.
   2. Loss of sensation of pressure, pain, or temperature—decreased awareness of developing decubitus ulcers or burns.
   3. Skin care.
      a. Clean and dry skin; avoid powder because it may cake.
      b. Massage with lotion around and toward bony prominences.
      c. Alternate air mattress and sheepskin pad.
      d. Keep linen from wrinkling; avoid mechanical friction against linen.

F. Maintain personal hygiene.
   1. Eye—loss of corneal reflex may contribute to corneal irritation, keratitis, blindness.
      a. Observe for signs of irritation.

b. Irrigate eyes, instill artificial tears or patch.
2. Nose—trauma or infection in nose or nasopharynx may cause meningitis.
   a. Observe for drainage of CSF.
   b. Clean and lubricate nares; do not clean inside nostrils.
   c. Change nasogastric tube at intervals.
3. Mouth—mouth breathing contributes to drying and crusting excoriation of mucous membranes, which may lead to aspiration and respiratory tract infections.
   a. Examine the mouth daily with a good light.
   b. Clean teeth, gums, mucous membranes, tongue, and uvula to prevent crusting and infection; lubricate lips.
   c. Inspect for retained food in the mouth of patients who have facial paralysis.
4. Ear—drainage of CSF from the ear indicates damage to the base of the brain and a danger of meningitis.
   a. Inspect ear for drainage of CSF.
   b. Loosely cover ear with sterile, dry dressing.
G. Promote adequate nutrition, fluid, and electrolyte balance.
   1. Intravenous fluids.
      a. Electrolyte solutions, hyperalimentation.
      b. Caution with IV rates if intracranial pressure is elevated.
   2. Tube feedings—high in proteins and calories.
      a. Position patient in semi-Fowler's position, slightly turned to right side.
      b. Check position of tube; aspirate and measure gastric contents; usually if greater than 50 to 100 cc, return and subtract that amount from feeding.
      c. Give feeding by gravity flow; flush tubing with water; prevent air from entering stomach via tubing.
      d. Monitor intake and output, and daily weight.
   3. Oral feedings.
      a. Check swallowing with ice chips.
      b. Put patient in semi-Fowler's position.

c. Have suction equipment available.
d. Give semi-liquid, soft, or blended foods.
H. Promote elimination.
   1. Catheter (Foley)—strict asepsis, catheter care.
   2. Cathartic—enema on a regular schedule.
   3. Bowel/bladder retraining if necessary.
I. Provide psychosocial support for patient and family.
   1. Assume that an unconscious patient can hear; frequently reassure and explain procedures to the patient.
   2. Encourage family interaction.

Glasgow Coma Scale

A. Comatose state based on three areas associated with level of consciousness.
B. Scoring system.
   1. Based on a scale of 1 to 15 points.
   2. Any score below 8 indicates coma is present.
C. Eye opening is the most important indicator.
D. Coma Scale. ❖ PROCEDURE ❖

1. Motor response.

	Points
Obeys	6
Localizes	5
Withdrawn	4
Abnormal flexion	3
Extensor response	2
Nil	1

2. Verbal response.

	Points
Oriented	5
Confused conversation	4
Inappropriate words	3
Incomprehensible sounds	2
Nil	1

3. Eye opening.

	Points
Spontaneous	4
To speech	3
To pain	2
Nil	1

Increased Intracranial Pressure

Etiology

Trauma, hemorrhage, tumors, abscess, hydrocephalus, edema, or inflammation.

Pathology

A. Cranial cavity is a solid compartment with relatively little room for expansion.
B. Increased intracranial bulk from blood, CSF, or brain tissue will increase intracranial pressure.
C. Increased pressure impedes cerebral circulation, absorption of CSF, and function of the nerve cells.
D. Increasing pressure if transmitted downward toward the brainstem can lead to eventual tentorial herniation, brainstem compression, and death.

Signs and Symptoms

A. See Basic Neurological Assessment, p. 122.
B. Level of consciousness (most sensitive indicator of increasing intracranial pressure) changes from restlessness to confusion to declining level of consciousness and coma.
C. Headache—tension, displacement of brain.
D. Vomiting.
E. Pupillary changes—unilateral dilation of pupil: slow reaction to light; fixed dilated pupil is ominous sign requiring immediate action.
F. Motor function—weakness, hemiplegia, positive Babinski, decerebrate, seizure activity.
G. Vital signs—rise in blood pressure; widening pulse pressure; reflex slowing of pulse; abnormalities in respiration, especially periods of apnea; temperature elevation.

Implementation

A. Elevate head of bed; avoid Trendelenburg's.
B. Limit fluid intake (1200 cc/day).
C. Administer medications as ordered: steroids, osmotic diuretics.
   1. Steroids (Decadron) decrease cerebral edema by their anti-inflammatory effect; decrease capillary permeability in inflammatory processes, thus decreasing leakage of fluid into tissue.
   2. Mannitol decreases cerebral edema; provides diuretic action by carrying out large volume of water through nephrons.
   3. Hypertonic IV solution administered because it is impermeable to blood-brain barrier; reduce edema by rapid movement of water out of ventricles into bloodstream.
D. Administer mechanical ventilation if ordered.
E. Prevent further complications.
   1. Monitor neurological dysfunction versus cardiovascular shock.
   2. Prevent hypoxia: avoid morphine.
   3. Monitor fluids: electrolyte and acid-base balance.
F. Surgical management.
   1. Ventriculoperitoneal shunt systems (most common). Designed to shunt cerebrospinal fluid from the lateral ventricles into the peritoneum.
   2. Postoperative care.
      a. Monitor closely for signs and symptoms of increasing intracranial pressure due to shunt failure.
      b. Check for infection (a common and serious complication). If present, removal of the shunt system is indicated in addition to appropriate chemotherapy.

Spinal Cord Injury

Definition: May include cervical injury leading to quadriplegia or respiratory failure; thoracic injury leading to flaccid/spastic paraplegia; or lumbar injury leading to flaccid paraplegia.

Pathophysiology

A. Neurological signs generally due to edema, concussion, compression, hemorrhage, partial or complete transection of cord, and disruption of sensory and motor pathways.

B. Spinal shock—initial flaccid paralysis, loss of sensation and reflexes, urinary and bowel retention, disturbed nerve supply to blood vessels, and hypotension.

C. Autonomic dysfunction—absence of sweating; decreased blood pressure and temperature in affected areas; poor response to reflex stimuli; paralytic ileus often occurs.

D. After spinal shock recedes—spastic paralysis and hyperreflexia; bowel and bladder control may be retained.

E. Lumbar injury (cauda equina)—persisting flaccid paralysis of lower extremities, bladder, and rectum; muscle atrophy.

Implementation

A. Direct efforts toward primary nursing goals: prevent further injury or complications and maintain optimal body functioning while patient is immobilized (see section on the unconscious or immobilized patient).

B. Maintain open airway and adequate ventilation—high cervical injuries can cause complete paralysis of muscles for breathing; observe for any signs of respiratory failure.

C. Immobilize patient as ordered, to allow fracture healing and prevent further injury.
   1. Stryker frame permits change of position between prone and supine.
      a. Maintain optimal body alignment.
      b. Place patient in center of frame without flexing or twisting.
      c. Position arm boards, footboards, canvas.
      d. Turn; reassure patient while turning.
      e. Free all tubings; secure bolts and straps.
   2. Regular hospital beds used in many rehabilitation centers.

3. Halo traction with body cast allows early mobilization.

4. Soft and hard collars and back braces used about six weeks postinjury.

5. Maintain skeletal traction if part of treatment.
   a. Cervical tongs for hyperextension (Crutchfield, Gardner-Wells, Vinke).
      (1) Apply traction to vertebral column by attaching weights to pair of tongs.
      (2) Insert tongs into outer layer of parietal area of skull.
   b. Facilitates moving and turning of patient while maintaining spine immobilization.
   c. Observe site of insertion for redness or drainage, alignment and position.

D. Monitor for potential complications. Neurological assessment should include watching for changes in muscle tone, motor movement, sensation, bladder/bowel function, presence/absence of sweating, and temperature.

E. Maintain optimal positioning.
   1. If turning permitted, logroll with firm support to head, neck, spine, and limbs.
   2. Maintain good body alignment with 10 degree flexion of knees, heels off mattress or canvas, and feet in firm dorsiflexion.
   3. Convalescence—cervical collar, tilt table, wheelchair, braces, parallel bars.

F. Maintain integrity of the skin.
   1. Do not administer IM medication below a lesion that is result of impaired circulation and potential skin breakdown.
   2. Provide elastic stockings to improve circulation in legs.

G. Promote adequate nutrition, fluid, and electrolyte balance.
   1. Provide diet high in protein, vitamins, calories.
   2. Avoid all citrus juices, which alkalize the urine and contribute to infection and renal calculi.

3. Avoid gas-forming and foods with high residue.
4. Monitor calcium, electrolyte, and hemoglobin levels.

H. Establish optimal bladder function.
   1. During spinal shock—bladder is atonic with urinary retention; danger of overdistention, stretching.
   2. Possible reactions:
      a. Hypotonic—retention with overflow.
      b. Hypertonic—sudden reflex voiding.
   3. Check for bladder distention, voiding, incontinence.
   4. Provide aseptic catheter care.
   5. Prevent urinary tract infection, calculi.
   6. Initiate bladder retraining.
      a. Hypertonic—sensation of full bladder, trigger areas, regulation of fluid intake.
      b. Hypotonic—the manual expression of urine (Credé).
   7. Administer medications to treat incontinence.
      a. Hypertonic—propantheline bromide, diazepam.
      b. Hypotonic—bethanechol chloride.

I. Establish optimal bowel function.
   1. Incontinence and paralytic ileus occur with spinal shock; later, incontinence, constipation, impaction.
   2. For severe distention, administer neostigmine methylsulfate and insert rectal tube, which decompresses intestinal tract.
   3. Initiate bowel retraining. ❖ Procedure ❖
      a. Record bowel habits before and after injury.
      b. Provide well-balanced diet with bulky foods.
      c. Encourage fluid intake.
      d. Encourage development of muscle tone, ability to sit in chair.
      e. Administer suppository as ordered.
      f. Emphasize importance of a regular, consistent routine.

J. Provide psychological support to patient and family.

1. Adjustment to paralysis may be very difficult as patient is usually young; may be inclined toward suicide.
2. Provide nonjudgmental atmosphere, security, sensory input.
3. Provide diversionary activities, socialization, independence, explanations, support.
4. Give encouragement and reassurance but never false hope.

K. Encourage optimal physical activity as tolerated by patient.
   1. Physical therapy exercises.
   2. Independent activity within limitations.
   3. Extensive program of rehabilitation and self-care.

Head Injury

Definition: Trauma to the skull by means of compression, tension, and/or shearing force resulting in varying degrees of injury to the brain.

Types

A. Brain concussion—violent jarring of brain within skull; temporary loss of consciousness.
B. Brain contusion—bruising, injury of brain.
C. Skull fracture—linear, depressed, compound, or comminuted.
D. Hemorrhage.
   1. Epidural hematoma—most serious; hematoma between dura and skull from tear in meningeal artery; forms rapidly.
   2. Subdural hematoma—under dura due to tears in veins crossing subdural space; forms slowly.
   3. Subarachnoid hematoma—bleeding into subarachnoid space.
   4. Intracerebral hematoma—usually multiple hemorrhages around contused area.

Assessment

A. Impaired level of consciousness, unconsciousness, confusion.

B. Headache, nausea, vomiting.

C. Pupillary changes.

D. Changes in vital signs, reflecting increased intracranial pressure or shock.

E. Rhinorrhea, otorrhea, nuchal rigidity.

F. Overt scalp/skull trauma.

Implementation

A. Direct efforts toward primary nursing goals: recognize, prevent, and treat complications (see section on the unconscious or immobilized patient, p. 125, for measures to maintain optimal body functioning).

B. Maintain open airway and adequate ventilation.

C. Awaken the patient as completely as possible to assess level of consciousness.

D. Assess and treat convulsions (see Convulsions, p. 134).

E. Control pain and restlessness.
1. Avoid morphine, a respiratory depressant, which will increase intracranial pressure.
2. Use codeine or other milder analgesic (use sparingly).

F. Prevent infection.
1. High risk of developing meningitis, abscess, osteomyelitis, particularly in presence of rhinorrhea, otorrhea.
2. Maintain strict asepsis.

G. Assess and treat other complications.
1. Shock—significant cause of death.
2. Cranial nerve paralysis.
3. Rhinorrhea (fracture ethmoid bone) and otorrhea (temporal).
   a. Check discharge—bloody spot surrounded by pale ring; positive test tape reaction for sugar.
   b. Do not attempt to clean nose or ears.
   c. Do not suction nose.
   d. Instruct patient not to blow nose.
4. Ear-drainage of CSF from the ear indicates damage to the base of the brain and a danger of meningitis.
   a. Inspect ear for drainage of CSF.
   b. Loosely cover ear with sterile, dry dressing.

Encephalitis

Definition: Severe inflammation of the brain caused by arboviruses or enteroviruses.

Assessment

A. Fever, headache, vomiting.

B. Signs of meningeal irritation.

C. Neuronal damage, drowsiness, coma, paralysis, ataxia.

Implementation

A. Monitor vital signs frequently.

B. Monitor neurological signs for alterations in condition.

C. Administer anticonvulsant medications as ordered: phenytoin.

D. Administer glucocorticoids as ordered: reduces cerebral edema.

E. Administer sedatives to relieve restlessness.

F. Manage fluid and electrolyte balance to prevent fluid overload and dehydration.

G. Position to maintain patent airway and prevent contractures. Provide passive or active range-of-motion exercises.

H. Promote adequate nutrition through tube feedings, and parenteral hyperalimentation if necessary.

I. Provide hygienic care, i.e., skin care, oral care, and perineal care.

J. Provide safety measures if patient is confused.

Cerebrovascular Accident (CVA)

Definition: Impaired blood supply in the brain caused by a hemorrhage or occlusion that results in a sudden focal neurological deficit. It is the most common cause of brain disturbance.

Pathophysiology

A. Causes.
   1. Thrombosis.
   2. Embolism.
   3. Hemorrhage.
   4. Compression or spasm.
B. Risk factors.
   1. Atherosclerosis.
   2. Hypertension.
   3. Anticoagulation therapy.
   4. Cardiac valvular disease.
   5. Synthetic valve and organ replacement.
   6. Atrial arrhythmias.
   7. Diabetes.
C. A transient ischemic attack (TIA) is a precursor symptom or warning of impending CVA.
   1. Rapid onset and short duration (30 minutes to 24 hours); by definition, must be resolved within this time period.
   2. Following resolution, no permanent neurological deficit.
   3. Most common symptoms: vision loss, diplopia, contralateral hemiparesis, aphasia, confusion, slurred speech, and vertigo.
D. Carotid endarterectomy is surgical procedure for carotid stenosis—often done following TIA or presence of bruit indicating stenosis.
   1. Procedure removes atherosclerotic plaque from arterial wall.
   2. Monitor closely first 24 hours for cerebral ischemia or thrombosis or intolerance from carotid clamping.
E. Cerebral anoxia longer than ten minutes to a localized area of brain causes cerebral infarction (irreversible changes).
F. Surrounding edema and congestion cause further dysfunction.
G. Lesion in cerebral hemisphere results in manifestations on the opposite side of the body.
H. Permanent disability unknown until edema subsides. Order in which function may return: facial, swallowing, lower limbs, speech, arms.

Assessment

A. Depend on site and size of involved area.
   1. Appear suddenly with embolism.
   2. More gradually with hemorrhage and thrombosis.
B. Generalized symptoms—headache; hypertension; changes in level of consciousness, convulsions; vomiting, nuchal rigidity, slow bounding pulse, Cheyne-Stokes respirations.
C. Focal—hemiparesis, hemiplegia, central facial paralysis, language disorders, cranial dysfunction, conjugate deviation eyes toward lesion, flaccid hyporeflexia (later, spastic hyperreflexia).
D. Residual manifestations.
   1. Lesion left hemisphere.
      a. Right hemiplegia; aphasia, expressive and/or receptive.
      b. Behavior is slow, cautious, disorganized.
   2. Lesion right hemisphere.
      a. Left hemiplegia.
      b. Behavior is impulsive, quick; unaware of deficits; poor judge of abilities, limitations; neglect of paralyzed side.
   3. General.
      a. Memory deficits; reduced memory span; emotional lability.
      b. Visual deficits; loss of half of each visual field.
      c. Apraxia (can move but unable to use body part for specific purpose).

Implementation

A. Strive for initial nursing goal: support life and prevent complications; long term goal is rehabilitation.
B. See section on the unconscious or immobilized patient, p. 125.
C. Maintain patent airway and ventilation—elevate head of bed 20 degrees unless patient is in shock.
D. Monitor clinical status to prevent complications.
   1. Neurological.
      a. Include assessment of recurrent CVA, increased intracranial pressure, bulbar involvement, hyperthermia.

b. Continued coma is a negative prognostic sign.
2. Cardiovascular—shock and arrhythmias, hypertension.
3. Lungs—pulmonary emboli.

E. Maintain optimal positioning.
1. During acute stages, quiet environment and minimal handling may be necessary to prevent further bleeding.
2. Upper motor lesion—spastic paralysis, flexion deformities, external rotation of hip.
3. Positioning schedule—2 hours on unaffected side; 20 minutes on affected side; 30 minutes prone, bid–tid.
4. Complications common with hemiplegia—frozen shoulder, footdrop.

F. Maintain skin integrity.

G. Maintain personal hygiene—encourage self-help.

H. Promote adequate nutrition, fluid, and electrolyte balance.
1. Encourage self-feeding.
2. Food should be placed in unparalyzed side of mouth.

I. Promote elimination.
1. Bladder control may be regained within three to five days.
2. Retention catheter may not be part of treatment regimen.
3. Offer urinal or bedpan every two hours day and night.

J. Provide emotional support.
1. Behavior changes as consciousness is regained—loss of memory, emotional lability, confusion, language disorders.
2. Reorient, reassure, and establish means of communication.

K. Promote rehabilitation to maximal functioning.
1. Comprehensive program—begin during acute phase and follow through convalescence.
2. Guidelines to assist patient with lesion left hemisphere.
a. Do not underestimate ability to learn.
b. Assess ability to understand speech.
c. Act out, pantomime communication; use patient's terms to communicate; speak in normal tone of voice.
d. Divide tasks into simple steps; give frequent feedback.
3. Guidelines to assist patient with lesion right hemisphere.
a. Do not overestimate abilities.
b. Use verbal cues as demonstrations; pantomimes may confuse.
c. Use slow, minimal movements and avoid clutter.
d. Divide tasks into simple steps; elicit return demonstration of skills.
e. Promote awareness of body and environment on affected side.

Cerebral Aneurysm

Definition: A dilation of the walls of a weakened cerebral artery leading to rupture from arteriosclerosis or trauma.

Assessment

A. Diplopia, eye pain, blurred vision, or ptosis.
B. Hemiparesis, nuchal rigidity.
C. Headache, tinnitus, nausea.
D. Irritability, seizure activity.

Implementation

A. Establish and maintain a patent airway.
B. Administer oxygen at 6 l/min. unless patient has COPD.
C. Place patient on bedrest in semi-Fowler's or side lying position.
D. Turn, cough, and deep breathe patient every two hours.
E. Suction only with specific order.
F. Provide darkened room without stimulation, i.e., limit visitors and lengthy discussions.
G. Avoid strenuous activity; provide range-of-motion exercises.

H. Provide diet low in stimulants such as caffeine. Restrict fluid intake to prevent increased intracranial pressure.

I. Monitor intake and output.

J. Monitor vital signs for hypertension or cardiac irregularities. Do not take rectal temperature due to vagal stimulation leading to cardiac arrest.

K. Observe for complications indicating rebleeding, clot formation, or increased size of aneurysm.

Hyperthermia

Definition: Increased temperature that has reached 41°C (106°F); associated with increased cerebral metabolism which may increase risk of hypoxia.

Treatment and Implementation

A. Induce hypothermia.
  1. External—cool bath, fans, ice bags, hypothermic blanket (most common).
  2. Drugs.
     a. Chlorpromazine—reduces peripheral vasoconstriction, muscle tone, shivering.
     b. Meperidine—relaxes smooth muscle, reduces shivering.
     c. Promethazine—dilates coronary arteries, reduces laryngeal and bronchial irritation.

B. Monitor hypothermia.
  1. Monitor temperature.
     a. Continuous probe or rectal thermometer.
     b. Read and record every 15 minutes.
  2. Prevent shivering.
     a. Shivering increases CSF pressure and oxygen consumption.
     b. Treatment: chlorpromazine.
  3. Prevent trauma to skin and tissue.
     a. Frostbite—crystallization of tissues with white or blue discoloration, hardening of tissue, burning, numbness.
     b. Fat necrosis—solidification of subcutaneous fat creating hard tissue masses.
     c. Initially give complete bath and oil the skin; during procedure, massage skin frequently with lotion or oil to maintain integrity of the skin.
  4. Prevent respiratory complications.
     a. Hypothermia may mask infection and cause respiratory arrest.
     b. Institute measures to maintain open airway and adequate ventilation.
  5. Prevent cardiac complications.
     a. Monitor cardiac status; hypothermia can cause arrhythmias and cardiac arrest.
     b. Have emergency equipment available.
  6. Monitor renal function.
     a. Insert Foley catheter.
     b. Monitor urinary output, BUN; may monitor specific gravity.
  7. Prevent vomiting and possible aspiration; patient may have loss of gag reflex and reduced peristalsis.
  8. Monitor changes in neurological function during hypothermia.

C. Effects of hypothermia.
  1. Reduces cerebral metabolism and demand for oxygen.
  2. Decreases cerebral and systemic blood flow.
  3. Reduces CSF pressure.
  4. Decreases endocrine, liver, and kidney function.
  5. Decreases pulse, blood pressure, and respiration; may affect cardiac pacemaker.

Convulsions

Definition: Forceful involuntary contractions of voluntary muscles; may be one component of a seizure.

Etiology

Cerebral trauma, congenital defects, epilepsy, infection, tumor circulatory defect, anoxia, metabolic abnormalities, excessive hydration.

Classification

A. Tonic convulsion—sustained contraction of muscles.

B. Clonic convulsion—alternating contraction/relaxation of opposing muscle group.

C. Epileptoid—any convulsion with loss of consciousness.

Implementation

A. Protect patient from further injury.

B. Observe and record characteristics of seizure activity.
   1. Level of consciousness.
   2. Description of aura, if present.
   3. Description of body position and initial activity.
   4. Monitor activity—initial body part involved, character of movements (tonic/clonic), progression of movement, duration, biting of the tongue.
   5. Respiration, color.
   6. Pupillary changes, eye movements.
   7. Incontinence, vomiting.
   8. Total duration of seizure.
   9. Postictal state—loss of consciousness; sleepiness; impaired speech, motor or thinking; headache; injuries.
   10. Post convulsion, neurological and vital signs.
   11. Frequency and number of convulsions.

C. Protect patient from trauma.
   1. Maintain patent airway.
   2. Keep padded tongue blade at bedside; use only with M.D.'s orders. Do not force between teeth if they are already clenched.
   3. Be sure side rails are padded and there is padding around head.
   4. Avoid use of any restraints.
   5. Remove any objects from environment that may cause injury.
   6. Remain with patient.

D. Care after the seizure.
   1. Maintain open airway—positioning, suction.
   2. Reorient to environment; give reassurance and support.

3. Monitor clinical status.
4. Administer anticonvulsants.
5. Maintain quiet environment.

Epilepsy

Definition: A combination of several disorders characterized by chronic seizure activity; a symptom of brain or CNS irritation. A seizure is an abnormal, sudden, excessive neuronal discharge of electrical activity within the brain.

Characteristics

A. Incidence in U.S. may be as low as 1 million or as high as 2.5 million.

B. Major problems may be an electrical disturbance (dysrhythmia) in nerve cells in one section of the brain.

C. Seizure are associate with changes in behavior, mentation and motor or sensory activity.

D. Causes may be genetic, trauma, brain tumor, circulatory or metabolic disorder, toxicity, or infection.

E. Diagnostic tests include CT to determine underlying CNS changes, EEG for a distinctive pattern, MRI, blood studies, etc.

Assessment

A. Tonic-clonic seizures, traditionally known as "grand mal."
   1. May begin with an aura, then a tonic phase—stiffening or rigidity of muscles, particularly arms and legs, followed by loss of consciousness.
   2. Clonic phase follows—hyperventilation with rhythmic jerking of all extremities.
   3. Full recovery may take several hours.

B. Absence seizures, formerly "petit mal."
   1. Brief, often just seconds, loss of consciousness; almost no loss or change in muscle tone.
   2. May occur 100 times/day. More common in children; may appear to be "day dreaming."

C. Myoclonic seizure.

1. Characterized by a brief, generalized jerking or stiffening of the extremities.
2. May occur singly or in groups; may throw person to the floor.

D. Atonic or akinetic seizures, also called "drop attacks."
   a. Characterized by sudden, momentary loss of muscle tone.
   b. Usually causes person to fall to the ground.

E. Assess for partial seizures (focal seizures).
   1. Simple partial seizure.
      a. Localized (confined to a specific area) motor symptoms, accompanied by sensory symptoms.
      b. Patient remains conscious throughout episode and may report an aura before seizure takes place.
   2. Complex partial (psychomotor) seizure.
      a. Area of brain most involved is temporal lobe (thus, this type of seizure is called psychomotor).
      b. Characterized by period of altered behavior and automatism (patient is not aware of behavior); evidenced by such mannerisms as lip smacking, chewing, picking at clothes, etc.
      c. Patient loses consciousness for a few seconds.

F. Idiopathic or unclassified seizures.
   1. This type of seizure accounts for half of all seizure activity.
   2. Occurs for no known reason and fits into no generalized or partial classification.

G. Assess for specific phases of seizure activity.
   1. Occurs without warning or following an *aura* (peculiar sensation that warns of an impending seizure—dizziness, visual or auditory sensation).
   2. Behavior at onset of seizure.

Implementation

A. Protect patient from injury or complication during seizure (see Convulsions p. 134).

B. Eliminate precipitating factors of seizure.

1. Accurate observation and recording of seizures.
2. Possible factors: drugs, alcohol, sleep, nutrition, loud noises, music, flickering lights, hyperventilation.
3. Treatment of underlying cause—tumor, infection.

C. Promote physical and mental health.
   1. Establish regular routines for activities of daily living.
      a. Diet, sleep, physical activity (activity tends to inhibit seizure activity).
      b. Provide appropriate safeguards during exercise and sports.
   2. Avoid alcohol, stress, exhaustion.
   3. Foster self-esteem and confidence; avoid overprotection of patient.
   4. Provide patient and family with facts regarding epilepsy.
      a. Control of the disorder.
      b. Recognition of impending seizure and care during seizure.
      c. Importance of carrying identification card in case of emergency.
      d. Organizations that provide services, such as the National Epilepsy League and the National Association to Control Epilepsy.

D. Administer and monitor effects of medications.
   1. Medication regimen may require periods of adjustment and/or a combination of drugs.
   2. Reinforce necessity for taking medication regularly as prescribed; observe response, any side effects or seizure activity.
   3. Administer anticonvulsants.
      a. Most common drugs: phenobarbital, diphenylhydantoin (Dilantin), mephenytoin (Mesantoin), primidone (Mysoline), paramethadione (Paradione), trimethadione (Tridione), ethosuximide (Zarontin).
      b. Usually used in combination—decreased dosage lessens side effects.
   4. Administer drugs as a preventative measure for further episodes.
      a. Phenytoin (Dilantin).

(1) Prevents seizures through depression of the motor areas of the brain.

(2) Side effects include GI symptoms, rash, and bleeding gums.

b. Diazepam (Valium).

(1) For relief of restlessness.

(2) To decrease seizure activity.

c. Phenobarbital (Luminal).

(1) Reduces responsiveness of normal neurons to impulses arising in the focal site.

(2) Side effects are drowsiness, ataxia, nystagmus.

(3) Toxic effects produce rash but usually no nausea and vomiting.

d. Carbamazepine (Tegretol).

(1) Inhibits nerve impulses by limiting influx of sodium ions across cell membranes.

(2) Give with meals; monitor for side effects—diplopia, blurred vision, ataxia, vomiting, leukopenia.

e. Clonazepam (Clonopin).

(1) Decreases frequency, duration and spread of discharge in minor motor seizures (absence, akinetic, myoclonic seizures).

(2) Side effects: lethargy, ataxia, vertigo thrombocytopenia—monitor CBC.

5. Monitor toxic side effects of drugs: drowsiness, skin rash, nervousness, nausea, ataxia, gum hyperplasia, blood dyscrasias.

6. Avoid sudden withdrawal of drugs—may precipitate status epilepticus.

E. Treatment of complicating status epilepticus.

1. Successive major convulsions without regaining consciousness between attacks are considered a medical emergency which may cause death.

2. Most frequent cause is sudden withdrawal of anticonvulsants; other factors include insulin, electroshock, acute infections, trauma, and metabolic disorders.

3. Management of complications.

a. Maintain open airway.

b. Terminate seizure with IV medications: phenobarbital, diphenylhydantoin, diazepam, paraldehyde.

c. Monitor patient's condition frequently for complications: cardiac, respiratory, and neurological status; arterial blood gases, glucose, calcium, electrolytes, renal and liver function.

Multiple Sclerosis

Definition: Chronic, slowly progressive, noncontagious, degenerative disease of the CNS.

Etiology

A. Definite cause unknown; autoimmunity or virus likely cause.

B. Incidence is greater in colder climate, equal in the sexes, and usually occurs between ages 20 to 40 years.

Pathophysiology

A. Demyelination of nerve fibers within long conducting pathways of spinal cord and brain.

B. Lesions (plaques) are irregularly scattered—disseminated.

C. Destruction of myelin sheath creates patches of sclerotic tissue, degeneration of the nerve fiber, and disturbance in conduction of sensory and motor impulses.

D. Initially the disease is characterized by periods of remission with exacerbation and variable manifestations but is followed by irreversible dysfunction.

E. Clinical course may extend over 10 to 20 years.

Assessment

A. Highly variable, depending on area of involvement: sensory fibers, motor fibers, brainstem, cerebellum, internal capsule.

B. Weakness, paralysis, incoordination, ataxia, intention tremor, bladder/bowel retention or incontinence, spasticity, numbness, tingling, analgesia, anesthesia, loss of position sense, impaired vision (diplopia, nystagmus), dysphagia, impaired speech, emotional instability, impaired judgment.

Implementation

A. Prevent precipitation of exacerbations.
   1. Avoid fatigue, stress, infection, overheating, chilling.
   2. Establish regular program of exercise and rest.
   3. Provide a balanced diet.
B. Administer and assess effects of medications.
   1. Steroids hasten remission. Prednisone is used for short-term therapy.
   2. Chlordiazepoxide for mood swings.
   3. Baclofen or dantrolene for spasticity.
   4. Bethanechol or oxybutynin to relieve urinary retention.
   5. Antibiotics, vitamin B, essential fatty acids.
C. Promote optimal activity.
   1. Moderation in activity with rest periods.
   2. Physical and speech therapy.
   3. Diversionary activities, hobbies.
   4. During exacerbation, patient is usually put on bed rest.
D. Promote safety.
   1. Sensory loss—regulate bath water; use caution with heating pads; inspect skin for lesions.
   2. Motor loss—avoid waxed floors, throw rugs; provide rails and walker.
   3. Diplopia—apply eye patch.
E. Encourage regular elimination—bladder/bowel training programs.
F. Provide education and emotional support to patient and family.
   1. Encourage independence and realistic goals; assess personality and behavior changes; observe for signs of depression.
   2. Provide instruction and assistive devices; provide information about services of the National Multiple Sclerosis Society.
G. Assess and prevent potential complications.
   1. Most common: urinary tract infection, calculi, decubitus ulcers.
   2. Contracture pain due to spasticity, metabolic or nutritional disorders, regurgitation, depression.

3. Common cause of death: respiratory tract infection, urinary tract infection.

Myasthenia Gravis

Definition: Myasthenia gravis is a neuromuscular disease characterized by marked weakness and abnormal fatigue of voluntary muscles.

Etiology

A. Unknown; question autoimmune reaction.
B. Patients with myasthenia have a high incidence of thymus abnormalities and frequently have systemic lupus erythematosus.

Pathophysiology

A. Basic pathology is a defect in transmission of nerve impulse at the myoneural junction, the junction of motor neuron with muscle.
B. Normally, acetylcholine is stored in synaptic vesicle of motor neurons to skeletal muscles.
C. Defect may be due to:
   1. Deficiency in acetylcholine/excess acetylcholinesterase.
   2. Defective motor-end plate and/or nerve terminals.
   3. Decreased sensitivity to acetylcholine.
D. Generally there is no muscle atrophy or degeneration; there may be periods of exacerbations and remissions.

Assessment

A. Symptoms are related to progressive weakness and fatigue of muscles when used; muscles generally are strongest in the morning.
B. Eyes are affected first: ptosis, diplopia, and eye squint.
C. Impaired speech; dysphagia; drooping facies; difficulty chewing, closing mouth, or smiling; breathing difficulty and hoarse voice.
D. Respiratory paralysis and failure.
E. Diagnosis confirmed with Tensilon test.
   1. Positive for myasthenia—improvement in muscle strength.

2. Negative—no improvement or even deterioration.

Implementation

A. Primary goals are to improve neuromuscular transmission and prevent complications.

B. Administer and assess effects of medications.
1. Anticholinesterase drugs increase levels of acetylcholine at myoneural junction.
   a. Neostigmine, pyridostigmine, ambenonium—main difference is duration of effect.
   b. Edrophonium (Tensilon)—is a rapid, brief-acting anticholinesterase used for testing purposes.
   c. Side effects.
      (1) Related to effects of increased acetylcholine in parasympathetic nervous system: sweating, excessive salivation, nausea, diarrhea, abdominal cramps; possibly bradycardia or hypotension.
      (2) Excessive doses lead to cholinergic crisis—atropine given as cholinergic blocker.
   d. Nursing measures.
      (1) Give medications exactly on time, 30 minutes before meals.
      (2) Give medication with milk and crackers to reduce GI upset.
      (3) Observe therapeutic or any toxic effects; monitor and record muscle strength and vital capacity.
2. Steroids.
   a. Suppress immune response.
   b. Usually the last resort after anticholinesterase and thymectomy.
3. The following drugs must be avoided.
   a. Streptomycin, kanamycin, neomycin, gentamicin are drugs that block neuromuscular transmission.
   b. Ether, quinidine, morphine, curare, procainamide, Innovar, sedatives—aggravate weakness of myasthenia.

C. Monitor patient's condition for complications.
1. Vital signs.
2. Respirations—depth, rate, vital capacity, ability to deep breathe and cough.
3. Swallowing—ability to eat and handle secretions.
3. Muscle strength.
4. Speech—provide method of communication if patient unable to talk.
5. Bowel and bladder function.
7. Psychological status.

D. Encourage optimal activity.
1. Plan short periods of activity and long periods of rest.
2. Time activity to coincide with maximal muscle strength.
3. Encourage normal activities of daily living.
4. Encourage diversionary activities.

E. Provide instruction and emotional support.
1. Instruct patient about medications and treatment regime and importance of adhering to medication schedule.
2. Instruct patient to avoid infection, stress, fatigue, and over-the-counter drugs.
3. Instruct patient to wear identification medal and carry emergency card.
4. Provide information about services of Myasthenia Gravis Foundation.

Myasthenic or Cholinergic Crisis

A. Myasthenic crisis.
1. Acute exacerbation of disease may be due to rapid, unrecognized progression of disease; failure of medication; infection; or fatigue or stress.
2. Myasthenic symptoms—weakness, dyspnea, dysphagia, restlessness, difficulty speaking.

B. Cholinergic crisis.
1. Cholinergic paralysis with sustained depolarization of motor-end plates is due to overmedication with anticholinesterase.
2. Symptoms similar to myasthenic state; restlessness, weakness, speaking difficulty, dysphagia, dyspnea.
3. Cholinergic symptoms—fasciculations, abdominal cramps, diarrhea, nausea, vomiting, salivation, sweating, increased bronchial secretion.

C. Tensilon test to differentiate crises, as symptoms are similar.
  1. Tensilon is given and if strength improves, it is symptomatic of myasthenic crisis and the patient needs more medication; if weakness is more severe, it is symptomatic of cholinergic crisis and overdose has occurred.
  2. Be prepared for emergency with atropine, suction, and other emergency equipment for respiratory arrest.
D. Crisis with respiratory insufficiency; patient cannot swallow secretions and may aspirate.
  1. Bed rest maintained.
  2. Endotracheal or tracheostomy tube to assist with ventilation may be required.
  3. Atropine given and anticholinesterase (cholinergic) may be held.
  4. Anticholinesterase (myasthenic) begun.

Parkinson's Disease

Definition: Degenerative disease of the brain resulting in dysfunction of the extrapyramidal system.

Etiology

A. Idiopathic.
B. Other possible causes: atherosclerosis, drug induction, postencephalitis.

Pathophysiology

A. Degeneration of basal ganglia due to depleted concentration of dopamine.
B. Depletion of dopamine correlated with degeneration of substantia nigra (midbrain structures which are closely related functionally to basal ganglia).
C. Loss in inhibitory modulation of dopamine to counterbalance cholinergic system and interruption of balance-coordinating extrapyramidal system.

D. Slowly progressive disease with high incidence of crippling disability; mental deterioration occurs very late.

Assessment

A. Appears in five stages: unilateral, bilateral, impaired balance, fully developed severe disease, and confinement to bed or wheelchair.
B. Symptoms.
  1. Tremor at rest—especially in hands and fingers (pill-rolling).
    a. Increases when stressed or fatigued.
    b. May decrease with purposeful activity or sleep.
  2. Rigidity—blank facial expression (mask-like).
    a. Drooling, difficulty with swallowing or speaking.
    b. Short, shuffling steps with stooped posture.
    c. Propulsive gait.
    d. Immobility of muscles in flexed position, creating jerky cogwheel motions.
    e. Loss of coordinated and associated automatic movement and balance.
  3. Akinesia—difficulty initiating voluntary movement.
  4. Autonomic dysfunction—lacrimation, incontinence, decreased sexual function, constipation.

Implementation

A. Strive for primary goals: reduce muscle tremor and rigidity and prevent complications.
B. Administer and assess effects of medications.
  1. Amantadine: used to treat patients with mild symptoms but no disability; side effect uncommon with usual dose.
  2. Anticholinergic drugs: most effective is Ethopropazine; used to treat tremors and rigidity, and inhibit action of acetylcholine; side effects include dry mouth, dry skin, blurring vision, urinary retention, and tachycardia.
  3. Levodopa (converted in body to dopamine).

a. Reduces akinesia, tremor, and rigidity.
b. Passes through blood-brain barrier.
c. Effectiveness may decline after 2–3 years.
d. Side effects.
   (1) Anorexia, nausea, and vomiting (administer drug with meals or snack; avoid coffee, which seems to increase nausea).
   (2) Postural hypotension, dizziness, tachycardia, and arrhythmias (monitor vital signs; caution patient to sit up or stand up slowly; have patient wear support stockings).
e. Contraindicated in patients with closed-angle glaucoma, psychotic illness, and peptic ulcer disease.

4. Sinemet—combination of carbidopa and levodopa; has fewer side effects than levodopa.
5. Antihistamines: reduce tremor and anxiety; side effect is drowsiness.
6. Antispasmodics (Artane, Kemadrin): improve rigidity but not tremor.
7. Bromocriptine (drug often used to replace levodopa when it loses effectiveness).
   a. Acts on dopamine receptors.
   b. Side effects: anorexia, nausea, vomiting, constipation, postural hypotension, cardiac arrhythmias, headache.
   c. Contraindicated in patients with mental illness, myocardial infarction, peptic ulcers, peripheral vascular disease.
8. Avoid the following drugs:
   a. Phenothiazines, reserpine, pyridoxine (vitamin B_6)—block desired action of levodopa.
   b. Monamine oxidase inhibitors—precipitate hypertensive crisis.
   c. Methyldopa—potentiates parkinsonian effects.

C. Provide appropriate nursing care following surgery.
1. Stereotaxic surgery to reduce tremor.
2. Implantation of electrodes through burr holes into target area of brain; creation of lesion with high frequency of coagulation probe.

D. Maintain regular patterns of elimination.
1. Constipation is often a problem due to side effects of medications, reduced physical activity, and muscle weakness.
2. Provide stool softeners, suppositories, mild cathartics.

E. Promote physical therapy and rehabilitation.
1. Provide preventive, corrective, and postural exercises.
2. Institute massage and stretching exercises, stressing extension of limbs.
3. Encourage daily ambulation; have patient lift feet up when walking and avoid prolonged sitting.
4. Facilitate adaptation for activities of daily living and self-care; encourage rhythmic patterns to attain timing; foster independence; utilize special aids and devices.
5. Remove hazards that might cause falls.

F. Provide education and emotional support to patient and family.
1. Remember, intellect is usually not impaired.
2. Assess changes in self-consciousness, body image, sexuality, moods.
3. Instruct patient to avoid emotional stress and fatigue, which aggravate symptoms.
4. Instruct patient to avoid foods high in vitamin B_6 and monamine oxidase.

Meningitis

Definition: Acute infection of the pia-arachnoid membrane.

Etiology

Organisms: meningococcus, staphylococcus, streptococcus, pneumococcus, Haemophilus influenzae, tuberculous.

Assessment

A. Painful, stiff neck—nuchal rigidity, Kernig's and Brudzinski's signs.
B. Severe headache, photophobia.

C. Fever.

D. Irritability, stupor, coma.

Implementation

A. Maintain open airway.

B. Treat the infective organism—antimicrobic therapy, intravenously.

C. Assess and treat increased intracranial pressure or seizures.

D. Control body temperature.

E. Provide adequate fluid and electrolyte balance.

F. Provide quiet environment.

CRANIAL NERVE DISORDERS

Trigeminal Neuralgia (Tic Douloureux)

Definition: Sensory disorder of the fifth cranial nerve, resulting in severe, recurrent paroxysms of sharp facial pain along the distribution of the trigeminal nerve. Etiology and pathology are unknown; incidence is higher in older women.

Assessment

A. Trigger points on the lips, gums, nose, or cheek.

B. May be stimulated by a cold breeze, washing, chewing, food/fluids of extreme temperatures.

Treatment and Implementation

A. Observe characteristics of attack and ways patient protects face from stimulus.

B. Avoid extremes of heat or cold; give small feedings of semiliquid or soft food.

C. Medical treatment.
   1. Massive doses of B_{12}.
   2. Inhalation: 10–15 drops of trichloroethylene on cotton.
   3. Anticonvulsants: Dilantin and Tegretol.

4. Alcohol injections to produce anesthesia of the nerve.

D. Surgical treatment.
   1. Peripheral—avulsion of supraorbital, infraorbital, or mandibular division.
   2. Intracranial.
      a. Division of the sensory nerve root for permanent anesthesia.
      b. Patient may experience numbness, stiffness or burning after surgery.
      c. Microsurgery allows for selective sectioning of the fifth nerve.
      d. Pain and temperature fibers are destroyed, and sensation of touch and corneal reflex are preserved.

E. Assess and treat complications after surgery.
   1. Facial paralysis.
   2. Irritation or ulceration of cornea due to loss of sensation.
   3. Local trauma to inside of mouth.

Bell's Palsy (Facial Paralysis)

Definition: Lower motor neuron lesion of the seventh cranial nerve, resulting in paralysis of one side of the face.

Assessment

A. Flaccid muscles.

B. Shallow nasolabial fold.

C. Inability to raise eyebrows, frown, smile, close eyelids, or puff out cheeks.

D. Upward movement of eye when attempting to close eyelid.

E. Loss of taste in anterior tongue.

Implementation

A. Palliative.

B. Analgesics, steroids, physiotherapy, support of facial muscles, protection of cornea.

C. Promote active facial exercises to prevent loss of muscle tone.

D. Instruct patient to chew food on unaffected side.

E. Present attractive, easy-to-eat foods to prevent anorexia and weight loss.

F. Provide special eye care to prevent keratitis.

G. Reassure and support.

Meniere's Disease

Definition: Dilatation of the endolymphatic system causing degeneration of the vestibular and cochlear hair cells.

Etiology

A. Etiology is unknown.

B. Possible causes may include allergies, toxicity, localized ischemia, hemorrhage, viral infection, and edema.

Treatment and Implementation

A. Direct care toward alleviating obstruction and reducing the pressure.

B. Surgical division of vestibular portion of the nerve or destruction of the labyrinth may be necessary for severe cases.

C. Maintain bedrest during acute attack.
   1. Prevent injury during attack.
   2. Provide side rails if necessary.
   3. Keep room dark when photophobia present.

D. Provide drug therapy.
   1. Vasodilators (nicotinic acid).
   2. Diuretics, antihistamines (Benadryl).
   3. Sedatives.

E. Monitor diet therapy.
   1. Low sodium.
   2. Lipoflavonoid vitamin supplement.
   3. Restricted fluid intake.

F. Assist with ambulation if necessary.

Guillain-Barré Syndrome

Definition: An acute infectious neuronitis of cranial and peripheral nerves. Immune system overreacts to an infection destroying the myelin sheath.

Characteristics

A. Etiology is unknown.

B. Occurs at any age but increased incidence between 30 and 50 years of age.

C. Both sexes equally affected.

D. Recovery is a slow process, taking two months to two years.

E. Diagnostic test results: CSF contains high protein, abnormal EEG.

Assessment

A. First report may be of a mild upper respiratory infection or gastroenteritis.

B. Initial symptom of weakness of lower extremities.

C. Gradual progressive weakness of upper extremities and facial muscles (24–72 hours); paresthesias may precede weakness.

D. Respiratory failure may occur.

E. Sensory changes—usually minor, but in some cases severe impairment of sensory information occurs.

F. Cardiac arrhythmias.

Implementation

A. No specific treatment available; supportive treatment includes monitoring for complications (respiratory, circulatory).

B. Carefully observe for respiratory paralysis and inability to handle secretions.

C. Provide chest physiotherapy and pulmonary toilet.

D. Maintain cardiovascular function.
   1. Monitor vital signs and cardiac rhythm.
   2. Vasopressors and volume replacement.

E. Prevent complications of immobility.
   1. Turn frequently.
   2. Provide skin care.

F. Provide appropriate diversion.

G. Reassure patient, especially during paralysis period.

H. Previous treatment included corticosteroids; this is now considered controversial.

Amyotrophic Lateral Sclerosis (Lou Gehrig's Disease)

Definition: The most common motor neuron disease of muscular atrophy. It is a rapidly fatal, upper and lower motor neuron deficit affecting the limbs.

Characteristics

A. May result from several causes.
   1. Nutritional deficiency related to disturbance in enzyme metabolism.
   2. Vitamin E deficiency resulting in damage to cell membranes.
   3. Metabolic interference in nucleic acid production by nerve fibers.
   4. Autoimmune disorders.
B. Inherited in 10 percent of the cases.
C. Occurs after age 40; most common in men.
D. Is fatal within 3–10 years after onset.
E. Diagnostic tests: EMG and muscle biopsy; increased protein in CSF.

Assessment

A. Atrophy and weakness of upper extremities.
B. Difficulty swallowing and chewing.
C. Respiratory excursion and breathing patterns.
D. Impaired speech.
E. Secondary depression.

Implementation

A. Assist with rehabilitation program to promote independence.
B. Monitor for complications.
   1. Prevent skin breakdown: reposition regularly, provide back care, and utilize pressure-relieving devices.
   2. Prevent aspiration of food or fluids: offer soft foods and keep patient in upright position during meals.
   3. Promote bowel and bladder function.
C. Provide emotional support.

INTRACRANIAL SURGERY

Preoperative and Postoperative Care

Preoperative Care

A. Observe and record neurological symptoms.
   1. Paralysis.
   2. Seizure foci.
   3. Pupillary response.
B. Prepare patient physically and psychologically for surgery.
   1. Prep and shave cranial hair (save hair).
   2. Apply scrub solution to scalp, as ordered.
   3. Avoid using enemas unless specifically ordered; the strain of defecation can lead to increased intracranial pressure.
   4. Explain postoperative routine orders such as neurological checks and headaches.
   5. Administer steroids or mercurial diuretics, as ordered, to decrease cerebral edema.
   6. Insert NG tube and/or Foley catheter as ordered.

General Postoperative Care

A. Observe neurological signs.
   1. Evaluate level of consciousness.
      a. Orientation to time and place.
      b. Response to painful stimuli.
      c. Ability to follow verbal command.
   2. Evaluate pupil size and reactions to light.
      a. Are pupils equal, not constricted or dilated.
      b. Do pupils react to light.
      c. Do pupils react sluggishly or are they fixed.
   3. Evaluate strength and motion of extremities.
      a. Are handgrips present and equal.
      b. Are handgrips strong or weak.
      c. Can patient move all extremities on command.
      d. Are movements purposeful or involuntary.

e. Do the extremities have twitching, flaccid, or spastic movements (indicative of a neurological problem).
4. Observe vital signs (TRP and BP).
   a. Keep patient normothermic to decrease metabolic needs of the brain.
   b. Observe respirations for depth and rate to prevent respiratory acidosis from anoxia.
   c. Observe blood pressure and pulse for signs of shock or increased intracranial pressure.
5. Evaluate reflexes.
   a. Babinski—positive Babinski is illicited by stroking the lateral aspect of the sole of the foot, backward flexion of the great toe or spreading of other toes.

Negative Babinski   Positive Babinski

   b. Romberg—when patient stands with feet close together, he or she falls off balance. If positive, may have cerebellar, proprioceptive, or vestibular difficulties.
   c. Kernig—patient is lying down with thigh flexed at a right angle; extension of the leg upward results in spasm of hamstring muscle, pain, and resistance to additional extension of leg at the knee (indicative of meningitis).
6. Watch for headache, double vision, nausea, or vomiting.
B. Provide for special needs.
   1. Maintain patent airway—oxygen deprivation and an increase of carbon dioxide may produce cerebral hypoxia and cause cerebral edema.
   2. Suction as necessary, but not through nose without specific order.
   3. Maintain adequate oxygenation and humidification.
   4. Place patient in semi-prone or semi-Fowler's position (or totally on side). Turn every two hours, side to side.
   5. Maintain fluid and electrolytes.
      a. Do not give fluid by mouth to semi-conscious or unconscious patient.
      b. Weigh to determine fluid loss.
      c. Monitor IV fluids; overhydration leads to cerebral edema.
   6. Record accurate intake and output.
   7. Take seizure precautions.
   8. Provide hygienic care, including oral hygiene.
   9. Observe dressing for unusual drainage (bleeding, cerebral spinal fluid).
   10. Prevent straining with bowel movements.

Medications

A. Steroids.
   1. Decrease cerebral edema by their anti-inflammatory effect.
   2. Decrease capillary permeability in inflammatory process, thus decreasing leakage of fluid into tissue.
B. Mannitol.
   1. Decrease cerebral edema.
   2. Diuretic action by carrying out large volume of water through the nephron.
C. Dilantin.
   1. Prevents seizures through depression of the motor areas of the brain.
   2. Side effects include gastrointestinal symptoms and rash.
D. Valium.
   1. Relieves restlessness.
   2. Decreases seizure activity.
E. Phenobarbital.
   1. Reduces responsiveness of normal neurons to the nervous impulses arising in the focal site.

2. Side effects are drowsiness, ataxia, nystagmus.
3. Toxic effects produce rash but usually no nausea and vomiting.

Precautions for Care of Neurosurgical Patient

A. Do not lower head in Trendelenburg's position or place in supine position.
B. Do not suction through nose without specific order.
C. Be careful when administering sedations and narcotics.
1. Cannot evaluate neurological status.
2. May cause respiratory embarrassment.
D. Do not give oral fluids unless patient fully awake.
E. Do not administer enemas or cathartics (may cause straining, therefore increasing intracranial pressure).
F. Do not place on operative side if large tumor or bone removed.

Neurosurgical Postoperative Complications

Increased Intracranial Pressure

A. Signs and symptoms.
1. Brain becomes compressed as intracranial pressure increases.
2. Change in level of consciousness.
3. Lethargy, slurring speech, and slow responses.
4. Changes in condition (often rapid).
   a. Patient becomes restless.
   b. Patient becomes confused.
   c. Increased drowsiness.
   d. Stupor to coma.
5. Changes in vital signs.
   a. Pulse changes—may decrease to 60 or occasionally increase above 100.
   b. Respiratory irregularities—progresses to Cheyne-Stokes and apnea can result.

c. Blood pressure increases with wide pulse pressure (difference between systolic and diastolic).
d. Moderately elevated temperature.
6. Headache.
7. Vomiting.
8. Pupil changes—increasing pressure or an expanding clot can displace the brain against the oculomotor or optic nerve.

B. Nursing care.
1. Inform physician of any vital sign changes or sensorium changes.
2. Observe intake and output for possible fluid overload leading to cerebral edema.
3. Observe surgical incision site for signs of edema.
4. Administer diuretics or steroids to decrease edema as ordered.
5. Administer anticonvulsant drugs as ordered.
6. Have spinal or ventricular puncture tray available to drain off cerebral spinal fluid as necessary.
7. Observe for level of consciousness—lethargy, slurred speech, slowed responses.

C. Precautions for care of neurosurgical patient.
1. Do not lower head in Trendelenburg's position or place in supine position.
2. Do not suction through nose without specific order.
3. Be careful when administering sedations and narcotics.
   a. Cannot evaluate neurological status.
   b. May cause respiratory embarrassment.
4. Do not give oral fluids unless patient fully awake.
5. Do not administer enemas or cathartics (may cause straining, therefore increasing intracranial pressure).
6. Do not place on operative side.

Seizures

A. Tonic–Clonic seizures—grand mal (see p. 135).
B. Treatment and nursing care.
1. Administer drugs as ordered (Dilantin, phenobarbital and other related drugs).

2. Provide safe environment.
   a. Pad side rails.
   b. Do not restrain during seizure.
   c. Only use tongue blade to prevent tongue from falling back into throat prior to seizure onset.
3. Observe and record.
   a. Activities preceding the seizure (aura, movements, etc.).
   b. Type of movements and area of body involved.
   c. Incontinence.
   d. Presence of unconsciousness during seizure.
   e. Length of seizure.
   f. Conditions following seizure.
      (1) Somnolent.
      (2) Continuation of previous activities.
      (3) Awareness of seizure activity.
4. Provide privacy during seizure.

Brain Abscess or Wound Infection

A. Signs and symptoms.
   1. Increased temperature unless abscess walled off, in which case temperature can be subnormal.
   2. Headache.
   3. Neurological deficits relative to area involved (focal seizures, blurred vision, etc.).
   4. Increased intracranial pressure.
B. Nursing care.
   1. Observe neurological signs.
   2. Decrease temperature: sponge bath, antipyretic drugs (Tylenol), cooling blanket.
   3. Administer appropriate antibiotics for causative agent.

POSITIONS FOR NEUROLOGICAL CONDITIONS

Condition	Position
Cerebral edema	Elevate head to promote venous return from brain to heart
Stroke with increased intracranial pressure	Head elevated—avoid neck flexion or severe head rotation; prone position impedes venous outflow from brain
CSF fistula, right- or left-sided dependent posturing	Head-up position to promote drainage and lower CSF pressure
Cerebrovascular accident (CVA)	Encourage flat in bed except for ADLs; prevent hip flexion deformities with padded splint at night, trochanter roll and footboard
Rupture of intracranial aneurysm with subarachnoid hematoma	30°–40° elevation, low-Fowler's to facilitate drainage from brain; bedrest
Subdural hematoma	Avoid sudden change in position; promote rest
Brain-Head injury	Low position at all times; semi-prone or lateral recumbent prevents aspiration and increases gaseous exchange; turn side to side to prevent stasis of secretions and skin excoriation
Cerebral aneurysm Cerebral concussion and contusion	Elevate head of bed; bedrest
Unconscious patient	Semi-prone position; prevent tongue from obstructing airway; encourage drainage of secretion and increased gaseous exchange
Intracranial Surgery	
Supratentorial surgery (above the cerebellum)	Head of bed elevated 45° with pillow under head and shoulders; lessens possibility of hemorrhage and improves circulation of CSF
Infratentorial surgery	Bed flat, small pillow under nape of neck and patient turned to either side; avoid flexion of neck causing brain stem compression and coughing and vomiting, since these increase ICP

EYE CONDITIONS AND SURGERY

Cataracts

Definition: Clouding or opacity of the lens that leads to blurring vision and eventual loss of sight.

Characteristics

A. Opacity is due to chemical changes of the fibers or chemical changes in protein of the lens—most often caused by the slow degenerative changes of age.

B. Surgical procedure is usually based on individual needs: that is, how much the patient can see out of the other eye.
   1. If any inflammation is present, surgery is not performed.
   2. Cataracts are removed under local anesthesia.
   3. Some simple cataracts are removed by use of alphachymotrypsin, which loosens the zonular fibers that hold the lens in position.
   4. Surgery is performed on one eye at a time.

C. Types of surgical extraction.
   1. Intracapsular—the lens is removed within its capsule.
   2. Extracapsular—the lens is lifted out without removing the lens capsule.
   3. Phacoemulsification (ultrasonic)—the lens is broken up by ultrasonic vibrations and extracted via extracapsular.

Implementation

A. Check that patient understands preoperative instructions.
   1. Patient must be transported to and from hospital.
   2. Patient must have someone at home following surgery.
   3. Patient should shampoo hair before surgery.
   4. Review instructions to decrease intraocular pressure. (Do not bend, cough, strain, or lift.)

B. Administer prescribed preoperative medications.
   1. Mydriatics (atropine sulfate)—note whether pupil dilates following drug instillation.
   2. Antibiotics or topical anti-infective (Gentamicin)—prevention of infection.
   3. Narcotics (meperidine)—for pain relief.
   4. Hyperosmotic agents (oral: glycerol or IV: Mannitol).
   5. Antiemetics (Compazine, Vistaril).

C. Provide postoperative care. Most procedures are done on outpatient basis.
   1. Instruct patient in postoperative drugs.
      a. Mydriatics (atropine sulfate)—two to six weeks after surgery.
      b. Miotic agents—prescribed for certain types of lens implants.
      c. Steroids (prednisolone suspension).
   2. Instruct in ways to alleviate symptoms that could result in complications.
      a. Nausea and vomiting.
      b. Restlessness.
      c. Coughing or sneezing.

Retinal Detachment

Definition: The retina is the part of the eye that perceives light; it coordinates and transmits impulses from its seeing nerve cells to the optic nerve. As the detachment extends and becomes complete, blindness occurs.

Assessment

A. Opacity of the eyes.

B. Flashes of light.

C. Floating spots—blood and retinal cells that are freed at the time of the tear and that cast shadows on the retina as they drift about the eye.

D. Progressive constriction of vision in one area.
   1. The area of visual loss depends on the location of detachment.
   2. When the detachment is extensive and rapid, the patient feels as if a curtain has been pulled over his eyes.

Preoperative Implementation

A. Keep patient on bed rest.

B. Cover both eyes with patches to prevent further detachment.

C. Position patient's head so the retinal hole is in the lowest part of the eye.

Surgical Procedure

A. Immediate surgery with drainage of fluid from subretinal space so that retina returns to normal position.

B. Retinal breaks are sealed by various methods that produce inflammatory reactions (chorioretinitis).
   1. Cryosurgery—cold probe applied to sclera causes chorioretinal scar—most common procedure.
   2. Laser beam seals small retinal tears—can also be used to produce the chorioretinitis.
   3. Diathermy—causes retina to adhere to choroid.

Postoperative Implementation

A. Maintain safe environment.
   1. Keep side rails up.
   2. Feed patient.
   3. Maintain bed rest for one or two days.
   4. Keep bed flat or in low-Fowler's position.

B. Prevent complications.
   1. Observe for hemorrhage, which is a common complication. Notify physician immediately of any sudden, sharp eye pain.
   2. Cover both eyes.
   3. Position so area of detachment is in dependent position. (If air bubble is present, position on abdomen.)
   4. Prevent clinical manifestations which can cause hemorrhage.
      a. Nausea and vomiting.
      b. Restlessness.
   5. Encourage patient to do deep breathing but to avoid coughing.
   6. Administer good skin care to prevent breakdown.
   7. Avoid external eye pressure.

C. Provide emotional support.
   1. Provide audible stimulation.
   2. Warn patient as you enter the room and always speak before touching.
   3. Orient to surroundings.

D. Provide patient instruction.
   1. During convalescent period.
      a. Wear patch at night to prevent rubbing of eyes.
      b. Wear dark glasses.
      c. Avoid squinting.
   2. During postconvalescent period.
      a. Avoid straining and constipation.
      b. Avoid lifting heavy objects for six to eight weeks.
      c. Avoid bending from the waist.

Glaucoma

Definition: Abnormally increased intraocular pressure, which may produce serious visual defects.

Characteristics

A. Chronic open-angle glaucoma.
   1. Results from an overproduction or obstruction to the outflow of aqueous humor.
   2. Ninety percent of all glaucoma cases are of this type.

B. Chronic closed-angle glaucoma follows an untreated attack of acute closed-angle glaucoma.

C. Acute narrowing-angle (closed-angle) glaucoma.
   1. Results from an obstruction to the outflow of aqueous humor.
   2. Caused by trauma, drugs, or inflammation.

D. Evaluate risk conditions.
   1. Over 40 years of age.
   2. Diabetic.
   3. Black patient.
   4. Hypertensive.
   5. Familial history of glaucoma.
   6. "Large-eyed" children.
   7. History of eye injury.

Assessment

A. Schiotz Tonometer Test (7 to 21 mmHg is normal).

B. Chronic open-angle.
1. Loss of peripheral vision and eventual loss of central vision.
2. Mild aching in the eyes.
3. Halos around lights.

C. Acute narrowing-angle (closed-angle) glaucoma.
1. Unilateral inflammation.
2. Pain.
3. Pressure over eye.
4. Moderate pupil dilation, nonreactive to light.
5. Cloudy cornea.
6. Blurring and decreased visual acuity.
7. Photophobia.
8. Halos around light.
9. Nausea and vomiting.

D. Chronic closed-angle glaucoma.
1. Usually no symptoms.
2. Halos around lights may occur.
3. Progresses to blindness.

Treatment and Implementation

A. For chronic open-angle glaucoma.
1. Aqueous humor production decreased through beta blockers.
2. Intraocular pressure lowered with epinephrine or diuretics.
3. Miotic eyedrops, such as pilocarpine, facilitate the outflow of aqueous humor.
4. Patient prepared for surgery—trabeculoplasty or trabeculectomy.

B. For acute closed-angle glaucoma.
1. Treated as an emergency problem.
2. Drugs administered to lower intraocular pressure.
3. Patient prepared for peripheral iridectomy.
   a. Part of iris is excised to reestablish aqueous humor outflow.
   b. Acetazolamide, mannitol administered.
   c. Pilocarpine given to constrict pupil and force iris away from trabecular, allowing fluid to escape.

C. For chronic closed-angle glaucoma.
1. Pilocarpine administered.
2. Patient is prepared for bilateral peripheral iridectomy.

D. Postoperative care.
1. Cycloplegic eyedrops to affected eye to relax the ciliary muscle and decrease inflammation.
2. Early ambulation.
3. Observe unaffected eye for symptoms of acute closed-angle glaucoma if cycloplegic drops are given by mistake.

Instilling Eye Drops. ❖ PROCEDURE ❖

A. Take medication to patient's room, and check room number against medication card or sheet.

B. Check patient's identaband and ask patient to state name.

C. Wash your hands.

D. Explain procedure to patient.

E. Tilt patient's head slightly backward.

F. Squeeze the prescribed amount of medication into eye dropper. Hold dropper with bulb in uppermost position.

G. Give tissue to patient for wiping off excess medication.

H. Expose lower conjunctival sac.

I. Drop prescribed medication into center of sac. (Do *not* place medication directly on cornea, since medication can cause injury to cornea.)

J. Ask patient to close eyelids and move eyes to distribute solution over conjunctival surface and anterior eyeball.

K. Remove excess medication from surrounding tissue.

Removal of Foreign Body From Eye. ❖ PROCEDURE ❖

A. Have patient look upward.

B. Expose and evert lower lid to expose conjunctival sac.

C. Wet cotton applicator with sterile normal saline and gently twist swab over particle and remove it.

D. If particle cannot be found, have patient look downward. Place cotton applicator horizontally on outer surface of upper lid.

E. Grasp eyelashes with fingers and pull upper lid outward and upward over cotton stick.

F. With twisting motion upward, loosen particle and remove.

Ophthalmic Drugs

A. Miotics: Pilocarpine HCl 1–6% solution; Carbamylcholine 1.5–3% solution.
   1. Action is contraction of ciliary muscle which increases flow of aqueous humor.
   2. Treatment for glaucoma and certain types of lens implants.
   3. Side effects: headache, conjunctiva irritation, and inflammation.

B. Mydriatics: Atropine sulfate 0.25–2% solution; Epinephrine HCl 0.1% solution; Cyclopentolate HCl 0.5–1%.
   1. Action is to block sphincter muscle response—dilates pupil.
   2. Treatment for ocular surgery and used in eye examinations.
   3. Side effects: headache, dizziness, dry mouth, flushing, and hyperemia.

C. Beta-blockers: Timolol maleate.
   1. Action is to reduce intraocular pressure by decreasing formation of aqueous humor or may facilitate outflow of aqueous humor.
   2. Treatment for glaucoma.
   3. Side effects: eye irritation.

D. Carbonic Anhydrase Inhibitors: Acetazolamide, PO or IV.
   1. Action is to restrict action of the enzyme necessary to produce aqueous humor—mild diuretic action.
   2. Treatment for glaucoma.
   3. Side effects: CNS disturbance, GI irritation, acidosis, hypokalemia.

E. Hyperosmotic agents: glycerol (oral) or Mannitol.
   1. Action is to increase blood osmolarity—reduce intraocular pressure.
   2. Treatment for cataract surgery as preoperative medication.
   3. Side effects: CNS—headache, confusion, blurred vision; GI irritability; nausea; dehydration.

EAR SURGERY

Stapedectomy

Definition: Surgery performed to correct otosclerosis; otosclerosis is a condition in which the normal bone of the middle ear is replaced by abnormal osseous tissue.

Surgical Procedure

A. An incision is made deep within the ear canal, close to the eardrum, so that the drum can be turned back and the middle ear exposed.

B. The surgeon frees and removes the stapes and the attached footplate, leaving an opening in the oval window.

C. The patient can usually hear as soon as this procedure has been completed.

D. The opening in the oval window is closed with a plug of fat or Gelfoam, which the body eventually replaces with mucous membrane cells.

E. A steel wire or a Teflon piston is inserted to replace the stapes.
   1. The wire is attached to the incus at one end and to the graft or plug at the other end.
   2. The wire transmits sound to the inner ear.

Implementation

A. Keep patient in low-Fowler's position unoperated side, or as ordered by physician.

B. Do not turn the patient.

C. Put side rails up.

D. Have patient deep breathe every two hours until ambulatory, but do not allow coughing.

E. Check for drainage; report excessive bleeding.

F. Prevent vomiting.

G. Give antibiotics as ordered.

H. Patient may have vertigo when ambulatory; stay with the patient and avoid quick movements.

I. Advise patient not to smoke.

Irrigation of External Auditory Canal.
❖ Procedure ❖

A. Remove any discharge on outer ear.

B. Place emesis basin under ear.

C. Gently pull outer ear upward and backward for adult, or downward and backward for child.

D. Place tip of syringe or irrigating catheter at opening of ear.

E. Gently irrigate with solution at 95° to 105°F, directing flow toward the sides of the canal.

F. Dry external ear.

G. If irrigation does not dislodge wax, instillation of drops will need to be carried out.

CARDIOVASCULAR SYSTEM

The heart and the circulatory system, both systemic and pulmonary, comprise one of the most essential parts of the body. Failure of the heart to function results in death of the organism. Blood, composed of cells and plasma, circulates through the body and is the means by which oxygen and nutritive materials are transported to the tissues and carbon dioxide and metabolic end products are removed from the tissues for excretion.

CARDIOVASCULAR ANATOMY

Gross Structure of the Heart

A. Muscular organ that functions as a pump.

B. Separated by a septum into a right, or venous, chamber and into a left, or arterial, chamber.

Layers

A. Pericardium.
   1. Fibrous pericardium—fibrous sac.
   2. Serous pericardium—allows for free cardiac motion.

B. Epicardium—covers surface of heart, extends onto great vessels, and becomes continuous with the inner lining of the pericardium.

C. Myocardium—muscular portion of heart.

D. Endocardium—thin, delicate inner layer of tissue which lines cardiac chambers and covers surface of heart valves.

Chambers

A. Right chambers.
   1. Right atrium (RA)—thin walled, distensible, low-pressure collecting chamber for systemic venous return (receives blood from superior vena cava, interior vena cava, and coronary sinus).

2. Right ventricle (RV)—thin walled, low pressure receiving chamber for blood from right atrium (pumps blood into low resistance pulmonary system).

B. Left chambers.
   1. Left atrium (LA)—thin-walled, low pressure collecting chamber for pulmonary venous system (receives oxygenated blood via the four pulmonary veins).
   2. Left ventricle (LV)—thick-walled, high-pressure chamber that propels blood into the high resistance systemic circuit (pumps oxygenated blood via aorta to all body tissues).

Valves

A. Strong membranous openings that operate to permit flow of blood only in one direction.

B. Classifications of valves.
   1. Atrioventricular valves, located as heart-guard openings between atria and ventricles, prevent backflow of blood from ventricles to atria during systole.
      a. Tricuspid—right heart valve.
         (1) Three cusps, or leaflets.
         (2) Free edges anchored to papillary muscles in right ventricle by chordae tendineae which contract when the ventricular walls contract.
      b. Mitral—left heart valve.
         (1) Two cusps, or leaflets.
         (2) Free edges anchored to papillary muscles in left ventricle by chordae tendineae which contract when the ventricular walls contract.
   2. Semilunar valves, located at blood's exit points inside pulmonary artery and aorta, prevent backflow from the aorta and pulmonary artery into the ventricles during diastole.
      a. Pulmonic—three cusps, or leaflets.
      b. Aortic—three cusps, or leaflets.

Coronary Blood Supply

A. Arteries.

1. Two arteries provide the myocardium with its own blood supply.
   a. Right coronary artery supplies mainly the right ventricle but also part of the left ventricle.
   b. Left coronary artery divides into two branches (left anterior descending artery and circumflex artery) and supplies mainly the left ventricle.
2. Coronary blood flow is regulated by oxygen needs of the myocardium.
3. Aortic pressure determines perfusion of myocardium.

B. Veins.
   1. Principle coronary veins empty into coronary sinus.
   2. Coronary sinus veins drain into right atrium.

Conduction System

A. Composed of specialized tissue that initiates rapid transmission of electrical impulses for orderly sequence of cardiac contraction.

B. Sinoatrial (SA) node.
   1. Main pacemaker of heart in which normal, rhythmic, self-excitatory impulse is generated.
   2. Normal heart elicits 60 to 100 electrical impulses/minute.
   3. External control is through autonomic nervous system.
      a. Sympathetic—speeds rate and increases force of contraction.
      b. Parasympathetic—slows rate and decreases force of contraction; has predominant control.

C. Internodal tracts—transmits electrical impulses through atria from sinoatrial node to atrioventricular node.

D. Atrioventricular (AV) node—contains delay tissue to allow atrial contraction to eject blood into ventricle before ventricular contraction.

E. Bundle of His—conducts the electrical impulse from the atria into ventricles.

F. Left and right bundles to Purkinje fibers—conduct impulses to all parts of the ventricles.

Gross Structure of Vasculature

Arteries

A. Arteries are elastic, muscular tubes that transport blood from the heart to the capillaries in the body tissue.

B. Strong, muscular walls of the arteries force blood onward to all parts of the body.

C. Blood flows rapidly to the tissues.

D. Factors influencing arterial flow.
   1. An adequate volume of blood (cardiac output).
   2. A closed system of unobstructive tubes.
   3. Set of heart valves to ensure flow of blood in one direction only.
   4. Resistance to flow, i.e., an increased thickness of blood causes slowing of blood flow.

Capillaries

A. Capillaries are minute passageways in which the exchange of blood and tissue fluid take place.

B. Capillary walls are thin and permeable to small substances.

C. Blood flow varies depending on type of tissue.

D. Capillaries permit rapid exchange of water and solutes.

Veins

A. Veins are thin-walled tubes that transport blood from tissues back to the heart.

B. Venous system.
   1. Pressure is low.
   2. Walls able to contract or expand, which permits storing of small or large amounts of blood.
   3. Many veins, particularly in the extremities, have valves which help to prevent backflow of blood.

C. Factors influencing venous return.
   1. Decrease in volume of circulating blood decreases venous return.
   2. Resistance in the venous system (such as occurs in CHF) decreases venous return.
   3. Muscle contraction increases venous return.
   4. Gravity.
   5. Respiration.
      a. Inspiration increases venous return.
      b. Expiration decreases venous return.
   6. Ability of right heart to handle venous return.

CARDIOVASCULAR PHYSIOLOGY

Function of Heart and Vessels

A. Heart supplies sufficient amounts of blood to meet the metabolic demands of body tissues.

B. Vessels provide the means of transporting blood to every part and organ of the body.

Regulation of Cardiac Activity

A. Properties of cardiac cells.
   1. Automaticity—ability to initiate an electrical impulse without external stimuli. Conduction of the impulse: SA node → AV node → bundle of His → Purkinje system.
   2. Conductivity—ability to transmit electrical impulses.
   3. Contractility—ability of muscle to shorten with electrical stimulation.
   4. Excitability—ability to be stimulated.

B. Cardiac cycle—cycle is one complete heart beat.
   1. Contraction (systole).
      a. Atria contract, AV valves close, ventricles pump out blood.
      b. "Lub" sound heard through stethoscope.
   2. Relaxation (diastole).
      a. Closure of semi-lunar valves, relaxation of atria and ventricles (volume of blood is constant in chambers).
      b. "Dub" sound heard through stethoscope.

C. Cardiac output (CO)—equals the volume of blood ejected from each ventricle in one minute.
   1. Stroke volume (SV) is the volume of blood ejected from each ventricle with each contraction.
   2. Calculation of cardiac output: stroke volume x heart rate = cardiac output.

Example: Stroke volume (SV) = 90 cc
Heart rate (HR) = 60 beats/minute
Then, 90 cc (SV) × 60 (HR) = 5400 cc (CO)

Cardiac Muscle Principles

A. Frank-Starling law states that, within physiological limits, the more the heart muscle is stretched by blood flow, the greater is the force of contraction.
   1. The heart can pump a large or a small amount of blood depending on the amount that flows into it from the veins.
   2. The heart can adapt to whatever the required load may be within the physiological limits of the total amount the heart can pump.
B. All or none principle states that cardiac muscle either contracts or does not contract when stimulated.

Compensatory Cardiac Mechanisms

A. Cardiac reserve—the difference between actual work being done and the maximum effort of which the heart is capable; a normal heart can increase its output four to six times.
B. Alterations in heart rate—a normal heart will increase its rate in response to increased oxygen need.
C. Dilatation—an increase in the length of the muscle fibers of the heart.
   1. Characterized by an increase in the *volume* of the heart chambers.
   2. There are physiological limits to dilatation.
D. Hypertrophy—an increase in the *diameter* of the muscle fibers of the heart.

1. Characterized by *thickening* of the walls of the heart chambers.
2. There are physiological limits to hypertrophy.

Pulse

A. Rhythmic dilation of an artery caused by contraction of the heart.
B. Palpated over any large surface artery.
C. Pulse deficit—difference between apical and radial pulse, which is due to weakened or ineffective contraction of the heart.

Blood Pressure

A. Pulse pressure—difference between systolic and diastolic pressure.
B. Factors influencing blood pressure.
   1. Force of heart contractions.
   2. Volume of blood (hemorrhage, for example, will cause decrease in blood pressure).
   3. Diameter and elasticity of blood vessels (arteriosclerosis, for example, will increase blood pressure).
   4. Viscosity of blood (polycythemia vera, for example, will increase blood pressure).

Nervous System Control

A. Control of the heart—impulses from the autonomic nervous system can modify the rate and strength of cardiac contractions.
   1. Sympathetic nervous system (adrenergic).
      a. Secretes epinephrine and norepinephrine.
      b. Increases heart rate.
      c. Increases force of contraction.
   2. Parasympathetic nervous system (cholinergic).
      a. Secretes acetylcholine.
      b. Exerts constant control as the "brake of heart."
      c. Slows heart rate.
      d. Decreases force of contraction.
B. Control of blood vessels.
   1. Sympathetic nervous system.

a. Causes vasoconstriction of blood vessels.

b. Causes *vasodilation* of coronary arteries.

2. Parasympathetic nervous system.

a. Causes vasodilation.

b. Has little direct effect on coronary arteries.

Blood Components

A. Plasma

1. Accounts for 55 percent of the total volume of blood.

2. Plasma composition.

a. Consists of 92 percent water and 7 percent proteins (proteins include serum, fibrinogen, albumin, gamma globulin).

b. Less than one percent organic salts, dissolved gases, hormones, antibodies, and enzymes.

B. Solid particles (blood cells and platelets).

1. Comprise 45 percent of the total blood volume.

2. Blood cells.

a. Erythrocytes (red blood cells).

(1) Normal count in an adult male is 4.6 million to 6.2 million cells, adult female is 4.2 million to 5.4 million cells/cu mm of blood.

(2) Contain hemoglobin which carries oxygen to cells and carbon dioxide from cells to lungs.

(3) Originate in bone marrow and are stored in the spleen.

(4) Average life span is 10 to 120 days.

b. Leukocytes (white blood cells).

(1) Normal count in an adult is 4500 to 11,000 cells per cu mm of blood.

(2) Primary defense against infection.

(3) Leukocyte types.

(a) Neutrophils play an active role in the acute inflammatory process and are phagocytic (able to destroy bacteria).

(b) Lymphocytes play an important role in immunologic responses.

(c) Monocytes are the largest of the leukocytes.

c. Platelets (thrombocytes).

(1) Normal count in an adult is 150,000 to 400,000 per cu mm of blood.

(2) Necessary for normal blood coagulation.

(3) Decreased platelet count leads to bleeding problems.

Spleen

A. Glandlike organ located in the left upper quadrant of the abdominal cavity.

B. Functions.

1. Stores blood.

2. Purifies blood by removing waste and infectious organisms.

3. Provides the primary source of antibodies in infants and children.

4. Produces lymphocytes, plasma cells, and antibodies in adults.

5. Produces erythrocytes in fetus.

6. Destroys erythrocytes when they reach the end of their life span.

Cardiovascular System Assessment

Patient History

A. Check for relevant signs and symptoms.

1. Pain.

a. Character.

b. Location.

c. Duration.

d. Intensity.

e. Precipitating, aggravating factors.

f. Relieving factors.

2. Respiratory problems.

a. Dyspnea—shortness of breath, feeling of inability to get enough air.

(1) Exertional dyspnea (DOE)—occurs while exercising.

(2) Paroxysmal nocturnal dyspnea (PND)—has sudden onset and interrupts patient's sleep.

b. Orthopnea—occurs while in recumbent position.

3. Fatigue.

4. Palpitations (heart feels like it's pounding).
5. Cerebral anoxia.
   a. Irritability.
   b. Restlessness.
   c. Confusion.
   d. Apprehension.
   e. Syncope.
6. Hemoptysis—coughing and spitting up of blood.
7. Edema—collection of fluid in interstitial spaces.
   a. Rales present in lungs.
   b. Ascites (abdominal cavity).
   c. Dependent (pedal).
8. Condition of extremities.
   a. Color.
   b. Temperature.
   c. Skin integrity.
   d. Presence of petechiae.
9. Syncope—transient loss of consciousness due to inadequate cerebral blood flow.
10. Neck vein distention.
11. Peripheral pulses.
    a. Presence or absence.
    b. Character.
    c. Rate.
12. Pulse deficit.
13. Blood pressure—lying, sitting and standing.
14. Lung sounds.
    a. Rales: fine, medium, coarse.
    b. Rhonchi: sibilant, sonorous.

B. Check for predisposing factors.
1. Hypertension.
2. Obesity.
3. Diabetes mellitus.
4. Hypercholesterolemia.
5. Smoking.
6. Sedentary life style.
7. Emotional stress.

DIAGNOSTIC PROCEDURES

A. Electrocardiogram—record of the heart's electrical activity as reflected by changes in electrical potential at skin level.

1. Purpose is to determine types and extent of heart damage, cardiac irregularities, and electrolyte imbalance.
2. Noninvasive and nonpainful, but procedure should be explained to patient.
3. Requires relaxation so as to reduce electrical interference from muscle movement.

B. Stress test—an electrocardiogram that is taken while the patient is exercising on a stationary bike or treadmill.
1. Purpose is to determine possible cardiac irregularities that may occur during exercise.
2. Test is monitored by physician.
3. Test is discontinued if electrocardiogram records change, if blood pressure increases, or if patient complains of angina.

C. Cardiac catheterization—insertion of a catheter into the heart and vessels surrounding the heart to examine one or both sides of the heart.
1. Purpose is to collect data such as pressure measurements of various chambers, blood oxygen measurement, cardiac output determination, and confirmation of the presence of coronary vessel disease.
2. Catheterization pathways.
   a. Right catheterization: venous system → superior vena cava → right atrium → right ventricle → pulmonary artery.
   b. Left catheterization: femoral artery → aorta → left atrium → left ventricle.
3. Possible complications/consequences.
   a. Fatigue, backache.
   b. Pain, bleeding, ecchymosis, swelling at insertion site.
   c. Thrombosis at insertion site.
      (1) Numbness, tingling, or coldness of extremity.
      (2) Loss of peripheral pulse.
   d. Arrhythmias with passage of catheters through ventricles, especially premature ventricular contraction and ventricular fibrillation.
   e. Perforation of heart (rare).
4. Nursing Care.
   a. Prior to procedure.
      (1) Give no food and fluids as ordered.

(2) Prep skin in areas of insertion site.

(3) Have patient rest quietly for three or more hours.

(4) Inform patient that there will be little or no pain, but that a fluttery sensation may be felt around heart as catheter is passed through vessels into heart.

   b. After the procedure.

(1) Provide bed rest for 12–24 hours as ordered.

(2) Take vital signs same as for any postop patient. Report blood pressure decreases of more than 10 percent or pulse increases of 10 percent.

(3) Check peripheral pulses distal to catheter insertion site (radial or pedal).

(4) Observe insertion sites for bleeding, swelling, infection, or thrombosis (pressure dressing may be in place).

(5) Elevate extremity if bleeding occurs.

(6) Instruct patient not to bend limb used for insertion site.

(7) Force fluids if not contraindicated.

(8) Observe for and report arrhythmias.

D. Routine chest films—for observation of silhouette of heart, chambers, and great vessels.

E. Fluoroscopy—examination of heart, lungs, and vessel movement as viewed on fluorescent screen in darkened room.

F. Coronary artery angiography—taking pictures of coronary circulation after injection of radiopaque dye.

G. Phonocardiogram—record produced by registering sounds produced by action of heart; sounds translated into electrical energy by a microphone.

H. Tests for serum enzymes levels.
1. Elevated following myocardial damage.
2. Serum enzyme studies include serum glutamic pyruvic transaminase (SGPT), lactic

dehydrogenase (LDH), and creatine phosphokinase (CPK), which is most definitive.

I. Echocardiography—records high frequency sound vibrations; assists in evaluating structures of the heart, dimensions of the chambers, and thickness of septum and walls.

J. Holter monitor—tape-recorded ambulatory electrocardiogram. Monitors cardiac cycle for 24 hours.

COMMON CARDIOVASCULAR DRUGS

Digitalis

A. Therapeutic effects.
1. Increases force of cardiac contraction.
2. Slows heart rate.
3. Slows conduction through AV node.
4. Increases automaticity which may cause many arrhythmias.

B. Used in congestive heart failure.
1. Increases contractility which reduces oxygen need.
2. Increases cardiac efficiency.
3. Reduces heart size.

C. Dosage individualized to patient and clinical situation (usually 0.25 mg qd).

D. Precautions.
1. Used with caution for patients with impaired renal or hepatic function.
2. Used with caution for patients with hypokalemia, which predisposes them to digitalis toxicity.

E. Side effects.
1. All types of cardiac arrhythmias.
2. Gastrointestinal effects.
   a. Anorexia.
   b. Nausea and vomiting.
   c. Diarrhea and/or constipation.
   d. Abdominal pain.
3. Central nervous system effects.
   a. Fatigue.
   b. Depression.

    c. Lethargy.

    d. Headache.

    e. Confusion, agitation.

  4. Ophthalmic effects.

    a. Disturbed color perception.

    b. Halos circling dark objects.

  5. Hypersensitivity.

    a. Pruritus.

    b. Urticaria.

F. Implications for nursing care.

  1. Take apical pulse for one full minute; notify physician if above 120 or below 60.

  2. Administer digitalis after meals to avoid gastric distress.

  3. Monitor for toxicity in the elderly as they are more sensitive to digitalis.

  4. Assist in designing instructional plan for patient.

    a. Drug action.

    b. Dosage.

    c. Keeping records.

    d. Method and timing for taking pulse.

  5. Store in tightly covered, light-resistant containers.

Calcium Blocking Agents

A. Therapeutic effects.

  1. Inhibits the influx of calcium ions across cell membrane.

  2. Decreases heart rate as conduction is slowed through SA and AV nodes.

  3. Increases myocardial oxygenation by causing coronary vasodilation.

  4. Decreases peripheral vascular resistance by causing vasodilation of peripheral arteries.

B. Used for angina, usually when beta blocker and nitrate therapy are not effective.

C. Drugs.

  1. Cardizem (diltiazem hydrochloride)—nausea, edema, arrhythmia, headache.

  2. Procardia (nifedipine)—vertigo, nausea, peripheral edema, headache, and flushing.

  3. Calan, Isoptin (verapamil hydrochloride)—hypotension, peripheral edema, vertigo. (Verapamil is also being used to treat supraventricular arrhythmias.)

Coronary Vasodilators

A. Therapeutic effects.

  1. Dilates vascular smooth vessels.

  2. Decreases peripheral arterial vascular resistance (afterload—calcium channel blockers and Apresoline).

  3. Decreases venous blood return to heart (preload—vasodilators, diuretics and digitalis drugs).

  4. Reduces myocardial oxygen consumption.

B. Used for angina.

C. Side effects.

  1. Flushed face.

  2. Headache.

  3. Vertigo and faintness.

  4. Postural hypotension.

D. Drugs.

  1. Short acting.

    a. IV—Tridil, Nitro-Bid, Nitrostat.

    b. Sublingual—nitroglycerin.

    c. Topical—Nitrol.

    d. Oral—Nitro-Bid.

  2. Long acting.

    a. Sublingual—Cardilate, Isordil.

    b. Oral—Peritrate, Sorbitrate.

    c. Topical disk—Nitrodisc, Nitro-Dur, Transderm-Nitro.

Antihypertensive Drugs

A. Therapeutic use—reduce blood pressure to normal or near normal without side effects.

B. Drugs.

  1. Thiazides—potentiates second drug when used in combination with other antihypertensive drugs.

  2. Hydralazine (Apresoline).

    a. Effect—adrenergic blocker.

    b. Side effects—headache, tachycardia, and postural hypotension.

  3. Methyldopa (Aldomet).

    a. Effect—decreases blood pressure.

    b. Side effects—postural hypotension.

  4. Ganglionic blocking agents—pentolinium tartrate (Ansolysen), mecamylamine (Inversine).

a. Effect: blocks parasympathetic and sympathetic ganglia.
b. Side effect: postural hypotension.
5. Postganglionic blocking agents—guanethidine (Ismelin).
a. Effect: blocks norepinephrine.
b. Side effect: postural hypotension.
6. Diazoxide (Hyperstat).
a. Effects: decreases peripheral vascular resistance in all circulatory beds; affects arterial smooth muscles.
b. Use: hypertensive crisis only.
c. Administration: IV, rapidly.
d. Side effects: hypotension (rarely severe), GI disturbances, angina, atrial and ventricular arrhythmias, palpitations, headache, hyperglycemia, fluid retention due to reabsorption of sodium, propranolol potentiates action.
7. Sodium nitroprusside (Nipride).
a. Effect: acts on vascular smooth muscle causing peripheral vasodilation. Effect occurs in two minutes but is transitory.
b. Administration: IV infusion.
c. Side effects: restlessness, agitation, muscle twitching, vomiting, or skin rash.
8. Captopril (Capoten).
a. Class of antihypertensive agents.
b. Effective for heart failure.
c. Works by suppressing the renin-angiotension-aldosterone system.
d. Serious adverse effects have been reported—must be used with discrimination under close medical supervision.
e. Warnings—proteinuria, agranulocytosis, hypotension.
C. Implications for nursing care.
1. May need to monitor blood pressure in lying, sitting, and standing position during dosage adjustment.
2. Observe for postural hypotension.
a. Change patient's position slowly.
b. Dangle patient's legs a few minutes before standing.
3. Monitor intake and output.
4. Weigh daily.

5. Encourage regular medical check-ups.

Diuretics

A. Therapeutic use—most diuretics block sodium and chloride reabsorption in ascending loop of Henle and distal tubule of the kidney and decrease ionic exchange of sodium in distal tubule, thereby excreting water.
B. Drugs.
1. Thiazides.
a. Common drugs—chlorothiazide (Diuril), hydrochlorothiazide (Hydrodiuril), chlorthalidone (Hygroton).
b. Administration—oral and parenteral.
c. Advantages—potent by mouth; effective antihypertensives.
d. Disadvantages or side effects—electrolyte imbalance; loss of potassium.
2. Potassium-sparing agents.
a. Common drugs—spironolactone (Aldactone), triamterene (Dyrenium).
b. Administration—oral only.
c. Advantages—conserve potassium.
d. Disadvantages—usually not effective when used alone (best used with thiazides), and electrolyte imbalance.
3. Potent diuretics.
a. Common preparations—furosemide (Lasix), ethacrynic acid (Edecrin).
b. Administration—oral and parenteral.
c. Advantages—rapid, potent action useful in cases of severe pulmonary edema and refractory edema.
d. Disadvantages—allergic reactions, severe electrolyte imbalance (potassium and chloride loss), and hypovolemia.
C. Implications for nursing care.
1. Time administration to avoid nocturia and sleep interruption.
2. Monitor intake and output.
3. Weigh daily.
4. Observe for postural hypotension.
5. Reduce potassium depletion by providing foods high in potassium (bananas, oranges).
6. Monitor for signs of fluid and electrolyte imbalance.

Anticoagulant Drugs

A. Heparin.
1. Therapeutic effects.
   a. Blocks conversion of prothrombin to thrombin and fibrinogen to fibrin.
   b. Prolongs clotting time.
2. Uses.
   a. Prophylaxis.
   b. Treatment of thrombi and emboli.
3. Dosage individualized according to patient's partial thromboplastin time.
4. Contraindications.
   a. Bleeding tendency.
   b. Severe liver or kidney disease.
   c. Following brain surgery.
5. Antagonist.
   a. Protamine sulfate.
   b. Effective within minutes.
6. Nursing care.
   a. Administer dosage ordered by physician according to patient's partial thromboplastin time (PTT at 50–80 seconds; normal is 39–53 seconds).
   b. Observe for any signs of bleeding in stools or urine or in emesis; report immediately.
   c. Utilize subcutaneous injection for administration.
      (1) Use lower abdominal skin area.
      (2) Do not pull back on plunger.
      (3) Do not massage area following injection.
   d. Observe for signs of toxicity.
      (1) Bruises or skin discoloration.
      (2) Frequent nosebleeds.
      (3) Hematuria.
   e. Instruct patient about precautions to take and observations to make when discharged.
B. Coumadin.
1. Therapeutic effects.
   a. Decreases prothrombin activity.
   b. Prevents utilization of vitamin K by the liver.
2. Uses.
   a. Oral use to decrease clotting activity.
   b. Takes 24 to 72 hours for action to develop and continues for 24 to 72 hours after last dose.
   c. Pro time kept at 18 to 30 seconds (normal is 12 to 14 seconds).
3. Antagonist.
   a. Vitamin K—aqua Mephyton IM or IV.
   b. Returns to hemostasis within six hours.
   c. Blocks action of Coumadin for one week.
4. Nursing care.
   a. Check pro time before giving.
   b. Give at same time each day.
   c. Teach patient to avoid foods high in vitamin K (cabbage, cauliflower, spinach, and leafy vegetables).

Antiarrhythmic Drugs

A. Therapeutic effects.
1. Increases recovery time of atrial and ventricular muscle.
2. Decreases myocardial excitability.
3. Increases conduction in cardiac muscle, Purkinje's fibers, and AV junction (exception: lidocaine).
4. Decreases contractility (exception: lidocaine).
5. Decreases automaticity.
B. Quinidine.
1. Uses—atrial fibrillation, atrial flutter, supraventricular and ventricular tachycardia, premature systoles.
2. Side effects.
   a. Hypersensitivity, thrombocytopenia.
   b. Cinchonism—nausea, vomiting, diarrhea, vertigo, visual disturbances, tinnitus.
   c. Sudden death from ventricular fibrillation.
   d. Congestive heart failure due to negative inotropism.
   e. Conduction disturbances.
C. Procainamide hydrochloride (Pronestyl).
1. Uses—premature ventricular systoles.
2. Side effects.
   a. Anorexia, nausea, vomiting, diarrhea.

b. Systemic lupus erythematosus and agranulocytosis.

c. Cardiac AV block.

D. Norpace.

1. Uses—premature ventricular contractions.

2. Side effects.

a. CNS—vertigo, syncope, fatigue.

b. CV—hypotension, edema, weight gain, SOB.

c. GI—nausea, vomiting, diarrhea.

d. GU—urinary retention.

E. Xylocaine (lidocaine).

1. Uses—ventricular tachyarrhythmias.

2. Side effects.

a. CNS disturbances—drowsiness, paresthesias, slurred speech, blurred vision, seizures, coma.

b. Cautious use in patients with liver disease or low cardiac output (metabolism of drug slowed).

Epinephrine (Adrenalin)

A. Effect: beta stimulation—increases heart rate and contractility.

B. Use: cardiac arrest most common.

Propanolol (Inderal)

A. Effect: blocks beta stimulation.

1. Decreases heart rate and contractility; that is, it decreases oxygen consumption.

2. Depresses automaticity of pacemakers and AV conduction.

3. Produces bronchoconstriction.

B. Uses.

1. Decreases ventricular rate from atrial flutter, fibrillation, and tachycardia.

2. Suppresses ectopic arrhythmias, especially ventricular arrhythmias.

3. Angina.

C. Side effects—should not be used in AV block, bradycardia, congestive heart failure, or lung disease (bronchospasm).

Atropine

A. Effects: anticholinergic.

1. Increases rate of SA node.

2. Increases conduction through AV node.

B. Uses.

1. Symptomatic sinus bradycardia.

2. Partial AV block.

C. Side effects.

1. Inability to void, especially with prostate enlargement.

2. Dry mouth, skin, flushing, dilation of pupil.

3. Decrease in bronchial secretions.

HEART DISORDERS

Coronary Artery Disease

Definition: Occurs as the result of accumulation of fatty materials (lipids, cholesterol being primary one), which narrows the lumen of coronary arteries. Clinical manifestations of disease reflect ischemia to myocardium, resulting from inadequate blood supply to meet metabolic demands.

Risk Factors

A. Diet—increased intake of cholesterol and saturated fats.

B. Hypertension—aggravates atherosclerotic process.

C. Cigarette smoking.

D. Diabetes mellitus—accelerates atherosclerotic process.

E. Lack of exercise; sedentary living.

F. Psychosocial tensions—may precipitate acute events.

G. Obesity—susceptibility to hypertension, diabetes mellitus, hyperlipidemia.

Assessment

A. Chest pain.

1. Angina, burning, squeezing, crushing tightness substernally or over precordial area.

2. May radiate down arms.

B. Nausea, vomiting.

C. Increased perspiration and cool extremities.

Treatment and Implementation

A. Monitor vital signs, particularly blood pressure and pulse.

B. Assist with EKG.

C. Administer nitrates if chest pain present (as ordered).

D. Evaluate chest pain—type, duration, relieved with medication.

E. Monitor breath sounds and signs of peripheral edema to detect early complications.

Angina

Definition: Severe chest pain due to temporary inability of coronary arteries to meet metabolic needs of myocardium. Pathophysiology involves narrowing of lumen of coronary artery, usually by atherosclerotic process. There is an interference with supply of oxygen to the heart.

Precipitating Factors

A. Exertion and effort.

B. Emotional upsets.

C. Tachyarrhythmias.

D. Overeating.

E. Extremes of temperature, especially cold.

F. Smoking.

Assessment

A. Pain.
  1. Location—precordial, substernal.
  2. Character—compressing, choking, burning, squeezing, crushing and heaviness.
  3. Radiation—left or right arm, jaw, neck, back.
  4. Duration—usually five to ten minutes; relieved by rest or nitroglycerin.

B. Dyspnea.

C. ECG changes; may not be evident at rest.

D. There are no physical signs 90 percent of the time.

Implementation

A. Instruct patient how to reduce frequency of attacks.
  1. Learn to live with moderation; physical activity should be sufficient to maintain general physical state, but short of causing angina.
  2. Avoid stress and emotional upset.
  3. Reduce caloric intake if overweight.
  4. Refrain from smoking.
  5. Decrease use of stimulants, e.g., coffee, tea, cola.
  6. Avoid heavy meals.
  7. Avoid extremes of temperature, especially cold.

B. Primary medication—nitroglycerin.
  1. Drug action.
     a. Dilates coronary arteries that are not atherosclerotic.
     b. Enhances blood flow to myocardium without increasing oxygen consumption.
  2. Use of drug is to relieve pain from myocardia ischemia.
  3. Side effects—hypotension, headache.
  4. Important considerations.
     a. Effective only sublingually.
     b. Dosage of one to two tablets may be repeated at five-minute intervals.
     c. Physician should be called if no relief in 15 minutes.
     d. No limit to number that may be taken in 24 hour period.
     e. Is not addictive.
     f. May be used prophylactically before engaging in activity known to precipitate angina.
     g. Avoid alcohol consumption with drug.
     h. Must be stored in closed, dark glass container to avoid light, heat, and moisture. Has only six-month shelf-life.

C. Instruct patient in use of nitroglycerin ointment. ❖ **PROCEDURE** ❖
  1. Apply directly to skin.

2. Wash off remaining ointment before new application.
3. Change skin placement with each application.

D. Other medications used.
  1. Long-acting nitrites (Isordil, Cardilate).
  2. Beta-blocker: propranolol (Inderal).
  3. Calcium blocking agents (Calan, Cardizem).

E. If medications ineffective, may require coronary artery bypass surgery.

Myocardial Infarction

Definition: Formation of destroyed tissue in cardiac muscle due to interruption of or insufficient blood supply for a prolonged period, resulting in sustained oxygen deprivation.

Etiology

A. Atherosclerotic heart disease.
B. Coronary artery embolism.
C. Decreased blood flow with shock and/or hemorrhage.
D. Direct trauma.

Assessment

A. Pain that is similar to angina but is usually more intense and has longer duration (30 minutes or longer).
  1. Location—left precordial, substernal.
  2. Character—crushing, viselike, tightening and burning.
  3. Radiation—jaw, back, arms.
B. Feeling of apprehension or doom.
C. Dyspnea or orthopnea.
D. Nausea and vomiting.
E. Diaphoresis.
F. Pallor or cyanosis.
G. Arrhythmias.
H. Signs of congestive heart failure.

Diagnosis

A. History (very important).
B. ECG changes.
C. Laboratory studies—serum enzymes (SGPT, LDH, CPK) released with death of tissue.
  1. CPK—isoenzymes, level rises in six hours—most valuable measurement.
  2. LDH—LDH_2, level rises in 6–8 hours.
D. Increase of white cell count.
E. Increased sedimentation rate.

Treatment and Implementation

A. Death-producing arrhythmias treated immediately with lidocaine.
B. IV or IM narcotic analgesics, as ordered, to relieve pain and anxiety.
C. Cardiac rhythm monitored continuously.
D. Lidocaine drip monitored.
E. Oxygen via cannula.
F. Monitored closely for signs of CHF (seen within first 24 hours).
G. IV nitroglycerin drip.
H. Swan-Ganz catheter with PAWP and CO readings.
I. Nursing care.
  1. Administer narcotic analgesics to relieve pain and anxiety.
  2. Administer oxygen with cannula.
  3. Observe for arrhythmias.
  4. Monitor vital signs, urine output.
  5. Observe for signs of congestive heart failure.
  6. Provide physical rest and emotional support.
    a. Sedation, graduated activity.
    b. Use of commode and self-feed.
  7. Maintain patient on stool softeners and soft diet to prevent increased workload on heart and prevent Valsalva maneuver.
  8. Provide low-fat, low-cholesterol, low-sodium diet.
  9. Rehabilitate patient to enable him to return to physical level according to cardiac capability.
    a. Plan exercise program.

b. Provide psychological support.

c. Avoid stressful environment.

d. Consider possible change of life style.

J. Rehabilitation: encourage patient to participate in organized cardiac rehabilitation program. Program usually consists of

1. Monitored exercise program based on METs.

2. Stress reduction classes.

3. Alterations in nutrition.

4. Sex counseling.

Complications

A. Arrhythmias.

B. Congestive heart failure.

C. Cariogenic shock.

D. Thrombophlebitis.

E. Pericarditis.

F. Ventricular aneurysm or rupture (late complication) due to weakened area of myocardium as result of myocardial infarction.

Heart Valve Stenosis

Definition: A progressive thickening of the valve cusps that results in the narrowing of the lumen of the valve opening.

Assessment

A. Predisposing factors.

1. History of congenital heart disease.

2. Rheumatic heart disease.

3. Arteriosclerosis.

B. May be asymptomatic.

C. May evidence mild symptoms.

1. Decreased cardiac output—tired and lethargic.

2. Dizziness and syncope.

3. Angina.

Implementation

A. Treat heart failure and arrhythmias.

B. Decrease cardiac workload.

C. Prevent and/or treat infections.

D. Monitor administration of anticoagulants for treatment and/or prevention of thrombi.

E. Provide emotional support.

F. Prepare patient for valvotomy if no calcification of valve or for surgical replacement of the valve.

G. Complications.

1. Atrial fibrillation.

2. Subacute bacterial endocarditis.

3. Thrombi formation.

4. Heart failure.

Congestive Heart Failure

Definition: A group of symptoms, not a disease, which results from decreased pumping effectiveness of the heart. Circulatory congestion occurs in response to the decreased or inadequate cardiac output.

Types of Heart Failure

A. Left heart failure—congestion occurs mainly in the lungs due to inadequate ejection of the blood into the systemic circulation.

B. Right heart failure—congestion occurs systemically due to inadequate pumping of the blood from the systemic circulation into the lungs.

Pathophysiology

A. Left heart failure.

1. Damage to myocardium of the left ventricle.

2. Left ventricle unable to pump adequate amount of blood; pressure increases in pulmonary vessels.

3. Backflow of blood into the lungs causes pulmonary congestion.

4. Symptoms are pulmonic in nature.

B. Right heart failure.

1. Increased pulmonary pressure.

2. Right ventricle unable to effectively pump blood to lungs.

3. Right side of heart becomes congested with blood.
4. Venous blood returning to right heart cannot be pumped quickly and efficiently.
5. Congestion of blood develops in the large veins leading to the right heart and, eventually, in the organs and tissues of the body.
6. Symptoms are systemic in nature.

Assessment of Left Heart Failure

A. Fatigue and weakness.
B. Dyspnea—orthopnea, PND, DOE.
C. Anxiety, apprehension, irritability, confusion, restlessness.
D. Cough—may be associated with blood-tinged, frothy sputum.
E. Wheezing.
F. Rales.
G. Cyanosis or pallor.
H. Arrhythmias.
I. Diaphoresis.

Assessment of Right Heart Failure

A. Peripheral edema in dependent parts—feet and legs; sacrum, back, buttocks.
B. Ascites.
C. Nausea, vomiting, anorexia.
D. Weight gain.
E. Hepatomegaly, liver congestion.
F. Oliguria during day; polyuria at night.
G. Arrhythmias.
H. Increased central venous pressure.
I. Jugular vein distention.

Implementation

A. Treat underlying cause.
B. Reduce pain and anxiety.
   1. Morphine sulfate.
   2. Physical and emotional rest.
C. Administer oxygen therapy as ordered; use cannula rather than mask because patient already feels he or she cannot breathe.

D. Reduce water and sodium retention.
   1. Diuretics.
   2. Restrict fluid intake.
   3. Moderate sodium restriction—1.5–2 gms.
   4. Bed rest in Fowler's position.
   5. Intake and output measure.
   6. Weigh daily.
   7. Special skin care to edematous areas.
E. Administer digitalis—increases strength of contraction and decreases rate.
F. Observe for arrhythmias.
G. Provide emotional support.
H. Instruct patient in principles of care.

Complications

A. Digitalis toxicity.
B. Electrolyte imbalance (especially hypokalemia) from diuretics.
C. Pulmonary embolism from bed rest.
D. Oxygen toxicity, especially COPD patients.
E. Acute pulmonary edema.

Acute Pulmonary Edema

Definition: An excessive quantity of fluid in the pulmonary interstitial spaces or in the alveoli usually following severe left ventricular decompensation.

Characteristics

A. The most common cause is greatly elevated capillary pressure resulting from failure of left heart and damming of blood in lungs.
B. Alveoli filled with fluid and bronchioles congested.
C. Retention of fluid resulting from reduced renal function.

Assessment

A. Moist rales and frothy sputum.
B. Severe anxiety, feelings of impending doom.
C. Marked dyspnea.

D. Stertorous breathing.

E. Marked cyanosis.

F. Profuse diaphoresis—cold and clammy.

G. Blood pressure and pulse changes.

Implementation

A. Place in high-Fowler's position.

B. Administer oxygen at 6 l/min if patient does not have COPD.

C. Administer medications (diuretics and digitalis) to improve myocardial contractility and reduce pulmonary and systemic blood volume.

D. Instruct patient in deep breathing and coughing exercises.

E. Monitor fluid intake and output, weigh daily.

F. Monitor vital signs.

G. Provide sedation with ordered medication. Observe respiratory rate and depth.

H. Administer drug therapy as ordered: nitroglycerin, nitroprusside, hydralazine.

I. Assist with rotating tourniquets on patient's extremities if ordered.
   1. Purpose.
      a. Reduce venous return to heart.
      b. Pool blood temporarily in extremities.
      c. Treatment for pulmonary edema.
   2. Complete procedure. ❖ **PROCEDURE** ❖
      a. Take blood pressure to determine midway between systolic and diastolic reading.
      b. Apply four pressure cuffs high up on all four extremities.
      c. Inflate three cuffs to pressure midway between systolic and diastolic pressure.
      d. Rotate the tourniquets every 15 minutes, using clockwise rotation.
      e. Release one tourniquet and then inflate the next tourniquet.
      f. Observe for presence of arterial blood flow by checking peripheral pulses. Arterial pulses should be present, venous pulses absent.
      g. Take frequent blood pressure readings to readjust cuff pressure.

h. Continue treatment for prescribed time, usually when diuretic has adequately functioned and signs of pulmonary edema lessened.

i. Discontinue tourniquets one at a time, continuing the cuff deflation in clockwise manner, and every 15 minutes.

Pacemaker Insertion

Definition: A temporary or permanent device to initiate and maintain heart rate when patient's pacemaker is nonfunctioning.

Conditions Requiring Pacemakers

A. Conduction defect following open heart surgery.

B. Heart block (usually third degree).

C. Tachyarrhythmias.

D. Stokes-Adams syndrome.

E. Bradyarrhythmias.

Types of Pacemakers

A. Demand—functions only if patient's own pacemaker fails to discharge.
   1. The pacemaker is set at a fixed rate and will discharge only if patient's own rate falls below it.
   2. Used mainly in Adams-Stokes or bradyarrhythmias or following cardiac surgery.

B. Asynchronous.
   1. Fixed rate—the pacemaker is set at a fixed rate and will fire regardless of patient's own rhythm.
   2. Variable rate—rate can be varied.

Pacemaker Placement

A. Epicardial.
   1. Electrodes are implanted on outside of left ventricle, and they barely penetrate myocardium.
   2. Battery pack is placed subcutaneously in a skin pocket.

B. Endocardial implantation—pacing electrode inserted through neck vein and placed near apex of right ventricle.
1. Permanent—battery is implanted beneath skin.
2. Temporary—battery is located outside of skin.

Implementation

A. Preplacement.
1. Assess vital signs for baseline data.
2. Evaluate heart sounds to determine arrhythmias for baseline data.
3. Assess lung sounds.
B. Postplacement.
1. Observe for battery failure (pacemaker not firing as set).
   a. Faints easily.
   b. Hiccoughs.
   c. Rhythm change.
2. Observe for hematoma at site of insertion.
3. Observe for arrhythmias.
4. Monitor vital signs.
5. Observe for pacemaker failure.
   a. Decreased urine output.
   b. EKG pattern changes.
   c. Decreased blood pressure.
   d. Cyanosis.
   e. Shortness of breath.
6. Check for complications.
   a. Hemorrhage and shock.
   b. Infection.

Inflammatory Diseases of the Heart

Definition: Conditions in which various microorganisms cause infection and inflammation of the structures of the heart. Damage to the valves of the heart is among the most serious consequences of inflammatory heart disease.

Types

A. Bacterial endocarditis—an infection of the lining of the heart.

B. Pericarditis—inflammation of the pericardium.
C. Myocarditis—inflammation of the muscle of the heart walls.
D. Rheumatic fever—a systemic disease of connective tissue which may involve the endocardium, myocardium, and pericardium.
E. Rheumatic heart disease—a chronic cardiac condition which usually follows one or more episodes of rheumatic fever with valvular damage.

Assessment

A. Signs of infection.
1. Fever.
2. Chills.
3. Diaphoresis.
4. Lassitude.
5. Anorexia.
B. Tachycardia.
C. Chest pain.
D. Dyspnea.

Implementation

A. Administer specific antibiotic therapy as ordered.
B. Provide bed rest.
C. Administer salicylates.
D. Provide adequate nutrition.

Complications

A. Mitral stenosis—progressive thickening of the valve cusps which results in the narrowing of lumen of mitral valve.
B. Mitral insufficiency—distortion of the valve that allows backward flow of blood from ventricle to atrium.
C. Aortic stenosis—narrowing of the aortic valve opening due to fibrosis and calcification.
D. Aortic insufficiency—occurrence of blood flow back into the ventricle from aorta.
E. Tricuspid stenosis—progressive narrowing of tricuspid valve lumen.

F. Tricuspid insufficiency—occurrence of blood flow back into atrium from ventricle.

PERIPHERAL VASCULAR DISORDERS

Hypertension

Definition: Sustained elevation of arterial pressure with systolic pressure greater than 140 mmHg and diastolic pressure greater than 90 mmHg. (35 million people have this disease in U.S.)

Types

A. Primary or essential—no known etiology (accounts for 85–90 percent).
B. Secondary hypertension—etiology (accounts for 5–10 percent).
   1. Renal disease.
   2. Endocrine disorders.
      a. Pheochromocytoma (adrenal tumor).
      b. Adrenal cortex lesions—aldosteronism, Cushing's syndrome.
   3. Toxemia of pregnancy.
   4. Increased intracranial pressure.
   5. Congenital heart disease.
   6. Increased workload of the heart.
      a. Congestive heart failure.
      b. Myocardial infarction.

Assessment

A. Asymptomatic in early stage.
B. Risk factors: age; race (two times more frequent in blacks); obesity; sex; stress.
C. Common symptoms.
   1. Headache, dizziness, tinnitus.
   2. Fatigue, insomnia.
   3. Epistaxis, blurred vision, spots before eyes.
D. Identify if target organ involvement is present.

   1. Eyes—narrowing of arteries, papilledema (malignant hypertension), visual disturbances.
   2. Brain—mental and neurologic abnormalities, encephalopathy, CVA.
   3. Cardiovascular system—left ventricular hypertrophy and failure, angina, aggravation and acceleration of atherosclerotic process in coronary arteries and peripheral vessels.
   4. Kidneys—renal failure.

Implementation

A. Treat causes of secondary hypertension.
B. Diet.
   1. Decrease sodium intake.
   2. Decrease calorie intake if overweight.
C. Drug therapy.
   1. Diuretics.
      a. Thiazides (Diuril, Esidrix, Enduron).
      b. Potassium sparing (Aldactone).
      c. Loop—potent diuretics (Lasix, Edecrin).
   2. Antihypertensives (Inderal, Aldomet, Catapres, Ismelin).
   3. Vasodilators—(Apresoline, Vasodilan).
D. Exercise—moderate; may increase when weight is reduced.
E. Help to relieve patient's environmental stress and anxiety.
F. Emphasize to patient the importance of following medical treatment regimen.
   1. Weight control.
   2. Low-sodium diet.
   3. Change in life style.
   4. Periodic medical checkups.

Thromboangiitis Obliterans (Buerger's Disease)

Definition: Chronic inflammation of arteries and veins, and secondarily, inflammation of nerves.

Assessment

A. Pain, temperature, and color changes (cyanosis); alterations in skin of lower extremities at rest and especially after exercise.

B. Intermittent calf claudication—severe calf cramping following exercise; relieved upon resting.

C. Decreased pulse rates.

D. Complications of swelling, ulceration, gangrene.

Treatment and Implementation

A. Cessation of smoking.

B. Bilateral sympathectomy.

C. Reduction of pain.

Raynaud's Disease

Definition: A vasospastic condition of arteries that occurs with exposure to cold or to strong emotion and affects fingers, toes, ears, nose, and cheeks.

Assessment

A. Raynaud's Disease—intermittent arteriolar vasoconstriction evidenced by pain or coldness; bilateral or symmetric numbness.

B. Raynaud's Phenomena—Intermittent pallor, cyanosis, rubor, and changes in skin temperature from cold or strong emotion; may be unilateral.

Implementation

A. Encourage patient to stop smoking—increases vasoconstriction.

B. Vasodilator drugs—calcium channel blocker—nifedipine (Procardia). Causes coronary vasodilation by increasing myocardial oxygenation.

C. Encourage patient to avoid precipitating factors such as cold temperature and emotional stress.

D. Wear warm clothing when in cold weather: boots, gloves, etc.

Deep Vein Thrombophlebitis

Definition: Formation of a clot in a vein—occurs most often in left leg.

Precipitating Causes

A. Stagnation of blood flow such as occurs from bed rest.

B. Change in clotting of blood.

C. Change in lining of blood vessel (trauma).

Assessment

A. In superficial vein.
   1. Vein hard to the touch.
   2. Skin reddened, hot, tender.

B. In deep vein.
   1. Affected area swollen, tender.
   2. Increased temperature, pulse, and white blood count.

C. Palpate peripheral pulses—presence of Homan's sign.

Implementation

A. Take preventive measures.
   1. Exercise.
   2. Nonconstrictive clothing.
   3. Foot-board walking.
   4. No "gatching" of bed.
   5. No pillow under knees.
   6. No calf massage.
   7. Adequate hydration.

B. Maintain strict bedrest 7–10 days.

C. Ensure proper fitting of elastic stockings.

D. Elevate affected limb slightly.

E. Administer anticoagulant drug therapy as ordered—check lab values before giving drug.

F. Apply heat to affected area if ordered.

Varicose Veins

Definition: A condition in which the veins are dilated because of incompetent valves.

A. Pregnancy.
B. Standing for long periods of time.
C. Poor venous return.
D. Heredity.
E. Obesity.
F. Poor posture.

Assessment

A. Aching of legs.
B. Swelling of ankles.
C. Browning of skin from blood which has escaped from overloaded veins.
D. Ulceration.

Implementation

A. Prevention.
B. Elevation of legs; wearing of nonconstrictive clothing and elastic stockings.
C. Surgery—vein ligation, stripping.

Nursing Care for Peripheral Vascular Problems

A. Limit disease and prevent complications.
B. Maintain adequate blood supply to affected areas.
   1. Warmth.
   2. Cleanliness.
   3. Infection control.
   4. Avoidance of heat and cold extremes.
C. Encourage patient to stop smoking.
D. Have patient wear nonconstrictive clothing and use body positions which protect affected areas from pressure.
E. Avoid emotional stress.
F. Teach patient to recognize an increase or extension of symptoms.
   1. Increase of pain in extremities.
   2. Changes in skin color.
   3. Ulceration.
   4. Change of temperature in extremities.

G. Lead patient to recognize limitations caused by disease.

Vein Stripping and Ligation

Definition: The ligation and removal of affected veins in the legs. Usually affects greater and lesser saphenous veins.

Preparation

A. Have patient scrub legs and lower abdomen once a day for three days prior to surgery.
B. Instruct on ambulation postoperatively.
C. Check that completion of preoperative scrub is done.
D. Observe for physician's marks on veins.
E. Take pulses for baseline data.

Implementation

A. Observe feet for edema, warmth, color (tight elastic bandages applied following surgery can impede circulation).
B. Take peripheral pulses.
C. Elevate feet above level of heart.
D. Position flat in bed or have patient walk. Do not allow to dangle legs or sit in a chair for at least one week.
E. Ambulate early—five minutes every hour.
F. Following bandage removal, utilize elastic stockings.

DISEASES OF THE BLOOD AND BLOOD FORMING ORGANS

Pernicious Anemia

Definition: A chronic and, if untreated, progressive anemia caused by the failure of gastric mucosa to provide an intrinsic factor essential for absorption of vitamin B_{12}.

Characteristics

A. Causes
1. Total gastrectomy.
2. Surgical resection of small intestine.
3. Atrophy of gastric mucosa.
4. Malabsorption disease—sprue.
5. Bacterial or parasitic infections.
B. May be autoimmune difficulty.
C. Genetic predisposition (especially in northern Europe).
D. Diagnostic tests.
1. RBC count megaloblastic maturation.
2. Bone marrow aspiration.
3. Upper GI series.
4. Schilling test (maintain NPO for 12 hours; collect 24-hour urine).
5. Gastric analysis—insertion of nasogastric tube, collection of aspirant, injection of histamine.

Assessment

A. Weakness, unsteady gait.
B. Dyspnea.
C. Palpitation, tachycardia.
D. Anorexia, dyspepsia.
E. Diarrhea.
F. Numbness and tingling of extremities.
G. Pallor, slight jaundice.
H. Glossitis.
I. Mild hepatomegaly (enlarged liver).
J. Splenomegaly (enlarged spleen).

Treatment and Implementation

A. Provide safety measures if neurological deficit is present—assist with ambulation.
B. Avoid pressure on lower extremities due to circulation deficit (foot cradle, etc).
C. Avoid extremes of heat and cold.
D. Administer B_{12} deep IM, as ordered.
E. Instruct in administration of B_{12}. This is a life-long therapy.
F. Provide support and explain behavior changes to patient and family.

Aplastic Anemia

Definition: Deficiency of circulating RBCs resulting from bone marrow suppression.

Characteristics

A. Causes.
1. Toxic action of drugs (Chloromycetin, sulfonarnides, Dilantin, alkylating agents, and antimetabolites).
2. Exposure to radiation.
3. Diseases that suppress bone marrow activity (leukemia and metastic cancer).
B. Pancytopenia frequently accompanies RBC deficiency.

Assessment

A. Increased fatigue.
B. Lethargy.
C. Dyspnea.
D. Cutaneous bleeding.
E. Low platelet and leukocyte count.

Treatment and Implementation

A. Medical treatment.
1. Bone marrow transplant and WBC transfusion are becoming more prevalent.
2. Splenectomy (especially in severe thrombocytopenia).
B. Administer androgens and/or corticosteroids as ordered.
C. Monitor transfusion of fresh platelets (RBC transfusion may be introduced also).
D. Administer antibiotics when infection occurs.
E. Carry out reverse isolation procedure.
F. Protect from infections.
G. Provide for adequate rest periods.
H. Observe for complications.
I. Provide physical comfort measures.
J. Provide emotional support for patient and family, especially while in isolation.
K. Educate public in use of toxic pesticides and chemicals.

Purpuras

Definition: The extravasation of blood into the tissues and mucous membranes.

Characteristics

A. Idiopathic thrombocytopenic purpura is characterized by platelet deficiency.
B. Vascular purpura is characterized by weak, damaged vessels, which rupture easily.

Assessment

A. Petechiae.
B. Postsurgical bleeding.
C. Increased bleeding time.
D. Abnormal platelet count.
E. Ecchymosis.

Treatment and Implementation

A. Identify underlying cause if possible.
B. Complete steps to control bleeding.
C. Monitor transfusion of platelets.
D. Monitor administration of corticosteroids.

Agranulocytosis

Definition: An acute, potentially fatal blood disorder characterized by profound neutropenia and most commonly caused by drug toxicity or hypersensitivity.

Assessment

A. Chills and fever.
B. Sore throat.
C. Exhaustion and depletion of energy.
D. Ulceration of oral mucosa and throat.

Implementation

A. Discontinue suspected chemical agents or drugs.
B. Isolate to reduce exposure to infections.

C. Administer corticosteroids if ordered.

Polycythemia Vera

Definition: A chronic disease of unknown etiology characterized by overactivity of bone marrow with overproduction of red cells and hemoglobin.

Assessment

A. Reddish-purple hue to the skin.
B. Increased blood volume.
C. Capillary engorgement.
D. Hemorrhage.
E. Venous thrombosis.
F. Arterial hypertension.
G. Hepatomegaly and splenomegaly.

Treatment and Implementation

A. Radiophosphorus in dosages based on body weight; initially IV, then orally.
B. Phlebotomy to remove 500–2000 ml of blood per week until hematocrit reaches 50 percent; repeated when hematocrit rises.

Leukemia

Definition: A disorder of blood-forming tissue characterized by proliferation of one type of white blood cell (granulocyte, lymphocyte, or monocyte), occurring in all races and developing at any age.

Characteristics

A. Increased proliferation process alters cell's ability to mature and/or function properly.
B. Forms of leukemia.
   1. Acute myelogenous leukemia (AML).
      a. Platelet deficiency, anemia present.
      b. Occurs usually after age 40.
   2. Chronic myelocytic leukemia (CML).
      a. Increase in granulocytes and platelet cells.

b. Disease of young adults—may be genetic.
3. Chronic lymphocytic leukemia (CLL).
   a. Decreased production of hematopoietic cells.
   b. Most common after age 50.
4. Acute lymphocytic leukemia (ALL).
   a. Lymphoblast cells increase and other blood cells are reduced.
   b. Appears before age 15; highest incidence in 3 to 4 year olds.

Assessment

A. Diagnostic tests: bone marrow aspiration and differential blood count.
B. Poor appetite; generalized discomfort.
C. Ulceration of the mouth and pharynx.
D. High fever.
E. Diarrhea.
F. Severe infection, e.g., pneumonia and septicemia.
G. Anemia with fatigue, lethargy, weakness, hypoxia, and pallor.
H. Bleeding gums, ecchymosis, and petechiae.
I. Splenomegaly, hepatomegaly, and lymphadenopathy.
J. Headache, disorientation, and convulsions.

Treatment and Implementation

A. Chemotherapeutic drugs, e.g., Methotrexate, Cytoxan, Lukeran.
B. Blood transfusions as required.
C. Steroids, such as prednisone, to decrease symptoms.
D. High calorie, high vitamin diet.
E. Prevent infections, ulcerations.

Hodgkin's Disease

Definition: A chronic, progressive, neoplastic, invariably fatal disease of unknown etiology, involving the lymphoid tissues of the body. It is most common between the ages of 20 and 40.

Signs and Symptoms

A. Painless enlargement of the lymph nodes.
B. Severe pruritus.
C. Irregular fever.
D. Splenomegaly and hepatomegaly.
E. Jaundice.
F. Edema and cyanosis of the face and neck.
G. Pulmonary symptoms including dyspnea, cough, chest pain, cyanosis, and pleural effusion.
H. Progressive anemia with resultant fatigue, malaise, and anorexia.
I. Bone pain and vertebral compression.
J. Nerve pain and paraplegia.
K. Laryngeal paralysis.
L. Increased susceptibility to infection.
M. Progresses in stages.
   1. Stage I: disease is restricted to single anatomic site, or is localized in a group of lymph nodes; asymptomatic.
   2. Stage II(a): two or three adjacent lymph nodes in the area on the same side of the diaphragm are affected.
   3. Stage II(b): symptoms appear.
   4. Stage III: disease is widely disseminated on both sides of diaphragm into the lymph areas and organs.
   5. Stage IV: involvement of bone, bone marrow, pleura, liver, skin, gastrointestinal tract, central nervous system, and gradually the entire body.

Treatment and Implementation

A. Radiation is used for stages I, II, and III in an effort to eradicate the disease.
B. Wide-field megavoltage radiation with doses of 3500 to 4000 roentgens over a four- to six-week period.
C. Chemotherapy with Cytoxan, nitrogen mustard, thiotepa, TEM, Velban, Oncovin, prednisone, and Matulane.
D. Diagnostic laparotomy.
E. Nursing care is supportive.
   1. Provide supportive relief from effects of radiation and chemotherapy.

a. Side effects include nausea and vomiting.
b. Controlled by premedication of sedatives and antiemetic agents.
2. Assist patient to maintain as normal a life as possible during course and treatment of disease.
3. Prevent infection as body's resistance is lowered.
4. Continually observe for complications: pressure from enlargement of lymph glands on vital organs.

Rupture of the Spleen

Definition: Traumatic bursting following violent blow or trauma to the spleen.

Assessment

A. Weakness due to blood loss.
B. Abdominal pain and muscle spasm particularly in the left upper quadrant.
C. Depression of abdominal bleeding.
D. Rebound tenderness.
E. Referred pain to left shoulder.
F. Palpable tenderness.
G. Leukocytosis well over 12,000.
H. Progressive shock with rapid, thready pulse; drop in blood pressure; and pallor.

Treatment

Splenectomy.

AUTOIMMUNE DISORDERS

Acquired Immunodeficiency Syndrome (AIDS)

Definition: Acquired immune deficiency diseases linked to HIV. A retrovirus, it primarily affects the helper T cells causing the immune system to collapse.

Characteristics

A. Specific etiology is unknown.
B. Risk factors.
   1. IV drug abusers.
   2. Homosexual males with multiple sexual partners.
   3. Hemophiliacs.
C. Incubation period may be as long as eight to ten years.
D. Individuals may have antibodies and be carriers but not exhibit AIDS.
E. Some individuals exhibit a mild version of immune system depression.
F. Transmission of virus is known to be through body fluids such as semen and blood products.
G. Disease is known to be lethal in a high proportion of persons, especially those with Kaposi's sarcoma.

Assessment

A. Initial symptoms indicative of syndrome onset.
   1. Weight loss, anorexia.
   2. Elevated temperature.
   3. Lymphadenopathy.
   4. Malaise.
   5. Dry, productive cough.
   6. Acute onset presents with overwhelming infection.
B. Lungs exhibit adventitious sounds (Pneumocystis carinii).
C. Purple lesions on skin (Kaposi's sarcoma).
D. Mucous membranes of mouth have fungus from candida albicans and ulcerating infections.

Implementation

A. Treatment is symptomatic or approved drugs: AZT or DDI.
B. Provide good skin care to prevent breakdown.
C. Provide respiratory care: turn, cough and deep breathe.
D. Place on secretion precaution.
E. Provide pain control.

F. Provide supportive care for patient who develops Pneumocystosis (an acute pneumonia caused by pneumocystis carinii).
   1. Disease occurs in about 60 percent of AIDS patients and is a major cause of death.
   2. There is an abrupt onset with fever, tachycardia, severe hypoxemia, and uncompensated respiratory alkalosis.

General Nursing Care Principles for Blood Disorders

Infections

A. Institute reverse isolation and meticulous medical asepsis.
B. Provide bed rest.
C. Provide protein, high vitamin, and high caloric diet.
D. Administer antibiotics as ordered.

Fatigue and Weakness

A. Conserve the patient's strength.
B. Provide frequent rest periods.
C. Institute ambulation activities as tolerated.
D. Decrease disturbing activities and noise.
E. Provide optimal nutrition.

Ulcerative Lesions

A. Provide nonirritating foods and beverages.
B. Provide frequent oral hygiene with mild, cool mouthwash and solutions.
C. Use applicators or soft-bristled toothbrush.
D. Lubricate the lips.
E. Give mouth care both before and after meals.

Dyspnea

A. Elevate the head of the bed.
B. Support the patient in the orthopneic position.
C. Administer oxygen when indicated.

D. Prevent unnecessary exertion.
E. Avoid gas-forming foods.

Bone and Joint Pains

A. Use cradle to relieve pressure of bedding.
B. Apply hot or cold compresses as ordered.
C. Immobilize joints when ordered.

Fever

A. Apply cool sponges.
B. Administer antipyretic drugs as ordered.
C. Encourage fluid intake unless contraindicated.
D. Maintain a cool environmental temperature.

Pruritus and/or Skin Eruptions

A. Keep patient's fingernails short.
B. Use soap sparingly, if at all.
C. Apply emollient lotions in skin care.

Anxiety

A. Explain the nature, the discomforts, and the limitations of activity associated with the diagnostic procedures and treatments.
B. Listen to the patient.
C. Treat the patient as an individual.
D. Allow the family to participate in the patient's care.
E. Encourage the family to visit with the patient; provide privacy for the family and patient.

RESPIRATORY SYSTEM

The respiratory system is a group of related organs that together perform pulmonary ventilation. The act of breathing involves an osmotic and chemical process by which the body takes in oxygen from the atmosphere and gives off end products, mainly carbon dioxide, formed by oxidation in the alveolar tissues.

ANATOMY AND PHYSIOLOGY

Ventilation Tract

Nose

A. Structure.
   1. Septum divides nose into two cavities.
   2. Ciliated mucous membrane lines the cavities.
   3. Four pairs of sinuses drain into nose.
B. Function.
   1. Serves as passage for air.
      a. Filters.
      b. Warms.
      c. Moistens.
   2. Serves as organ of smell.
   3. Aids in phonation.

Pharynx

A. Structure.
   1. Tubelike structure.
   2. Composed of muscle.
   3. Ciliated mucous membrane lines the cavity.
   4. Divides into three areas.
      a. Nasopharynx—contains adenoids.
      b. Oropharynx—contains tonsils.
      c. Laryngopharynx.
B. Function.
   1. Serves as passage for air and food.
   2. Aids in phonation.

Larynx

A. Structure.
   1. Composed largely of cartilage held together by muscles.
   2. Major cartilages.
      a. Thyroid (forms Adam's apple).
      b. Epiglottis.
      c. Cricoid.
   3. Ciliated mucous membrane lines the structure.
   4. Contains vocal cords.
B. Function.
   1. Passage for air.
   2. Produces sound.

Trachea

A. Structure.
   1. Cylindrical structure.
   2. Walls consist of smooth muscle and C-shaped rings of cartilage.
   3. Divides at lower end into two primary bronchi.
B. Function—passage for air.

Pulmonic Organs

Lungs

A. Structure.
   1. Medial surface is roughly concave to allow room for mediastinal structures.
   2. Bronchi enter through slits (hili) in each lung.
   3. Left lung is partially divided by fissures into two lobes (upper and lower).
   4. Right lung is partially divided by fissures into three lobes (upper, middle, and lower).
   5. Visceral pleura covers outer surfaces.
   6. Interior consists of bronchial tree.
B. Function.
   1. Distribute air to alveoli.
   2. Exchange gas between air and blood.

Bronchi

A. Structure.
1. Right mainstem bronchus (RMSB)—slightly larger and more vertical than left bronchus; most frequent route for aspirated materials.
2. Left mainstem bronchus (LMSB)—branches off the trachea at a 45 degree angle.
3. Walls contain incomplete cartilaginous rings at site where they enter lungs.
4. Ciliated mucous membrane lines the structures.
5. Primary bronchi divide into smaller branches (secondary bronchi) just past site of lung entry.
6. Secondary bronchi continue to branch, forming small bronchioles.
7. Bronchioles subdivide into smaller and smaller tubes and terminate into alveolar ducts and their several alveolar sacs.
B. Function—distribute air to lung's interior.

Alveoli

A. Structure—makes up the walls of alveolar sacs composed of single layer of tissue.
B. Function—gas exchange between air and blood.

Thorax

A. Structure.
1. The thorax (chest) is divided into three divisions, separated by partitions of pleura.
   a. Pleural divisions—each division occupied by a lung.
   b. Mediastinum—occupied by esophagus, trachea, large blood vessels, and heart.
2. Pleura.
   a. Parietal layer lines entire thoracic cavity.
      (1) Adheres to internal surface of ribs, superior surface of diaphragm.
      (2) Partitions off mediastinum.
   b. Visceral layer covers outer surface of each lung.

c. The two layers, separated only by a potential space (pleural space), contain just enough pleural fluid for lubrication.
B. Function—pleura allows for changes in chest size required for inspiration and expiration.

Principles of Pulmonary Ventilation

Respiratory Cycle Mechanics

A. Inspiration—active process.
1. Diaphragm descends, external intercostal muscles contract.
2. Chest expands, allowing air volume into the lungs as alveolar pressure decreases.
B. Expiration—passive process.
1. Diaphragm ascends, external intercostal muscles relax.
2. Chest becomes smaller, air moves out of lungs.
C. Atmospheric pressure—intrapulmonic pressure.
1. Air moves into and out of the lungs because of the differences in air pressure inside and outside of the lung. (Atmospheric pressure—760 mmHg.)
2. During inspiration, air moves into the lungs. Intrapulmonic pressure (pressure within the lungs) is lower than atmospheric pressure.
3. During expiration intrapulmonic pressure is higher than atmospheric pressure.

Exchanged Air Volumes

A. Total lung capacity (TLC)—total volume of air that is present in the lungs after maximum inspiration.
B. Vital capacity (VC)—volume of air that can be expelled following a maximum inspiration.
C. Tidal volume (TV)—volume of air exhaled after a normal inspiration.
D. Expiratory reserve volume (ERV)—largest additional volume of air that can be forcibly expired after tidal air expiration.

E. Inspiratory reserve volume (IRV)—amount of air that can be forcibly inspired over and above a normal inspiration.

F. Residual volume (RV)—amount of air remaining in lung following maximal expiration.

Exchange of Gases

A. In lungs.
1. Air and blood exchange gases through membrane of capillaries around alveoli.
2. Oxygen enters blood from the alveolar air.
3. Carbon dioxide enters alveolar air from the blood.

B. In tissues.
1. Takes place between arterial blood flowing through tissue capillaries and cells.
2. Oxygen diffuses out of the arterial blood into the cells.
3. Carbon dioxide diffuses out of the cells into the blood.

Transportation of Gases in Blood

A. Oxygen combines with hemoglobin, the means of transportation, in blood to form oxyhemoglobin.

B. Half of the carbon dioxide is carried in the plasma as bicarbonate ions.

C. About one third of blood carbon dioxide combines with the hemoglobin to form carbominohemoglobin.

Regulation of Respiration

A. Chemoreceptors—cells sensitive to changes in carbon dioxide concentrations in arterial blood.
1. Above normal range (35–45 mmHg) concentrations of carbon dioxide stimulate respirations.
2. Below normal concentrations of carbon dioxide slow respirations.
3. A decrease in arterial blood pH stimulates respirations.

B. Arterial blood pressure.

1. A sudden rise in arterial blood pressure results in reflexive slowing of respirations.
2. A sudden drop in arterial blood pressure results in reflexive increase in rate and depth of respirations.

C. Conditions that decrease lung compliance.
1. Atelectasis—collapse of the alveoli as a result of obstruction or hypoventilation.
2. Pneumonia—inflammatory process involving the lung tissue.
3. Pulmonary edema—accumulation of fluid in the alveoli.
4. Pleural effusion—accumulation of pleural fluid in the pleural space compressing lung on the affected side.
5. Pulmonary fibrosis—scar tissue replacing necrosed lung tissue as a result of infection.
6. Pneumothorax—air present in the pleural cavity; lung is collapsed as volume of air increases.

Surfactant

A. Surface-active material that lines the alveoli and changes the surface tension, depending on the area over which it is spread.

B. Surfactant in the lungs allows the smaller alveoli to have lower surface tension than the larger alveoli.
1. Results in equal pressures within both and prevents collapse.
2. Production of surfactant depends on adequate blood supply.

C. Conditions that decrease surfactant.
1. Hypoxia.
2. Oxygen toxicity.
3. Aspiration.
4. Atelectasis.
5. Pulmonary edema.
6. Pulmonary embolus.
7. Mucolytic agents.
8. Hyaline membrane disease.

Compliance

A. Relationship between pressure and volume: elastic resistance. This is determined by dividing the tidal volume by peak airway pressure

(V_t PAP). Total compliance equals chest wall complains plus lung compliance.

B. Conditions that decrease chest wall compliance.
1. Obesity—excess fatty tissue over chest wall and abdomen.
2. Kyphoscoliosis—marked resistance to expansion of the chest wall.
3. Scleroderma—expansion of the chest wall limited when the involved skin over the chest wall becomes stiff.
4. Chest wall injury—as in crushing chest wall injuries.
5. Diaphragmatic paralysis—as a result of surgical damage to the phrenic nerve, or disease process involving the diaphragm itself.

DIAGNOSTIC PROCEDURES

A. Pulmonary function tests.
1. Measurement of blood gases.
   a. An effective way to evaluate lung function and lung adequacy.
   b. Measure oxygen tension (arterial) (PaO_2) and carbon dioxide tension (arterial) ($PaCO_2$).
2. Measurement of lung air.
   a. Analyzes physical phenomena involved with the movement of the air in and out of the chest.
      (1) Vital capacity—measurement of the maximum amount of air that can be expired following a maximal inspiration.
      (2) Maximum breathing capacity—measurement of airway resistance within the lungs.
      (3) Timed vital capacity—the pattern of vital capacity as related to time.
   b. Measures the effectiveness of the mechanical processes and blood gases.

B. Chest x-ray.
1. Necessary in the assessment of respiratory disorders.

2. The view may be taken back to front (posteroanterior), side (lateral), or at an angle (oblique).
3. No specific preparation is necessary.

C. Bronchoscopy.
1. A direct visual examination of the trachea, two major bronchi, and multiple smaller bronchi.
2. A hollow instrument (bronchoscope) is passed into the trachea, under local anesthesia.
3. A biopsy of tissue or sample of secretions can be obtained.
4. Preparation of patient.
   a. NPO 8 to 12 hours before procedure.
   b. Remove dentures.
   c. Provide mouth care.
   d. Explain process to patient so that he or she can relax and cooperate during procedure.
   e. Administer sedative for relaxation.
5. Postprocedural care.
   a. NPO for several hours, until gag reflex returns.
   b. Encourage patient to expectorate.
   c. Advise patient to smoke and talk as little as possible; procedure may cause throat irritation.

D. Bronchography.
1. Specialized x-rays of the bronchi and bronchioles.
2. Catheter introduced into the trachea and positioned above the bifurcation, under local anesthesia.
3. Radio-opaque oil injected by catheter into the trachea, and patient is tilted in various positions so that the dye flows throughout the bronchial tree.
4. Preparation of patient.
   a. Same as for a bronchoscopy.
   b. May require postural drainage to remove thick bronchial secretions.
5. Postprocedural care.
   a. Same as for a bronchoscopy.
   b. May require postural drainage to remove excess oil.

E. Sputum examination.

1. A microscopic examination of the cells of the sputum.
2. Sputum should be raised from deep within the bronchi such as sputum first expectorated in the morning.
3. If culture is to be grown, specimens need to be collected in a sterile container.
4. May require a 24-hour specimen.
5. Patient's mouth should be first washed out to remove food particles.
6. Note color, consistency, odor and quantity of sputum.

F. Gastric analysis.
   1. Laboratory examination of stomach contents may include bronchial secretion the patient previously swallowed.
   2. A gastric tube is inserted and stomach contents are aspirated.
   3. Patient is NPO 8 to 12 hours prior to the procedure.

G. Thoracentesis.
   1. Removal of fluid from chest cavity.
   2. Under local anesthesia an aspiration needle inserted into the pleura.
   3. Purpose is both diagnostic and therapeutic.
   4. Nursing care.
      a. Assist patient to proper position.
      b. During procedure, observe patient for change of skin color and for changes in pulse and/or respiratory rate.
      c. After procedure, observe patient for change in respiratory rate and for coughing, expectoration of blood, or blood-tinged sputum.

H. Lung scintigraphy: measures concentration of gamma rays from lung after intake of isotope.

I. Perfusion studies: outline pulmonary vascular structures after intake of radioactive isotopes IV.

J. Biopsy of respiratory tissue
   1. May be done by needle, via bronchoscope, or an open lung procedure biopsy.
   2. Nursing care: observe for hemothorax and/or pneumothorax.

K. Tuberculin skin test
   1. Mantoux intradermal test (more reliable).
      a. Tuberculin injected intradermal, intermediate PPD.
      b. Test read 48 to 72 hours postintradermal wheal production.
      c. Erythema not important.
      d. Area of induration more than 10 mm: indicates positive reaction (patient has had contact with the tubercle bacillus).
      e. Reactions of 5 to 9 mm require retest.
   2. Tine test.
      a. Not recommended for diagnosis.
      b. Test read on third day.
      c. Mantoux test if induration more than 2 mm.

Respiratory System Assessment

A. Check for airway patency.
   1. Clear out secretions.
   2. Insert oral airway if necessary.
   3. Position patient on side if there is no cervical spine injury.

B. Listen to lung sounds.
   1. Absence of breath sounds: indicates lungs not expanding, due either to obstruction or deflation.
   2. Rales (crackling sounds): indicate vibrations of fluid in lungs.
   3. Rhonchi (coarse sounds): indicate partial obstruction of airway.
   4. Decreased breath sounds: indicate poorly ventilated lungs.
   5. Detection of bronchial sounds that are deviated from normal position: indicates mediastinal shift due to collapse of lung.

C. Determine level of consciousness; decreased sensorium can indicate hypoxia.

D. Observe sputum or tracheal secretions; bloody sputum can indicate contusions of lung or injury to trachea and other anatomical structures.

E. Evaluate vital signs for temperature, respiratory rate, pulse, and changes in skin color.

F. Evaluate for tightness or fullness in chest.

G. Determine degree of pain patient is experiencing.

H. Assess for respiratory complications.
1. Assess for abnormal breathing patterns.
   a. Dyspnea—labored or difficult breathing.
   b. Hyperpnea—abnormal deep breathing.
   c. Hypopnea—reduced depth of breathing.
   d. Orthopnea—difficulty breathing in other than upright position.
   e. Tachypnea—rapid breathing.
   f. Stridor—noisy respirations as air is forced through a partially obstructed airway.
2. Evaluate cough.
   a. Normally a protective mechanism utilized to keep the tracheobronchial tree free of secretions.
   b. Common symptom of respiratory disease.
3. Assess bronchospasm.
   a. Bronchi narrow and secretions may be retained.
   b. Condition may lead to infection.
4. Observe for hemoptysis—expectoration of blood or blood-tinged sputum.
5. Assess for cyanosis—late sign of hypoxia, due to large amounts of reduced hemoglobin in the blood (PaO_2 of about 50 mmHg).
6. Observe for hypoxia (anoxia)—a deficiency of oxygen in body tissues.
7. Evaluate for hypercapnia.
   a. Occurs when carbon dioxide is retained.
   b. High levels of oxygen depress and/or paralyze the medullary respiratory center.
   c. Peripheral chemoreceptors (sensitive to oxygen) become the stimuli for breathing.
8. Assess for presence of respiratory alkalosis or acidosis.
I. Assess for other system complications.
1. Evaluate for polycythemia—increase in RBCs as a compensatory response to hypoxemia.
2. Observe for clubbing of fingers. Pathogenesis is not well understood.

3. Evaluate for cor pulmonale—enlargement of the right ventricle as a result of pulmonary arterial hypertension following respiratory pathology.
4. Evaluate for chest pain.
5. Assess for atelectasis.
6. Check for abdominal distention.
7. Assess for hypertension.

CHRONIC OBSTRUCTIVE PULMONARY DISEASES (COPD)

Definition: A broad category applied to respiratory disorders that obstruct normal ventilation pathways.

Chronic Asthma

Definition: Recurrent paroxysms of dyspnea with a characteristic wheezing due to an inherited allergic tendency.

Assessment

A. Dyspnea, orthopnea.
B. Sense of tightness in the chest; feeling of impending suffocation.
C. Wheezing.
D. A slight dry cough.
E. Anxious expression.
F. Perspires freely.

Treatment and Implementation

A. Administer bronchodilators (epinephrine, Aminophylline), antihistamines, corticosteroids.
B. Humidify inspired air.
C. Provide oxygen therapy only after a long attack and occurrence of cyanosis.
D. Manage environment so that it is as free as possible from contributive factors to respiratory infection.
E. Protect patient from feeling closed in.

F. Provide rest.

G. Encourage fluids—3000 ml daily.

H. Watch for toxic effects of drugs.

Chronic Bronchitis

Definition: The hypersecretion of mucus by the bronchial glands; a chronic or a recurrent respiratory infection often following a long history of bronchial asthma or an acute respiratory infection.

Assessment

A. Cough is usually the earliest symptom; most marked on arising in the morning and just prior to going to bed.

B. Expectoration of thick, white, stringy mucus.

C. As the disease progresses, the sputum may become purulent, copious, and occasionally streaked with blood.

D. Possible sensation of heaviness in the chest.

E. Characteristic appearance is drawn, anxious, pale, and markedly dyspneic.

F. Speech characterized by short, jerky sentences.

G. Upright position often leaning slightly forward.

H. Distention of veins in neck during expiration.

Treatment and Implementation

A. Provide prompt and effective treatment of predisposing factors; good treatment directly related to the control of cigarette smoking and air pollution.

B. Increase pulmonary ventilation by reducing bronchospasms—bronchodilators.

C. Administer expectorants, intermittent antibiotic therapy.

D. Monitor oxygen therapy.

E. Postural drainage—chest physiotherapy.

F. Force fluids to 3000 ml.

G. Provide intermittent positive pressure breathing (IPPB).

H. Maintain mouth care.

Emphysema

Definition: The permanent overdistention of the alveoli with resulting destruction of the alveolar walls. (Emphysema is a Greek word meaning "overinflated.")

Signs and Symptoms

A. Cough—may be present many years before dyspnea.

B. Dyspnea—chief complaint.

C. Increased sputum production.

D. Weight loss.

E. Hypoxia, hypercapnia.

F. Barrel chest.

G. Prolonged expiratory phase.

H. Wheezes, forced expiratory rhonchi.

I. Complications.
  1. Pulmonary hypertension.
  2. Right-sided heart failure.
  3. Spontaneous pneumothorax.

Implementation

A. Monitor for signs of impending hypoxia.

B. Monitor for alterations in lung sounds.

C. Teach pursed lip breathing exercises.

D. Administer low concentration oxygen. Usually 2 l/min.

E. Monitor for signs of carbon dioxide narcosis.

F. Provide hydration.
  1. Necessary to liquefy secretions present, or to prevent formation of thick, tenacious secretions.
  2. Hydration methods.
    a. Oral intake of fluids.
    b. IV administration of fluids.
    c. Humidification via face mask or aerosol mask.

G. Implications of humidification.
    a. Relief of bronchospasm and mucosal edema.
    b. Mobilization of secretions.
    c. Administration of medications.

H. Provide chest physiotherapy.

Specialized Nursing Care

Chronic Pulmonary Disease

A. When progress is slow, be patient, give attention to detail, and maintain interest and hope.

B. Give instruction for general health care.
1. Principles of optimum nutrition for patient and family.
2. A plan for adequate rest, recreation, and suitable work.
3. The value of treatment program.
4. Instructions concerning medications, breathing exercises, and avoidance of infection.

C. Observe and record symptoms.
1. Amount of coughing, amount and character of sputum, degree of dyspnea and/or wheezing.
2. Color, weight, and appetite of patient.
3. Attitudes and sense of well-being.
4. Complications and progression of illness.

D. Help adjust activities for the patient within framework of his or her tolerance.

E. Positions for Chest Physiotherapy.
❖ **PROCEDURE** ❖
1. To affect RUL and LUL, place patient upright.
2. To affect RML, position patient on left side with head slanted down, right shoulder one-quarter turn onto pillow. Cup anteriorly over left nipple.
3. To affect lingula LL, position patient on right side with head slanted down, left shoulder one-quarter turn onto pillow. Cup anteriorly over right nipple.
4. To affect RLL and LLL, place patient in Trendelenburg's position, alternating sides, or prone.

Administration of Oxygen ❖ PROCEDURE ❖

A. Conditions requiring oxygen therapy
1. Atmosphere hypoxia: oxygen therapy will correct depressed level of oxygen.

2. Hypoventilation hypoxia: 100% oxygen will yield five times more oxygen into the alveoli than normal air.

B. Conditions where oxygen therapy is not corrective.
1. Hypoxia caused by anemia, carbon monoxide poisoning, or abnormal hemoglobin transport.
2. Inadequate tissue use of oxygen (cyanide poisoning).
3. Chronic obstructive lung disease requires that oxygen be used with caution since oxygen could suppress respiratory drive and result in respiratory arrest.

C. Symptoms of hypoxia.
1. Early symptoms.
a. Restlessness.
b. Headache.
c. Visual disturbances.
d. Slight confusion.
e. Hyperventilation.
f. Tachycardia.
g. Hypertension.
h. Dyspnea.
2. Advanced symptoms.
a. Hypotension.
b. Bradycardia.
c. Metabolic acidosis (production of lactic acid).
d. Cyanosis.
3. Chronic hypoxia.
a. Polycythemia.
b. Clubbing of fingers and toes.
c. Thrombosis.

D. Properties of oxygen.
1. Colorless, odorless, and tasteless gas.
2. Supports combustion.

E. Methods of administration.
1. Nasal catheter (used infrequently)—produces oxygen concentration of 30–50%.
a. Insert so tip of catheter is visible immediately behind the uvula.
b. Change every 8–12 hours.
c. Apply nonoily lubricant to irritated or dry nasal mucous membrane.
2. Face mask—produces oxygen concentration of 30 to 65%.

a. May cover nose and mouth or nose only.

b. May have rebreathing bag so patient inhales part of the air previously exhaled.

3. Cannula—produces oxygen concentration of 35–40%.
   a. Fit small prongs into each nostril.
   b. Remove and clean every eight hours.

4. Tent—produces oxygen concentration of 50–60%.
   a. Cover either entire or upper third of the bed.
   b. Used infrequently.

Implementation

A. Check equipment.
   1. Eliminate kinks in tubing.
   2. Maintain proper positioning.
   3. Check water supply in humidification bottle.
   4. Adjust to proper liter flow.

B. Maintain safety measures.
   1. No smoking or fire of any kind.
   2. No materials that produce static electricity.
   3. No electrical equipment; however, some hospital equipment may be safely used.

C. Monitoring a patient with oxygen.
   ❖ **PROCEDURE** ❖
   1. Check order for type of therapy, use of catheter or cannula, and desired liter flow.
   2. Place patient in semi- or high-Fowler's position to ensure adequate lung expansion.
   3. Turn and reposition patient frequently to prevent skin decubiti.
   4. Encourage deep breathing and coughing exercises unless directed otherwise.
   5. Ensure adequate hydration, especially if secretions are thick and tenacious.
   6. Assess patient's progress by frequently checking vital signs, color, and level of consciousness.
   7. Remain with patients who are frightened or anxious until they feel secure.
   8. Use oxygen very conservatively on anyone with chronic lung disease—high levels of oxygen will knock out carbon dioxide center and lead to respiratory arrest.

D. Using an Oxygen Analyzer. ❖ **PROCEDURE** ❖
   1. Calibrate analyzer with room atmosphere prior to each reading.
   2. Open tubing to the air, and compress two full times to fill analyzer.
   3. Depress button. Analyzer should read 20% for room air. Adjust dial as necessary to obtain this reading.
   4. Place tubing close to patient's nose.
   5. Compress bulb three to six times, depress button, and read findings.
   6. Based on reading, adjust oxygen flow.
   7. Check analyzer with 100% oxygen at least one time per day.

E. Using pulse oximetry.
   1. Allows for continual monitoring of arterial blood gas (ABGs).
   2. Sensor is applied to skin (noninvasive) and photodetector registers light passing through vascular bed.
   3. Oxygen saturation level can be read on digital monitor.
   4. Rotate site of clip-on probe every four hours.

ACUTE PULMONARY DISEASES

Common Cold (Coryza)

Definition: An infectious viral disease of the upper respiratory tract. It has a duration of 4–14 days and is endemic throughout the world.

Assessment

A. Sneezing.

B. Chills and slight fever.

C. Headache.

D. Watery eyes.

E. Dry, scratchy, sore throat.

F. Copious nasal discharge.

Treatment and Implementation

A. Encourage bed rest or extra sleep.
B. Advise avoidance of contact with others.
C. Force fluids.
D. ASA (aspirin) to relieve discomforts.
E. Instruct patient in proper use of tissues and preventive measures for spread of infection.

Pneumonia

Definition: Inflammation of the lungs due to infection caused by virus, bacteria, or fungus. Inflammation leads to replacement of air in the alveolar sacs by fluid or tissue.

Assessment

A. Complaint of tightness or fullness in chest.
B. Cough, dyspnea, or shortness of breath.
C. Increased vital signs, particularly temperature and respiratory rate.
D. Restlessness.

Treatment and Implementation

A. Administer antibiotics.
B. Administer oxygen therapy (see section on administration of oxygen, p. 184).
C. Monitor IVs or force fluids.
D. Elevate head of bed.
E. Monitor vital signs.
F. Encourage bed rest with frequent position change.
G. Monitor urinary output.
H. Check frequency of bowel movement.
I. Isolate patient if required.
J. Encourage expectoration.

Atelectasis

A. Collapse of pulmonary alveoli, caused by mucous plug or inadequate ventilation.
B. Signs and symptoms.
　1. Asymmetrical chest movement.

　2. Decreased or absent breath sounds over affected area.
　3. Shortness of breath leading to cyanosis.
　4. Painful respirations.
　5. Increased vital signs: temperature, respiration, pulse.
　6. Anxiety and restlessness.

Pleurisy

Definition: Inflammation of the pleura that is usually a complication of pulmonary diseases.

Types

A. Acute fibrinous (dry pleurisy)—only small amounts of exudate are formed during the inflammatory process.
B. Pleurisy with effusion—large amounts of fluid are secreted and collect in the space between the pleural layers.

Assessment

A. Very sharp pain during respiration.
B. Pain gradually subsides as fluid is formed in pleural space.
C. Dry cough.
D. Fatigue.
E. Possible shortness of breath.

Treatment and Implementation

A. Thoracentesis performed to remove fluid if condition is severe.
B. Encourage bed rest.
C. Ventilate room well but maintain warmth.
D. Encourage coughing.
E. Position patient on side of the effusion.
F. Apply heat to painful area.

Influenza

Definition: Infectious epidemic disease of short duration that is caused by a virus.

Assessment

A. Sudden onset with variable individual symptoms.
B. Chills, high fever.
C. Severe headache, muscular aches.
D. Anorexia, weakness, apathy.
E. Sneezing, dry cough.
F. Sore throat, nasal discharge.

Treatment and Implementation

A. Administer ASA for muscle aches and headache, and codeine to control cough.
B. Cool vapor steam inhalation.
C. Encourage bed rest.
D. Ventilate room well.
E. Take TPR every four hours during temperature elevation.
F. Provide large amounts of fluid.

Pulmonary Tuberculosis (TB)

Definition: An infectious disease of the parenchyma of the lung, bronchi, bronchioles, alveoli, pleurae, and bronchopulmonary lymph nodes that is characterized by the formation of tubercles. It is caused by the organism *Mycobacterium tuberculosis* (Koch's bacillus). It is acquired by inhalation of disseminated air droplets of excretions from the nose, mouth, throat, and lungs of infected individuals.

Assessment

A. Insidious onset, early symptoms mild and nonspecific.
B. Fatigue.
C. Anorexia, weight loss.
D. Elevated temperature, particularly in the late afternoon and the evening.
E. Night sweats.
F. Initial nonproductive cough that later becomes productive of mucopurulent and blood-streaked sputum.
G. Hemoptysis (expectoration of blood from respiratory tract or lungs).
H. Mantoux skin test: positive.
   1. PPD tuberculin injected intradermal.
   2. Test read in 48–72 hours. Induration of 10 mm or more means patient has had contact with the disease.

Treatment and Implementation

A. Maintain respiratory precautions.
   1. Strict isolation for 2–4 weeks or coughing has ceased or negative sputum.
   2. Masks necessary only for uncooperative patient.
B. Administer medications in single daily dose and on time.
C. Current drug regimen.
   1. Isoniazid (300 mg daily), pyrazinamide and Rifampin (600 mg daily) for two months.
   2. Followed by four months of isoniazid and rifampin.
   3. Ethambutol (15 mg/kg daily) and streptomycin (500 mg daily) are usually part of the initial treatment regimen.
   4. Six months of drug therapy is usually sufficient to kill tubercle bacilli.
D. Chemoprophylaxis—isoniazid and vitamin B_6 therapy for six months to one year.
E. Compliance is major problem in eliminating TB—work with patient to adhere to drug regimen.

CHEST INJURIES

Emergency Assessment of Respiratory Function

A. Check for airway patency and ventilation.
B. Inspect thoracic cage for injury.
   1. Inspect for contusions, abrasions, and deep open wounds.
   2. Watch for movement of chest; asymmetrical movement indicates tension pneumoth-

orax, hemothorax, fractured ribs, and/or flail chest.

C. Observe color; cyanosis indicates decreased oxygenation.

D. Observe type of breathing; stertorous breathing usually indicates obstructed respiration.

E. Listen to lung sounds.
   1. Absence of breath sounds indicates lungs not expanding, due to either obstruction or deflation.
   2. Rales (crackling sounds) are produced by vibrations of fluid and indicate fluid in lungs.
   3. Rhonchi (coarse rattlings) indicate partial obstruction of airway.
   4. Decreased breath sounds indicate poorly ventilated lungs.
   5. Bronchial sounds, deviated from normal position, indicate mediastinal shift due to collapse of lung.

F. Determine level of consciousness; decreased sensorium may indicate hypoxia.

G. Observe sputum or tracheal secretions; bloody sputum may indicate contusions of lung or injury to trachea and other anatomical structures.

Emergency Implementation

A. Take brief history from patient (or individual accompanying patient) to aid in total evaluation of his or her condition.

B. Assist with electrocardiogram to establish if there is associated cardiac damage.

C. Maintain patent airway.
   1. Place hand over nose and mouth to detect breathing; maintain adequate ventilation.
   2. Clear out secretions; suction.
   3. Insert either oral airway or endotracheal tube as necessary.

D. Position patient on side if no spinal injury.

E. Seal off open chest wound immediately with pressure dressing to prevent air from entering thoracic cavity.

F. Maintain fluid and electrolyte balance.

1. When replacing blood and fluid loss, watch carefully for fluid overload as it can lead to pulmonary edema.
2. Record intake and output.

G. Maintain acid-base balance; assist with frequent blood gas determination as acid-base imbalances occur readily with compromised respirations or with mechanical ventilation.

H. Provide for relief of pain.
   1. Use analgesics with caution as they depress respirations. (Demerol is drug of choice.)
   2. Avoid atropine or morphine sulfate and barbiturates.
   3. Nerve block used as necessary.

Open Wounds of the Chest

Pathophysiology

A. Air that enters the pleural cavity from the atmosphere causes collapse of lung.

B. Air entering and leaving the wound during inspiration and expiration can be detected.

C. Intrapleural negative pressure is lost, thereby embarrassing respirations. If not corrected promptly, this leads to hypoxia and death.

Implementation

A. Apply vaseline gauze to wound with pressure dressing.

B. Place patient on assisted ventilation if necessary.

C. Prepare for insertion of chest tubes.

D. Place patient in high-Fowler's position (unless contraindicated) to help provide adequate ventilation.

Hemothorax or Pneumothorax

Definition: Hemothorax is an accumulation of blood within the pleural space. Pneumothorax is an accumulation of air within the pleural space. The

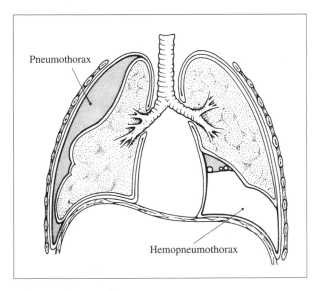

Anatomical View of Lungs

blood or air accumulation builds up positive pressure in the pleural space and collapses the lung.

Assessment

A. Pain.
B. Decreased breath sounds.
C. Tracheal shift to unaffected side.
D. Dyspnea and respiratory embarrassment.

Treatment and Implementation

A. A number 18 needle may be inserted into the second intercostal space, midclavicular line, followed by aspiration of the fluid or air by means of a thoracentesis (emergency treatment).
B. Chest tubes may be inserted and connected to closed-chest drainage.
C. Observe vital signs continuously for shock and cardiac failure complications.

Fractured Ribs

Definition: Fracture varies from simple to severe multiple breaks with flail chest and internal injuries; rib fracture is the most common chest injury.

Assessment

A. Pain and tenderness over fracture area.
B. Bruises at injury site.
C. Respiratory distress resulting from bone splinters that have punctured lung, causing pneumothorax.
D. Shallow respirations, from splinting of chest, can cause a reduction in lung compliance as well as respiratory acidosis.

Treatment and Implementation

A. Administer mild analgesic (small dose of Demerol) for relief of pain. (*Caution:* Narcotics can depress respiration and the cough reflex.)
B. Encourage deep breathing and coughing to prevent respiratory complications such as atelectasis and pneumonia.
C. Observe for signs of hemorrhage and shock.
D. Intercostal nerve block is administered, if necessary, to decrease pain.

Flail Chest

Definition: Unstable chest wall with respiratory impairment resulting from multiple rib fractures.

Assessment

A. Pain.
B. Dyspnea leading to cyanosis.
C. Detached position of flail chest moving in opposition to other areas of chest cage and lung.
  1. On inspiration, the affected chest area is depressed; on expiration, it is bulging outward.
  2. Opposing chest movement causes poor expansion of lungs and leads to carbon dioxide retention and respiratory acidosis.

D. Inability to cough effectively, which leads to accumulation of fluids and respiratory complications such as pneumonia and atelectasis.

E. Cardiac failure due to impaired filling of blood to the right side of the heart caused by the high venous pressure built up by paradoxical breathing.

F. Rapid, shallow, and noisy respirations.

Treatment and Implementation

A. Prepare for tracheostomy with a cuffed tracheostomy tube.

B. Place patient on volume-controlled respirator (MA-1, Bear 5, Servo 90), which delivers the same amount of tidal volume with each breath independent of patient's respirations.

C. Suction frequently to prevent respiratory complications.

D. Prevent pain by administering nerve block or Demerol as ordered.

E. Observe for signs of shock and hemorrhage. For patient on ventilator, use nasogastric tube to prevent abdominal distention and emesis, which can lead to aspiration.

F. Assist patient not on mechanical ventilator.
   1. Encourage turning, coughing, and hyperventilating every hour.
   2. Administer oxygen.
   3. Maintain IPPB therapy.
   4. Suction as needed.

RESPIRATORY TRACT SURGICAL PROCEDURES

Submucous Resection (SMR)

Definition: Removal of part of deflected nasal septum.

Procedure

A. Lay back flap of mucous membrane.

B. Excise portion of septum.

C. Rationale.
   1. Restore normal breathing space.
   2. Permit more adequate sinus drainage.

Treatment and Implementation

A. Provide routine postoperative care.

B. Observe respiration.

C. Pack nasal cavity.

D. Apply mustache dressing.

Laryngectomy

Definition: Partial or total removal of larynx (epiglottis, thyroid cartilage, hyoid bone, cricoid cartilage, and part of trachea); may sometimes include removal of neck tissue.

Procedure

A. Bring out stump of trachea and suture to neck skin.

B. Close portion of pharynx.
   1. Procedure is permanent.
   2. Breathing through nose is eliminated.

C. If neck tissue and lymph nodes involved, radical neck resection performed.

D. Rationale: removal of benign or malignant tissue, tumors, or lymph nodes, if involved.

Treatment and Implementation

A. Suction frequently with sterile technique until area has healed; then use clean technique.

B. Observe for hemorrhage from surgical site.

C. Instruct patient regarding means for communication.
   1. Patient will not be able to speak immediately after surgery.
   2. Inform patient of available speech rehabilitation after healing has occurred.

D. Feed through nasogastric tube.

E. Encourage normal eating patterns after healing has occurred.

F. Instruct patient how to care for opening.

G. Possibly refer patient to the Lost Cord Club.

Tracheostomy

Definition: Creation of an external opening into the trachea for insertion of a breathing tube.

Procedure

A. Position patient so trachea is prominent.

B. Midline incision for tubal insertion.

C. Rationale.
1. Remove tracheobronchial secretions for patient unable to adequately cough.
2. Use with mechanical ventilators.
3. Use as emergency measure for unconscious patients.

Treatment and Implementation

A. Care for and maintain cuffed tracheostomy tube. ❖ PROCEDURE ❖
1. Release of cuff pressure five minutes out of every hour. (If high volume/low pressure cuff is used, cuff is not routinely deflated.)
2. Hyperventilation of patient before and after cuff is deflated with ambu bag.
3. Suction airway before deflating or inflating cuff.
   a. Always apply oral or nasal suction first, so that when cuff is deflated, secretions will not fall into lung from area above cuff.
   b. Catheter must be changed before tracheostomy suctioning.
4. Humidification with tracheostomy mist mask if patient not on ventilator.

B. Observe for hemorrhage from tracheostomy site.

C. Change dressings (nonraveling type) and cleanse surrounding area with hydrogen peroxide at least every four hours.

D. Care for and maintain silver tracheostomy tube.

1. Removal of inner cannula for soaking in hydrogen peroxide solution to loosen mucus accumulation.
2. Cleansing of inner and outer aspects of tube with brush.
3. Sterile saline or water rinse.
4. Suction of outer cannula before reinsertion.
5. Special orders for tube care.
   a. Disinfect tube by boiling for five minutes.
   b. Leave tube in disinfectant solution for varying lengths of time.
   c. Inner cannula is usually replaced by an interchangeable part every four hours.

THORACIC CAVITY SURGICAL PROCEDURES

Types of Procedures

A. Exploratory thoracotomy is an incision of the thoracic wall for locating bleeding, injuries and/or tumors.

B. Thoracoplasty is the removal of ribs or portions of ribs to reduce the size of the thoracic space.

C. Pneumonectomy is the removal of entire lung.

D. Lobectomy is the removal of a lobe of the lung.

E. Segmented resection is the removal of one or more segments of the lung.

F. Wedge resection is the removal of a small, localized area of disease near the surface of the lung.

Postoperative Implementation

A. Employ closed chest suction for all surgeries but pneumonectomy.
1. In pneumonectomy, it is desirable that the fluid accumulate in empty thoracic space.

2. Eventually the thoracic space fills with serous exudate which consolidates, preventing extensive mediastinal shifts.

B. Maintain patent chest tube; drain by chest tube stripping.

C. Maintain respiratory function.
   1. Patient to turn, cough, and deep breathe.
   2. Suction if necessary.
   3. Oxygen therapy.
   4. IPPB therapy.
   5. Mechanical ventilation if necessary.

D. Ambulate patient to enhance adequate ventilation and prevent postoperative complications.

E. Provide range-of-motion exercises to all extremities for promotion of adequate circulation.

F. Monitor for signs of increased central venous pressure which indicates impaired venous return to heart.

G. Positioning of patient.
   1. Semi-Fowler's position to facilitate lung expansion when vital signs are stable.
   2. Specific positions that require readjustment every one to two hours.
      a. Pneumonectomy.
         (1) Position on operated side for back care only.
         (2) Position on back or unoperated side only. (Some physicians will allow positioning on either side after 24 hours.)
      b. Segmental resection or wedge resection.
         (1) Position on back or unoperated side.
         (2) Position enhances expansion of remaining pulmonary tissue.
      c. Lobectomy.
         (1) Turn to either side.
         (2) Expands lung tissue on both sides.

H. Encourage postoperative arm and shoulder exercises.
   1. Affected arm should be put through both active and passive range of motion every four hours.

2. Exercises should start within four hours after surgery when patient has returned to room.
3. Exercising prevents formation of adhesions.

Postoperative Complications

Respiratory Complications

A. Causes.
   1. Inadequate ventilation.
   2. Airway obstructed by accumulation of secretion.
   3. Atelectasis (collapsed or airless lung) from underexpansion of lungs and anesthetic agents during surgery.
   4. Hypoventilation and carbon dioxide build-up from incisional splinting as a result of pain.
   5. Depression of CNS from overuse of medications.

B. Tension pneumothorax.
   1. Air leak through pleural incision lines.
   2. Mediastinal shift can occur.

C. Pulmonary embolism.

D. Bronchopulmonary fistula.
   1. Subcutaneous emphysema from escape of air into pleural space which is then forced into subcutaneous tissue around incision.
   2. Inadequate closure of bronchus during resection.
   3. Alveolar or bronchiolar tears in surface of lung (particularly following pneumonectomy).

E. Atelectasis and/or pneumonia from airway obstruction or as result of anesthesia.

F. Possible respiratory arrest.

Circulatory Complications

A. Hypovolemia from loss of fluid or blood; can result in cardiac arrest.

B. Arrhythmias from underlying myocardial disease; can result in cardiac arrest.

C. Pulmonary edema from fluid overload of circulatory system.

MANAGEMENT OF THORACIC SURGICAL EQUIPMENT

Chest Tubes

General Principles

A. Purpose is the removal of air and serosanguineous fluid from pleural space following thoracic surgery.
B. Tubes are placed in pleural cavity and attached to water seal suction to maintain closed system.
C. Tubes are attached to water seal suction to maintain closed system.
   1. All connectors are taped.
   2. Bottle stoppers should fit tightly.
   3. Bottles kept below level of bed.
   4. Suction level maintained where ordered (be sure that bubbling is not excessive in the pressure-regulating bottle).
   5. Water level maintained in bottle.
D. Mechanics of system.
   1. Used after some intrathoracic procedures.
   2. Chest tubes placed intrapleurally.
   3. Breathing mechanism operates on principle of negative pressure.
      a. Pressure in chest cavity is lower than pressure of atmosphere.
      b. An injury that breaks into chest cavity (such as stab wound) will cause atmospheric air to then rush into the cavity.
      c. Vacuum must be applied to chest to reestablish negative pressure when chest has been open.
   4. Closed water seal drainage is method of reestablishing negative pressure.
      a. Water acts as a seal and keeps the air from being drawn back into pleural space.

Disposable water-seal suction equipment (Pluer-Evac).

      b. Open drainage system would allow air to be sucked back into chest cavity and cause collapse of lung.
   5. Closed drainage is established by placing catheter into pleural space and allowing it to drain under water.
      a. The end of the drainage tube is always kept under water.
      b. Air will not be drawn up through catheter into pleural space when tube is under water.
   6. Drainage can be accomplished with one, two, or three bottles.
   7. Some physicians do not allow clamping or milking of chest tubes. Follow physician's orders.

Implementation ❖ PROCEDURE ❖

A. Assist physician in placement of tubes.
   1. Tubes placed in pleural cavity following thoracic surgery.

2. Provides for removal of air and serosan-guineous fluid from pleural space.
B. Attach to water-seal suction—maintains closed system.
   1. Tape all connectors.
   2. Ensure that all stoppers in bottles are tight fitting.
C. Apply suction.
   1. Keep bottles below level of bed.
   2. Keep suction level where ordered (be sure that bubbling is not excessive in the pressure-regulating bottle).
   3. Maintain water level in bottle.
D. Maintain patency—strip chest tubes only with physician's orders.
   1. If ordered, milk chest tubes every 30 to 60 minutes if clots or debris present.
      a. Milk away from patient toward the drainage receptacle.
      b. Alternately compress and release drainage tubing between thumb and forefinger—this method prevents pressure changes.
      c. Continue going down tube in this method until reaching drainage receptacle.
   2. Milking may be ordered— stripping should be avoided.
E. Maintain safety.
   1. Keep rubber-tipped hemostats at bedside so that tube can be clamped off near to chest insertion site. Clamping is controversial—check hospital policy.
   2. Clamp only to locate source of air leak when bubbling occurs in water-seal chamber; to prevent air from entering pleural space; to verify patient is ready for chest tube removal.
F. Monitor intake and output.
   1. With Pleur-evac suction equipment, visually measure chest drainage (holds up to 2800 to 3000 cc drainage). With two or three-bottle suction, tape or bottle markings may approximate the amount of drainage (similar to Pleur-evac).
   2. Change equipment only when the drainage chamber is full.

Water-Seal Chest Drainage

Assessment

A. Assess patient's respiratory rate, rhythm, and breath sounds for signs of respiratory distress.
B. Check that all connections on tubing are airtight and suction control is connected.
C. Examine system to see if it is set up and functioning properly.
D. Identify any malfunctions in system, i.e., air leaks, negative pressure, or obstructions.

Implementation

A. Maintain water-seal suction system.
B. Cessation of fluctuations indicates reexpansion of lung.
C. Chest tubes are used for lung reexpansion, bubbling will occur in the water-seal bottle.

One-Bottle Suction System

1. There is only one bottle; it functions as a collection bottle for drainage as well as to prevent air from leaking into pleural cavity.
2. As the drainage increases in amount, the water-seal tube (immersed in the drainage) is pulled up slightly to decrease the amount of force that is required to permit the fluid to be drained from the pleural space.
3. The depth to which the water-seal tube is immersed below the fluid in the bottle determines the pressure exerted by the water.
4. Vent is used to prevent pressure build-up and to allow continuous air removal.

Two-Bottle Suction System

1. Two-bottle suction.
   a. Drainage bottle (bottle number one) is connected from patient and is between the patient and the water-seal bottle (or bottle number two).
      (1) Short tube goes from patient into drainage bottle (not to extend below drainage level).

     (2) Short tube with rubber tubing goes from the drainage bottle to water-seal bottle.

     (3) This tube extends below water level in the water-seal bottle.

  b. Mark drainage level on outside of bottle.

2. Bottle number two.

  a. The long tube extends below water level about 2 cm.

  b. A second short tube provides an air vent.

  c. Water in this bottle goes up the tube when patient inhales and down the tube when patient exhales. Fluctuates 5–10 cm.

  d. Water in this bottle should not bubble constantly.

Three-Bottle Suction System

1. One bottle is connected to suction motor—called a pressure regulator bottle.

2. Bottle number three regulates the amount of pressure in the system. (Bubbles constantly.)

3. Three tubes.

  a. Short tube, above water level, comes from water-seal bottle.

  b. Short tube connected to suction motor.

  c. Third tube, below water level in bottle, opens to the atmosphere outside of bottle.

  d. The depth to which third tube is submerged in the water determines the pressure within the drainage system.

4. When control bottle fluid becomes too low, outside air is sucked into the system. Depth of control tube under water determines suction level of system.

5. Whenever the motor is off, drainage system must be open to the atmosphere.

  a. Intrapleural air can escape from the system.

  b. Vent prevents pressure build-up which interferes with drainage from patient.

Comparison of one, two, and three bottle suction.

Site for Pneumothorax

Site for Hemothorax

Floor

Provide a straight line of tubing from chest tube to collection system. Keep collection system below level of chest tube insertion site (on the floor).

Suctioning Equipment

A. Nasotracheal.
  1. Equipment needed.
     a. Sterile suction catheter, usually No. 14 or No. 16 French.
     b. Sterile saline.
     c. Suction machine.
     d. Sterile gloves.
  2. Procedure. ❖ **PROCEDURE** ❖
     a. Preoxygenate 1–2 minutes before beginning procedure.
     b. Lubricate catheter with normal saline.
     c. Insert catheter 6–8 inches into the nose.
     d. Do not apply suction while introducing catheter.
     e. When advanced as far as possible, begin suctioning by withdrawing catheter slowly, rotating it with pressure applied. (Usually a whistle tip catheter or Y connector tube is used to apply pressure.)
B. Tracheostomy.
  1. Equipment needed.
     a. Same equipment as for nasotracheal.
     b. Sterile syringe (5 ml) and sterile saline for instillation into tracheostomy tube.
  2. Procedure. ❖ **PROCEDURE** ❖
     a. Be sure that suction catheter is not more than half the diameter of the tracheostomy tube.
     b. Preoxygenate before beginning procedure.
     c. Lubricate with sterile saline.
     d. Insert catheter through tracheostomy tube for 8–12 inches with suction turned off.
     e. Suction for no more than ten seconds.
     f. Rotate catheter while withdrawing it.
     g. Do not repeat procedure for at least three minutes, unless necessary to withdraw more secretions to permit adequate ventilation.
     h. If secretions are very tenacious, 3–5 ml of sterile saline may be inserted through tube and allowed to remain for a few seconds before suctioning (this increases viscosity of secretions and facilitates removal).

i. To remove secretions from right bronchus, turn patient's head to left; vice versa for left bronchus.

Common Respiratory Drugs

Bronchodilators Commonly Used

A. Aminophylline.
   1. Relaxes smooth muscle of the tracheo-bronchial tree.
   2. Intravenous, oral, elixir.
   3. Should be taken on an empty stomach since it is not absorbed well in an alkaline medium.
   4. Side effects.
      a. Gastric irritation.
      b. Nausea.
      c. Cardiac arrhythmias (tachycardia, ventricular ectopy).
B. Ephedrine.
   1. Relaxes smooth muscle of the tracheo-bronchial tree, reduces congestion, and acts as a vasoconstrictor.
   2. Tablet, parenteral.
   3. Side effects.
      a. Anxiety, tremulousness, palpitations.
      b. Insomnia.
      c. Difficulty of urination.
      d. CNS stimulation.
C. Isuprel.
   1. Relaxes smooth muscle of the tracheo-bronchial tree, relieves bronchospasm, and acts as a cardiac stimulant (increases cardiac output and venous return to the heart).
   2. Mistometer, solution for nebulization, IV (requires ICU).
   3. Caution necessary for patients with existing cardiac arrhythmias associated with tachycardias.
      a. It may result in aggravation of arrhythmias.
      b. Should not be used with epinephrine since both are cardiac stimulants and the combined effect may produce serious arrhythmias.
   4. Side effects.
      a. Tachycardia, nervousness, palpitations.
      b. Arrhythmias.
      c. Nausea.
      d. Headaches.
      e. Flushing, tremor, dizziness.
      f. Weakness.
      g. Diaphoresis.
      h. Chest pain.
D. Bronkosol.
   1. Relaxes smooth muscle of the tracheo-bronchial tree.
      a. Acts as bronchovasoconstrictor and reduces congestion.
      b. Less effective than Isuprel in its bronchodilating effect, but more potent than epinephrine.
   2. Hand nebulizer and solution for aerosolization.
   3. Precautions are the same as for Isuprel, but the side effects seem to appear less frequently.
E. Choledyl.
   1. Relaxes smooth muscle of the tracheo-bronchial tree.
      a. Relieves bronchospasm.
      b. Useful in long-term therapy of bronchospasm.
   2. Tablet, elixir.
   3. Concomitant use with other bronchodilators may increase side effects, especially CNS stimulation.
   4. Side effects.
      a. Gastric distress.
      b. Palpitations.
      c. CNS stimulation.

General Respiratory Drugs

A. Epinephrine.
   1. Acts directly on beta cells of the bronchi, increases tidal volume, and relieves congestion in bronchial mucosa and constricting pulmonary vessels.
   2. Used in anaphylaxis and asthma.
   3. Subcutaneous injection.

4. Strong cardiotonic.
5. Vital signs should be monitored during use.
6. Side effects.
   a. Palpitations and tachycardia.
   b. Headache.
   c. Tremor, weakness, and vertigo.

B. Corticosteroids.
1. Used in conjunction with bronchodilators for treatment of bronchospasms. Aerosol use prevents systemic side effects of steroids.
2. Routes:
   a. Prednisone p.o.
   b. Methylprednisolone, hydrocortisone IV.
   c. Beclomethasone diproprionate (Beclovent, Vanceril) MDI (metered dose inhalant).
   d. Triamcinolone (Azmacort) MDI.
3. Instruct patient to rinse mouth after use to prevent oral candidiasis.
4. Side effects include increased appetite, euphoria and psychosis.

Mucokinetic Agents

A. Mucomyst.
1. Reduces viscosity of purulent and nonpurulent secretions by breaking disulfide bond; assists in removal of secretions.
2. Inhalation medication.
3. Inactivates many antibiotics, including penicillin.
4. Side effects.
   a. Stomatitis.
   b. Hemoptysis.
   c. Nausea.

B. Potassium iodide.
1. Expectorant liquefies tenacious bronchial secretions.
2. Enseal (enteric-release) capsule.
3. Not used in acute bronchitis.
4. Thyroid abnormalities can occur with use.

GASTROINTESTINAL SYSTEM

The alimentary tract's primary function is to provide the body with a continual supply of nutrients, fluids, and electrolytes for tissue nourishment This system has three components: a tract for ingestion and movement of food and fluids; secretion of digestive juices for breaking down the nutrients; and absorption mechanisms for the utilization of foods, water, and electrolytes for continuous growth and repair of body tissues.

ANATOMY AND PHYSIOLOGY

Alimentary Tract

A. Mouth.
1. Cheeks.
2. Hard and soft palates.
3. Muscles.
4. Maxillary bones (jaw).
5. Tongue—aids in chewing, swallowing, and speaking; contains taste buds.
6. Salivary glands.
   a. Constant secretions form saliva.
   b. Three pairs of glands located in the mucous membrane of the oral cavity.
      (1) Parotid—below the ear.
      (2) Submaxillary—floor of mouth.
      (3) Sublingual—floor of mouth.
7. Teeth—assist in mastication and in mixing saliva with food.
8. Digestive process starts in the mouth.

B. Pharynx.
1. Tubal structure that extends from the base of the skull to the esophagus.
2. Serves as a passageway for air from nasal cavity to larynx and for food from mouth to esophagus.
3. Parts.
   a. Nasopharynx.
   b. Oropharynx.

    c. Laryngopharynx.

C. Esophagus.
1. Muscular canal.
2. Extends from pharynx to stomach.

D. Stomach.
1. Distensible pouch located between the esophagus and the duodenum.
2. Divisions.
    a. Fundus which forms upper portion is located immediately below the cardiac sphincter.
    b. Body which forms the largest and central portion.
    c. Pylorus forms the lower portion.
3. Sphincters.
    a. Cardiac sphincter is muscle around the lower end of the esophagus where it opens into the stomach.
    b. Pyloric sphincter is muscle around the lower end of the stomach where it opens into the duodenum.
4. Curvatures.
    a. Lesser curvature.
    b. Greater curvature.
5. Layers.
    a. Serous coat is the outer layer which forms the visceral peritoneum; the peritoneum folds and forms the omentum, which hangs over the intestines like an apron.
    b. Muscular layer formed of three directional (circular, longitudinal, and oblique) muscle fibers.
    c. Submucous layer contains blood vessels and lymphatics.
    d. Mucous layer contains microscopic glands which assist in digestion.
6. Glands.
    a. Mucous gland secretes mucus.
    b. Gastric gland secretes gastric juice containing hydrochloric acid and digestive enzymes.
7. Function.
    a. Mechanical digestion.
      (1) Most digestion occurs near pyloric area where peristalsis is more forceful.
      (2) Peristalsis is stimulated by the vagus nerve.
    b. Chemical digestion—excretes gastric juice containing hydrochloric acid and enzymes.

E. Small intestine.
1. Convoluted tube approximately 23 feet in length.
2. General functions.
    a. Digestion and absorption.
    b. Receives bile and pancreatic juices.
3. Segments.
    a. Duodenum begins at the pylorus and connects with the jejunum where it ends; it is approximately ten inches long.
    b. Jejunum is the middle portion which is approximately eight feet long and lies coiled around the umbilical region.
    c. Ileum is the terminal section which joins the colon at the ileocecal valve; it is approximately 12 feet long.
4. Folds.
    a. Extend around the intestinal lumen; most numerous in the duodenum but disappear in the lower ileum.
    b. Contain numerous villi through which products of digestion are absorbed. Each villus has an arteriole, venule and lymph vessel.
    c. Folds provide a large surface area which assists digestion, secretion, and absorption.

F. Large intestine.
1. Extends from the ileocecal valve to the anus; it is five to six feet long and is wider than the small intestine.
2. Segments.
    a. Cecum connects with the ileum at the ileocecal valve; appendix attaches to the distal end.
    b. Ascending colon continues up the right side of the abdomen to lower borders of the liver where it turns.
    c. Transverse colon continues from the ascending colon across the abdomen

(front of stomach) to lower border of the spleen.

    d. Descending colon continues from the transverse colon down the left side of the abdomen to the brim of the pelvis.

    e. Sigmoid colon is the S-shaped portion which extends to the rectum.

    f. Rectum is six to eight inches long and ends at anus.

  3. General functions.

    a. Reabsorption of fluids, electrolytes, glucose, and urea.

    b. Mechanical digestion.

    c. Peristalsis and defecation.

    d. Elimination of wastes.

Accessory Organs

A. Liver.

  1. Located in the right upper abdomen and protected by lower ribs.

  2. Largest organ in the body.

  3. General functions.

    a. Metabolism of carbohydrates, fats, and proteins.

    b. Detoxification of harmful substances in the blood.

    c. Breakdown of old blood cells.

    d. Constant secretion of bile, which drains from the liver through the hepatic duct into the common duct to the small intestine; bile is stored in the gallbladder.

    e. Stores glycogen and vitamins A, B, B_{12}, and K.

    f. Produces and stores heparin and fibrinogen.

B. Gallbladder.

  1. Small sac of smooth muscle located in a depression at the edge of the visceral surface of the liver.

  2. Functions as a reservoir for bile.

    a. Bile from the hepatic duct enters the gallbladder through the cystic duct for storage.

    b. Stored bile leaves the gallbladder through the cystic duct to flow through the common duct into the small intestine.

    c. Bile activates the pancreas to release its digestive enzymes and an alkaline fluid.

C. Pancreas.

  1. Soft, pinkish-white organ that is six inches long and one inch wide; it adheres to the middle portion of the duodenum.

  2. Composed of exocrine and endocrine tissue.

    a. Exocrine cells secrete juices containing digestive enzymes.

    b. Endocrine cells secrete glucagon and insulin.

DIAGNOSTIC PROCEDURES

Upper Gastrointestinal Roentgenography

A. Purpose.

  1. For visualizing GI tract.

    a. Structure and function of the esophagus.

    b. Size and shape of the right atrium.

    c. Size and shape of the stomach.

    d. Motility of the stomach.

    e. Ulcerations, tumor formations, and anatomic abnormalities of the stomach and small intestines.

    f. Emptying time of the stomach.

  2. For documenting in permanent records.

B. Procedure.

  1. Ingestion of barium or other contrast medium.

  2. Pass x-rays through the body so that GI tract will stand out in silhouette on film.

C. Preparation of the patient.

  1. NPO after midnight prior to the day of the test.

  2. Withhold medications.

  3. Explain procedure to the patient.

Barium Enema

A. Purpose.
   1. For visualizing the lower intestinal tract.
   2. For revealing abnormalities of structure and motility of the cecum and appendix.
B. Procedure.
   1. Barium enema given.
   2. X-ray film taken.
C. Preparation of the patient.
   1. Evacuate the intestinal tract by enema, laxatives, or suppositories until returning solution is clear.
   2. NPO after midnight (some methods allow clear liquids for breakfast).
   3. Explain procedure to patient.

Endoscopy

A. Purpose.
   1. For visualizing inside of body cavity to detect lesions.
   2. For taking biopsy.
   3. Secure washings for cytologic examination.
B. Preparation of the patient.
   1. NPO after midnight.
   2. Premedicate the patient.
   3. Give patient support during exam.
   4. Assist the physician.
   5. Topical anesthetic may be used to facilitate passage of the scope into the esophagus during exam. The anesthetic depresses the gag reflex.
C. Nursing care following an esophagogastroduodenoscopy (EGD).
   1. Withhold fluids or food by mouth until swallowing reflex returns.
   2. Observe carefully for swelling.
   3. Prevent aspiration if vomiting occurs.

Gastric Analysis

A. Purpose.
   1. For analyzing stomach contents for acid-fast bacilli, for volume, and for free acid.
   2. For detecting gastric bleeding.

B. Procedure.
   1. Insertion of nasogastric tube to aspirate stomach contents.
   2. Specimens obtained at varying times.
C. Preparation of the patient.
   1. NPO six to eight hours prior to exam.
   2. Collect specimens as ordered; label and send to lab.
   3. Remove nasogastric tube and provide oral hygiene.

Stool Analysis

A. Purpose.
   1. For examining amount, consistency, color, shape, blood, fecal urobilinogen, fat, nitrogen, parasites, food residue, and other substances.
   2. For culturing bacteria and viruses.
B. Procedure.
   1. Collect fresh, warm stool specimen for parasite analysis.
   2. Collect specimen in small amount for occult blood analysis (guaiac).
   3. Obtain a 24-hour collection for chemical analysis.
   4. Collect specimen in sterile container for C&S.
C. Stool characteristics.
   1. Color.
      a. Foods (spinach, cocoa) produce dark red.
      b. Medicines (senna) produce yellow.
      c. Iron produces black.
      d. Upper GI bleeding produces tarry black.
      e. Fresh, lower tract bleeding produces bright red.
   2. Stool abnormalities.
      a. Steatorrhea may be indicated by bulky, greasy, foamy, and foul-odored stools.
      b. Biliary obstruction may be indicated by light gray or clay-colored stools.
      c. Ulcerative colitis may be indicated by loose stools with copious amounts of mucus and/or pus.

d. Constipation or obstruction may be indicated by small, hard-massed stools.

GASTROINTESTINAL DISORDERS

Anorexia

Definition: Loss or lack of appetite for food.

Causes

A. Anxiety, depression.
B. Improper fit of dentures.
C. Illness, physical discomfort.
D. Constipation.
E. Intestinal obstruction.

Implementation

A. Become familiar with patient's eating habits, i.e., likes and dislikes in food, cultural and religious beliefs regarding food.
B. Permit, when possible, patient to choose own food.
C. Show interest, but don't force patient to eat.
D. Provide a pleasant and inviting environment.
E. Serve small portions of attractively prepared food.

Nausea and Vomiting

Definitions: Nausea is the distressing feeling that is felt when nerves ending in stomach and other body parts are irritated; may lead to vomiting. Vomiting is ejection of stomach contents through mouth.

Causes

A. Stress, fear, and depression.
B. Pain.
C. Acute febrile illness.
D. Medications.
E. Anesthesia.
F. Diseases of the stomach.
G. Intestinal obstruction.
H. Pregnancy.
I. Head injury.

Implementation

A. Administer relief-giving drugs.
B. Monitor fluid and electrolyte replacement.
C. Protect the patient from unpleasant sights, sounds, and smells.
D. Attempt to keep the stomach empty.
E. Promptly remove used equipment; change soiled linens and dressings.
F. Ventilate room and use unscented air fresheners.
G. Observe and record the character and quantity of emesis.

Constipation and Diarrhea

Definitions: Diarrhea is the rapid movement through intestines of loose, watery stools resulting from increased peristalsis. Constipation is the delay in the evacuation of feces, with passage of hard and dry fecal material.

Causes

A. Diarrhea—fecal impaction, ulcerative colitis, intestinal infections, drugs, or neurosis.
B. Constipation—lack of regularity, psychogenic causes, drugs, inadequate fluid intake, mechanical obstruction, lack of dietary bulk, or lack of exercise.

Implementation

A. Administer laxatives for constipation; antidiarrheals for diarrhea.

B. Observe stools for color, odor, shape, consistency, amount, presence of mucus, blood, or pus.

C. Provide perirectal skin care.

Oral Infections

Definitions: Stomatitis is an inflammation of the mouth. Glossitis is an inflammation of the tongue. Gingivitis is an inflammation of the gums.

Causes

A. Mechanical trauma.

B. Foods, drinks, allergies, or medications.

C. Poor oral hygiene.

D. Pathogens.

Assessment

A. Anorexia.

B. Excessive salivation.

C. Foul breath (halitosis).

Treatment and Implementation

A. Remove causative factor.

B. Provide frequent, soothing oral hygiene.

C. Apply topical medications and administer systemic antibiotics.

D. Provide soft, bland diet.

E. Administer analgesic (may be topical application) 30 minutes before meals.

Malignant Tumors of the Mouth

Definition: Cancer of the mouth that usually affects the lips, tongue, or the mouth floor.

Predisposing Factors

A. Poor oral hygiene.

B. Chronic irritation.

C. Chemical and thermal trauma, i.e., tobacco, alcohol, and hot-spiced foods.

Treatment

A. Surgical removal of tumor.

B. Radiation therapy.

Esophageal Disorders

Definition: Local or systemic infection or chemical irritation from reflux of gastric juices into the lower esophagus.

Assessment

A. Heartburn.

B. Intolerance of spices.

C. Alcohol and caffeine intolerance.

D. Dysphagia.

Treatment and Implementation

A. Give oral antacids.

B. Provide bland diet.

C. Elevate head of bed; do not recline after meals.

Esophageal Varices

Definition: Tortuous dilation of veins in the lower esophagus caused by portal hypertension and often associated with cirrhosis of liver.

Treatment and Implementation

A. Placement of Sengstaken-Blakemore tube to exert pressure against ruptured vessels.
   1. Maintain pressure in balloon.
   2. Do not deflate balloon.

B. Administer vitamin K.

C. Observe for hemorrhage and shock.

D. Provide frequent oral hygiene.

Cancer of Esophagus

Definition: Malignant tumors of the esophagus; carcinomas, constituting four percent of all malignant tumors along the GI tract, are the most common form of tumor.

Assessment

A. Dysphagia (most common).
B. Substernal pressure.

Treatment and Implementation

A. Radiation therapy.
B. Gastrostomy tube.
C. Watch for complications (rupture, hemorrhage).

Esophageal Hernia (Hiatus Hernia)

Definition: Protrusion of a portion of the stomach through the diaphragm and into the thorax.

Causes

A. Congenital weakness of the diaphragm.
B. Trauma.
C. Relaxation of the muscles.
D. Intra-abdominal pressure (obesity, ascites, pregnancy).

Assessment

A. Heartburn and pain.
B. Dysphagia.
C. Vomiting.
D. Regurgitation (especially after large meals or ingestion of spicy foods).

Implementation

A. Provide small frequent meals (avoid highly seasoned foods).
B. Maintain patient in upright position during and after meals.
C. Administer antacids after meals and at bedtime.
D. Elevate head of bed to avoid regurgitation during sleep.
E. Avoid anticholinergic drugs which delay emptying of stomach.
F. Advise patient against constrictive clothing around the waist.
G. Advise patient against sharp and forward bends.

Dyspepsia (Indigestion)

Definition: Imperfect digestion symptomatic of other GI diseases or disorders; characterized by heartburn and other abdominal discomforts.

Causes

A. Rapid ingestion.
B. Disease.
C. Altered gastric secretions.
D. Emotional problems.

Implementation

A. Provide bland diet.
B. Administer antispasmodics, tranquilizers, and antacids.
C. Advise patient to modify current eating habits.

Acute Gastritis

Definition: Inflammation of the stomach.

Causes

A. Ingestion of corrosive or erosive substances, (alcohol, aspirin, or contaminated food).
B. Acute systemic infections.
C. Radiotherapy or chemotherapy.
D. Infection.

Assessment

A. Epigastric burning and pain.
B. Nausea and vomiting.
C. Malaise.
D. Hemorrhage.
E. Anorexia.
F. Headache.

Treatment and Implementation

A. Attempt to eliminate the cause; treat symptomatically.
B. Administer antacids and phenothiazines.

Principles of Nursing Care for Gastrointestinal Surgery

Preoperative Care

A. Psychological care.
  1. Allay fears regarding postoperative concerns.
  2. Familiarize the patient with hospital procedures.
    a. Show method for getting in and out of bed.
    b. Teach leg exercises.
    c. Teach deep breathing and coughing exercises.
    d. Explain pain medication schedule.
    e. Discuss recovery room routines.
  3. Encourage questions and feedback to determine what patient actually understands.
  4. Include family in preoperative explanations.
B. Physical care.
  1. Report any change in vital signs.
  2. Check and record each item on preoperative check list.
  3. Give enema to cleanse the lower colon.
  4. Remove all prostheses.
  5. Encourage patient to void.
  6. Administer preoperative medication (it will dry secretions and promote sense of well-being).
  7. Put side rails up.
  8. Remove valuables and place in safekeeping.

Postoperative Care

A. Check airway for obstruction.
B. Evaluate the need for pain medication.
C. Check for presence and patency of tubes.
D. Monitor IV.
  1. Check flow rate and contents of bottle.
  2. Check insertion site for pain and signs of inflammation.
E. Examine dressing for color and amount of drainage; record in nurse's notes.
F. Check vital signs frequently.
G. Observe for signs of hypovolemic shock.
  1. Drop in blood pressure.
  2. Increase in pulse or respirations.
  3. Change in color.
  4. Dyspnea.
H. Observe for first passage of flatus on all GI surgical patients. Bowel sounds or flatus indicate the return of peristalsis.
I. Record the time and amount of first voiding.
J. Turn patient every two hours.
  1. Encourage coughing and deep breathing.
  2. Support abdominal incision with pillow, hands, or blanket during patient coughing to reduce strain on incision and increase patient comfort.
K. Assist in ambulation as ordered.
L. Encourage taking of food as ordered and tolerated.
M. Follow general principles of nasogastric tube care.

Management of Postoperative Pain

A. Evaluate need for medication every three to four hours for the first 24 hours; give freely.

B. Do not give morphine to patients with biliary or pancreatic disorders as it results in spasms of the smooth muscle.

Management of Nasogastric Intubation and Decompression

A. Purpose of intubation.
 1. Prevent postoperative vomiting after GI surgery.
 2. Provide feedings.
 3. Relieve abdominal distention as a result of bowel obstruction or paralytic ileus.
 4. Provide rest for the GI tract.
B. Tubal types.
 1. Stomach tubes—flexible tubes introduced by way of nose to decompress stomach after surgery or for feedings.
    a. Salem sump—remove fluid accumulation.
    b. Levin tube—gastroduodenal catheter.
 2. Intestinal tubes—tubes placed in intestinal tract by way of nose to relive gas pressure.
    a. Miller-Abbott—double-channel intestinal tube.
    b. Cantor tube—used for intestinal decompression.
C. Nursing care.
 1. Provide frequent oral and nasal care.
 2. Maintain patency of tubes with irrigation of normal saline as ordered.
 3. Check for placement of tubes before irrigation by listening with stethoscope for air bubble insertion via syringe.
 4. Observe color and amount of drainage.
 5. Record intake and output.
 6. Be alert to fact that vomiting or abdominal distention is an indication of obstruction.

Peptic Ulcer Disease (PUD)

Definition: Ulceration in the mucosal wall of the stomach, pylorus, or duodenum.

Predisposing Factors

A. Emotional and physical stress.
B. Irregular, hurriedly ingested meals.
C. Seasonal factor (spring and fall).
D. Excessive smoking.
E. Drugs, e.g., salicylates, phenylbutazone, and steroids.
F. Hereditary factors.

Assessment

A. Boring, aching, gnawing or burning epigastric pain.
B. Pain usually occurring one half to three hours after eating.
C. Weight loss from reduced intake or weight gain from excessive intake in effort to relieve pain.
D. Vomiting which may result from pain or from pyloric obstruction due to ulcerations and to scarring that accompanies healing.
E. Occult blood in stool from bleeding.

Implementation

A. Promote healing process by preventing complications.
B. Provide symptomatic relief.
C. Eliminate irritating factors, e.g., alcohol, smoking, stress, and salicylates.
D. Administer histamine H_2 receptor antagonists (Tagamet, Zantac), antacids, anticholinergics, iron, and antibiotics.
E. Observe emesis and/or stool closely (iron preparations may also result in dark stools).
F. Provide diet that eliminates gas-producing foods—three meals per day.
G. Observe and report significant physical and emotional responses to therapy.
H. Observe for indications of complications (i.e., hemorrhage, perforation).
I. Gastric surgery may be required if medical treatment is ineffective.

Gastric Surgical Procedures

A. Vagotomy—interruption of vagal innervation to reduce stimulation of hydrochloric acid production.

B. Gastrectomy or partial gastrectomy—removal of stomach portion that produces hydrochloric acid; anastomosis between remaining portion of stomach and small bowel (gastroenterostomy).

C. Gastrostomy, jejunostomy—creation of opening into the stomach or jejuneum for general purpose of maintaining nutritional status of patient when conditions make use of normal food route not feasible.

Postoperative Implementation

A. Provide routine care.
  1. Observe and record vital signs.
  2. Observe for signs of shock.
  3. Check dressing for abnormal drainage or bleeding.
  4. Provide bed rest.
  5. Record intake and output.
  6. Turn patient and encourage cough and deep breathing exercises every 2 hours.

B. Manage accessory equipment.
  1. Foley and IV tubes.
  2. Nasogastric tube.
    a. Ensure patency.
      (1) Irrigate with normal saline.
      (2) Maintain proper suction pressure.
      (3) Maintain correct position.
    b. Observe and record color, consistency, amount, and unusual odor of gastric contents.

C. Raise bed to semi-Fowler's position.

D. Following removal of NG tube provide diet of warm liquids; provide soft diet.

E. Control pain but avoid irritating medications such as salicylates.

F. Change incisional dressings as needed.

G. Prevent constipation.

H. Ambulate first postoperative day unless specified otherwise.

I. Discourage smoking.

J. Protect patient from stressful situations.

Postoperative Complications

A. Hemorrhage.
  1. Indications.
    a. Emesis with coffee-grounds color.
    b. Tarry black stools (melena).
    c. Hematemesis (vomiting of bright-red blood).
  2. Treatment—possible surgical procedure.

B. Perforation—erosion through stomach muscle into peritoneum.
  1. Indications.
    a. Acute onset of severe, persistent pain that may be referred to shoulder or between the scapulae.
    b. Tender, boardlike rigidity of the abdomen.
    c. Thready, rapid pulse.
  2. Treatment—surgical procedure.

C. Pyloric obstruction (scarring, edema, or inflammation at the pylorus from healing of chronic ulcerations).
  1. Indications.
    a. Nausea and projectile vomiting.
    b. Pain.
    c. Weight loss.
    d. Constipation.
  2. Treatment—gastric decompression or surgical repair to relieve the stenosis (narrowing).

D. "Dumping syndrome" (rapid emptying of large amounts of food into small bowel following gastrectomy).
  1. Indications.
    a. Weakness, faintness.
    b. Diaphoresis.
    c. Palpitations.
  2. Nursing care.
    a. Serve frequent meals of small proportions.
    b. Encourage drinking liquids between meals instead of with meals.

c. Provide nutrients that are low in carbo-hydrates, high in proteins, and moderate in fats.

d. Encourage 30 minute rest period after meals.

e. Discourage use of table salt and sugars.

Gastric Cancer

Definition: Malignant tumor of the stomach, a common cancer of the digestive tract.

Assessment

A. *Early stage of carcinoma produces no symptoms.*

B. Weight loss.

C. Vague feeling of fullness and sensation of pressure.

D. Anemia as a result of blood loss.

E. Occult blood in stools.

F. Vomiting if pylorus becomes obstructed.

G. Late stage produces symptoms that include ascites, palpable mass, metastatic pain.

Treatment

A. Surgical resection.

B. Radiation therapy.

C. Chemotherapy.

Diverticulitis

Definition: Inflammation of diverticula (blind pouches) formed in the intestinal mucosa and walls of the sigmoid. Diverticulosis is the presence of multiple diverticula. Confirmed by upper-lower GI series and sigmoidoscopy.

Assessment

A. Cramplike pain.

B. Flatulence.

C. Nausea and fever.

D. Bowel irregularity.

E. Irritability, spasticity of intestine.

Implementation

A. Provide high residue diet that is high in protein, calories, vitamins, and iron. Low residue diet used in inflammatory phase of diverticulitis.

B. Administer antispasmodics.

C. Establish normal bowel habits for patient who has deviated from normal patterns.

D. Performance of surgery as necessary.

Ulcerative Colitis

Definition: Chronic ulcerous and inflammatory disease of the colon and rectum which commonly begins in the rectum and sigmoid colon and spreads upward; characterized by periods of exacerbation and remission.

Cause

A. Specific cause is unknown.

B. Autoimmune factors, allergic reactions and emotional instability are potential causative factors.

C. Bacterial infections may be causal factor.

Assessment

A. Anemia and malnutrition.

B. Frequent stools that contain mucus, blood, and pus.

C. Anorexia, weight loss.

D. Cramplike pain.

E. Abdominal tenderness.

Treatment and Implementation

A. Relieve anxiety, i.e., provide quiet environment, remove stress factor, and give medication.

B. Administer antibiotics for secondary bowel inflammation.

C. Administer steroid therapy for inflammation, toxicity, and emotional symptoms.

D. Administer anticholinergic drugs to relieve cramps and control diarrhea.

E. Provide high protein, high caloric diet with vitamin and iron supplements.

F. Allow patient to ventilate his or her feelings; extend acceptance to patient.

G. Administer no cathartics in acute stage; condition contraindicates cathartics.

H. Administer IV therapy during acute phase.

I. Bed rest during acute phase.

J. Surgical treatment is indicated if medical management fails.

Complications

A. Dehydration.

B. Anemia and malnutrition (iron and vitamin K deficiency).

C. Magnesium and calcium imbalance.

D. Perforation, peritonitis, and hemorrhage.

E. Abscesses and strictures.

F. Hemorrhoids and anal fissures.

G. Tendency to bleed.

Intestinal Obstruction

Definition: Impairment of the forward flow of intestinal contents by partial or complete blockage.

Causes

A. Adhesions (fibrous bands of abdominal scar tissue which may become looped over a portion of the bowel).

B. Incarcerated or strangulated hernias.

C. Volvulus (twisting of the bowel).

D. Intussusception (telescoping of bowel upon itself).

E. Tumors.

F. Hematoma.

G. Fecal impaction.

H. Ileus (ineffective peristalsis due to toxic or traumatic disturbance of innervation to the bowel).

I. Loss of blood supply to the bowel with resulting necrosis.

Assessment

A. Nausea and vomiting.

B. Reverse peristalsis with possible fecal vomiting.

C. Abdominal distention.

D. Absence of stools.

Treatment and Implementation

A. Intestinal decompression tube may be inserted to remove gas and fluid.

B. Monitor parenteral fluids and electrolytes.

C. Administer antibiotics.

D. Note and record in chart.
   1. Extent and nature of pain.
   2. Characteristics, amount, and frequency of stools, emesis, and flatus.
   3. Amount of intake and output.
   4. Vital signs.

E. Possible performance of surgery if medical therapy ineffective.

Colon Surgery

A. Ileostomy.
   1. Procedure—creation of opening into ileum brought through abdominal wall for purpose of eliminating bowel contents. Large intestine may or may not be removed.
   2. Conditions that may lead to ileostomy.
      a. Ulcerative colitis.
      b. Crohn's disease.
   3. Postoperative care.
      a. Observe and record vital signs.
      b. Need not irrigate for evacuation as stool is always in liquid state.

c. Watch for excoriation of skin around stoma; condition may occur with ileostomy because of enzymatic action.

d. Increase fluid intake because reabsorption in large bowel is absent.

e. Provide low residue, high calorie diet; avoid foods that increase peristalsis or produce flatus.

B. Colostomy. ❖ **Procedure** ❖

1. Procedure—creation of abdominal stoma for bowel evacuation following removal of portion of lower (large) intestine.

2. Conditions indicating colostomy.

   a. Cancer—usually requires permanent colostomy.

   b. Traumatic injury—may require permanent or temporary colostomy.

   c. Diverticulitis or obstruction—usually requires temporary colostomy.

3. Preoperative care.

   a. Explain to patient the use of apparatus to be utilized in care of the colostomy.

   b. Reassure patient that nurse will give assistance in learning to care for the colostomy.

   c. Accept the patient's feelings about consequence of procedure; observe for depression, anxiety, and frustration.

   d. Provide high calorie, low residue diet for several days.

   e. Administer intestinal antiseptics with sulfa and neomycin (PO) to decrease bacterial content of colon and to soften and decrease bulk of contents of colon.

   f. Cleanse bowel by administering laxatives and enemas.

   g. Provide adequate fluids and electrolytes.

4. Postoperative care.

   a. Depends on which part of colon involved; contents are liquid to formed.

   b. Patient has no voluntary control of bowel evacuation.

   c. Ascending colostomy is hard to train for evacuation.

   d. Evacuate bowel every 24 to 48 hours.

   e. Control with diet and/or irrigation.

f. Maintain skin care around stoma.

g. Assure proper fit and placement of appliance.

h. Increase fluid intake.

i. Support and guide patient in learning to care for body function which henceforth will be accomplished differently.

Appendicitis

Definition: Inflammation of appendix as a result of bacterial infection.

Assessment

A. Rebound tenderness (major symptom).

B. Generalized and severe abdominal pain.

C. Nausea and vomiting.

D. Elevated temperature.

E. Anorexia.

Surgical Procedure Appendectomy.

A. Preoperative care.

1. Raise bed to semi-Fowler's position to relieve strain on abdomen.

2. Give nothing by mouth.

3. Insert nasogastric tube.

B. Postoperative care—routine for abdominal surgery.

C. Complications.

1. Rupture.

2. Peritonitis.

   a. Indications.

      (1) Severe abdominal pain localized in right lower quadrant.

      (2) Elevated temperature.

      (3) Elevated white cell count.

   b. Treatment.

      (1) Massive antibiotics.

      (2) GI decompression.

      (3) Bed rest.

      (4) High-Fowler's position to localize infection.

      (5) Nothing by mouth.

Hernia

Definition: Protrusion of part of an organ through the structures normally containing it.

Types

A. Inguinal—occurring in the groin as result of increased abdominal pressure.
B. Femoral—occurring in the femoral canal.
C. Umbilical—occurring at the umbilicus.
D. Incisional—occurring at incisional site as a result of improper healing.

Classifications

A. Reducible hernia—can be replaced in normal cavity.
B. Irreducible hernia—cannot be replaced in the normal cavity.
C. Incarcerated—resulting edema of the affected structures.
D. Strangulated—gangrenous condition results due to trapped blood supply.

Treatment and Implementation

A. Surgical repair—hernioplasty; herniorrhaphy.
B. Advise patient not to cough following surgical repair.
C. Take measures to prevent urinary retention.
D. Encourage patient to ambulate soon after surgery to prevent postoperative complications.

Hemorrhoids

Definition: Dilated varicose veins of the anal canal that cause discomfort and bleeding.

Types

A. Internal—occurs above the internal sphincter, covered by mucous membrane.
B. External—occurs outside the external sphincter, covered by anal skin.
C. Thrombosed—infected, clotted, and painful.

Causes

A. By straining to evacuate when constipated.
B. Irritation and diarrhea.
C. Increased venous pressure from congestive heart failure.
D. Increased abdominal pressure as occurs in pregnancy.
E. Habitual toilet sitting (reading of magazines in the bathroom).

Assessment

A. Anal itching.
B. Painful bowel evacuation.
C. Bleeding with bowel evacuation.

Treatment and Implementation

A. Treat constipation and other causes of increased pressure.
B. Relieve pain with heat, astringents, and topical and systemic analgesics.
C. Internal hemorrhoids ligated with rubber bands—tissue necroses and drops off.
D. Postoperative care of hemorrhoidectomy.
   1. Make routine observations including vital signs.
   2. Maintain meticulous perineal and rectal cleanliness.
   3. Apply topical anesthetics; give sitz baths for comfort.
   4. Maintain prone or on-side positions to prevent pressure and provide comfort.
   5. Administer medications before first postoperative bowel movement.
   6. Increase liquids and bulk with administration of stool softeners to decrease discomfort of first bowel movement.
   7. Give ordered enema with caution.
      a. Administer medications to relieve pain before giving enema.
      b. Use well-lubricated tip.
      c. Introduce tip with gentleness.

DIAGNOSTIC PROCEDURES FOR LIVER, GALLBLADDER, AND PANCREAS DISORDERS

Radiologic Techniques

A. Cholecystogram.
1. Purpose—visualize gallbladder by means of radiopaque dye given intravenously few minutes prior to exam or by means of Telepaque given orally the evening prior to exam.
2. Preprocedural nursing care (using Telepaque)
   a. Give patient low-fat meal evening prior to exam.
   b. Give Telepaque according to body weight at three to five minute intervals with 240 ml of water (minimum).
   c. Give nothing by mouth after midnight.
B. Cholangiography.
1. Purpose—visualize bile ducts by means of contrast radiopaque injected directly into biliary tree.
2. Preprocedural nursing care.
   a. Restrict fluids to concentrate dye.
   b. Cleans intestinal tract.
C. Liver scan—visualize liver tissue by means of administered radioiodine (^{131}I) or similar substances and scintiscan to reveal its concentration in the liver.

Liver Biopsy

A. Purpose—facilitate diagnosis by sampling liver tissues with needle aspiration to determine tissue changes.
B. Preprocedural nursing care.
1. Obtain baseline vital signs.
2. Maintain NPO regimen.
3. Assemble equipment, position patient, and assist the physician.
C. Postprocedural nursing care.
1. Position patient on right side over biopsy site to prevent hemorrhage.
2. Observe for complications (hemorrhage, shock).
3. Measure and record vital signs.

Laboratory Examination

A. Serum bilirubin level—abnormal amounts indicate biliary and liver disease leading to jaundice.
B. Carbohydrate metabolism—glucose tolerance levels should return to normal within one to two hours.
C. Blood ammonia—level rises in liver failure because liver converts ammonia to urea.
D. Enzyme production—elevation of enzymes reflects organ damage (SGPT, SGOT, LDH).
E. Prothrombin time—clotting ability reduced in liver cell damage.

DISORDERS OF THE LIVER, GALLBLADDER, AND PANCREAS

Jaundice

Definition: Symptom of liver disorder characterized by yellow pigmentation of the skin and due to accumulation of bilirubin pigment in the blood. The degree of jaundice is best detected in the sclera of the eyes.

Indications

A. Rapid rate of red blood cell destruction (hemolytic jaundice).
B. Diseased liver cells.
C. Viral liver cell necrosis or cirrhosis of the liver.
D. Obstruction due to inflammation, tumors, or cholestatic agents.

Implementation

A. Relieve pruritus with starch baths, lotions, antihistamines, and mild sedatives.
B. Provide emotional support.

C. Prepare family for patient's altered skin and eye color.

D. Remove mirrors from patient's line of sight.

E. Encourage bed rest.

Viral Hepatitis

Definition: Inflammation of the liver caused by a virus.

A. Type A hepatitis (infectious hepatitis).
   1. Transmitted by excreta, infected blood transfusion, contaminated syringes and needles, contaminated food products, and possibly by way of respiratory tract.
   2. Signs and symptoms.
      a. Headache and fever.
      b. Nausea, anorexia, and vomiting.
      c. Abdominal pain with tenderness.
      d. If jaundiced, patient produces dark urine and clay-colored stools.
      e. Maculopapular rash.
   3. Nursing care.
      a. Isolate to prevent transmission of disease.
      b. Use disposable equipment.
      c. Provide high caloric, well-balanced diet.
      d. Encourage adequate rest.
      e. Stress the importance of continuing medical supervision after hospitalization.
      f. Advise patient never to be blood donor.
      g. Advise against use of alcoholic beverages.
      h. Encourage gamma globulin as preventive measure when in close contact with others.

B. Type B hepatitis (serum hepatitis, viral).
   1. Transmitted by oral, parenteral, or sexual route by means of infusion or ingestion from the blood or secretions of an infected person; and by contaminated equipment, such as needles, syringes, and dental instruments.
   2. Signs and symptoms are similar to but more severe than infectious hepatitis.

   3. Treatment and nursing care.
      a. Encourage bed rest until symptoms have decreased in severity.
      b. Provide well-balanced diet supplemented with vitamins.
      c. Administer antacids for gastric acidity.

C. Type C—formerly non-A, non-B.
   1. Transmitted by contaminated blood.
   2. Incidence noted following gamma globulin injection.
   3. Incubation period 7–8 weeks.
   4. May not show jaundice.

Hepatic Coma

Definition: Hepatic coma results from brain cell alterations due to build-up of ammonia levels.

Assessment

A. Impaired memory, attention, concentration, and rate of mental response.

B. Confusion, inappropriate behavior, and depressed level of consciousness.

C. Untidy appearance.

D. Flapping tremor upon dorsiflexion of the hand.

E. Disorientation leading to eventual coma.

Implementation

A. Observe, measure, and record neurologic status daily (ability to perform simple task such as writing one's signature diminishes as the blood ammonia level increases).

B. Weigh patient daily because liver function decreases and ascites and edema increase.

C. Measure and record intake and output.

D. Administer sedatives and analgesics sparingly because failing liver unable to detoxify them.

E. Eliminate protein from the diet temporarily because the ammonia formed from the breakdown of proteins cannot be converted into urea for excretion.

Cirrhosis

Definition: Progressive disease of the liver characterized by diffuse damage (degeneration) to the cells which cannot be recovered or reversed.

Types

A. Alcoholic (nutritional).
B. Postnecrotic (e.g., precipitated by viral hepatitis).

Assessment

A. Gastrointestinal distress, fatigue, low resistance to infection, gradual failing health.
B. Emaciation and ascites due to malnutrition.
C. Edema of lower extremities.

Implementation

A. Provide diet adequate in proteins and carbohydrates, low in salt, and multivitamins (especially B).
B. Avoid administering sedatives and opiates.
C. Prevent infection by providing adequate rest and environmental control.
D. Provide good skin care and control pruritus resulting from elevated BUN.
E. Measure and record and compare vital signs to previous measurement.
F. Evaluate level of consciousness and be alert to personality changes and signs of increasing stupor.

Cholecystitis with Cholelithiasis

Definition: Inflammation of the gallbladder caused by cholelithiasis (presence of gallstones).

Assessment

A. Pain in upper right quadrant of abdomen that is moderate to severe with passage of stones.
B. Nausea and vomiting.
C. Intolerance to fat.
D. Fever.
E. Jaundice will occur if common bile duct obstructed with stones.
F. Edema from inflammation.

Treatment and Implementation

A. Administer drugs for control of pain (Demerol—morphine sulfate may increase pain).
B. Insert nasogastric tube for suction.
C. Give nothing by mouth (low fat diet may be possible).
D. Measure and record intake and output.
E. Stones removed with shock wave lithotripsy—lithotriptor sends waves through a water bag.
F. Postoperative nursing care for cholecystectomy.
   1. Maintain T-tube which provides for bile drainage from liver, allowing some of the bile to enter into the common duct. T-tube provides independent drainage.
      ❖ **PROCEDURE** ❖
      a. Ensure patency and avoid stress on the tube; carefully position after dressings are changed.
      b. Use measures to control infection.
      c. Note character and amount of drainage.
      d. Clamp and release regimen as initial step in preparation for T-tube removal.
   2. Prevent infection (patients are often obese and may have delayed healing).
   3. Observe for indications of biliary obstruction, such as clay-colored stool, jaundiced sclera and/or skin.
   4. Advise patient to remain on low-fat diet for at least two to three months. Also avoid alcohol and gas-forming foods.
G. Endoscopic cholecystectomy—removal of gallbladder through small puncture hole in abdomen.
   1. Laser disects gallbladder.
   2. Patient discharged day of surgery—recovery 2–3 days.

Acute Pancreatitis

Definition: Inflammation of the pancreas. Cause is unknown, although alcoholic indulgence or biliary tract disease are thought to be predisposing factors.

Assessment

A. Constant abdominal pain radiating to the back and flank.
B. Nausea and vomiting.
C. Low-grade temperature.
D. Jaundice (observe stool for fat or clay color).
E. Abnormal glucose levels.

Treatment and Implementation

A. Give nothing by mouth.
B. Insert nasogastric tube for nausea and vomiting—low suction.
C. Provide skin care.
D. Administer medications.
    1. Demerol for pain—avoid opiates—may cause spasms.
    2. Anticholinergics to reduce pancreatic secretion.
    3. Sodium bicarbonate to reverse metabolic acidosis.
E. Monitor glucose levels with Clinitest and blood tests—may give regular insulin to treat hyperglycemia.
F. Measure and record intake and output—maintain fluids and electrolytes.
    1. Hypocalcemia—treated with calcium gluconate.
    2. Hypokalemia—treated with potassium.
G. Maintain quiet, nonstressful environment.
H. Observe and record vital signs.
I. Weigh and record patient's weight.

Chronic Pancreatitis

Definition: Gland is fibrosed and ducts are obstructed following repeated attacks of acute pancreatitis.

Assessment

A. Pain—persistent epigastric and left upper quadrant pain.
B. Anorexia, nausea, vomiting, and constipation.
C. Disturbance of protein and fat digestion.

Treatment and Implementation

A. Monitor drugs.
    1. Antacids.
    2. Histamine antagonists (Tagamet and Zantac).
    3. Anticholinergics.
    4. Pancreatic replacements.
B. Provide low protein, low fat, high carbohydrate, bland diet.
C. Report any diabetic symptoms.

GENITOURINARY SYSTEM

This system—the kidneys and their drainage channels—is essential for the maintenance of life. The organs of the GU system are responsible for excreting the end products of metabolism as well as regulating water and electrolyte concentrations of body fluids.

ANATOMY AND PHYSIOLOGY

Kidneys

A. Paired glandular organs located to the right and left of the midline, lateral to lower thoracic vertebrae, that have the ability to adapt to the body's changing needs for elimination of various substances.
B. Major functions.
  1. Excrete most of the end products of body metabolism.
  2. Maintain body acid-base and plasma electrolyte equilibrium.
  3. Produce enzymes that act on plasma substance which is capable of raising blood pressure.
C. Composition.
  1. Nephrons—microscopic filtering units.
  2. Glomerulus—capillary clusters within nephron capsule; filtering unit of the nephron.
  3. Tubule—collecting channel in nephron that converts the fluid to urine as it goes to the pelvis of the kidneys.
  4. Pelvis—collecting funnel; leads into ureter.
D. Urine.
  1. Composed of excess water and other soluble waste materials that are not reabsorbed into the tubules.
  2. Characteristics of normal urine.
    a. Can be diluted or concentrated.
    b. Clear.
    c. Yellow-amber in color.
    d. Slightly acid.
    e. Specific gravity 1.015 to 1.025.
    f. Negative for bacteria, albumin, sugar, blood, ketones, or bilirubin.

Ureter

A. Paired tubes lined with mucosa connecting the kidneys with the bladder.
B. Conducts urine by rhythmic contractions.

Bladder

A. Round, hollow, membranous sac with muscular walls, located in the pelvis.
B. Extraperitoneal; however, peritoneum adheres to dome of bladder.
C. May hold 1000 cc in volume if outflow obstructed.

Urethra

A. Single tube which allows passage of urine from bladder to outside of body.
B. Female urethra approximately 3 to 5 cm in length.
C. Male urethra approximately 20 cm in length.

DIAGNOSTIC PROCEDURES

A. Blood chemistry—blood urea nitrogen (BUN) analysis will indicate the ability of the kidney to excrete waste products.
B. Intravenous pyelogram (IVP)—injection of contrast dye for visualization on x-ray film of absence, presence, location, size, and configuration of each kidney, the filling of the renal pelvis, and outlines of the ureters.
C. Phenolsulfonphthalein (PSP)—a dye that tests the excretory function of the kidney.
D. Renal biopsy—needle inserted through renal tissue to extract tissue cells that are examined for evidence of malfunction; test can indicate the presence of disease, confirm a diagnosis,

indicate prognosis, or give evidence of response to treatment.

E. Cystoscopy—direct visualization by cystoscope for purposes of inspection, biopsy, treatment, or removal of stones.

F. Retrograde pyelogram—insertion of cystoscope and placement of ureteral catheters followed by injection of contrast dye into the catheters for visualization on x-ray film of ureters and kidneys.

DISORDERS OF THE KIDNEY

Nonspecific Assessment

A. Retention—inability to expel urine from the bladder due to obstruction or loss of innervation.

B. Incontinence—loss of voluntary control in discharge of urine.

C. Residual urine—urine remaining in bladder after voiding.

D. Anuria—suppression or failure of kidney to produce sufficient urine.

E. Oliguria—amount and frequency of urination are diminished.

F. Hematuria—blood in the urine, usually caused by infection or trauma.

Principles of Implementation

A. Maintain accurate measurement of intake and output.

B. Force or restrict fluids as ordered.

C. Observe and record characteristics of urine and times of voiding.

D. Record specific urinary complaints, e.g., urgency, burning, pain, frequency, bladder spasms, and inability to void (retention).

E. Strain all urine and take specimen to lab (if ordered) if renal lithiasis (stones) are suspected.

F. Maintain comfort of patient; position and provide analgesics and external heat for renal colic.

Specialized Catheter Care ❖ PROCEDURE ❖

A. Maintain patency of catheters.

B. Types of urinary tract catheters.
   1. Foley catheter—designed with inflatable balloon which, upon inflation, anchors catheter within bladder.
   2. Three-way Foley catheter—provides for drainage of urine, balloon for anchoring, and a third channel to allow for irrigation of the bladder.
   3. Straight catheter—a simple rubber catheter that is inserted into bladder for drainage and then removed.
   4. Ureteral catheters—very small-gauge catheters inserted directly into ureters during cystoscopy for drainage of urine from the pelvis of the kidney or for injection of dye for diagnostic purposes; if left inserted, they are usually anchored with a Foley.

Acute Renal Failure

Definition: Sudden loss of kidney function caused by failure of renal circulation or tubular or glomerular damage.

Causes

A. Dehydration.

B. Shock.

C. Traumatic injury.

D. Toxic agents, e.g., sulfonamides, arsenic.

E. Infection.

Assessment

A. Decreased urine output (volume of less than 400 to 500 ml/24 hours).

B. Hypertension may develop.

C. Nausea, vomiting, diarrhea, and convulsions leading to coma.

Treatment and Implementation

A. Treat cause of failure immediately.
B. Monitor body fluid volume and electrolytes.
C. Monitor urinary output (hourly basis may be indicated).
D. Weigh patient daily.
E. Follow diet restrictions: limited protein and sodium, with vitamin supplements.
F. Observe for complications of fluid overload, electrolyte disturbances, and CHF.

Chronic Renal Failure

Definition: Progressive impairment of kidney function which, without intervention, ends fatally in uremia.

Assessment

A. Weakness, fatigue, and headaches.
B. Anorexia, nausea, and vomiting.
C. Hypertension with renal and heart failure.
D. Anemia.
E. Central nervous system signs (i.e., irritability, convulsions).

Treatment and Implementation

A. Monitor intake and output.
B. Weigh patient daily.
C. Provide diet low in salt and altered amounts of protein; prepare as attractively as possible.
D. Monitor blood pressure closely.
E. Provide emotional support because chronicity of disease may precipitate depression.
F. Assist with hemodialysis.
   1. Procedure permits passage through a semipermeable membrane of substances, such as urea, creatinine, and uric acid, which diffuse through the pores of the membrane in the machine.
      a. The blood, which contains the waste products, flows from the patient into the dialysis machine where it comes into contact with the dialysate.
      b. The waste products are removed through contact of the blood as it flows into the machine and comes in contact with the dialysate.
   2. In essence, the dialysis machine becomes the patient's "kidney."
G. Peritoneal dialysis.
   1. A method of separating substances by interposing a semipermeable membrane. The peritoneum is used as the dialyzing membrane and substitutes for kidney function during failure.
   2. Procedure allows for infusion of dialysate through a peritoneal catheter for "dwell time" in order that waste products in the blood may diffuse into the solution.
   3. The dialysate is in direct contact with blood supply of mesentery.
   4. After "dwell time" fluid is drained by gravity into receptacles, and sample is sent to laboratory for testing. The volume returned by gravity should equal or be in excess of the volume of the infusion.

Pyelonephritis

Definition: An acute or chronic infection and inflammation of one or both kidneys that usually begins in the renal pelvis.

Assessment

A. Attacks of chills and fever, with malaise.
B. Tenderness and dull, aching pain in the back.
C. Frequency and burning with urination.

Treatment and Implementation

A. Record characteristics, frequency, and amount of voiding.
B. Provide diet high in calories and vitamin supplements and low in protein.
C. Give sufficient liquids to maintain urine volume of 1500 ml/24 hrs.
D. Observe for edema and signs of renal failure.

E. Teach principles of optimum personal hygiene to prevent further infections.

Acute Glomerulonephritis

Definition: Inflammatory disease of both kidneys that interferes with glomerular filtration; most commonly caused by repeated streptococcal infections in childhood.

Assessment

A. Headache, malaise, and weakness.
B. Oliguria and puffiness around the eyes.
C. Hematuria.
D. Moderate to marked hypertension.
E. Tenderness at costovertebral angle is common.
F. Diagnostic urinalysis indicates erythrocyte casts.

Treatment and Implementation

A. Administer antibiotics and antihypertensives.
B. Encourage bed rest.
C. Provide diet low in protein, low in sodium, high in carbohydrates, and high in vitamins.
D. Restrict fluids based on previous day's output.
E. Do not permit increase of activity until blood pressure and BUN are normal for one to two weeks.
F. Record intake and output.
G. Weigh patient daily.
H. Observe for signs of overhydration, hypertension, and renal failure.

KIDNEY SURGERY

Nephrectomy

Definition: Surgical removal of a kidney.

Indications

A. Severe injury producing irreparable damage to cells.
B. Chronic disease.
C. Permanent loss of kidney function.
D. Renal donor.

Implementation

A. Measure and record intake and output.
B. Encourage patient to take fluids.
C. Observe for signs of hemorrhage and shock.
D. Provide care for incision and Penrose drain.
E. Encourage postoperative exercises and early ambulation.
F. Control environment against infection from visitors and personnel.

Nephrostomy

Definition: Creation of surgical opening into kidney and placement of a catheter in the renal pelvis for urinary drainage.

Implementation

A. Record characteristics of drainage and urine.
B. Check for bleeding at surgical site as this is major complication.
C. Unless ordered, do not clamp catheter.
D. Unless ordered, do not irrigate (never irrigate with force; use only 5 to 10 cc of sterile solution; be especially careful not to contaminate).
E. In bilateral nephrostomy, maintain separate outputs.
F. Maintain patency of tubes when positioning patient and when changing dressings.

Urolithotomy

Definition: Removal of stones (calculi) formed in the urinary system (urolithiasis).

Types

A. Ureterolithotomy—removal of calculi from ureter which may be accomplished with use of cystoscope and stone crusher.

B. Pyelolithotomy—removal of stone from kidney pelvis.

Implementation

A. Force fluids.

B. Strain all urine.

C. Measure and record intake and output.

D. Observe and record characteristics of urine and time of voiding.

E. Prevent infection.

F. Observe for perforation of bladder, abdominal rigidity, anuria, chills, fever, and urine retention.

BLADDER DISORDERS AND SURGERY

Cystitis

Definition: Inflammation of the bladder from infection or from obstruction of the urethra.

Assessment

A. Frequency and urgency of urination.

B. Burning sensation in urethra during urination.

C. Suprapubic discomfort.

D. Dark and odorous urine.

E. Urinalysis reveals presence of bacteria and blood cells.

Treatment and Implementation

A. Attempt to remove cause of the infection.

B. Administer antibiotic therapy.

C. Collect uncontaminated urine specimen (catheterized or mid-stream).

D. Maintain adequate fluid intake.

E. Decrease patient's activity during the acute stage.

F. Teach principles of optimum personal hygiene to prevent recurrent infection.

Suprapubic Cystostomy

Definition: Creation of surgical opening and placement of catheter into bladder for urinary drainage.

Implementation

A. Change dressings frequently, and give skin care (avoid reinforcing and creating bulky, wet, odorous dressings that cause excoriation to the skin).

B. Maintain patency of catheter when applying dressing or positioning patient.

C. Provide clamp and release regimen until patient can void voluntarily.

Cystectomy

Definition: Removal of bladder (due to presence of tumors) with diversion of ureters into "bladder" constructed from loop of ileum which is brought through abdominal wall as an ileostomy opening.

Implementation

A. Provide routine postoperative care.

B. Maintain nasogastric tube.

C. Care for stoma with ileostomy procedure.

D. Measure and record intake and output.

E. Observe for development of fistula or dehiscence.

F. Refer patient to enterostomy therapist and a visiting nurse association.

Prostatectomy

Definition: Removal of prostate gland.

Indications

A. Enlargement of prostate (benign prostatic hypertrophy) which interferes with free urinary bladder flow.

B. Malignancy of prostate gland.

Symptoms of Enlargement

A. Recurring infection.

B. Urine stasis.

C. Nocturia.

D. Frequency.

E. Dysuria.

F. Straining to void.

Treatment

A. Medical regimen.
   1. Estrogen therapy may be given to slow rate of growth and extension of tumor.
   2. Radiation to local lesion to reduce tumor: external beam radiation or implant.

B. Surgical options.
   1. Transurethral resection (TUR) most common intervention—removal of prostatic tissue by instrumentation through urethra.
   2. Suprapubic prostatectomy—removal of prostate by abdominal incision with bladder incision.
   3. Retropubic prostatectomy—abdominal incision without opening bladder.
   4. Perineal prostatectomy—perineal incision.

Postoperative Implementation

A. Maintain adequate bladder drainage via catheter.
   1. Suprapubic catheter used following suprapubic prostatectomy.
   2. Continuous bladder irrigation (or triple lumen catheter) is used following transurethral resection. ❖ **PROCEDURE** ❖
      a. One lumen is used for inflating bag (usually 30 cc bag), one for outflow of urine, and one for irrigating solution instillation.
      b. Run solution in rapidly if bright red drainage or clots are present; when drainage clears, decrease to about 40 drops/minute.
      c. If clots cannot be rinsed out with irrigating solution, irrigate with syringe as ordered.

B. Provide fluids to prevent dehydration (2 to 3 liters every 24 hours).

C. Provide high protein, high vitamin diet.

D. Observe for signs of hemorrhage and shock.

E. Traction is applied to Foley catheter (if not connected to three-way drainage) to help in hemostasis.
   1. Catheter is pulled on and taped to leg.
   2. Do not release traction without order (traction released after bright red drainage has diminished).

F. Instruct patient in perineal exercises to regain urinary control.
   1. Tense perineal muscles by pressing buttocks together; hold for as long as possible.
   2. Repeat this process ten times every hour.

G. Ambulate early (after urine has returned to nearly normal color).

H. Observe for complications.
   1. Epididymitis (most frequent).
   2. Gram negative sepsis.

I. Administer urinary antiseptics or antibiotics as ordered to prevent infection.

J. Provide wound care for suprapubic and retropubic prostatectomies (similar to that for abdominal surgery).

K. Provide sitz bath and heat lamp treatments to promote healing.

ENDOCRINE SYSTEM

The endocrine system is one of the integrative body systems that regulates body functions. It is made up of a series of glands which function individually or conjointly to integrate and control innumerable metabolic activities of the body. These glands automatically regulate various body processes by releasing chemical signals called hormones.

ANATOMY AND PHYSIOLOGY

Endocrine Glands

A. Secrete hormones directly into the bloodstream.
B. Located in various parts of the body.
C. Each gland has a specific function; actions of glands are also interrelated, influencing one another.
   1. Tropic hormones.
      a. Secreted by anterior lobe of pituitary gland.
      b. Influence several other glands' secretion of hormones.
   2. Target glands—those glands affected by tropic hormones.
      a. Thyroid.
      b. Adrenal cortex.
      c. Gonads.
D. Also called *ductless glands* since they secrete directly into the bloodstream.
E. See Appendix 1 for a tabulation of gland function, hormones, and glandular disorders.

Hormones

A. Secreted in minute amounts but exert powerful influence on the body.
   1. Growth and development.
   2. Metabolism.
   3. Reproduction.
   4. Development of personality.
B. Influence is integrative and regulating; they control rate, but do not initiate cellular processes.
C. Effect of hormone on the body may occur in area far removed from secreting gland.

Endocrine System Assessment

A. Assess for growth imbalance.
   1. Excessive growth.
      a. Pituitary or hypothalamic disorders.
      b. Excess adrenal, ovarian, or testicular hormone.
   2. Retarded growth.
      a. Endocrine and metabolic disorders; difficult to distinguish from dwarfism.
      b. Hypothyroidism.
B. Evaluate obesity.
   1. Sudden onset suggests hypothalamic lesion (rare).
   2. Cushing's syndrome (with characteristic buffalo hump).
C. Assess abnormal skin pigmentation.
   1. Hyperpigmentation may coexist with depigmentation in Addison's disease.
   2. Thyrotoxicosis may be associated with spotty brown pigmentation.
   3. Pruritus is a common symptom in diabetes.
D. Check for hirsutism.
   1. Normal variations in body occur on nonendocrine basis.
   2. First sign of neoplastic disease.
   3. Indicates changes in adrenal status.
E. Evaluate appetite changes.
   1. Polyphagia is a common sign of uncontrolled diabetes.
   2. Indicates thyrotoxicosis.
   3. Nausea and weight loss may indicate Addisonian crisis or diabetic acidosis.
F. Check for polyuria and polydipsia.
   1. Symptoms usually of nonendocrine etiology.
   2. If sudden onset, suggest diabetes mellitus or insipidus.
   3. May be present with hyperparathyroidism or hyperaldosteronism.
G. Assess mental changes.

1. Though often subtle, may be indicative of underlying endocrine disorder.
   a. Nervousness and excitability may indicate hyperthyroidism.
   b. Mental confusion may indicate hypopituitarism, Addison's disease, or myxedema.
2. Mental deterioration is observed in untreated hypoparathyroidism and hypothyroidism.

H. Assess for coma state.
   1. Drowsiness.
   2. Hyperpnea.
   3. Tachycardia.
   4. Subnormal temperature.
   5. Fruity odor to breath.
   6. Acetone in urine (test done if over 2+ sugar in urine).
   7. Stupor leading to coma.

DIAGNOSTIC PROCEDURES

Radioactive Iodine (RAI) Uptake Radioiodine ^{131}I)

A. Purpose: measures the absorption of the iodine isotope to determine how the thyroid gland is functioning.
B. Drug given by mouth or IV.
C. Results.
   1. Normal values: 5 to 35 percent in 24 hours (recently lowered values in United States due to increased ingestion of iodine).
   2. Elevated values indicate: hyperthyroidism, thyrotoxicosis, hypofunctioning goiter, iodine lack, excessive hormonal losses.
   3. Depressed values indicate: low T_4, antithyroid drugs, thyroiditis, myxedema, or hypothyroidism.

T_3 and T_4 Resin Uptake Tests

A. Purpose: both of these are used as screening tests for diagnosis in thyroid disorders. T_4 is 90 percent accurate in diagnosing hyperthyroidism and hypothyroidism.
B. Results.
   1. Normal values:
      a. T_4: 3.8 to 11.4%.
      b. T_3: 25 to 35%.
   2. T_4.
      a. Elevated: hyperthyroidism, early hepatitis, exogenous T_4.
      b. Decreased: hypothyroidism, abnormal binding, exogenous T_3.
   3. T_3.
      a. Elevated: hyperthyroidism, T_3 toxicosis.
      b. Decreased: advancing age.

DISORDERS OF THE PITUITARY GLAND

Acromegaly

Definition: Overproduction of growth-stimulating hormone by the anterior lobe, occurring in adulthood after closure of the epiphyses of the long bones.

Assessment

A. Excessive growth of short, flat bones.
   1. Large hands and feet.
   2. Thickening and protrusion of the jaw and orbital ridges.
   3. Coarse facial features.
   4. Pain in joints.
B. Increased diaphoresis.
C. Oily, rough skin.
D. Increased hair growth over the body.
E. Menstrual disturbances; impotence.
F. Symptoms associated with local compression of brain by tumor.
   1. Headache.
   2. Visual disturbances; blindness.
G. Related hormonal imbalances may develop.
   1. Diabetes mellitus.

2. Cushing's syndrome.

H. Increased growth-stimulating hormone level as indicated by laboratory tests.

Treatment and Implementation

A. Provide emotional support.
1. Encourage expression of patient's feelings.
2. Avoid situations which may be embarrassing to the patient.
3. Encourage family to give support to and to communicate with the patient.
B. Give frequent skin care.
C. Provide proper positioning and support for painful joints.
D. Test urine for sugar and acetone.
E. Be of possible needed treatment.
1. Irradiation of the tumor.
2. Hypophysectomy.
3. Lifelong replacement of hormones as a result of above treatments.

Hypophysectomy

Definition: Excision of the pituitary gland.

A. General preoperative care.
1. Emotional support.
2. Explanation of procedure to be performed.
B. General postoperative care.
1. Signs of related hormonal disturbances and deficiencies.
   a. Adrenal insufficiency.
   b. Hypothyroidism and acute thyroid crisis.
   c. Diabetes insipidus.
   d. Severe hypoglycemia.
2. Education.
   a. Importance of continual medical supervision.
   b. Safe self-administration of replacement hormones.
      (1) Cortisone.
      (2) Thyroid.
      (3) Sex hormones.
      (4) Vasopressin tannate.
   c. Avoidance of over-the-counter drugs.

d. Measures to prevent infections; prompt reporting to physician if infections appear.
e. Recognition of stress and avoidance of stress-producing situations.
f. Importance of medic-alert band and carrying emergency medications.
g. Avoidance of forceful blowing of nose and of coughing.
3. Need for emotional support and involvement of family in ongoing care.

Gigantism

Definition: Overproduction of growth-stimulating hormone by the anterior lobe, occurring in childhood prior to closure of the epiphyses of the long bones.

Assessment

A. Symmetrical overgrowth of the long bones.
B. Increased height in early adulthood of eight to nine feet.
C. Deterioration of mental and physical processes, which may occur in early adulthood.

Treatment

A. Irradiation of pituitary.
B. Hypophysectomy.

Dwarfism

Definition: Underproduction of growth-stimulating hormone by the anterior lobe.

Signs and Symptoms

A. Severe retardation of physical growth.
B. Premature body-aging processes.

Implementation

A. Human growth-stimulating hormone injections (HGH).

B. Given if the imbalance is diagnosed and treated in early stage.

Diabetes Insipidus

Definition: Antidiuretic hormone (ADH) deficiency resulting from damage or tumors occurring in the posterior lobe of the pituitary gland.

Assessment

A. Severe polyuria.
B. Severe polydipsia.
C. Dehydration.
D. Weight loss; muscle weakness.
E. Laboratory values-low urinary specific gravity (1.001 to 1.005).

Treatment and Implementation

A. Administer vasopressin tannate (Pitressin Tannate) IM or nasal spray.
B. Administer benzothiadiazide diuretics for mild cases.
C. Be aware that hypophysectomy may be required if tumor is present.
D. Provide adequate fluids; avoid fluids with diuretic-type actions.
E. Measure intake, output, and weight.
F. Advise patient of importance of wearing medic-alert band.

DISORDERS OF THE ADRENAL GLAND

Addison's Disease

Definition: Hypofunction of adrenal cortex of adrenal gland, resulting in deficiency of steroid hormones (glucocorticoids, mineralocorticoids, and androgens).

Assessment

A. Slow and insidious onset: eventually fatal if untreated.
B. Lassitude, lethargy, and generalized weakness.
C. Gastrointestinal disturbances, e.g., nausea, diarrhea, and anorexia.
D. Hypotension.
E. Increased pigmentation of the skin.
F. Emotional disturbances.
G. Weight loss.
H. Elevated serum potassium, decreased serum sodium, elevated BUN levels, and low blood sugar.

Treatment and Implementation

A. Be aware that lifelong replacement therapy with synthetic corticosteroid drugs will be required.
B. Provide emotional support.
C. Weigh patient daily; monitor vital signs qid.
D. Observe for side effects of replacement hormones.
   1. Cortisone and hydrocortisone side effects.
      a. Sodium and water retention.
      b. Potassium depletion.
      c. Drug-induced Cushing's syndrome.
      d. Gastric irritation (give medication with meal or antacid).
      e. Mood swings.
      f. Local abscess at injection site when given IM (inject deeply into gluteal muscle).
      g. Addison's crisis, which might be produced by sudden withdrawal of medication.
   2. Fludrocortisone acetate side effects—the same as for cortisone and hydrocortisone, particularly sodium retention and potassium depletion.
   3. Deoxycorticosterone acetate side effects—sodium retention and potassium depletion.
E. Protect patient from exposure to infection and from stress.
F. Provide high carbohydrate, high protein diet in frequent small feedings.

G. Maintain strict intake and output records.

Addisonian Crisis

Definition: Condition caused by adrenal insufficiency, which may be precipitated by infection, trauma, stress, surgery, or diaphoresis with excessive salt loss.

Assessment

A. Severe headache; abdominal, leg, and lower back pain.
B. Extreme, generalized muscular weakness.
C. Severe hypotension and shock.
D. Irritability and confusion.
E. Death from shock, vascular collapse, or hyperkalemia.

Treatment and Implementation

A. Monitor IV fluid replacement to restore fluid and electrolyte balance.
B. Steroid replacement.
C. Monitor vital signs and intake and output continually and closely until crisis passes.
D. Take measures to protect patient from infection.
E. Do not allow patient to do anything for self and encourage remaining as quiet as possible; perform no unnecessary nursing procedures.

Cushing's Syndrome

Definition: Disease produced by hyperfunction of the adrenal cortices of the adrenal glands, resulting in hypersecretion of the glucocorticoid steroid hormones.

Assessment

A. Abnormal adipose tissue distribution.
   1. Moonlike fullness of face.
   2. Buffalo hump (fatty swellings on body).
   3. Obese trunk with thin extremities.
B. Reddish purple striae of skin stretched with fat tissue.
C. Fragile skin; easily bruised.
D. Osteoporosis; susceptible to fractures.
E. Hyperglycemia; may eventually develop diabetes mellitus.
F. Mood swings from euphoria to depression.
G. High susceptibility to infections; diminished immuno-response to infections once they occur.
H. Lassitude and muscular weakness.
I. Masculine characteristics in females.
J. Potassium depletion.
K. Sodium and water retention.
L. Elevated blood sugar and glycosuria.
M. Elevated white blood count with depressed hyperkalemia.
N. Elevated plasma cortisone levels.
O. Elevated 17-hydroxycorticosteroids in urine.

Treatment and Implementation

A. Take measures to protect from infections.
B. Protect patient from accidents or falls.
C. Give meticulous skin care, avoiding harsh soaps.
D. Provide low caloric, high protein, high potassium diet.
E. Provide emotional support.
   1. Encourage ventilation of patient's feelings.
   2. Avoid reacting to patient's appearance.
   3. Anticipate the needs of the patient.
   4. Explain to patient that changes in body appearance and emotional lability should improve with treatment.
F. Measure intake and output; test for urinary sugar; weigh daily.
G. Provide specialized care if adrenalectomy is necessary.
   1. General preoperative care.
   2. Postoperative care.
      a. Frequent monitoring of vital signs and intake and output.
      b. Careful administration of parenteral fluids and medications as ordered.

c. Strict adherence to sterile techniques when changing dressings.

d. Observation for shock, hypoglycemia.

H. Be aware that chemotherapy may be administered for inoperable, cancerous tumors.

DISORDERS OF THE THYROID GLAND

Myxedema

Definition: Adult form of decreased synthesis of thyroid hormone resulting in a hypothyroid state.

Assessment

A. Occurs primarily in older age group, five times more frequent in women than in men.

B. Slowed rate of body metabolism.
1. Lethargy, apathy, and fatigue.
2. Intolerance to cold.
3. Hypersensitivity to sedatives and barbiturates.
4. Weight gain.
5. Cool, dry, rough skin.
6. Coarse, dry hair.

C. Personality changes.
1. Forgetfulness and loss of memory.
2. Complacency.

D. Anorexia, constipation, and fecal impactions.

E. Interstitial edema.
1. Nonpitting edema in the lower extremity.
2. Generalized puffiness.

F. Decreased diaphoresis.

G. Menstrual disturbances.

H. Cardiac complications.
1. Coronary heart disease.
2. Angina pectoris.
3. Myocardial infarction and congestive heart failure.

I. Anemia.

J. Below normal test results.

1. PBI.
2. ^{131}I.
3. T_3 and T_4.

K. Elevated serum cholesterol level.

Treatment and Implementation

A. Administer thyroid replacement (initial small dosage, increased gradually).

B. Individualize maintenance dosage.
1. Desiccated thyroid.
2. Sodium levothyroxine (Synthroid Sodium).
3. Triiodothyronine (Cytomel).

C. Observe for symptoms of overdosage in thyroid preparations.
1. Myocardial infarction, angina, and cardiac failure, particularly in patients with cardiac problems.
2. Restlessness and insomnia.
3. Headache and confusion.

D. Provide time for patient to complete activities.

E. Provide warm environment with extra blankets and other modes of warming.

F. Give meticulous skin care.

G. Orient patient as to date, time, and place.

H. Take measures to prevent constipation.

I. Administer sedatives or narcotics as ordered by physician. (Usually one-half to one-third normal dosage is ordered.)

Hyperthyroidism (Thyrotoxicosis)

Definition: A result of increased synthesis of thyroid hormone often accompanied by exophthalmic goiter (Graves' disease).

Assessment

A. Occurs four times more frequently in women than in men; usually occurs between 20 to 40 years of age.

B. Increased rate of body metabolism.
1. Weight loss despite ravenous appetite and ingestion of large quantities of food.
2. Intolerance to heat.

3. Nervousness, jitters, and fine tremor of hands.
4. Smooth, soft skin and hair.
5. Tachycardia and palpitation.
6. Diarrhea.

C. Personality changes.
1. Irritability and agitation.
2. Exaggerated emotional reactions.
3. Mood swings from euphoria to depression.

D. Enlargement of the thyroid gland (goiter).

E. Exophthalmos.
1. Fluid collects around eye sockets, causing eyeballs to protrude.
2. Condition not always in evidence.
3. Usually does not improve with treatment.

F. Cardiac complications common.

G. Above normal test results.
1. PBI.
2. ^{131}I.
3. T_3 and T_4.

H. Relatively low serum cholesterol.

Treatment and Implementation

A. Administer drugs if ordered by physician.
1. Antithyroid drugs.
   a. Most common are propylthiouracil and methimazole (Tapazole).
   b. Possible side effect of agranulocytosis.
2. Iodine preparations.
   a. Saturated solution of potassium iodide (SSKI).
   b. Lugol's Solution.
3. Radioiodine therapy.
   a. Useful for patients who are poor surgical risks.
   b. Uptake of ^{131}I by thyroid gland results in destruction of thyroid cells.
   c. Myxedema may occur as complication.

B. Provide for adequate rest.
1. Bed rest.
2. Calming diversionary activities.

C. Provide cool, quiet, stable environment.

D. Maintain diet high in calories, protein, and vitamins; no stimulants.

E. Weigh daily.

F. Provide emotional support to patient.
1. Be aware that exaggerated emotional responses are a manifestation of hormone imbalance.
2. Be sensitive to patient's needs.
3. Avoid stress-producing situations.

G. Adhere to regular schedule of activities.

H. Provide specialized care if thyroidectomy (subtotal or total removal of thyroid gland) is required.
1. Ensure that patient is in required preoperative state.
   a. Return of thyroid function tests to normal.
   b. Adequate nutritional status.
   c. Marked decrease in signs of thyrotoxicosis.
   d. Absence of cardiac problems.
2. Provide postoperative care.
   a. Monitor vital signs carefully.
   b. Observe closely for signs of complications.
      (1) Hemorrhage.
      (2) Respiratory distress.
      (3) Laryngeal nerve injury.
      (4) Tetany and hypocalcemia.
      (5) Thyroid "storm."
   c. Have tracheostomy tray suction equipment, and oxygen equipment at bedside.
   d. Raise bed to semi-Fowler's position; avoid strain to suture line.
   e. Encourage head and neck range-of-motion exercises when ordered.

Thyroid Storm or Thyroid Crisis

Definition: Acute, potentially fatal hyperthyroid condition which may occur as a result of surgery, inadequate preparation for surgery, severe infection, or from stress.

A. High fever (may rise to 106°F) and dehydration.

B. Tachycardia.

C. Irritability and restlessness leading to delirium and coma.

Treatment and Implementation

A. Administer drugs and take special measures as ordered.
   1. Hypothermic measures.
   2. Hydration.
   3. Antithyroid drugs and iodine preparations.
   4. Adrenergic and catecholamine blocking agents.
   5. Corticosteroids.
B. Monitor vital signs, intake and output.
C. Take safety measures if agitated or comatose.
D. Provide calm, quiet environment.
E. Protect from infection.

DISORDERS OF THE PARATHYROID GLANDS

Hypoparathyroidism

Definition: Condition caused by acute or chronic and deficient hormone production by the parathyroid gland.

Signs and Symptoms

A. Acute hypocalcemia.
   1. Numbness, tingling, and cramping of extremities.
   2. Acute, potentially fatal tetany.
      a. Painful muscular spasms.
      b. Seizures.
      c. Irritability.
      d. Positive Chvostek's sign.
      e. Positive Trousseau's sign.
      f. Laryngospasm.
      g. Cardiac arrhythmias.
B. Chronic hypocalcemia.
   1. Poor development of tooth enamel.
   2. Mental retardation.
   3. Muscular weakness with numbness and tingling of extremities.
   4. Loss of hair and coarse, dry skin.
   5. Personality changes.

   6. Cataracts.
   7. Cardiac arrhythmias.
   8. Renal stones.
C. Laboratory values.
   1. Low serum calcium levels.
   2. Increased serum phosphorus level.
   3. Low urinary calcium and phosphorus output.
   4. Increased bone density on x-ray examination.

Treatment and Implementation

A. General care.
   1. Frequently check for increasing hoarseness.
   2. Observe for irregularities in urine.
   3. Force fluids as ordered.
B. Acute care.
   1. Prepare for administration of IV calcium gluconate solution.
   2. Administer anticonvulsants and sedatives.
   3. Prepare for tracheostomy if laryngospasm has caused obstruction.
C. Chronic care.
   1. Administer oral calcium salts and vitamin D preparations.
   2. Provide high calcium, low phosphorus diet.

Hyperparathyroidism

Definition: Abnormal, excessive hormone production by the parathyroid gland.

Assessment

A. Bone demineralization with deformities, pain, high susceptibility to fractures.
B. Hypercalcemia.
   1. Calcium deposits in various body organs such as eyes, heart, lungs, and kidneys (stones).
   2. Gastric ulcers.
   3. Personality changes, depression, and paranoia.

4. Nausea, vomiting, anorexia, and constipation.
5. Polydipsia and polyuria.

Treatment and Implementation

A. Be aware that subtotal surgical resection of parathyroid glands may be necessary.
B. Administer additional oral calcium as ordered, for bone rebuilding processes may be required for several months.
C. Force fluids (include juices to make urine more acidic).
D. Take safety measures to prevent accidents and injury.
E. Provide a diet high in phosphorus.
F. Measure intake and output.
G. Observe urine closely for stones.
H. Observe for digitalis toxicity if patient is taking digitalis.

DISORDERS OF THE PANCREAS

Diabetes Mellitus (Type I, Type II)

Definition: A group of disorders that have a variety of genetic causes, but have glucose intolerance as a common thread. Condition is caused by absence or lack of insulin or inability of cells to use insulin effectively.

Characteristics

A. Classifications.
1. Type I—insulin dependent diabetes mellitus (IDDM).
2. Type II—noninsulin dependent diabetes mellitus (NIDDM).
3. Gestational (GDM)—increased blood glucose levels during pregnancy.
4. Impaired glucose tolerance (IGT). Plasma glucose levels vacillate between normal or increased (formerly latent, borderline, and subclinical diabetes).

B. Distinguishing features of Type I and Type II diabetes.
C. Risk factors.
1. Patient history—hereditary predisposition.
2. Weight—presence of obesity.
3. High stress levels.
D. Results of laboratory values.
1. Elevated fasting blood sugar; postprandial blood sugar; glucose tolerance test or tolbutamide (Orinase) tests.
2. Clinitest and Testape.
a. Indicate presence of sugar in urine, i.e., 1+ to 4+.
b. Clinitest: 2-drop and 5-drop method: from no sugar (blue) to 4+ or 2 percent (orange-rust).
c. Values of the two tests are not interchangeable.
3. Acetest and Ketostix—may be positive for presence of acetone in urine.
4. Elevated cholesterol and triglyceride levels.
5. Capillary blood glucose (finger stick).
6. Glycosylated hemoglobin test.
a. Abnormally high in diabetes with chronic hyperglycemia.
b. Values.
(1) Normal 3.5–6.2%.
(2) Good control less than 7.5%.
(3) Fair control 7.6–8.9%.
(4) Poor control more than 9.0%.

Assessment

A. Early symptoms.
1. Common to both Type I and Type II.
a. Polyuria.
b. Polydipsia.
c. Polyphagia.
d. Blurred vision.
e. Fatigue.
f. Abnormal sensations (prickling, burning).
g. Infections (vaginitis).
2. Type I.

a. Anorexia.
b. Nausea, vomiting.
c. Weight loss.
3. Type II.
a. Obese.
b. Slow wound healing.

Complications

A. Ketoacidosis.
1. Onset.
a. Acute or over several days.
b. Result of stress, infection, surgery, or lack of effective insulin.
c. Overeating may contribute to but does not cause onset.
d. Life-threatening situation.
2. Hyperglycemia, glucosuria, ketosis, ketonuria, and low CO_2, combining power.
3. Polyuria, polydipsia, and dehydration.
4. Nausea, vomiting, and anorexia.
5. Flushed, warm skin.
6. Blurred vision.
7. Acetone odor (sweet) on breath.
8. Kussmaul respirations (rapid, deep).
9. Cardiac failure and coma.
B. Infections.
C. Vascular disease.
1. Microangiopathy—affects basement membrane of almost all small blood vessels throughout body.
a. Retinopathy; nephropathy.
b. Tight control of blood sugar—using smaller and more frequent doses of insulin will reduce complications by 50–60 percent.
2. Large vessel.
a. Coronary heart disease.
b. Atherosclerosis, arteriosclerosis.
D. Neuropathy.
E. Cataracts.

Treatment

A. Diet.
1. The cornerstone of management, interdependent with medication and exercise.
2. Attainment of normal weight may reduce symptoms.
3. Total calories are individualized.
a. Stress high-carbohydrate foods.
b. Water-soluble fiber (oat bran, pectin) important.
c. Protein intake between 60–85 grams.
4. ADA exchange diet.
a. Seven exchange lists.
b. Prescribed as to total calories and number of exchanges from each group.
c. Calories divided into:
(1) 60% CHO.
(2) 20% Fat.
(3) 20% Protein.
B. Medications.
1. Insulin.
a. Types.
(1) Short acting.
(a) Regular.
(b) Semilente.
(c) Humulin.
(2) Intermediate acting.
(a) NPH.
(b) Lente.
(c) Humulin.
(3) Long acting.
(a) PZI.
(b) Ultralente.
(4) Available in U100.
b. Concentration.
(1) Two types commonly available.
(2) U100 insulin has 100 units of insulin in each cc of liquid.
(3) U40 insulin has 40 units in each cc.
(4) Syringe must correspond to insulin type.
c. Insulin pump—a battery operated device worn on a belt—delivers low-dose insulin at a continuous rate through a needle inserted in sub q tissue.
2. Oral hypoglycemic drugs.
a. Sulfonylureas.
(1) Thought to stimulate beta cells to increase insulin release.
(2) Tolbutamide (Orinase), short acting.

(3) Chlorpropamide (Diabinese), long acting.

(4) Acetohexamide (Dymelor), intermediate acting.

(5) Tolazamide (Tolinase), intermediate acting.

b. Second generation sulfonylureas.

(1) Glyburide, intermediate acting.

(2) Glipizide, short acting.

C. Exercise.

1. Decreases body's need for insulin.

2. Regular, ongoing activities important.

3. Administer 10 gm CHO before exercise.

Common Problems in Regulation

A. Somogyi or rebound effect: insulin caused hypoglycemia at midnight which rebounds to hyperglycemia in early morning.

1. Symptoms: night sweats, restlessness, early morning nausea, headaches, and confusion.

2. Treated by gradually lowering insulin dosage while monitoring blood glucose.

B. Dawn phenomenon: blood glucose is normal until 3 a.m. and then begins to rise in early morning.

Implementation

A. Give meticulous skin care, particularly of lower extremities.

B. Take measures to protect patient from infection, injury, stress.

C. Observe for signs of insulin reaction and ketoacidosis.

D. Take second voided specimen for accurate sugar and acetone urine test.

E. Measure intake and output.

F. Provide emotional support.

1. Encourage patient to verbalize feelings.

a. Necessity for changes in life style, diet, and activities.

b. Possible change in self-image and self-esteem.

c. Fear of future and complications.

2. Encourage involvement of family.

G. Educate patient in effective self-management.

1. Determine patient's current status.

a. Level of knowledge.

b. Cultural, socioeconomic, and family influences.

c. Daily dietary and activity patterns.

d. Emotional and physical status and effect on current ability to learn.

2. Inform patient about insulin and insulin injections.

a. Keep insulin at room temperature; refrigerate extra supply of insulin.

b. Rotate insulin bottle gently prior to drawing up insulin.

c. Use sterile injection techniques.

d. Rotate injection sites.

e. Watch for signs of under- and overdosage.

3. Advise patient about oral medications.

a. Take medications regularly.

b. Watch for hypoglycemic reactions occurring with sulfonylureas.

c. Be aware that alcohol ingestion in conjunction with sulfonylureas produces Antabuse effects.

4. Advise patient to take all possible measures to prevent infection and injury.

a. Report infection or injury promptly to physician.

b. Maintain meticulous skin care.

c. Maintain proper foot care.

d. Be aware that insulin requirements may need to be increased when suffering from infections.

e. Be prepared for impairment of healing process.

f. Avoid tight-fitting garments and shoes.

g. Avoid "bathroom surgery" for corns and calluses.

5. Stress the importance of diet.

a. No variation in meal times.

b. Importance of patient's individual dietary goals.

c. Incorporation of diet into life style, cultural and socioeconomic food patterns, and daily activities.

d. Need for increase of intake when vigorously exercising.

6. Stress the importance of exercise.

a. Regularity and amount of exercise important.
b. Sporadic, vigorous activities should be avoided.
c. With careful planning, participation in most activities and sports is possible.
d. Increased or decreased food intake might be required according to anticipated level of activity.
7. Advise patient to wear medic-alert band or carry other identification regarding diabetic status.
8. Advise patient to carry a form of concentrated sugar at all times.

Functional Hyperinsulinism (Hypoglycemia)

Definition: Condition that is the result of excess secretion of insulin by the beta cells of the pancreas gland.

Assessment

A. Personality changes.
1. Tenseness.
2. Nervousness.
3. Irritability.
4. Anxiousness.
5. Depression.
B. Excessive diaphoresis.
C. Excessive hunger.
D. Muscle weakness and tachycardia.
E. May be associated with "dumping syndrome" following gastrectomy.
F. May occur prior to development of diabetes mellitus.
G. Laboratory values—low blood sugar during hypoglycemic episodes.

Treatment and Implementation

A. Provide high protein, low carbohydrate diet.
B. Take measures to reduce anxiety and tenseness; may be attained through counseling.

Ketoacidosis

Definition: The two major metabolic problems that are the source of this condition are hyperglycemia and ketoacidemia, both due to insulin lack associated with hyperglucagonemia.

Assessment

A. Ketoacidotic coma is usually preceded by a few days of polyuria and polydipsia with associated symptoms.
1. Fatigue.
2. Nausea and vomiting.
3. Mental stupor.
B. Physical assessment indicates dehydration, rapid breathing, and fruity order of acetone to breath.

Treatment and Implementation

A. Maintain fluid and electrolyte balance.
1. Normal saline IV until blood sugar reaches 250–300 mg; then a dextrose solution is started.
2. Potassium added to IV after renal function is evaluated and hydration is adequate.
B. Provide insulin management.
1. Give ½ dose IV and ½ dose sub q.
2. Give with small amounts of albumin as insulin adheres to IV tubing.
3. Hourly dosage depends on S & A and blood sugar levels.
C. Provide patent airway and adequate circulation to brain.
D. Obtain hourly sugar and acetone urine tests.
E. Test blood sugar level q 1–2 hours. Keep sugar and acetone at 1+.
F. Maintain personal hygiene.
G. Protect from injury if comatose.

Table 1. Insulin Treatment

Category	Types	Onset	Peak	Duration	Times and Symptoms of Untoward Reaction
Rapid acting	Regular	30–60 min.	2–5 hours	6–8 hours	15 min to 4–5 hours; hunger, trembling, visual disturbance, cold perspiration, weakness, coma
	Semilente	1–2 hours	3–8 hours	10–16 hours	
	Humulin R	30–60 min.	2–3 hours	5–7 hours	
Intermediate acting	NPH	1–2 hours	6–12 hours	18–26 hours	4–6 hours; majority of attacks occur in early morning or evening—extreme fatigue may be only symptom
	Lente	1–3 hours	6–8 hours	18–24 hours	
	Humulin R	1 ½–3 ½ hours	8–12 hours	18–24 hours	
Slow acting	Protamine	4–8 hours	10–20 hours	36 hours	12–24 hours: usually early morning, gradual onset, sleeplessness, nausea, headache, confusion
	Zinc (PZI)	4–6 hours	8–24 hours	24–36 hours	
	Ultralente				

Table 2. Complications Associated with Diabetes

Clinical Manifestations	Diabetic Hypoglycemia	Hyperglycemic Hypersmolar Ketoacidosis (DKA)	Nonketotic Coma (HHNK)
	Type I	*Type I*	*Type II*
Cause	Too much insulin or too little food	Absence or inadequate insulin	Uncontrolled diabetes or oral hypoglycemic drugs
Onset	Rapid (within minutes)	Slow (about 8 hours)	Slow (hours to days)
Appearance	Exhibits symptoms of fainting	Appears ill	Appears ill
Respirations	Normal	Rapid and deep, shortness of breath	Rapid and deep; absence of Kussmaul's
Breath odor	Normal	Sweetish due to acetone	Normal
Pulse	Tachycardia	Tachycardia	Tachycardia
Blood pressure		Lowered blood pressure	Decreased blood pressure
Hunger	Hunger pangs in epigastrium	Loss of appetite	Hunger
Thirst	None	Increased	Increased, dehydration
Vomiting	Nausea; vomiting rare	Common	Common
Eyes	Staring, double vision	Appear sunken	Visual loss
Headache	Common	Occasionally	Occasionally
Skin	Pallor, perspiration, chilling sensation	Hot, dry skin	Hot, dry skin
Muscle action	Twitching common, unsteady gait	Twitching absent	Twitching absent
Pain in abdomen	None	Common	Common
Mental status	Confusion, erratic, change in mood, unable to concentrate	Malaise, drowsy, confusion, coma	Confused, dull, coma

Table 2. Complications Associated with Diabetes (*Continued*)

Clinical Manifestations	Diabetic Hypoglycemia	Hyperglycemic Hypersmolar Ketoacidosis (DKA)	Nonketotic Coma (HHNK)
	Type I	*Type I*	*Type II*
Lab findings			
Sugar in urine	None after residual is discarded	Present	Present
Blood sugar	Below 50–70 mg/dl blood	High, 350–900 mg/dl	Very high, 800 mg/dl up to 2400 mg/dl
Ketones	Absent	High	Absent
Ketones in blood plasma	Absent	4+ present	Absent

INTEGUMENTARY SYSTEM

The integumentary system comprises the enveloping membrane or skin of the body. It consists of the outer epidermis and inner layer of dermis. The hair, nails, and various glands are outgrowths of the skin. The skin performs many vital body functions that include protection against negative elements in the environment and reception of temperature, touch, and pressure.

ANATOMY AND PHYSIOLOGY

Skin

A. Skin comprises about 15 percent of the body weight and forms a barrier between the internal organs and the external environment.
B. The epidermis, dermis, and subcutaneous tissue compose the skin's three layers.
C. Skin is the largest sensory organ of the body. It contains nerves and specialized sensory organs sensitive to pain, touch, pressure, heat, and cold.
D. Chief pigment is melanin, produced by basal cells.
E. Skin harbors bacterial flora.
   1. Bacteria normally present in varying amounts.
   2. Organisms are shed with normal exfoliation of skin; bathing and rubbing may also remove bacteria.
   3. Normal pH of skin (4.2 to 5.6) retards growth of bacteria.
   4. Damaged areas of skin are potential points of entry for infection.
F. Functions of skin.
   1. Protection.
   2. Temperature regulation.
   3. Sensation.
   4. Storage.

Hair

A. Keratinous structures growing out of tubular invaginations of the epidermis called hair follicles.
B. Hair goes through cyclic changes of growth, atrophy, and rest.
C. Melanocytes present in the bulb of each hair account for color.
D. All parts of the body except the palms, soles of the feet, distal phalanges of fingers and toes, and the penis are covered with some form of hair.

Sweat Gland

A. Aggregate of cells that produce a liquid (perspiration) salty to the taste and with a pH ranging from 4.5 to 7.5.
B. Contains duct that opens out at the surface of the skin.
C. Chief components of sweat are water, sodium, potassium, chloride, glucose, urea, and lactate.

System Assessment

A. Assess color.
   1. Assess color of skin, including deviations from the normal range within individual's race.
      a. Use a nonglare daylight or 60-watt bulb.
      b. Note especially the bony prominences.
      c. Observe for pallor (white), flushing (red), jaundice (yellow), ashen (gray), or cyanosis (blue) coloration.
      d. Check mucous membranes to be accurate.
   2. Observe for increased or decreased areas of pigmentation.
   3. Observe for various skin discolorations: ecchymosis, petechiae, purpura, or erythema.
B. Evaluate skin temperature.
   1. Palpate skin (especially areas of concern) for temperature.
   2. Note changes in different extremities.

C. Assess turgor.
   1. Observe skin for its ease of movement and speed of return to original position.
   2. Observe for excessive dryness, moisture, wrinkling, flaking and general texture.
   3. Observe for a lasting impression or dent after pressing against and removing finger from skin—indicates edema or fluid in the tissue.
D. Assess skin sensation.
   1. Ability to detect heat, cold, gentle touch, and pressure.
   2. Note complaints of itching, tingling, cramps, or numbness.
E. Observe cleanliness.
   1. Observe general state of hygiene. Note amount of oil, moisture, and dirt on the skin surface.
   2. Note presence of strong body odors.
   3. Investigate hair and scalp for presence of body lice.
F. Assess integrity (intactness of skin).
   1. Note intactness of skin. Observe for areas of broken skin (lesions) or ulcers.
   2. Assess any lesion for its location, size, shape, color(s), consistency, discomfort, odor, and sensation associated with it.
G. Assess skin conditions (see Appendix 1 for types of skin lesions).

General Implementation

A. Determine type of lesion or area of altered tissue (see Appendix 1 for types of skin lesions).
   1. Primary lesion is initial, or first, lesion.
   2. Secondary lesion is a result of a change or complication that involves a primary lesion.
B. Provide psychological support.
   1. Encourage patient to express feelings.
      a. May be embarrassed about appearance.
      b. May be fearful of scarring.
      c. May be depressed about long duration and chronicity of disorder.
   2. Accept patient as he or she is; nonverbal communication is therapeutic (touch).
C. Take measures to prevent damage to healthy skin.

1. Prevent scratching.
   a. Keep fingernails smooth and short.
   b. Encourage patient to wear cotton gloves as reminder not to scratch.
   c. Restrain if ordered.
2. Use hot and cold applications with caution.
D. Take measures to prevent secondary infections.
   1. Use medical aseptic technique.
   2. Maintain isolation if lesions are infectious.
   3. Careful handwashing.
E. Take measures to reverse inflammatory process.
   1. Relieve symptoms.
      a. Control room temperature and humidity.
      b. Decrease local irritation.
   2. Give medication and treatment as needed.

ALLERGIC REACTIONS

Contact Dermatitis

Definition: Skin reaction caused by contact with a substance to which the skin is sensitive. Reaction is characterized by inflammation as evidenced by itching, redness, and skin lesions.

Causes

A. Contact with chemicals.
   1. Clothing (especially woolens).
   2. Cosmetics.
   3. Household products (especially detergents).
   4. Industrial substances (paints, dyes, cements).
B. Contact with toxic irritants: poison oak, poison ivy, or poison sumac.

Assessment

A. Papules.
B. Vesicles.

C. Severe itching (pruritus).

Preventive Measures

A. Avoid irritant or remove irritating clothing.
B. Do not use detergent.
C. Wear rubber gloves for household chores.
D. Make request of industry to provide protective clothing; or allow change of job site for highly sensitive individuals.

Treatment and Implementation

A. Cleanse skin of plant oils.
B. Apply lotion.
C. Administer steroids for severe reactions.
D. Apply cold wet dressings of Burrow's Solution to relieve itching.

Eczema

Definition: Superficial inflammatory process involving primarily the epidermis.

Assessment

A. Local eruptions.
   1. Erythema, papules, vesicles may be present.
   2. Area may be edematous, weeping, eroded, and/or crusted.
B. Swelling of regional lymph nodes.
C. May occur at any age, but particularly common in infancy.
D. Runs a chronic course with remission and exacerbation.
   1. Patient usually becomes irritable.
   2. Skin may be thickened, scaled, and fissured.

Treatment and Implementation

A. Seek the cause which may be foods, emotional problems, or familial tendencies.
B. Do not allow the patient to be vaccinated for smallpox; isolate from individuals recently vaccinated.

C. Control skin eruptions.
   1. Encourage patient to withhold scratching.
   2. Apply wet dressings or give therapeutic baths (no soaps during acute stages).
   3. Apply mild lotion (calamine) when no oozing or vesiculation is present.
   4. Apply cornstarch paste to remove crusts.
   5. Rub cornstarch into bed linen, and do not use woolen blankets.

BACTERIAL INFECTIONS

Impetigo

Definition: Bacterial disease caused by streptococcal, staphylococcal, or combined infection.

Assessment

A. Local vesicles.
B. Pustules evolving from vesicles that become crusted.

Treatment and Implementation

A. Prevent the spread of disease.
B. Dry the lesions by exposure to air (use compresses of Burrow's Solution to remove the crusts so as to allow better exposure to air).
C. Apply local antibiotic ointments or bland emollients to prevent cracking and fissures as directed by physician.
D. Caution family to use only hexachlorophene soap, to use other hygienic care materials, and to use separate towels to prevent the spread of the disease.

Furuncle (Boil)

Definition: Bacterial inflammation of skin caused by staphylococcal infection of a hair follicle.

Assessment

A. Onset is sudden; the skin becomes red, tender, and hot around the hair follicle.
B. The center forms pus, and the core may be extruded spontaneously or by excision and manipulation.

Treatment and Implementation

A. Isolate towels, soap, and clothing; necessary to maintain scrupulous cleanliness.
B. Administer systemic antibiotics if a series of furuncles occur and if ordered.
C. Check for presence of diabetes mellitus. Should be ruled out only after tests prove negative.

VIRAL INFECTIONS

Herpes Simplex

Definition: Infectious condition (cold sore) caused by a virus that may occur on lips, face, or genitalia.

Assessment

A. Local burning, tingling, itching.
B. Local erythema.
C. Vesicles appear later.

Implementation

A. Keep lesion dry and clean.
B. Advise patient to avoid sexual or direct contacts.
C. Encourage patient to request physician to periodically reexamine lesion.

Herpes Zoster

Definition: Acute infectious process caused by viral invasion of central nervous system.

Assessment

A. Pain and discomfort.
B. Cutaneous lesions usually located along major nerve root.

BURNS

Definition: Destruction of skin layers by thermal, chemical, or electrical agents.

Classification of Burns

A. Degree of burn—determined by layers involved.
   1. First degree—superficial partial thickness.
      a. Involves epidermis.
      b. Area is red or pink.
      c. Moderate pain.
      d. Spontaneous healing.
   2. Second degree—partial thickness.
      a. Involves epidermis and dermis to the basal cells.
      b. Blistering.
      c. Severe pain.
      d. Regeneration in one month.
      e. Scarring may occur.
   3. Third degree—full thickness.
      a. Involves epidermis, dermis, and subcutaneous tissue and may extend to the muscle in severe burns.
      b. White, gray, or black in appearance.
      c. Absence of pain.
      d. Edema of surrounding tissues.
      e. Eschar formation.
      f. Grafting needed due to total destruction of dermal elements.
   4. Fourth degree.
      a. Involves muscle and bone.
      b. Increased destruction of RBCs.
B. Classification according to the percentage of body area destroyed.
   1. Critical burns—30 percent or more of the body has sustained second degree burn and 10 percent has sustained third degree

burn; further complicated by respiratory involvement, smoke inhalation, fractures, and other tissue injury.

    2. Moderate burns—less than 10 percent of the body has sustained third degree burn and 15 to 30 percent has sustained second degree burn.

    3. Minor burns—less than 15 percent of the body has sustained second degree burn and less than 2 percent has sustained third degree burn.

    4. Estimation of percentage of total body surface involved with "Rule of Nines" (see Appendix 2).

C. Classification according to cause.

    1. Thermal burns: flame burns, scalding with hot liquids, or radiation.

    2. Chemical burns: strong acids or strong alkali solutions.

    3. Electrical burns.

      a. Most serious type of burn.

      b. Body fluids may conduct an electrical charge through body (look for entrance and exit area).

      c. Cardiac arrhythmias may occur.

      d. Toxins are created postburn that injure kidneys.

      e. Voltage and ampere information important in history taking.

Problems Associated with Burns

A. Fluid and electrolyte imbalance.

    1. Edema appears around the wound as a result of damage to capillaries.

    2. There is a loss of fluid at the burn area.

B. Pulmonary changes from inhalation injury.

    1. Pulmonary edema.

    2. Obstruction of the air passages from edema of the face, neck, trachea, and larynx.

    3. Restriction of lung mobility from eschar on chest wall.

C. Renal changes.

    1. In burns of 15 to 20 percent of the body surface, there is a decreased urinary output, which must be avoided or reversed.

    2. Urinary tract infections are frequent.

D. Gastrointestinal changes.

    1. Acute gastric dilation.

    2. Paralytic ileus.

    3. Curling's ulcer that produces "coffee ground" aspirant.

E. Factors which determine seriousness of burn.

    1. Age.

      a. Below 18 months.

      b. Above 65 years.

    2. General health.

    3. Site of burn.

    4. Associated injuries (fractures).

    5. Causative agents.

Treatment and Implementation

A. Maintain patent airway.

B. Maintain aseptic area.

C. Provide fluid replacement therapy.

    1. Shock phase.

      a. First 24 to 48 hours postburn, fluid shifts from plasma to interstitial space.

      b. Potassium levels rise in plasma.

      c. Blood hemoconcentration and metabolic acidosis occur.

      d. Fluid loss is mostly plasma.

      e. Nursing responsibilities.

        (1) Monitor vital signs frequently.

        (2) Monitor urinary output (50 to 100 cc/hour).

        (3) Give one half of total fluids in first eight hours.

    2. Postshock phase (diuretic phase).

      a. Capillary permeability stabilizes and fluid begins to shift from interstitial spaces to plasma.

      b. Hypokalemia, hypernatremia, hemodilution, and pulmonary edema are potential dangers.

      c. Nursing responsibilities.

        (1) Monitor CVP.

        (2) Observe lab values.

        (3) Maintain adequate urine output.

D. Relieve pain with morphine sulfate as ordered. Give small doses frequently. Give IV.

E. Assess peripheral circulation.

F. Provide adequate heat to maintain patient's temperature.

G. Promote good body alignment: begin range of motion early.

H. Administer antacids to prevent stress ulcer.

I. Maintain reverse isolation.

J. Maintain wound care.
1. Initial excision: mainly for electrical burns.
2. Occlusive dressings.
   a. Painful and costly.
   b. Decreases water loss.
   c. Limits range-of-motion exercises.
   d. Helps to maintain functional position.
   e. Advent of topical antibiotics has led to decreased use.
3. Exposure method.
   a. Allows for drainage of burn exudate.
   b. Eschar forms protective covering.
   c. Use of topical therapy.
   d. Skin easily inspected.
   e. Range-of-motion exercises easier to perform.

K. Apply topical preparations to wound area.
   ❖ **PROCEDURE** ❖
1. Mafenide (Sulfamylon).
   a. Exerts bacteriostatic action against many organisms.
   b. Penetrates tissue wall.
   c. Dressings not needed when used.
   d. Breakdown of drug provides heavy acid load. Inhibition of carbonic anhydrase compounds situation. Individual compensates by hyperventilating.
   e. Alternate use with Silvadene.
2. Silvadene.
   a. Broad antimicrobial activity.
   b. Effective against yeast.
   c. Inhibits bacteria resistant to other antimicrobials.
      (1) Not usually used prophylactically.
      (2) Given for specific organism.
      (3) Not helpful first 48 hours due to vessel thrombosis.
   d. Can be washed off with water.
3. Silver nitrate—used for many years but decreasing in use.

L. Administer systemic antibiotics.

M. Debridement and eschar removal daily.

N. Provide long-term care.

1. Maintain good positioning to prevent contractures.
2. Provide adequate rest.
3. Prevent infection.
4. Maintain adequate protein and caloric intake to promote healing.
5. Monitor hydration status.
6. Protect skin grafts.
7. Provide psychological support (as important as physical care).
   a. Deal with the patient's fear of disfigurement and immobility from scarring.
   b. Provide constant support, as plastic repair is lengthy and painful.
   c. Involve the family in long-term planning and day-to-day care.

Isolation Protocol ❖ PROCEDURE ❖

A. Protocol for entering isolation room
1. Put on cap.
2. Put on and tie mask.
3. Put on gown and tie.
4. Wash hands and put on gloves.

B. Protocol for leaving isolation room
1. Untie gown at waist.
2. Take off gloves.
3. Wash hands.
4. Take off cap.
5. Untie gown at neck.
6. Pull gown off and place in laundry hamper.
7. Take off mask.
8. Leave room and wash hands.

SKIN DISORDERS AS MANIFESTATION OF INTERNAL DISEASE

Lupus Erythematosus

Definition: Collagen disease of the connective tissue that leads to a skin rash. The disease may involve any organ of the body.

Assessment

A. Discoid eruption—a chronic, localized scaling erythematous skin eruption over nose, cheeks, and forehead producing characteristic "butterfly" appearance.

B. Fever, malaise and weight loss.

C. Exacerbation and remission of symptoms.

D. Sensitivity to sunlight (photophobia).

E. Systemic (disseminated) lupus erythematosus may involve multiple organs and lead to death.

Treatment and Implementation

A. Protect patient from sunlight and avoid antibiotic ointments that may spread the lesions.

B. Administer steroid treatment to prevent progression of the disease.

C. Advise patient that strict personal hygiene is an absolute requirement.

D. Be aware that there is no development of immunity and recurrence is common.

Syphilis

Definition: Contagious venereal disease that leads to many structural and cutaneous lesions caused by the spirochete *Treponema pallidum*. The disease is transmitted by direct, intimate contact or in utero.

Stages

A. Primary stage.
   1. Incubation period is ten days to three weeks.
   2. Characteristic lesion is red, eroded, indurated papule; the sore or ulcer at the site of the invasion by the spirochete is called a chancre.
   3. Accompanied by enlarged lymph node in drainage area of chancre.
   4. May be painless or painful.
   5. This stage is highly infectious.

B. Secondary stage.
   1. Develops if the individual is not treated in the primary stage.
   2. May be mild enough to pass unnoticed or it may be severe, with a generalized rash on skin and mucous membrane.

Characteristics

A. Fever and sore throat.

B. Malaise may be present.

C. Transmitted most commonly by sexual intercourse, but infants may become infected during the birth process.

D. No age or race is immune to the disease.

E. Diagnosed by serum studies and/or dark field examination of secretions of the chancre.

Treatment and Implementation

A. Administer, if ordered, long-acting Bicillin as primary treatment.

B. Advise patient to avoid sexual contact until clearance is given by physician.

MALIGNANT TUMORS OF SKIN

Basal Cell Epithelioma

Definition: Tumor arising from the basal layer of the epidermis. Lesion is a small, smooth papule with telangiectasis and atrophic center.

Assessment

A. Starts as a papule and grows slowly.

B. Central area may become depressed and ulcerated, forming a classic rodent ulcer.

C. Locally invasive and seldom metastasizes.

Treatment and Implementation

A. Surgical excision is preferred.

B. Radiation therapy is administered for lesions of the eyelid and nose.

C. Watch for potential malignancy in other locations.

Squamous Cell Carcinoma

Definition: Tumor of the epidermis that frequently arises out of keratosis and is considered an invasive cancer. The lesion begins as erythematous macules or plaques with indistinct margins; surface often becomes crusted.

Assessment

A. Lesions enlarge more rapidly than in basal-cell epithelioma and may metastasize.
B. A nodular tumor usually appears on the lower lip, tongue, head, or neck.

Treatment

A. Excision is preferred.
B. Irradiation.

Melanoma

Definition: Malignant pigmented tumor that arises out of melanocytes and is often fatal. May arise from so-called blue-black mole.

Treatment

A. Surgical excision preferred.
B. Cancer-destroying drugs may be used.

APPENDIX 1. TYPES OF SKIN LESIONS

Primary lesions

Bulla	Large vesicle; elevation of filled with serous fluid.
Erythema	Form of macula showing redness over skin.
Lichenification	Thickening of affected tissue
Macule	Flat, discolored patch on skin of various colors and shapes
Papule	Raised, solid elevation of skin usually smaller than 1 cm.
Pustule	Small elevation of skin filled with purulent fluid.
Telangiectasis	Dilation of capillary, producing visible, red, irregular line.
Vesicle	Elevation of skin filled with clear, serous fluid; "blister."
Wheal	Irregularly shaped elevation that is caused by edema.

Secondary lesions

Crust	Dried serum from open lesion mixed with surface dirt and dead cells; "scab."
Scale	Flake of shed dry epidermis.

APPENDIX 2. "RULE OF NINES"

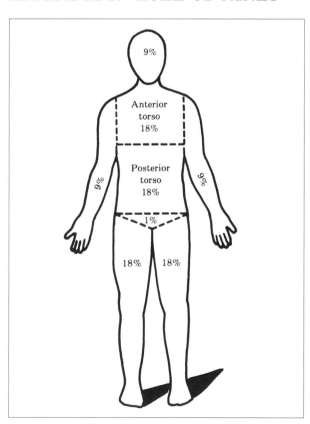

MUSCULOSKELETAL SYSTEM

Skeleton provides body with support and protection. The skeleton is used in locomotion but requires muscles to supply source of power and added support. Musculoskeletal system assists in unifying actions of whole body and helps it adjust to environmental changes.

ANATOMY AND PHYSIOLOGY

Skeletal System

A. System of separate bones (206) bound together by ligaments.
B. System responsible for supporting, moving, and giving shape to the body.
   1. Supports surrounding tissues and provides body with framework.
   2. Protects vital organs and soft tissues.
   3. Provides leverage and source of attachment for skeletal muscles.
   4. Forms erythrocytes, granular leukocytes, and thrombocytes in red marrow of bone.
   5. Stores calcium and other minerals.

Classification

A. According to body region.
   1. Axial skeleton—includes head and trunk which form central axis to which appendicular skeleton is attached.
      a. Composed of 80 bones.
      b. Includes skull, spine, ribs, sternum, and hyoid bone.
   2. Appendicular skeleton—includes shoulder girdle, arm bones, pelvic girdle, and leg bones.
      a. Composed of 126 bones.
      b. Shoulder (pectoral girdle from which arms hang).
         (1) Consists of two clavicles (collarbones).
         (2) Consists of two scapulae (shoulder blades), which are attached to clavicle.
      c. Arm bones.
         (1) Humerus (upper arm bone) is connected at elbow to ulna and radius (lower arm bones).
         (2) Carpals make up wrist.
         (3) Metacarpals form hand palm.
         (4) Phalanges form finger bones.
      d. Pelvic girdle (hip).
         (1) Pelvis formed from pelvic girdle, plus bones of sacrum and coccyx.
         (2) Encircles and protects genitourinary organs.
         (3) Sockets in girdle fit femur leg bone.
      e. Leg bones.
         (1) Constructed similarly to arm bones but heavier and stronger.
         (2) Femur (thigh bone) extends from pelvis to knee.
         (3) Tibia and fibula extend from knee to ankle.
         (4) Knee is separate bone (patella).
         (5) Ankle bones (tarsals); foot bones (metatarsals); toe bones (phalanges).
B. According to shape.
   1. Longbones—made up of a shaft (diaphysis) and two flared ends (epiphyses); include radius and femur.
   2. Short bones; include carpals and tarsals.
   3. Flatbones; include ribs and skull.
   4. Irregular bones; include vertebrae.

Development

A. The bonelike tissue of very young is mostly cartilage.
B. Cartilage is replaced by bone tissue through process of ossification.
   1. Calcium collects in cartilage and becomes hardened.
   2. Some cartilage cells break loose so that channels develop in bone shaft.
   3. Blood vessels enter channels carrying small cells of connective tissue; some tissue cells (osteoblasts) form true bone.

a. Osteoblasts enter hardened cartilage, forming layers of hard bone.
b. Other cells work to tear down old bone structure (osteoclasts) so osteoblasts can rebuild with new bone.

C. Bone-growth process occurs by mechanism of cartilage formation followed by replacement of cartilage with hard material.
1. Cartilage grows over hardened bone.
2. Cartilage hardens with addition of calcium.
3. Process continues until full growth of body is reached.

D. Amount of calcium deposited and reabsorbed into blood is regulated by the parathyroid and thyroid glands.

Structure

A. Bone is formed of dense connective tissue.
1. Tissue consists of bone cells (osteocytes).
2. Cells embedded in matrix made up of calcified intercellular substance.
3. Bone consists of 50 percent water and 50 percent solid matter.
4. Calcium phosphate is the basic bone chemical that gives hardness and strength.

B. Bone is comprised of concentric cylindrical layers.
1. Periosteum (the exterior covering, outer layer)—thin, tough membrane of fibrous tissue.
   a. Supports tendons connecting muscle to bone.
   b. Serves as protective sheath.
   c. Serves to extend blood supply to bone.
2. Compact bone layer—dense hard layer of bone tissue.
   a. Fibrous composition to give resiliency to bone.
   b. Compact tissue tunneled by central canal or hollow cavity.
      (1) Marrow (soft tissue, medulla) contained in compact bone hollow.
      (2) Contains fine branching canals (haversian system) through which small blood vessels and lymphatics run.

(3) Porous bone layer—spongy (cancellous) tissue that contains sponge-like hollows.

Joints

A. Articulation is a union or junction of two or more bones.
B. Function of joint is skeletal flexibility and motion.
C. Classification—according to structural variations that allow for different kinds of movement.
1. Diarthroses—joint is freely movable.
   a. This type of joint is a cavity enclosed by a capsule lined with synovial membrane that secretes a lubricant.
   b. Capsule is reinforced by ligaments.
   c. Articular cartilage covers ends of bones.
   d. Types of joint movement make for structural variations.
      (1) Hinge type allows single directional movement (elbow).
      (2) Ball-and-socket type allows bending (hip).
      (3) Saddle type allows multidirectional shifting (thumb).
      (4) Pivot type allows rotary movement.
      (5) Gliding type allows limited sliding of bones against each other (wrist, ankle, invertebral joints).
      (6) Ellipsoidal type.
2. Synarthroses—joint is immovable.
   a. Tissue grows between articulating surfaces.
   b. Includes suture lines of skull.
3. Amphiarthroses—joint with minimal movement.

Muscular System

A. System of fibers (more than 600) attached to bones and marked by striation.
B. System allows body movement under control of voluntary nervous system.
1. Provides for body movement, locomotion.
2. Provides support for the body.

3. Performs body functions such as partial production of heat.

Classification

A. According to location—posterior tibial allows inversion of foot.
B. According to direction of fibers—muscle of tongue allows for change in shape for eating.
C. According to action—flexor muscle of toe allows toe to bend on itself, extensor muscle of toe allows extension of toe.
D. According to size and shape—trapezius of neck and shoulder allows for elevation and rotation of shoulder.
E. According to number of origin heads—biceps of arm allow for flexing and turning arm upward.
F. According to points of attachment—sternocleidomastoid allows for flexion and rotation of head.

Cell Structure

A. Fibers of voluntary muscles grouped together in sheath of connective tissue.
B. Each bundled group of muscle fibers surrounded by connective tissue sheath.
C. Sheath tissue may be continuous with fibrous tissue that extends from the muscle as a tendon.

Properties

A. Excitability—capacity of muscle to respond to stimulus without intervention of motor nerves.
B. Contractility—ability of muscle to shorten, tighten, and contract.
C. Tonicity—ability of muscle to maintain steady contraction which determines its firmness.
D. Extensibility—ability of muscle to stretch in response to applied force.
E. Elasticity—ability of strained muscle to regain original size and shape when applied force is removed.

Contraction

A. For muscle contraction and other fine movements to occur, muscle tissue must be stimulated.
   1. Each fiber receives own neural impulse from somatic motor neuron.
   2. Signal of impulse along nerve muscle fiber changes chemical to mechanical energy.
   3. Each fiber has stored supply of fuel for contraction energy source.
      a. Stimulus releases calcium to cause fiber filament movement.
      b. Nerve stimulates breakdown of ATP.
B. Area where motor neuron ends in muscle fiber is called myoneural junction.

Movement

A. Skeletal muscles produce body movement by pulling on bones.
B. Bones serve as levers, and joints serve as fulcrums of these levers.
   1. Each muscle has a point of origin and a point of insertion that are usually attached to bone.
   2. The point of origin is the more fixed point of attachment.
   3. The point of insertion is the more movable end.
C. Muscles that move a body part usually do not extend over that part.
D. Skeletal muscles usually perform with group action; some contract while others relax.
   1. Prime movers are muscles responsible for the primary movement of contraction.
   2. Antagonists are muscles that exert an action opposing that of prime mover.
   3. Synergists are muscles that enhance action of prime mover.
E. Accessory parts.
   1. Ligaments—cordlike connective tissue that holds bones together.
   2. Tendons—attach muscles to bones.

MUSCULOSKELETAL DISORDERS

Fractures

Definition: A break in the continuity of bone.

A. Direct application of force at site.
B. Distant application of force but transmitted to fracture site.
C. Sudden muscle contraction.
D. Spontaneous break as result of disease.

Classification

A. According to severity.
1. Simple (closed)—a break is present but no external wound in skin.
2. Compound (open)—a break is present and there is external wound in skin over or leading to fracture site.
3. Comminuted—bone has splintered into fragments.
4. Greenstick—one side of the bone broken but the opposite side is bent.
B. According to direction and location.
1. Oblique—break runs in slanting direction.
2. Spiral—break coils around bone.
3. Extracapsular—break occurs outside the joint.
4. Intracapsular—break occurs inside the joint.

Assessment

A. Deformity.
B. Loss of power or movement.
C. Pain, tenderness, and muscle spasm over fracture site.
D. Edema.
E. Discoloration from bruising.
F. Possible shock.

Emergency Implementation

A. Keep limb or part stable until immobilized.
B. Take measures to prevent shock.
C. Cover open wound with dry and clean or sterile dressing.

Treatment

A. Objectives.
1. Regain correct alignment through reduction.
2. Maintain alignment.
3. Regain function of affected part.
B. Fractures treated by reduction; broken ends pulled into alignment and continuity of bone established so healing can occur.
1. Methods of reduction.
a. Closed—fractured bone brought into alignment by manual manipulation; no incision made.
b. Open—surgical incision made and bone aligned under direct visualization; also performed to cleanse open fracture or to stabilize alignment with inserted fixators.
2. Forms of alignment.
a. Closed—application of cast, splint, and/or traction.
b. Open—fixation with metallic pins, wires, screws, plates, nails, or rods.

Principles of Cast Care ❖ PROCEDURE ❖

A. After application of cast, allow 24 to 48 hours for drying.
1. Cast will change from dull to shiny substance when dry.
2. Heat can be applied to assist in drying process.
B. Do not handle cast during drying process as indentations from fingermarks can cause skin breakdown under cast.
C. Keep extremity elevated to prevent edema.
D. Provide for smooth edges surrounding cast.
1. Prevents crumbling and breaking down of edges.
2. Stockinet can be pulled over edge and fastened down with adhesive tape to outside of cast.

E. Observe casted extremity for signs of circulatory impairment. Cast may have to be cut if edematous condition continues.

F. If there is an open, draining area on affected extremity, a window (cut out portion of cast) can be utilized for observation and/or irrigation of wound.

G. Keep cast dry; it can break down when water comes in contact with plaster. Plastic bags or plastic coated bed Chux can be utilized during the bath or when using bedpan, to protect cast material.

H. Utilize isometric exercises to prevent muscle atrophy and to strengthen the muscle.

I. Position patient with pillows to prevent strain on unaffected areas.

J. Turn every two hours to prevent complications. Encourage to lie on abdomen four hours a day.

The Immobilized Patient

A. Prevent respiratory complications.
   1. Have patient cough and deep breathe every two hours.
   2. Turn every two hours if not contraindicated.
   3. Provide suction if needed.

B. Prevent thrombus and emboli formation.
   1. Apply antiembolic stockings.
   2. Initiate isometric and isotonic exercises.
   3. Start anticoagulation therapy, if indicated.
   4. Turn every two hours.
   5. Observe for signs and symptoms of pulmonary and/or fat emboli.

C. Prevent contractures.
   1. Start range-of-motion exercises to affected joints qid, all joints bid.
   2. Provide foot board and/or foot cradle.
   3. Position and turn every two hours.

D. Prevent skin breakdown.
   1. Massage with lotion once a day to prevent drying.
   2. Use alcohol for back care to toughen skin.
   3. Massage elbows, coccyx, heels bid.
   4. Turn every two hours.

   5. Alternate pressure mattress, sheepskin.
   6. Use Stryker boots or heel protectors.
   7. Use elbow guards.

E. Prevent urinary retention and calculi.
   1. Force fluids.
   2. Monitor intake and output.
   3. Administer urinary antiseptic (Mandelamine, etc.).
   4. Offer bedpan every four hours.

F. Prevent constipation.
   1. Force fluids.
   2. Provide high fiber diet.
   3. Administer laxative or enema.
   4. Offer bedpan at same time each day—encourage to establish good bowel habits.

G. Provide psychological support.

Traction

A. Traction is force applied in two directions.

B. Purpose is to reduce and/or immobilize a fracture, to provide proper bone alignment and regain normal length, or to reduce muscle spasm.

Skeletal Traction

A. Mechanical—applied to bone, using pins (Steinmann), wires (Kirschner), tongs (Crutchfield).

B. Most often used in fractures of femur, tibia, humerus.

C. Nursing care.
   1. Observe pin or tong insertion site for drainage, odors, erythema, edema (usually indication of inflammatory process or infection).
   2. Watch for skin breakdown if bandage is used to apply traction.
   3. Cover end of pins or wires with rubber stoppers or cork to prevent puncture of nursing personnel or patient.
   4. Cleanse area surrounding insertion site of pin or tongs with hydrogen peroxide or Betadine. Some physicians order antibiotic ointments to be applied to area.

Balanced Suspension Traction

A. Thomas' splint with Pearson attachment is used in conjunction with skin or skeletal traction (used particularly with skeletal traction for fractured femur).

B. Balanced suspension traction is produced by a counterforce other than the patient.

C. Nursing care. ❖ **PROCEDURE** ❖
   1. Maintain proper alignment.
   2. Protect skin from excoriation, particularly around the top of Thomas' splint. Pad with cotton wadding or ABDs.
   3. Prevent pressure points around the top of Thomas' splint by keeping patient pulled up in bed.
   4. Maintain at least 20-degree angle from thigh to the bed.
   5. Provide foot plate to prevent foot drop.
   6. Keep heels clear of Pearson attachment to prevent skin breakdown and decubitus.
   7. Position patient frequently from side to side (as ordered).
   8. Unless contraindicated, head of bed can be elevated for comfort and facilitating adequate respiratory functions.
   9. Place overbed table on unaffected side.

Skin Traction

A. Traction applied by use of elastic bandages, moleskin strips, or adhesive.

B. Used most often in alignment or lengthening (for congenital hip displacement, etc.).

C. Most common types.
   1. Russell traction.
   2. Buck's extension (most common).
      ❖ **PROCEDURE** ❖
      a. Pull is exerted in one plane.
      b. Used for temporary immobilization.
      c. Apply moleskin or adhesive material to leg. Follow with application of ace wrap.
      d. Attach a foot block with a spreader and rope which goes into a pulley.

   e. Attach weight to pulley and hang freely over edge of bed. (Not more than eight to ten pounds of weight can be applied.)
   f. Observe and readjust bandages for tightness and smoothness (can cause constriction which leads to edema or even nerve damage).

3. Cervical traction (used for whiplashes and cervical spasm). ❖ **PROCEDURE** ❖
   a. Use head harness (or halter).
      (1) Pad chin.
      (2) Protect ears from friction rub.
   b. Elevate head of bed and attach weights to pulley system over head of bed.
   c. Observe for skin breakdown.
      (1) Powder areas encased in the halter.
      (2) Place back of head on padding.

4. Pelvic traction (used for low back pain). ❖ **PROCEDURE** ❖
   a. Apply girdle snugly over patient's pelvis and iliac crest; attach to weights.
   b. Observe for pressure points over iliac crest.
   c. Keep patient in good alignment.
   d. May raise foot of bed slightly (12 inches) to prevent patient from slipping down in bed.

D. Care of traction apparatus. ❖ **PROCEDURE** ❖
   1. Weights should hang freely and not touch the floor.
   2. Pulleys should not be obstructed.
   3. Ropes in the pulley should move freely.
   4. Knot should be secured in rope to prevent slipping.
   5. Proper body alignment (up in bed, in direct line with traction) and proper countertraction should be maintained.
   6. Weights should not be removed or lifted without specific order. (Exceptions are pelvic and cervical traction that patients can remove at intervals.)
   7. Sharp edges from traction apparatus should be covered with hollowed out rubber balls to prevent injury to nursing personnel if they bump into equipment.

APPENDIX 3. TYPES OF TRACTION

Type	Position	Purpose
Skin Traction		
Cervical	Head of bed elevated 30°–40°	Relieve muscle spasms and compression in upper extremities and neck
Buck's	Foot of bed elevated	Immobilize hip when fractured, relieve muscle spasms before hip surgery
Bryant's	Flat with 90° hip flexion	Stabilize fractured femur; correct congenital hip in young children
Russell's	Foot of bed slightly elevated	Stabilize fractured femur prior to surgery
Pelvic	Head of bed elevated, knee gatch elevated to same level (William's position)	Relieve low back, hip, or leg pain; reduce muscle spasm
Skeletal Tongs		
(Blackburn, Gardner-Wells, Crutchfield, Vinke Tongs)	Spine immobilized	Provide for hyperextension; traction allows vertebrae to slip back into position
Halo Vest	Flat, low-Fowler's in bed, ambulate, or sit up	Stabilize fractured or dislocated cervical vertebrae
Balanced Suspension		
Steinmann pin, Kirschner wires, used with Thomas' splint and Pearson attachment	Low-Fowler's, either side or back	To approximate fractures of femur, tibia, fibula

E. Care of patient in traction. ❖ **PROCEDURE** ❖
   1. Maintain correct alignment.
   2. Maintain counterbalance or correct pull.
      a. Pull is exerted against traction in opposite direction (balanced suspension).
      b. Pull is exerted against a fixed point.
      c. Bed is elevated under area involved to provide the countertraction.
   3. Provide firm mattress or bedboards.
   4. Observe for complications.
   5. Provide range-of-motion exercises for unaffected extremities.
   6. Observe for circulatory impairment.
      a. Blanching of nailbeds (color should return quickly when nailbeds are depressed).
      b. Extremity should be pink and warm.
      c. Check for edema in affected extremity.
      d. Patient should be able to wiggle finger or toes.
      e. Patient should not have tingling or loss of sensation in affected extremity.
   7. Prevent foot drop.
      a. Provide footplate.
      b. Encourage dorsiflexion exercises.
   8. Provide overhead trapeze to allow patient to assist in activities (turning, moving up in bed, using bedpan, etc.)
   9. Prevent postoperative complications.

Hip (Proximal) Fracture

Definition: Bone discontinuity of proximal end of femur, intracapsular or extracapsular, which occurs most frequently in elderly women.

Preoperative Implementation

A. Provide care similar to patients in skin traction.
B. Give special care if patient's increased age is a factor.
C. Observe for elimination regularity.
D. Encourage proper exercises.
E. Maintain proper positioning.
F. Assist patient with eating; nourishing diet essential for healing process.

Operative Procedure

A. Surgical fixation with nails, plates, or screws.
B. Possible prosthesis.

Postoperative Implementation

A. Turn patient from unaffected side to back as routine; a physician's order is required to turn from side to side.
B. Turn patient with hip prosthesis by always placing pillows between legs to avoid adduction.
C. Elevate head (may be limited to 30 to 40 degrees) to avoid acute hip flexion.
D. Introduce quadricep and gluteal setting muscle exercises; encourage use of overhead trapeze for assistance in moving.
E. Take measures to protect patient when moving from bed to chair (patient not to bear weight on affected leg).
F. Provide routine postoperative measures to ensure patient's comfort.
G. Take measures as necessary to prevent complications.

Hip Arthroplasty (Total Hip Replacement)

Definition: Amputation of femoral head with implantation of a steel ball and stem and placement of polyethylene or metal cupin for the acetabulum; its purpose is the alleviation of pain and the restoration of movement for those with osteoarthritis or rheumatoid arthritis.

Postoperative Implementation

A. Keep operative leg in abduction to prevent flexion by use of pillows or abductor splints.
   1. Positioning is important (every two hours).
   2. Turn patient about 45° with aid of trapeze and pillows. Do not elevate bed more than 30° to 45°.
   3. Do not turn to affected side unless specific orders.
B. Keep Hemovac in place until drainage has substantially decreased (24 to 96 hours).
   1. Check dressing to ensure patency of Hemovac.
   2. Observe drainage for signs of hemorrhage or infection.
C. Prevent edema.
   1. Readjust antiembolic stockings at least every four to eight hours.
   2. Change position frequently by raising and lowering head of bed. When ordered, tilt bed to change positions.
D. Ambulate patient carefully at bedside—first or second postoperative day.
   1. Do not allow patient to bear weight on affected hip.
   2. Up with walker second postoperative day.
   3. Avoid positions with 60° to 90° flexion, such as sitting straight up in a chair.

Arthrotomy (Knee Surgery)

Definition: Incision of joint for removal of cartilage.

Implementation

A. Encourage and assist with bed exercises.
B. Begin quad setting, straight-leg raising exercises (should be done for five minutes every half hour).

1. Quad-setting exercises—tightening or contracting the muscles of anterior thigh (knee cap is drawn up toward thigh).
2. Straight-leg raising—lifting leg straight off the bed, keeping knee extended and foot in neutral position.

C. Encourage and assist with dorsiflexion and plantar flexion of feet and ankles.
D. Apply ice bags to knee to reduce edema as necessary.
E. Help patient out of bed first postoperative day (use three point crutch walking gait without weight-bearing).
F. Give routine postoperative care as necessary.

Total Knee Replacement

Definition: Implantation of a metallic upper portion which substitutes for the femoral condyle and a lower, high polymer plastic, portion which substitutes for the tibial joint surfaces.

Implementation

A. CPM may be ordered postop—moderate flexion and extension.
B. Provide quad setting and straight-leg raising exercises every hour; encourage general bed exercises.
C. Patient usually has a cast or splint—provide care.
D. Do not dangle leg; may result in dislocation.
E. Insert hemovac to drain excessive blood and drainage.
1. Record and measure intake and output accurately.
2. Observe for hemorrhage and infection.
F. Instruct patient how to walk with crutch—will be out of bed in 2–3 days.
G. Provide general postoperative care.

Amputation

Definition: Surgical removal of part or all of an extremity; connecting bones may be separated at joint (disarticulation).

Types

A. Closed, or flapped—skin closed over bone end of stump.
B. Open, or guillotine—skin not closed over stump end in order that drainage can occur.

Preoperative Implementation

A. Support patient emotionally and listen to patient's expressed concerns regarding limb loss.
B. Help patient strengthen muscles of upper extremity (if lower extremity affected) as preparation for crutch walking.
1. Extend and flex arms while holding weights.
2. Do push-ups if condition permits.
C. Inform patient of possible occurrence of phantom pain following surgery. The sensation may last from a few hours to a longer period of time.

Postoperative Implementation

A. Delayed fitting of prosthesis.
   ❖ **PROCEDURE** ❖
1. Observe stump for excessive bleeding (keep tourniquet ready in event of hemorrhage).
   a. Reinforce or change dressing only if ordered.
   b. Observe drainage especially if Penrose drain inserted.
2. Elevate extremity.
   a. Elevation of bed is preferred.
   b. If pillow used, remove within 48 hours to avoid flexion contracture.
3. Turn patient to prone position first postoperative day for brief period and gradually increase time.
4. Exercise all extremities.
5. Assist with transfer of patient to wheelchair.
6. Assist with and encourage crutch walking several days postoperatively.
7. Apply ace bandage properly (avoid tightness while maintaining tension); helps to condition stump.

8. Observe for signs of depression; listen to patient's expression of feelings.
9. Encourage physical and psychological progress.

B. Immediate fitting of prosthesis.
1. Immediate fitting causes less pain and hastens healing.
2. Immediately following surgery, sterile dressing is applied to stump followed by rigid plastic dressing.
3. Prosthetic device is attached.
4. If cast falls off, wrap stump immediately with ace bandage and call physician; normally, cast will be changed and reapplied 10 to 14 days postoperatively.
5. Observe for drainage and mark site with pen.
6. Elevate extremity stump for only 24 hours.
7. Assist patient in dangling and walking first day postoperatively (first use parallel bars, then crutches).
8. Be aware that exercises are usually not required because of early ambulation.

Laminectomy

Definition: Removal of posterior arch of vertebrae (lamina) to expose the spinal cord; performed on the cervical or lumbar area of vertebra for removal of spinal cord tumors or herniated disc.

Postoperative Implementation

A. Observe neurovascular signs.
B. Monitor dressing for clear or bloody drainage.
C. Place pillow between patient's legs and turn patient from side to side as a unit (log roll) every two hours.
D. Head of bed is usually kept flat for lumbar laminectomy but elevated for cervical laminectomy.
E. Roll patient onto bedpan (as used with fractures), supporting back with pillow.
F. Give assistance in preparation for ambulation.
   ❖ **PROCEDURE** ❖
   1. Turn patient on side.

2. Reach under shoulder that is resting on bed.
3. Help raise patient as he or she uses arms to push up from bed.
4. Help patient swing over edge of bed.

G. Instruct patient in proper movement and position.
1. Turn as a unit.
2. Sit with back straight.
3. When necessary to reach floor with hands, squat and maintain straight back.

H. Give routine postoperative care.

Spinal Fusion

Definition: Removal of bone from iliac crest for fusing with spinal vertebrae.

Postoperative Implementation

A. Keep patient supine for first 8 hours to reduce possibility of compression ordered by physician (most physicians order patient to be off back first 48 hours.)
B. Monitor both surgical sites.
C. Brace is applied when patient is ambulated; beginning of ambulation varies from three to four days to eight weeks, depending on extent of fusion.
D. Patient is not to lift, bend, stoop, or sit for prolonged periods for at least three months.
1. Grafts are stable by one year.
2. Some limitation to flexion of spine, depending on extent of fusion.
E. Provide routine care as for postlaminectomy.

Osteoarthritis

Definition: Degeneration of articular cartilage in the joints resulting from prolonged wear and tear on joint surfaces.

Predisposing Factors

A. Aging.

B. Faulty body posture, joint trauma.

C. Familial tendency.

D. Being female (females more frequently affected than males).

E. Obesity.

Assessment

A. Onset usually insidious and gradual.

B. Stiffness of joints.

C. Aching of joints (more noticeable after exercise).

D. Limited joint movement.

E. Nodular bony enlargements on the distal joints of fingers (Heberden's nodes).

F. Occurs usually in hip, knee, vertebra, and finger joints.

Treatment and Implementation

A. Arrange for weight reduction if indicated.

B. Provide rest periods; avoid excessive exercise of joints.

C. Apply warm moist packs; give tub baths and paraffin dips.

D. Assist with exercise program to improve posture.

E. Provide range of motion exercises.

F. Administer medications as ordered.
   1. Anti-inflammatory drugs, e.g., phenylbutazone, acetylsalicylic acid.
   2. Analgesics, e.g. acetylsalicylic acid.
   3. Corticosteroid intraarticular injections.

G. Be aware of possible need for surgical procedure (synovectomy, arthrodesis, or arthroplasty).

H. Instruct patient in use of proper body mechanics.

I. Advise patient to avoid emotional stress to lessen strain on muscles and joints.

J. Encourage patient to engage in prescribed exercises, to take prescribed medications, and to avoid being overweight.

Rheumatoid Arthritis

Definition: Chronic systemic disease affecting any or all of the body systems and characterized by recurrent inflammation involving the linings of the joints; joint capsule progressively changes and ankylosis occurs. Actual cause is unknown; suspected causes may be an autoimmune disorder or hereditary factors.

Assessment

A. Easily fatigued.

B. Loss of weight.

C. Joint pain and stiffness, especially in the morning.

D. Painful and stiff joints that become swollen, reddened, and tender.

E. Subcutaneous nodules over bony prominences.

F. Anemia.

G. Periods of remission and exacerbation.

Treatment and Implementation

A. Encourage adequate rest periods; extent of rest depends on current status of disease.
   1. During day as necessary.
   2. Use of firm mattress and no pillows; improper positioning of joints can result in contracture.
   3. Use of splints for supporting joints.
   4. Relief from emotional stress.

B. Administer medications as ordered.
   1. Anti-inflammatory analgesics (see osteoarthritis medications).
   2. Corticosteroids, e.g., prednisone.
   3. Intraarticular corticosteroid injections into joint.
   4. Gold salts.

C. Apply moist heat, i.e., baths, packs, paraffin dips.

D. Encourage exercise of joints within limits of tolerance.

E. Be aware of possible need for surgery (see osteoarthritis).

F. Discuss aspects of the disease with the patient in a realistic and optimistic manner.

G. Assist patient in maintaining independence.

H. Advise patient to call on physician for any problems; caution against promises for quick cures, whatever the source.

Osteoporosis

Definition: Decrease in the amount of bone capable of maintaining structural integrity of the skeleton. Etiology is unknown.

Assessment

A. Backache with pain radiating around trunk.

B. Skeletal deformities.

C. Pathologic fractures.

D. Lab findings.
   1. Serum calcium, phosphorus and alkaline phosphatase are usually normal.
   2. Parathyroid hormone may be elevated.

Treatment and Implementation

A. Provide pain control.

B. Prevent fractures.
   1. Instruct in safety factors—watch steps, avoid use of scatter rugs.
   2. Keep side rails up to prevent falls.
   3. Move gently when turning and positioning.
   4. Assist with ambulation if unsteady on feet.

C. Administer medications as ordered.
   1. Estrogen—decreases rate of bone resorption.
   2. Calcium and vitamin D—support bone metabolism.

D. Instruct in regular exercise program.
   1. Range-of-motion exercises.
   2. Ambulation several times per day.

E. Instruct in good use of body mechanics.

F. Provide diet high in protein, calcium, vitamin D.

APPENDIX 1. SURGICAL POSITIONS AND AMBULATION

System	Postop Position	Ambulation
Neurosurgical		
Craniotomy		
Surgery involving: posterior fossa	Supine or low-Fowler's (10°) side to side only	Evening or first day
Anterior or middle fossa	Low-or semi-Fowler's; side to back to side unless bone flap removed, then nonoperative side and back only	Evening or first day
Ventriculoperitoneal shunt	Supine, back to unoperative side	First to second day
Respiratory		
Laryngectomy	Semi-Fowler's; side-back-side	First or second day, depends on extent of surgery
Tracheostomy	Semi-Fowler's; side-back-side	Evening of surgery
Nasal surgery	Submucous resection	Rhinoplasty
	Semi-Fowler's back	First day

System	Postop Position	Ambulation
Tonsillectomy	Semi-Fowler's if local anesthesia used; modified Trendelenburg's, side-lying or prone with head turned to side if general anesthesia used	Evening of surgery
Lung surgery Lobectomy Segmental resection Thoracotomy	Semi-to high-Fowler's; side-back-side	Evening of surgery or first day
Pneumonectomy	Semi- to high-Fowler's back to operative side	First day
Circulatory		
Open-heart surgery for atrial and ventricular septal defects	Low-Fowler's or supine; turn side-back-side	First to third day
Valve replacement surgery	Supine or low-Fowler's until vital signs stable; turn side-back-side	First to second day
Coronary artery bypass	Supine or low-Fowler's until vital signs stable; turn side-back-side	First to second day
Ear		
Stapedectomy	Low-Fowler's; unoperative side only	Evening of surgery or first day
Eye		
Cataract removal	Low-Fowler's; unoperative side only	Day of surgery; usually within 2–4 hours post-op
Repair of detached retina	Varies with site of detachment; unoperative side only or as ordered	Evening of surgery or first day
Enucleation	High-Fowler's; unoperative side only or as ordered	First day
Gastrointestinal		
Gastric resection Ileostomy Colostomy Colon resection Appendectomy Cholecystectomy	Minimum low-Fowler's; turn side-back-side	Evening of surgery or first day
Small bowel resection Portacaval shunt Partial pancreatectomy	Low-Fowler's; turn side-back-side	First day
Hemorrhoidectomy	Supine; turn side to side	First day
Radical neck	Fowler's, side lying either side	First to second day

APPENDIX 1. SURGICAL POSITIONS AND AMBULATION (*Continued*)

System	Postop Position	Ambulation
Genitourinary		
Nephrostomy	Semi- to high-Fowler's; unoperative side only	Evening of surgery
Nephrolithotomy Nephrectomy Transplant	Semi- to high-Fowler's; unoperative	Evening of surgery
Ureterolithotomy TURP Orchiectomy	Low-Fowler's; side-back-side	Evening of surgery
Cystectomy and ileal conduit Bladder suspension	Low-Fowler's; side-back-side	First day
Gynecologic		
Hysterectomy Oopherectomy	Low-Fowler's; side-back-side	Evening of surgery
Radical hysterectomy Pelvic exenteration Vulvectomy	Supine or low-Fowler's; side-back-side	Third day
Mastectomy	Fowler's; unoperative side or back	Evening of surgery
Musculoskeletal		
Amputation	Low-Fowler's; unoperative side and back, prone once per shift after first day	Evening of surgery; use adaptive devices, i.e., crutches
Open reduction and internal fixation	Fowler's; side-back-side	Evening of surgery or first day
Hip prosthesis	Low-Fowler's; back or unoperative side only. DO NOT FLEX hips, abduction and external rotation keep in	First to third day, nonweight-bearing
Hip nailing Total knee replacement	Low-Fowler's; unoperative side and back only	First day, nonweight-bearing
Total hip replacement	Supine or side to side with orders; DO NOT FLEX hips, keep in abduction and external rotation	First to third day, nonweight-bearing
Laminectomy	Low-Fowler's; turn side to side, may position on back, log roll	Evening of surgery or first day
Spinal fusion	Flat, side to side only, not on back, log roll	Second or third day with brace

8

ONCOLOGY NURSING

Oncology is the area of nursing that focuses on the patient with cancer. Cancer is second only to cardiovascular disease as the leading cause of death in the United States. As such, it is an area that will demand more nursing care and involvement in the future. This chapter focuses on cancer as a disease, its treatment, and oncology nursing concepts .

Cancer Incidence and Trends

A. Cancer—a definition.
  1. Term represents a group of more than 100 neoplastic diseases that involve all body organs.
  2. One or more cells lose their normal growth-controlling mechanism and continue to grow uncontrolled.
B. Second leading cause of death in U.S. after heart disease.
  1. Ranks fourth for males and first for females as cause of death; second after accidents as cause of death for children.
  2. Greatest increase seen in lung cancer—consistent with smoking patterns.
C. Incidence rate:
  1. Five million in U.S. diagnosed with cancer.
  2. Number of cancer deaths increased by 11 percent during past 40 years.

Identified Causes and Risk Factors

A. Multiplicity theory: multiple factors lead to the development of cancer; 60–90 percent thought to be related to environmental factors.
B. Carcinogens: agents known to increase susceptibility to cancer.
  1. Chemical carcinogens: asbestos, benzene, vinyl chloride, by-products of tobacco, etc.
  2. Iatrogenic chemical agents: DES; chemotherapy; hormone treatment; immunosuppressive agents.
  3. Radiation carcinogens: x-rays; sunlight (ultraviolet light); nuclear radiation.
  4. Viral factors: herpes simplex; Epstein-Barr; Hepatitis B and retroviruses.

5. Genetic factors: hereditary or familial tendencies.
6. Demographic and geographic factors.
7. Dietary factors: obesity; high-fat diet; diets low in fiber; diets high in smoked or salted foods; preservatives and food additives; alcohol.
8. Psychological factors: stress.

Preventive Measures

A. Optimal Dietary Patterns.
  1. Avoid obesity (at 40 percent overweight, there is a 55 percent increased risk of cancer in females and 33 percent in males).
  2. Decrease fat intake of both saturated and unsaturated fats—maximum 30 percent of total calories.
  3. Increase total fiber in diet—decreases risk of colon cancer.
  4. Increase vitamin A—reduced incidence of larynx, esophagus, and lung cancers.
  5. Increase vitamin C—aids tumor encapsulation and promotes longer survival time.
  6. Increase vitamin E—inhibits growth of brain tumors, melanomas, and leukemias.
  7. Decrease alcohol consumption.
  8. Avoid salt-cured, smoked, or nitrate-cured foods.
B. Minimize exposure to carcinogens.
  1. Avoid smoking—thought to be a cause of 75 percent lung cancers in U.S.
  2. Avoid oral tobacco—increases incidence of oral cancers.
  3. Avoid exposure to asbestos fibers and constant environmental dust.
  4. Avoid exposure to chemicals.
  5. Avoid radiation exposure and excessive exposure to sunlight.
C. Obtain adequate rest and exercise to decrease stress.
  1. Chronic stress associated with decreased immune system functioning.
  2. Strong immune system responsible for destruction of malignant cells as they develop.

Early Detection Methods

A. Risk Assessment (see Risk Factors).
B. Health history and physical assessment.
C. Screening methods.
   1. Tests such as a mammography, Pap test, sigmoidoscopy, etc.
   2. Self-care practices: breast self-examination (BSE); testicular self-examination (TSE); skin inspection.
D. Teaching patient the seven early warning signs of cancer.
   1. Change in bowel or bladder habits.
   2. Any sore that does not heal.
   3. Bleeding or unusual discharge.
   4. Lump or thickening in breast or elsewhere.
   5. Indigestion or difficulty swallowing.
   6. Obvious change in wart or mole.
   7. Nagging cough or hoarseness.

Characteristics

A. Benign Neoplasms: usually encapsulated, remain localized, and are slow-growing.
B. Malignant Neoplasms; not encapsulated, will metastasize and grow, and exert negative effects on host.
C. Categories of malignant neoplasms:
   1. Carcinomas—grown from epithelial cells; usually solid tumors (skin, stomach, colon, breast, rectal tumors).
   2. Sarcomas—arise from muscle, bone, fat, or connective tissue—may be solid.
   3. Lymphomas—arise from lymphoid tissue (infection-fighting organs).
   4. Leukemias and myelomas—grow from blood-forming organs.
D. Mechanisms of metastasis.
   1. Metastasis occur via lymphatics—spreads along lymph channels to mass in lymphs nodes (e.g., breast to axillary nodes) or spread diffusely.
   2. The bloodstream may carry cells from one site to another (e.g., liver to bone, etc.).
   3. Direct spread of cancer cells (seeding) where there are no boundaries to stop the growth (e.g., ovary and stomach).

Comparison of Benign and Malignant Tumors

Malignant	Benign
Cell Type	
Abnormal from those of tissues	Close to those of original original tissues
Growth	
Rapid; infiltrates surrounding tissues in all directions	Slow and noninfiltrating
Encapsulated	
Infrequent	Frequent
Metastasis	
Through blood, lymph, or new tumor sites	Remains localized
Effect	
Terminal without treatment	Can become malignant or obstruct vital organs

   4. Transplantation is the transfer of cells from one site to another.

Diagnosis

A. Laboratory and radiologic tests often identify a problem first.
   1. Radiographic procedures (e.g., tomography, CT, contrast studies).
   2. Ultra sonography.
   3. Radioisotopic Scanning Studies (e.g., brain scan, Gallium imaging).
   4. Magnetic Resonance Imaging (MRI).
   5. Biologic response markers (useful for diagnosing primary tumors).
   6. Other laboratory tests (enzyme tests, such as acid phosphatase).
B. Biopsy: definitive diagnosis of cancer.
   1. Excisional biopsy—removes all suspicious tissue.
   2. Incisional biopsy—removes a sample of tissue from a mass.
   3. Needle aspiration—aspiration of small amount of core tissue from a suspicious area.

4. Exfoliative cytology—cells in tissue or secretions are evaluated by PAP method.
C. Tissue specimens are evaluated by frozen or permanent sections by a pathologist.
D. Results from biopsy and other diagnostic procedures (blood tests, x-ray studies, endoscopic procedures) will determine extent of disease-staging.

Staging: How Cancer is Classified

A. Staging describes the extent or metastasis of a malignant tumor; also quantifies severity of disease.
B. A useful system of staging for carcinomas is the TNM system.
   1. T: Primary tumor.
   2. N: Regional nodes.
   3. M: Metastasis.
C. The extent to which malignancy has increased in size:
   1. TO: no evidence of primary tumor.
   2. TIS: carcinoma in situ.
   3. T_1, T_2, T_3 T_4: progressive increase in tumor, size, and involvement.
   4. TX: tumor cannot be assessed.
D. Involvement of regional nodes.
   1. NO: regional lymph nodes not abnormal.
   2. N_1 N_2, N_3, N_4: increasing degree of abnormal regional lymph nodes.
   3. NX: regional lymph nodes cannot be assessed clinically.
E. Metastatic development.
   1. MO: no evidence of distant metastasis.
   2. M_1 to M_3: increasing degree of distant metastasis.

Treatment Methods

A. Broad goals.
   1. Goal of therapy is to cure the patient—eradicate the tumor.
   2. When cure is not possible, controlling or arresting tumor growth becomes the goal—to prolong survival.
   3. Palliation or alleviation of symptoms is a third goal.
B. The major forms of cancer treatment include surgery, radiation therapy, chemotherapy, and combined approaches.

Surgery

A. Useful as primary treatment for localized cancer (breast, colon, melanoma of skin, etc.).
   1. Highest rate of cure for localized disease.
   2. Disadvantage—deforming or debilitating to patient.
B. Types of treatment.
   1. Local excision: simple surgery with small margin of normal tissue surrounding tumor.
   2. En bloc dissection or wide excision: removal of tumor, tissues, and any contiguous structures.
   3. Surgery on cancer in situ.
      a. Electrosurgery—application of electrical current to cancerous cells.
      b. Cryosurgery—deep freezing with liquid nitrogen.
      c. Chemosurgery—applied chemotherapeutic agents layer by layer with surgical excision.
      d. CO_2 laser—use of laser for local excision.
   4. Palliative surgery—promotes comfort and quality of life without cure.

Implementation

A. Preoperative care.
   1. Promote health status prior to surgery.
      a. Malnourished patient is at risk for infection, delayed wound healing, and dehiscence.
      b. Mental status may impact results of surgery.
   2. Provide emotional support prior to surgery.
      a. Encourage talking about fears and anxieties.
      b. Provide accurate information—clarify levels of knowledge.

c. Assess family needs and provide information and support.
B. Postoperative care.
  1. Provide traditional post-op care (see page 54).
  2. Provide for physical comfort.
     a. Enteral feeding.
     b. Pain relief.
     c. Positioning and activity.
     d. Wound care and healing.
  3. Provide emotional support.
     a. Allow for grief process—encourage expression of fears.
     b. Discuss change in body image—support increase in self-esteem.
     c. Provide accurate information.
  4. Support rehabilitation process.
     a. Encourage family involvement.
     b. Refer clients and families to appropriate resources.
     c. Complete discharge planning.

Radiation Therapy

A. Definition: use of high energy moving through space or medium to treat disease.
B. Indications.
  1. Used to treat solid tumors—ionizing radiation transfers energy to molecules present in cancer cell.
  2. Different tissues have different radiosensitivities—rapidly dividing tissues (testes, ovaries, lymphoid tissues, and bone marrow) are more sensitive.
C. Types of radiation.
  1. Electromagnetic—radiation in wave form.
     a. X-rays—linear accelerators.
     b. Electrons—delivered by machines.
     c. Gamma rays—delivered by machines that contain radioactive sources (Cobalt-60, Cesium-137) or radioactive substances (seeds, threads, or liquids).
  2. Particulate—radiation in the form of heavy particles.
     a. Beta particles—high speed electrons (Phosphorus-32; Strontium-90).

b. Neutrons and Pions—currently used experimentally.

External Radiation

A. Teletherapy—external source of radiation. (Machine is a distance from patient.)
B. Types.
  1. Natural radioactive source—gamma rays delivered via machine to lesion.
  2. Machine is the linear accelerator—high voltage electric current delivers electrons to patient.
C. Side effects: fatigue—major systemic effect; headache; nausea and vomiting; skin irritation or injury; scaling, erythema; dryness.

Implementation

A. Offer psychological support.
  1. Tell patient what to expect from treatment.
  2. Explain radiotherapy room.
  3. Tell patient of possible side effects and ways to minimize them.
B. Promote diet: high protein, high carbohydrate, fat free, and low residue.
  1. Foods to avoid: tough, fibrous meat; poultry; shrimp; all cheeses (except soft); coarse bread; raw vegetables; irritating spices.
  2. Foods allowed: soft-cooked eggs, ground meat, pureed vegetables, milk, cooked cereal.
  3. Increase fluids.
  4. Diet supplement to increase calorie and fluid intake.
  5. Remind patient not to eat several hours before treatment.
C. Administer medications.
  1. Compazine—nausea.
  2. Lomotil—diarrhea.
D. Provide skin care—radiodermatitis occurs three to six weeks after start of treatment.
  1. Avoid creams, lotions, perfume to irradiated areas.
  2. Wash with lukewarm water, pat dry (some physicians allow mild soap).

3. Avoid exposure to sunlight or artificial heat such as heating pad.
4. Cornstarch may be used for itchy skin.
E. Observe for "wet" reaction.
   1. Weeping of skin due to loss of upper layer.
   2. Promote rest after therapy.
   3. Cleanse area with warm water and pat dry bid.
   4. Apply antibiotic lotion or steroid cream if ordered.
   5. Expose site to air.

Internal Radiation

A. Implantation of radioactive substance within a patient.
B. Types.
   1. Unsealed sources: isotopes (^{131}I and ^{32}p.).
      a. Liquid and administered orally.
      b. Half-life generally short but varies with isotope.
      c. Precautions important during high risk period (usually first four days).
   2. Sealed sources: radium needles, radon seeds, and ^{137}Cs.
      a. Radioactive substance encased in metal capsule placed in body cavity.
      b. Delivers radiation directly to tumor.
      c. Even though implant is sealed, special precautions are instituted.
C. Side effects.
   1. Occur when normal cells are damaged.
   2. Acute side effects occur during or shortly after radiation therapy; chronic effects occur months or years following therapy.
   3. Common side effects from radiation therapy: alopecia (hair loss); mouth dryness; mucositis; esophagitis; nausea and vomiting; diarrhea; cystitis; erythema; and dry and wet desquamation.
   4. Factors influencing degree of side effects.
      a. Body site irradiated.
      b. Radiation dose—higher dose given, the more potential side effects.
      c. Extent of body area treated (larger area, more potential for side effects).
      d. Method of radiation therapy.

Implementation

A. Maintain bed rest when radiation source in place.
   1. Restrict movement to prevent dislodging radiation source.
   2. Do not turn or position patient except on back (when cesium needle in tongue or cervix).
B. Administer range-of-motion exercise qid.
C. Avoid direct contact around implant site; avoid washing areas, etc.
D. Take vital signs every four hours (report temperature over 100°F).
E. Observe for dehydration or paralytic ileus (if cervical implant).
F. Observe and report skin eruption, discharge, abnormal bleeding.
G. Provide clear liquid diet (low residue is sometimes ordered) and force fluids.
H. Insert Teflon Foley catheter as ordered (radiation decomposes rubber) to avoid necessity of bedpan.
I. Observe frequently for dislodging of radiation source (especially linen and dressings).
   1. When radiation source falls out, do not touch with hands. Pick up source with foot-long applicator.
   2. Put source in lead container and call head nurse–physician.
   3. If unable to locate source, call head nurse–physician immediately and bar visitors from room.
J. After source is removed.
   1. Administer Betadine douche as ordered if cervical implant.
   2. Give Fleets enema.
   3. Patient may be out of bed.
   4. Avoid direct sunlight to radiation areas.
   5. Administer cream to relieve dryness or itching.
K. Instruct that patient may resume sexual intercourse within seven to ten days.
L. Notify head nurse if nausea, vomiting, diarrhea, frequent urination or bowel movements, or temperature above 100°F is present.

Radiation Safety Measures

A. General guidelines for radiation safety measures.
  1. Wear radiation badges to monitor total amount of radiation exposure. Cumulative dose (measured in millirems) not to exceed 1250 every 3 months.
  2. Observe for displacement or dislodgement of radiation source every four to six hours.
  3. Check that sealed lead container is kept in patient's room in case of accidental dislodgment.
  4. Collect body waste until it can be determined radiation source is not dislodged.
  5. Radiation source removed at prearranged time—after removal, patient is no longer radioactive.
  6. Do not allow persons under 18 or pregnant women to visit or care for patients with radioactive implant.
  7. Never touch a dislodged sealed source—use long-handled tongs or contact radiation safety personnel.
  8. Mark patient's room and chart with radiation safety precautions.
B. Follow special principles of time, distance, and shielding.
  1. Minimize time.
    a. Radiation exposure proportional to amount of time spent with patient.
    b. Care planned to be delivered in shortest amount of time to meet goals—be efficient with time.
    c. Review procedures before beginning them.
  2. Maximize distance.
    a. Intensity of radiation related to distance from patient.
    b. Duration of safe exposure increases as distance is increased; work as far away from source as possible.
  3. Utilize shielding.
    a. Use lead shields or other equipment to reduce transmission of radiation.
    b. Store radioactive material in lead-shielded container when not in use.

C. Follow radiation precautions for isotope implant.
  1. All body secretions considered contaminated—use special techniques for disposal.
  2. If patient vomits within first four hours—everything vomitus touches is considered contaminated.
  3. Use disposable gown, dishes, etc.
  4. Limit contact with hospital personnel and visitors.

Chemotherapy

Characteristics

A. The medical management of cancer includes the use of chemotherapy. First used in the early 50s, there are now more than 80 effective drugs available.
  1. Chemotherapy is method of choice when there is suspected or confirmed spread of malignant cells.
  2. Method used when the risk of recurrence systemically is high.
  3. May be used as palliative measure to relieve pain or increase comfort.
B. Mechanism of action—chemotherapeutic agents eradicate cells, both normal and malignant, that are in the process of cell reproduction.

Drug Classification

A. Drugs classified by group into those that act on a certain phase of cell reproduction (cell cycle specific) or those that do not (cell cycle nonspecific).
B. Cell cycle specific agents: antimetabolites and mitotic inhibitors.
  1. Act on the cell during a particular phase of reproduction.
  2. Most effective in tumors where a large number of cells are dividing.

3. Divided doses produce greater cytotoxic effects (not all cells will be in the same phase at the same time).
4. Antimetabolites—Methotrexate, 6-mercaptopurine, 5-fluorouracil, Azacytidine, Cytarabine.
5. Mitotic inhibitors—plant alkaloids—vincristine, vindesine, vinblastine, teniposide.

C. Cell cycle nonspecific drugs: alkylating agents, antitumor antibiotics, and nitrosoureas.
1. Act on cells during any phase of reproduction—some drugs will attack cells in the resting phase (not actively dividing).
2. Agents are dose-dependent—the more drug given, the more cells destroyed.
3. These drugs are more toxic to normal tissue because they are less selective.
4. Alkylating agents—Cytoxan, Myleran, melphalan (L-PAM), Thiotepa, etc.
5. Antitumor antibiotics—Adriamycin, Cosmegen, Dactinomycin.
6. Nitrosoureas—streptozocin, methyl CCNU, BCNU.

D. Other miscellaneous agents (such as Procarbazine) are used in the chemotherapy group, but their exact mechanism of action is unknown.

E. Hormones (estrogens, androgens, progestins) are used in therapy to affect the hormonal environment.
1. Affect the growth of hormone-dependent tumors.
2. Antihormones (Tamoxifen) block tumor growth by depriving the tumor of the necessary hormones.

F. Combination chemotherapy.
1. Drugs used in combination for synergistic activity.
2. Many protocols represent three or four drugs. (Example: the protocol for Hodgkin's lymphoma is based on four drugs, called MOPP.)

Chemotherapeutic Administration

A. Chemotherapeutic agents are administered through a variety of routes.

1. Oral route—used frequently. Safety precautions must be observed.
2. Intramuscular and sub q used infrequently as drugs are not vesicants.
3. Intravenous is the most common route.
   a. Provides for better absorption.
   b. Potential complications: infection, phlebitis.
4. Central venous catheter infusion—used for continuous or intermittent infusions.
5. Venous Access Devices (VADs)—used for prolonged infusions.
6. Intraarterial route—delivers agents directly to tumor in high concentrations while decreasing drug's systemic toxic effect.
7. Intraperitoneal—used for ovarian and colon cancer. High concentration of agents delivered to peritoneal cavity via a catheter, then drained.

B. Factors for deciding dosage and timing of drugs.
1. Dosage calculated on body surface area and kilograms of body weight.
2. Time lapse between doses to allow recovery of normal cells.
3. Side effects of each drug and when they are likely to occur.
4. Liver and kidney function, as most antineoplastics are metabolized in one of these organs.

Chemotherapy Safety Guidelines

A. Antineoplastic drugs are potentially hazardous to personnel and may have teratogenic and/or carcinogenic effects.

B. Safety guidelines have been issued by the Occupational Safety and Health Administration (OSHA).
1. Obtain special training for drug administration.
2. Wear surgical latex gloves and a disposable, closed, long-sleeved gown.
3. Use Luer-Lok syringes.
4. Label all prepared drugs appropriately.
5. Double bag chemotherapy drugs once prepared, before transport.

6. Have equipment ready to clean up any accidental spill.
7. Dispose of all materials in marked containers labeled hazardous waste.
8. Dispose of all needles and syringes intact.

Side Effects of Chemotherapy

A. Side effects occur primarily due to the mechanism of action of potent drugs on normal cells.
B. Skin and mucosa, protective linings of the body, are damaged; mucositis (cells of the mucosa are affected)—may extend from oral cavity and stomatitis through GI tract.
C. Alopecia, or hair loss, caused by damage to rapidly dividing cells of the hair follicles.
   1. Hair loss begins 2–3 weeks after chemotherapy and continues through the cycles of chemotherapy; regrowth occurs following the course of therapy.
   2. Scalp hypothermia (ice cap) and scalp tourniquet reduces the amount of drug reaching the hair follicle and may prevent hair loss.
D. Nausea, vomiting and anorexia are common.
   1. Support changes in food preferences, additional or less seasoning, small and more frequent meals.
   2. Offer high calorie and protein supplements.
   3. Diarrhea is related to toxicity of the drugs on the mucosal lining; diet bland and low residue.
E. White blood cell and platelet disruption.
   1. White blood cell suppression—leukopenia (less than 5,000/mm^3 when normal white blood cell is 5,000–10,000/mm^3).
   2. Platelet suppression to below normal (less than 150,000/mm^3 when normal is 150,000–4000,000/mm^3.
      a. A number less than 50,000/mm^3 makes the patient susceptible to bleeding gums, nose, easy bruising, heavier menstrual flow, etc.
      b. Tell patient precautions: soft toothbrush, avoidance of douches and enemas, care with trimming nails.

Cancer Nursing

A. Key stress periods for patient with cancer are: time of diagnosis, period of hospitalization, and release from the hospital.
   1. Shock and fear are the major reactions.
   2. Severe depression is experienced by some patients.
   3. The emotional pain of the diagnosis initially outweighs the physical component of the cancer.
B. Adjustment to cancer depends on past life experiences.
C. Phases of psychological adaptation to terminal illness include: denial, anger, bargaining, depression, and acceptance.
D. The patient will experience a range of feelings and defense mechanisms.
   1. Denial may occur initially with the diagnosis; this is a protective mechanism necessary until the diagnosis can be confronted.
      a. Allow patient to be in denial until he or she is ready to face reality.
      b. Provide opportunities for the patient to confront her illness—be open to questions and clarification.
   2. Fear and anxiety may manifest in physical symptoms: insomnia, nausea, vomiting, diarrhea, headaches, etc.
   3. Anger and resentment, especially in the initial phases of the disease, may be a healthy way of expressing feelings.
   4. Depression may be considered normal for a period of time following surgery.
      a. Observe for the signs of depression.
      b. Because suicide is always a risk with depression, interventions should be aimed at safety for the patient.

Psychosocial Aspects of Caring for the Cancer Patient

A. Talk with the patient so that he or she will not feel they have to cope alone—provide emotional support to help allay fears and anxieties.

B. Always be honest with the patient—provides the foundation for a nurse-patient relationship.
1. Accurate information can be followed by an open discussion of disease, prognosis, the patient's feelings, etc.
2. Knowing the truth enables patient to begin to accept situation.

C. Assist patient to cope with pain.
1. Stay with patient, especially when the pain is severe.
2. Respect patient's response to pain and believe what patient tells you.

D. Provide general comfort measures.
1. Position for proper alignment.
2. Use touch and massage for painful areas.
3. Exercise extremities gently to maintain range of motion.
4. Maintain patency of tubes and keep free of infection using meticulous handwashing and aseptic techniques.

5. Preserve the patient's energy by prioritizing activities.
6. Assist the patient to obtain adequate rest at night and during the day to reduce fatigue.

E. DO NOT undermedicate for cancer pain.
1. Undertreatment with analgesics has been identified as a major problem (70 to 80 percent) for cancer patients—and nursing has a crucial responsibility to correct this problem.
2. Two forms of undertreatment: physicians underprescribe and nurses routinely administer less than half the amount patients could receive.

F. Support family of patient as they move through the grieving process.

G. Introduce the hospice concept—provides care for the terminally ill patient and family.

9

EMERGENCY NURSING

EMERGENCY AND FIRST AID NURSING

Disasters

Definition: A catastrophe which may be either natural or man-made in origin.

A. General guidelines: keep calm, take time to think, then take appropriate action.

B. First steps to take in a disaster—gather the following items:
1. Water.
2. Canned or sealed packaged foods that do not require refrigeration or cooking.
3. Medicines needed by family members.
4. First aid kit.
5. Blankets or sleeping bags.
6. Flashlights.
7. Battery-powered radio.
8. Covered containers for toilet and/or garbage.

C. Precautions after a disaster.
1. Use caution in entering a building or working indoors.
2. Check for gas leaks.
3. Stay away from fallen or damaged electrical wires.

Water, Food, and Sanitation Principles

A. Care and use of water.
1. Allocate one quart of water per day per person.
2. Strain rusty water through a paper towel or several thicknesses of clean cloth.
3. Methods of purifying water.
a. Boil three to five minutes.
b. Add four purifying tablets per gallon of water.
c. Add eight drops chlorine to one gallon of water, and let stand for 30 minutes.
d. Add ten drops bleach to one gallon of water, and let stand for 30 minutes.
e. Use 12 drops tincture of iodine per one gallon of water.

B. Care and use of food.
1. One-half normal intake is adequate except for growing children and pregnant women.
2. Store in covered containers.

C. Sanitation.
1. Emergency toilet facility can be made by using a watertight container with snug-fitting cover.
2. After each use, pour or sprinkle household disinfectant to decrease odor and germs.

D. Garbage—dispose of garbage by wrapping in newspaper and placing in air-tight container.

E. Insect control.
1. Maintain cleanliness.
2. Spray with insect repellent if available.

First Aid Care

Definition: Immediate care given to a person who has been injured or suddenly taken ill, when medical assistance is not available.

A. First aid training can mean the difference between life and death, temporary and permanent disability, and rapid recovery and long hospitalization.

B. General directions for giving first aid.
1. Decisions and actions vary according to:
a. Circumstances.
b. Number of persons involved.
c. Immediate environment.
d. Availability of medical assistance.
e. Availability of equipment and supplies.
2. Improvise—make do with what is available.
3. Set priorities.
a. Sorting of casualties.
(1) Sorting is done by most responsible person.
(2) Rapid initial evaluation of the victims general condition to determine most seriously injured person.
b. Priorities of treatment.
(1) First priority is victim needing immediate attention in order to survive.

(2) Second priority is victim needing immediate surgery.

(3) Third priority is victim who requires surgery but can tolerate a delay.

4. Cardinal rules.
    a. Establish airway.
    b. Stop bleeding.
    c. Treat for shock.
    d. Preserve function of injured area.
    e. Give comfort.
    f. Preserve cosmetic appearance.
5. When calling for assistance, give following information.
    a. Identify problem.
    b. Relate what is currently being done.
    c. Give your name and name of victim.
    d. Give location of accident.
    e. Relate number of persons involved.
    f. Give phone number you are calling from.
6. Once first aid is begun, remain with victim until qualified persons arrive or victim is able to care for self.
7. Do not make a diagnosis.

C. Dressings—applied over wounds.
    1. Function.
        a. Assist in controlling bleeding.
        b. Absorb blood and wound secretions.
        c. Prevent additional contamination.
        d. Ease pain.
    2. Sterilizing dressings.
        a. Place in moderate oven (350°) for three hours.
        b. Press clean cloth with iron.

D. Bandage—used to hold dressing or splint in place.
    1. Material used.
        a. Usually gauze, cloth, or elastic.
        b. Emergency—handkerchief, belt, tie.
    2. General principles for applying bandages.
        a. Snug but not so tight as to interfere with circulation.
        b. Leave fingertips and toes exposed when splint or bandage applied.
        c. Check for swelling, color changes, and coldness in extremities.

COMMON EMERGENCIES

Wounds

Definition: Break in the continuity of the tissue of the body, either internal or external.

A. Classification.
    1. Open-break in the skin or mucous membrane.
    2. Closed-injury to underlying tissues without a break in the skin or mucous membrane.

B. Types of open wounds.
    1. Incised.
    2. Contused.
    3. Lacerated.
    4. Punctured.

C. First aid for open wounds. ❖ **PROCEDURE** ❖
    1. Stop bleeding immediately.
    2. Protect wound from contamination and infection.
    3. Provide shock care.
    4. Obtain medical attention.

D. Techniques to stop severe bleeding. ❖ **PROCEDURE** ❖
    1. Direct pressure.
    2. Elevation.
    3. Pressure on supplying artery.
    4. Tourniquet.

E. Characteristics of closed wounds.
    1. No break in skin.
    2. Blood loss may be from outer openings of body cavities.
    3. Usually caused by an external force.
    4. Victim demonstrates signs of internal bleeding.

F. First aid for closed wounds.
    1. Check for fractures and other internal injuries.
    2. Treat for shock.
    3. Do not give fluids by mouth if internal injuries are suspected.
    4. Apply ice to small areas of closed wounds.

G. Measures to prevent contamination or infection of wounds.

1. Do not remove cloth pad initially placed on wound.
2. Do not cleanse deep wounds which require medical attention.
3. Use sterile dressing or cleanest dressing available.
4. Do not remove deeply embedded objects.

Shock States

Definition: An abnormal physiological state in which there is insufficient circulating blood volume for the size of the vascular bed, thereby resulting in circulatory failure and tissue anoxia.

Classifications of Shock States

A. Hypovolemic.
   1. Definition: decreased intravascular fluid volume.
   2. Etiology.
      a. Blood loss (hematogenic)—from trauma, surgery, etc.
      b. Plasma and/or fluid loss.
         (1) Plasma loss—burns.
         (2) Fluid loss—diarrhea, vomiting, diabetes.
B. Neurogenic.
   1. Definition: massive vasodilation and pooling of blood due to failure of sympathetic nerve impulses to produce vasoconstriction.
   2. Etiology.
      a. Drug overdose, especially narcotics.
      b. Severe pain.
      c. Damage to medulla.
      d. Deep anesthesia.
C. Vasogenic.
   1. Definition: massive vasodilation and pooling of blood due to failure of peripheral vessels to react to neural stimuli.
   2. Etiology.
      a. Antigen—antibody reaction causes anaphylactic shock.
         (1) Insect stings.

      (2) Allergies to drugs, particularly antibiotics.
      (3) Blood transfusions.
      (4) Vaccines.
   b. Bacterial invasion causes gram negative sepsis (septic shock).
      (1) Following urinary tract instrumentation.
      (2) Overwhelming bacterial invasion of an "at risk" patient.
D. Cardiogenic.
   1. Definition: left ventricular pump failure which results in circulatory inadequacy.
   2. Etiology.
      a. Myocardial infarction.
      b. Congestive heart failure.
      c. Cardiac arrest.

Early Shock

A. Early stages, regardless of cause.
   1. Decreased tissue perfusion.
   2. Cellular hypoxia.
   3. Increased sympathetic nervous system activity.
B. Oliguria—usually the first sign of shock.
   1. Decreased blood volume through kidneys.
   2. Decreased urine output; hyperkalemia can be a problem.
C. Hypotension.
   1. Due to compensatory peripheral vasoconstriction (not evident initially, but it does appear in late shock).
   2. Narrowing pulse pressure—due to systolic pressure falling and diastolic pressure being maintained.
   3. Traditional criteria—systolic blood pressure below 70 mmHg.
D. Tachycardia—due to heart's responding to increased sympathetic activity.
E. Tachypnea.
   1. Medulla is stimulated by buildup in lactic acid through anaerobic metabolism.
   2. As blood pH is lowered, the respiratory rate increases in an effort to blow off excess carbon dioxide and return body to acid-base balance.

F. Cool, dry or moist skin is present.
   1. Caused by peripheral vasoconstriction.
   2. Blood is supplied to vital organs rather than to skin.
G. Sensorium changes—due to brain cell hypoxia.
   1. Restlessness.
   2. Apprehension and anxiety.
   3. Lethargy.
   4. Confusion.
   5. Semiconsciousness to coma.
H. Excess thirst is present due to loss of fluids or blood volume as well as peripheral vasoconstriction, which decreases salivary secretions.
I. Fatigue and muscle weakness—result of shift from aerobic to anaerobic metabolism leading to lactic acid buildup.

Severe Shock

A. Blood pressure: below 70 mmHg and narrowing of pulse pressure (body loses ability to compensate and blood pressure drops rapidly).
B. Shallow, irregular respirations.
C. Tachycardia.
D. Level of unconsciousness: progresses to coma as blood supply to brain cell decreases.
E. Dilated, fixed pupils due to decreased oxygen to brain.
F. Anuria as blood supply to kidneys decreases sharply.
G. Cyanotic skin, mucous membranes, and nailbeds.

Hypovolemic Shock

Degrees of Shock

A. Slight: approximately 20 percent of blood volume is lost.
B. Moderate: approximately 35 percent of blood volume is lost.
C. Severe: approximately 45 percent of blood volume is lost.

Treatment and Implementation

A. Monitor patency of IV for drug (vasodilator), plasma expanders, IV fluid, or blood replacement.
B. Start IV fluid with D_5W. When adequate kidney function is assessed, Ringer's lactate (more isotonic) is used.
C. Place in supine position with feet and/or head slightly elevated (Trendelenburg's position compromises venous return as well as respirations).
D. Provide oxygen via nasal catheter, mask, or cannula.
E. Record vital signs every 15 minutes. Changes take place slowly except when massive hemorrhage occurs.
   1. Blood pressure.
      a. Decreased BP is usually late sign of shock.
      b. Orthostatic hypotension develops before systemic hypotension.
      c. Systolic BP below 80 mmHg indicates inadequate coronary artery blood flow.
      d. Progressive drop in BP with a thready, increasing pulse indicates fluid loss.
      e. Decreased BP with strong, irregular pulse indicates heart failure.
   2. Respirations.
      a. Become rapid and shallow early in shock (compensation for tissue anoxia).
      b. Slow breathing (below four per minute) appears late in shock after compensatory failure.
      c. Emergency respiratory equipment (ventilator, trach tubes, etc.) should be available.
   3. Temperature.
      a. Below normal with hemorrhagic shock.
      b. Gradually increasing temperature indicates sepsis.
   4. Central venous pressure.
F. Insert Foley catheter for hourly urine volumes.
   1. Record intake and output.
   2. Notify physician if total urine output is below 30 ml/hour.
G. Monitor skin changes.

1. Change in skin temperature and color reflect changes in tissue oxygenation and perfusion.
   a. Cold, clammy skin indicates peripheral vascular constriction.
   b. Flushing and sweating reflects over-heating, which indicates increased metabolic rate and the need for oxygen.
   c. Pallor and cyanosis indicate tissue hypoxia.
2. Observe for restlessness—indication of hypoxia.

H. Place enough light covering over patient to prevent chilling, but not enough to cause vasodilatation.

I. Treat the cause of the shock (stop bleeding, prepare for surgery, etc.)

Cardiogenic Shock

Assessment

A. Cardia arrhythmias leading to cardiac arrest.
B. Heart failure symptoms.
   1. Orthopnea.
   2. Cyanosis.
   3. Dyspnea.
   4. Pitting edema.
   5. Distended neck veins.
   6. Pulmonary congestion.
C. Acidosis.
D. Hypokalemia.

Treatment and Implementation

A. Administer digitalis preparation in addition to diuretics.
B. Watch for hypokalemia and arrhythmias.
C. Administer vasodilators or vasopressors, as ordered.
D. Check arterial blood gases frequently.
E. Monitor intra-aortic balloon.
F. Follow interventions for hypovolemic shock for additional nursing care.

Vasogenic Shock

Septic Shock (Toxic Shock)

A. Mortality—60 to 82 percent.
B. Caused by bacterial toxins (gm – or +); leads to vasodilatation.
C. Conditions leading to septic shock.
   1. Peritonitis.
   2. Urinary tract manipulations.
   3. Gas gangrene.

Assessment

A. Mild infection.
   1. Fever; warm, pink face.
   2. Perspiration.
   3. Weakness, generalized aching.
B. Severe infection.
   1. High temperature (over 104°) and sudden violent chills.
   2. Hemorrhage into tissue.
   3. Muscular pain.
   4. Rapid, deep respirations.
   5. Confusion and disorientation is present.
   6. Warm, dry skin.

Implementation

A. Administer broad spectrum antibiotics and then organism specific antibiotics.
B. Provide systemic supportive nursing management.

Anaphylactic Shock

A. Caused by hypersensitivity to allergen (allergic reaction to medication, bee sting, etc.).
B. Antigen—antibody reaction.
C. Increased cell membrane permeability—histamine is released, causing marked vasodilatation.
D. Bronchiolar constriction.
E. Pooling of blood, causing decreased venous return.
F. Decreased cardiac output and hypoxia.

Assessment

A. Local edema.

B. Urticaria (occasional).

C. Flushed face.

D. Apprehension is present.

E. Dyspnea, respiratory difficulty, cyanosis, wheezing.

F. Vertigo, decreased blood pressure, increased pulse.

Treatment and Implementation

A. Identify causative agent.

B. Position for optimal cerebral perfusion (flat or 30-degree elevation if dyspneic).

C. Maintain patent airway.

D. Administer epinephrine, sub q.
   1. Dilates bronchioles, constricts arterioles.
   2. Side effects: tachycardia, CNS stimulation.
   3. Rapid acting.

E. Administer oxygen.

F. Administer antihistamine (Benadryl).
   1. Relieves itching, wheals, congestion of nasal mucosa.
   2. Side effect: dries mucous membranes.

G. Maintain IV of D_5W—as much as 2000 ml in one hour.

H. Administer corticosteroids.
   1. Reduce formation of cellular proteins and decrease edema.
   2. Side effects: same as any steroids.

I. Administer aminophylline—bronchodilator; controls bronchospasms.

Snake Bite

Assessment

A. Assess extent of envenomation: Rattlesnakes, copperheads, cottonmouths (pit vipers) are responsible for 98 percent of venomous bites.

B. Signs:
   1. Blood oozing from wound.
   2. One or two distinct puncture wounds.
   3. Edema and discoloration.
   4. Numbness around bite within 5 to 15 minutes.
   5. Painful and enlarged lymph nodes.

C. Reactions to poisonous snakes occur within 30 to 60 minutes.

D. Advanced signs indicating shock.
   1. Nausea, vomiting.
   2. Ecchymosis, blebs, blisters.
   3. Bleeding.
   4. Weakness, vertigo, clammy skin.

Treatment and Implementation

A. Emergency treatment: within 30 to 60 minutes of medical help.
   1. Immobilize area with support or sling.
   2. Apply tourniquet.
   3. Do not allow patient to physically exert self as this hastens spread of venom.
   4. Seek medical help immediately.

B. Emergency treatment: when medical help is not available within 30 to 60 minutes.
   ❖ **PROCEDURE** ❖
   1. Apply nonocclusive tourniquet or constriction band 5 to 13 cm above wound.
      a. Adjust to allow for venous and lymphatic flow restriction but allow for arterial flow.
      b. Loosen, but do not remove, for 1½ minutes every 15 minutes.
   2. Wash around bite with alcohol, hydrogen peroxide, or soap and water.
   3. Sterilize knife with match flame, alcohol, or soap and water, make longitudinal incision (not cross marks) 0.3 to 0.6 cm long and no more than 0.3 cm deep through each fang mark.
   4. Apply suction over incision site.
   5. Procedure must be done within 10 minutes of bite. After 30 to 60 minutes, little venom will be extractable.

C. In-hospital treatment.
   1. Within 30 to 60 minutes, make incisions and use suction intermittently for at least one hour.
   2. Test for sensitivity to horse serum.

3. Judge severity of envenomation before giving antivenin.
    a. Minimal pit viper bite: 1 to 5 ampules of antivenin (Crotalidae) IM.
    b. Moderate bite: 5 to 9 ampules IV drip.
    c. Severe bite: 9 ampules IV drip immediately and up to 20 ampules over next 4 to 24 hours, until edema ceases and symptoms improve.
4. Administer tetanus toxoid.
5. Administer analgesics for pain.
    a. ASA for mild pain.
    b. Codeine or Demerol for severe pain.
6. Administer antibiotics.
    a. Initial dose: ampicillin, erythromycin, or tetracycline 500 mg.
    b. Maintain 250 mg every 4 hours for 24 hours.

Bee Sting

Assessment

A. Generalized itching.
B. Erythema and hives.
C. Feeling of heat throughout body.
D. Weakness, vertigo.
E. Nausea, vomiting, abdominal cramps.
F. Tightness in chest, difficulty swallowing or breathing.

Treatment and Implementation
❖ PROCEDURE ❖

A. Remove stinger with tweezers or by scraping motion with fingernail. Do not squeeze venom sac.
B. Immediately administer epinephrine 1:1000 solution sub q as ordered.
    1. Adult: 0.25 to 0.3 ml at sting site and same amount in unaffected arm.
    2. Child: 0.01 ml/kg (maximum 0.25 ml at each site).

C. Repeat injections as ordered one to three times at 20 minute intervals until blood pressure and pulse rise toward normal.
    1. Adult: 0.3 to 0.4 ml.
    2. Child: less than 20 kg, 0.10 to 0.15 ml; over 20 kg, 0.15, to 0.3 ml.
D. Apply tourniquet above sting on an extremity. Loosen every three to five minutes to allow venom to slowly enter circulation.
E. Cleanse sting area and apply ice to relieve pain and edema.
F. Administer pressor agents as ordered if blood pressure does not stabilize following 2 to 3 sub q injections of epinephrine.
    1. Aramine or Levophed drugs of choice.
    2. Administer IV drip at 30 to 40 drops per minute.
G. Monitor IV solution of D_5W with 250 mg aminophylline and 30 to 40 mg Solu-Cortef to support circulation and prevent shock.
H. Observe for signs of laryngospasm or bronchospasm. Be prepared to assist with a tracheostomy.
I. Keep patient warm and positioned supine with head and feet slightly elevated.
J. Administer a rapid-acting antihistamine: Benadryl 50 mg IM as ordered.

Choking

Definition: Temporary or permanent asphyxia due to obstruction of the airway.

A. Signs and symptoms.
    1. Violent choking.
    2. Alarming attempts at inhalation.
    3. Cyanosis of face, neck, and hands.
    4. Cessation of breathing.
    5. Inability to speak.
    6. Unconsciousness.
B. First aid measures.
    1. Remove object if possible.
    2. Allow victim to assume position of comfort.
    3. Encourage coughing.
    4. Heimlich maneuver (see page 279).

5. Artificial respirations if breathing ceases.
6. Obtain medical assistance.

Poisoning

Definition: Introduction into the body or onto the skin surface of any solid, liquid or gas that tends to impair health or to cause death.

A. First aid treatment.
   1. Call doctor or poison control center. Give the following information.
      a. Age of victim.
      b. Name and amount of poison taken.
      c. Whether or not victim vomited.
   2. If victim is conscious, give antidote, if known.
   3. Induce vomiting (syrup of ipecac) if material ingested is not strong acid or petroleum product (activated charcoal).
   4. If inhaled gases, remove victim to fresh air.
   5. If contact poison, wash exposed areas.
B. Follow-up treatment as prescribed.

Frostbite and Cold Exposure

A. Signs and symptoms.
   1. White or grayish-yellow skin.
   2. Pain.
   3. Blisters.
   4. Area cold and numb.
   5. Mental confusion.
B. First aid treatment.
   1. Cover area.
   2. Rewarm area quickly.
   3. Do not rub.
   4. Elevate affected area.

Heat Exhaustion

Definition: Response to heat characterized by fatigue and weakness; occurs when intake of water cannot compensate for loss of fluids through sweating.

A. Signs and symptoms.

   1. Pale, clammy skin.
   2. Profuse perspiration.
   3. Headache.
   4. Nausea.
   5. Dizziness.
   6. Fainting.
B. First aid treatment.
   1. Offer victim sips of salt water—½ glass every 15 minutes for one hour.
   2. Have victim lie down and elevate feet.
   3. Place in cool environment.
   4. Apply cool, wet cloths.

Heat Stroke

Definition: Response to heat characterized by extremely high body temperature due to disturbance in sweating mechanism.

A. Signs and symptoms.
   1. High body temperature—104° or higher.
   2. Hot, red, dry skin.
   3. Rapid, strong pulse.
B. First aid treatment—cool body quickly.

Burns

Definition: Injury of the skin, subcutaneous tissue muscle, and/or bones caused by heat, chemical agent, or radiation.

A. Classification of burns.
   1. First degree—red skin, mild swelling and pain, rapid healing.
   2. Second degree—red or mottled skin, blisters, considerable swelling, wet appearance due to loss of plasma, and severe pain.
   3. Third degree—deep tissue destruction, white or charred appearance, complete loss of all layers of skin. Skin graft needed for healing.
B. First aid treatment for first degree burn.
   ❖ **PROCEDURE** ❖
   1. Apply cold water or submerge in cold water.
   2. Prevent contamination.

3. Avoid greasy substances.

C. First aid treatment for second degree burn.
1. Immerse burn, if fairly small area, in cold water for one to two hours.
2. Apply clean cloths.
3. Blot area dry.
4. Do not break blisters.
5. Do not apply antiseptic preparations or home remedies.
6. Elevate affected extremities.
7. Seek medical attention.

D. First aid treatment for third degree burns.
1. Do not attempt to remove clothing from burned area.
2. Cover burn with sterile dressing.
3. Elevate involved extremities.
4. Do not immerse burn in water or apply ice water to it.
5. If medical help is not quickly available, and victim is conscious and not vomiting, give victim, at 15 minute intervals, a solution of ½ teaspoon of salt and ½ teaspoon of soda in a quart of water.

Fracture

Definition: A break or crack in a bone.

A. Types of fractures.
1. Open—bone ends protrude through skin.
2. Closed—bone cracked or broken but does not protrude through skin.

B. Signs and symptoms.
1. Victim heard or felt bone snap.
2. Abnormal or false motion in body area.
3. Differences in shape and length of corresponding bones.
4. Obvious deformities.
5. Swelling.
6. Discoloration.
7. Pain or tenderness to touch.

C. First aid measures.
1. Prevent motion of injured parts and adjacent joints.
2. Elevate involved extremities.
3. Apply splints.

D. Splinting—device used to immobilize extremity or trunk when a fracture is suspected.
❖ **PROCEDURE** ❖
1. Purpose.
a. Immobilize part.
b. Decrease pain.
c. Reduce chance of shock.
d. Protect against further injury during transportation.
2. Principles.
a. Ensure splint is long enough to extend past joint on either side of suspected fracture.
b. Place pad between splint and skin.
c. Immobilize joints above and below location of suspected fracture.
d. Apply splint to extremity; do circulation checks to fingers/toes.

Sprain

Definition: Injury to a joint ligament or a muscle tendon in region of a joint.

A. Signs and symptoms.
1. Swelling.
2. Tenderness.
3. Pain on motion.
4. Discoloration.

B. First aid measures.
1. Do not allow walking if ankle or knee sprained.
2. Elevate limb for 24 hours.
3. Apply ice first 24 hours.
4. If swelling and pain persist, seek medical attention.

Strain

Definition: Injury to a muscle as a result of over-stretching.

A. Signs and symptoms.
1. Pain on motion.
2. Discoloration.

B. First aid measures.
1. Bed rest.

2. Heat.
3. Bed board (with back sprain).

Dislocation

Definition: Injury to capsule and ligaments of a joint that results in displacement of a bone end at a joint.

A. Signs and symptoms.
1. Swelling.
2. Obvious deformity.
3. Pain upon motion.
4. Tenderness to touch.
5. Discoloration.
B. First aid measures.
1. Splint and immobilize affected joint in position as found.
2. Do not reduce dislocation or correct deformity near a joint.
3. Apply sling if appropriate.
4. Elevate affected part if possible.

EMERGENCY TREATMENTS

Cardiopulmonary Resuscitation (CPR)

Suspect Unconsciousness

A. Call for help.
B. Quickly approach victim.
C. Check responsiveness.
1. Shake shoulders.
2. Shout "Are you OK?"
D. Position properly.
1. Victim: flat on firm surface.
2. Rescuer: next to victim at approximately the same level.

Respiratory Management

A. Airway obstruction.

1. Food or other foreign body aspirant (if known cause of unconsciousness).
   ❖ **PROCEDURE** ❖
   a. Tilt head—hyperextend neck and chin forward.
   b. One attempt to ventilate will not be successful if obstructed.
   c. If not successful, reposition head and reattempt to ventilate.
   d. If not successful, presence of foreign body is assumed.
   e. Turn patient to one side and finger-probe for obstruction only if patient is *not* breathing.
   f. If this method proves unsuccessful, institute Heimlich maneuver.
2. Heimlich maneuver—abdominal thrust.
   ❖ **PROCEDURE** ❖
   a. Place patient in sitting or standing position. Stand behind and place arms around waist of patient.
   b. Make a fist and place it halfway between xiphoid and umbilicus.
   c. Place other hand on top of fist and perform a quick upward thrust.
   d. Repeat this maneuver three more times before returning to first method of removing a foreign body.
   e. Repeat entire procedure until open airway is obtained or advanced life support service is available.
3. Oral airway obstructants that are blood, emesis, mucus or water.
   a. Turn head to side.
   b. Suction (if available).
   c. Perform finger swoops.
B. Open airway.
1. Adult.
   a. Apply head-tilt method.
   b. Apply jaw-thrust or chin-lift method (if neck injury even remotely possible).
2. Infant or toddler.
   a. Tilt head back without hyperextension.
   b. Use normal, horizontal alignment, flat surface.
C. Evaluate respiratory function.
1. Maintain open airway.
2. Observe for respiratory activity.

a. Put ear down near mouth.

b. Look for chest movement.

c. Feel for air flow with cheek.

d. Listen for exhalation.

D. Administer ventilations. ❖ **PROCEDURE** ❖

1. Maintain open airway.

2. Form tight seal.

3. Adult management.

   a. Replace victim's dentures (if any).

   b. Pinch off nostrils.

   c. Fit mouth-to-mouth seal.

4. Infant or toddler management.

   a. Encircle nose and mouth.

   b. Maintain tight seal.

   c. Take fresh breath; do not allow complete deflation of lungs (stairstep volume).

   d. Maintain position.

   e. Assess volume: adult—800 ml minimum; infant—cheek full puffs.

5. Administer two full long breaths (1-1½ per second).

   a. Give breaths slowly to allow time for chest to expand.

   b. Between breaths, release seal for exhalation.

Circulatory Management ❖ PROCEDURE ❖

A. Take major pulse.

1. Adult—carotid preferably (check for 5-10 seconds) and femoral as alternate.

2. Palpate one side, with two fingers, for five seconds.

B. If pulse absent begin CPR.

1. For adults.

   a. Place hand on midline, lower half of sternum, two finger-widths above xiphoid.

   b. Place heel of one hand on sternum, other hand superimposed.

   c. Interlace fingers or extend off rib cage.

   d. Rate 80 to 100 per minute, depth 1½ to 2 inches.

   e. Count compressions: one-and, two-and, three-and, etc.

   f. Release pressure between compressions for cardiac refilling.

g. Do not take hands off chest between compressions.

2. For children.

   a. Place hand on midline sternum, midway between xiphoid process and cricothyroid notch.

   b. Use heel of one hand only.

   c. Rate 80 per minute, depth 1–1½ inches.

3. For infants.

   a. Place fingers on midline sternum, midway between xiphoid process and cricothyroid notch.

   b. Use two fingers only.

   c. Rate 100 per minute, depth ½ to 1 inch.

   d. Count compressions: one, two, three, four.

C. CPR protocol.

1. Shake and shout.

2. Open airway.

3. Look, listen, and feel for breathing.

4. Call code.

5. Ventilate patient with two slow breaths.

6. Check carotid pulse for 5 to 10 seconds.

7. Initiate CPR at 15 cardiac compressions to two ventilations at rate of 80–100 compressions per minute.

8. Check for carotid pulse after one minute. If absent, continue CPR.

Interpolation (Compressions: Ventilations)

A. Lone rescuer: (15:2 for adults; 5:1 for infants).

B. Two rescuers: (5:1 adults).

C. Changing roles. ❖ **PROCEDURE** ❖

1. Compressor sets pace (one, one thousand, two, one thousand, three, one thousand, four, one thousand, breath).

2. Compressor observes for need and institutes change.

3. Compressor states, "Change, one-thousand; two, one-thousand."

4. Rescuer giving breaths gets into position to give compressions.

5. Rescuer giving compressions moves to victim's head after fifth compression, counts pulse for five seconds.

6. If no pulse, rescuer checking pulse states, "No pulse, start CPR," gives a breath, and CPR is begun again.

CPR Evaluation

A. In process. ❖ **PROCEDURE** ❖
   1. Check major pulse after one minute of CPR.
      a. Equal to 4 sets of 15:2 by one rescuer.
      b. Equal to 12 sets of 5:1 by two rescuers.
   2. Check major pulse every four to five minutes thereafter.
   3. Check pupil every four to five minutes; optional if third trained person present (not always a conclusive indicator).
   4. Observe for abdominal distention (all age groups).
      a. If evident, reposition airway and reduce force of ventilation.
      b. Maintain a volume sufficient to elevate ribs.
   5. Ventilator must check carotid pulse frequently between breaths to evaluate perfusion.
   6. Ventilator must observe each breath for effectiveness.
   7. If respiratory arrest only, check major pulse after each minute (12 breaths) to ensure continuation of cardiac function.

B. After termination.
   1. Diagnosis made (no pulse, no respirations) and intervention instituted within one minute after unconsciousness.
   2. Assistance summoned and entry into Emergency Medical System done promptly and efficiently.
   3. Proper CPR performed until acceptable termination.
   5. No delay in CPR longer than five seconds for extraordinary circumstances (intubation, transportation down stairs).
   6. Victim outcome.
      a. Condition.
      b. Potential for cardiac rehabilitation.
      c. Secondary complications (fractured ribs, ruptured spleen, lacerated liver, etc.).

Termination of CPR

A. Successful resuscitation.
   1. Spontaneous return of adequate life support.
   2. Assisted life support.
B. Transfer to emergency vehicle (other trained rescuers assume care).
C. Pronounced dead by physician.
D. Exhaustion of rescuer(s).

10

GERIATRIC NURSING

GENERAL CONCEPTS

General Principles

Terminology

A. Geriatrics—concerned with the diseases and care of patients with diseases of old age.
B. Gerontology—study of normal aging process.
C. Aging—natural continuous process.
 1. Begins at birth.
 2. Is common to all living organisms.
D. Old age.
 1. Over 65 years of age.
 2. After retirement.
E. Frail elderly—75 years or over.
F. Ageism—negative attitude toward elderly.

Profiles

A. Those over 65 in 1980.
 1. Make up about 10% of the population.
 2. Most live in urban or rural settings.
 3. Yearly income of 15–25% is at or below the poverty level.
 4. About 50% are high school graduates.
 5. About 50% have convenient access to senior service centers but a low number use these centers.
 6. 2–10% are alcohol abusers.
B. Cost of health care for the aged.
 1. Only 5% are institutionalized.
 2. 25% of all prescription drugs are for the elderly.
 3. Diseases may be multiple and chronic (over 40% have more than one illness concurrently).
 4. Disability results more readily when an aging person becomes ill.
 5. Response to treatment is diminished.
 6. Resistance is lower due to the aging process so person is more susceptible to disease.
 7. The aged have less resistance to stressors: mental, environmental, and physical.

8. Poor health care is prevalent.
 a. Less than ⅓ have annual checkups.
 b. Many see health care as a service to be used only during life crisis.
 c. Many see more than one doctor, so care is fragmented.
C. Increased life expectancy.
 1. Advanced health care.
 2. Decreased infant/child mortality.
 3. Improved nutrition and sanitation.
 4. Increased infectious disease control.
D. Causes of death.
 1. Heart disease is major cause.
 2. Cancer is second.
 3. Stroke/CVA is third.
E. Major fears of the aged.
 1. Physical and economic dependency.
 2. Chronic illness.
 a. Arthritis 44%.
 b. Hypertension 39%.
 c. Hearing deficit 28%.
 d. Heart disease 27%.
 3. Loneliness.
 4. Boredom resulting from not being needed.

Aging Process

Theories of Aging

A. Individualized process.
 1. Each person ages at a different rate.
 2. Each person ages in a different manner.
 3. No single factor has been found to cause or prevent aging.
B. Biological theories.
 1. Genetic programming and/or mutations.
 2. "Wear and tear"—overexertion and stress cause body cells to wear out.
 3. Cellular changes caused by free radical oxidation.
 4. Increased amounts of collagen in tissue.
 5. Exposure to radiation, pathogens, nutritional deficiencies.
 6. Autoimmune reactions.
C. Psychosocial theories.
 1. Activity.

a. Aging will increase in direct proportion to decrease in activity.
b. Optimum pattern is to continue in lifestyle of middle age.
2. Personality-continuity—basic personality or behavior patterns are unchanged by aging.
3. Disengagement—society and individual withdraw from each other.

Factors That Influence Aging

A. Heredity.
B. Nutrition.
C. Health status.
D. Life experiences.
E. Environment.
F. Stress.

Physiological Changes

A. Cells.
1. Fewer in number.
2. Larger in size.
3. Decreased total body fluid due to decreased intracellular fluid.
B. Nervous system.
1. Decreased speed of nerve conduction.
2. Delay in response and reaction time, especially with stress.
3. Diminution of sensory faculties.
a. Decreased vision.
b. Loss of hearing.
c. Diminished sense of smell and taste.
d. Greater sensitivity to temperature changes with low tolerance to cold.
C. The ear.
1. Presbycusis.
a. Progressive hearing loss in inner ear.
b. High frequency tones are lost first.
c. Sounds are distorted; difficulty understanding words when other noises in background.
d. 50% of those over age 65.
2. Tympanic membrane atrophic, sclerotic.
3. Cerumen accumulates; may impact due to increased amount of keratin.

D. The eye.
1. Pupil sphincter sclerosis with loss of light responsiveness.
2. Cornea more spherical.
3. Lens more opaque.
4. Increased light perception threshold.
a. Adapt to darkness more slowly.
b. Difficult to see in dim light.
5. Loss of accommodation.
6. Decreased visual field; less peripheral vision.
7. Decreased color discrimination on blue/green end of scale.
E. Cardiovascular system.
1. Heart valves thicken and become rigid.
2. Cardiac output decreases 1% per year after age 20 due to decreased heart rate and stroke volume.
3. Vessels lose elasticity.
a. Less effective peripheral oxygenation.
b. Position change from lying to sitting or sitting to standing can cause blood pressure to drop up to 65 mmHg.
4. Blood pressure increases due to increased peripheral vessel resistance.
a. Systolic may normally be 170.
b. Diastolic may normally be 95.
F. Respiratory system.
1. Respiratory muscles lose strength and become rigid.
2. Ciliary activity decreases.
3. Lungs lose elasticity.
a. Residual capacity increases.
b. Larger on inspiration.
c. Maximum breathing capacity decreases; depth of respirations decreases.
4. Alveoli increase in size, reduce in number.
5. Arterial blood oxygen pO_2 decreases to 75 mmHg.
6. Arterial blood carbon dioxide pCO_2 unchanged.
7. Coughing ability is reduced.
G. Gastrointestinal system.
1. Tooth loss.
a. Periodontal disease major cause of loss after 30 years of age.
b. Other causes include poor dental health, poor nutrition.

2. Taste sensation decreases.
   a. Chronic irritation of mucous membranes.
   b. Atrophy of up to 80 of taste buds.
   c. Lose sensitivity of those on tip tongue first: sweet and salt.
   d. Lose sensitivity of those on sides later: salt, sour, bitter.
3. Esophagus dilates.
4. Stomach.
   a. Hunger sensations decrease.
   b. Secretion of gastric acid decreases.
   c. Emptying time decreases.
5. Peristalsis weakens and constipation is common.
6. Absorption function is impaired.
   a. Body absorbs less nutrients due to reduced intestinal blood flow and atrophy of cells on absorbing surfaces.
   b. Decrease in gastric enzymes affects absorption.
7. Liver.
   a. Smaller with decreased storage space.
   b. Decreased blood flow.

H. Genitourinary system.
1. Kidneys.
   a. Smaller due to nephron atrophy.
   b. Renal blood flow decreases 50%.
   c. Glomerular filtration rate decreases 50%.
   d. Tubular function diminishes.
      (1) Less able to concentrate urine; lower specific gravity.
      (2) Proteinuria 1+ is common.
      (3) Blood urea nitrogen BUN increases to 21 mg%.
   e. Renal threshold for glucose increases.
2. Bladder.
   a. Muscle weakens.
   b. Capacity decreases to 200 ml or less causing frequency.
   c. Emptying is more difficult, causing increased retention.
3. Prostate enlarges in some degree in 75% of men over 65.
4. Vulva atrophies.
5. Vagina.

a. Mucous membrane becomes dryer.
b. Elastic tissue decreases so surface is smooth.
c. Secretions become reduced, more alkaline.
d. Flora changes.
6. Sexuality.
   a. Older people are sexual beings also.
   b. There is no particular age at which a person's sexual functioning ceases.
   c. Frequency of genital sexual behavior (intercourse) may tend to decline gradually in later years, but capacity for expression and enjoyment continue far into old age.

I. Endocrine system.
1. Production of most hormones is reduced.
2. Parathyroid function and secretion are unchanged.
3. Pituitary.
   a. Growth hormone present but in lower blood levels.
   b. Reduced ACTH, TSH, FSH, LH production.
4. Reduced thyroid activity.
   a. Decreased basal metabolic rate.
   b. Reduced I^{131} uptake.
5. Reduced aldosterone production.
6. Reduced gonadal secretion of progesterone, estrogen, testosterone.

J. Integumentary system.
1. Wrinkles due to loss of subcutaneous fat.
2. Scalp hair thins and grays.
3. Hair in nose and ears thickens.
4. Skin pigmentation increases due to clustering of melanocytes.
5. Elasticity lessens due to decreased hydration and vascularity.
6. Fingernails become hard and brittle.
7. Toenails become overgrown and horny.
8. Sweat glands decrease in number and function.

K. Musculoskeletal system.
1. Bone loses density, brittleness increases.
2. Kyphosis with backward tilt of head occurs.
3. Hips, knees, wrists flex.
4. Discs thin so height decreases.

5. Joints enlarge and stiffen.
6. Tendons shrink and sclerose with decrease in tendon jerks.
7. Muscle fibers atrophy.
   a. Person moves more slowly.
   b. Muscle cramps and/or tremors occur.

Psychological Changes

A. Factors that influence these changes.
   1. Physiological changes primarily, especially those of the sense organs.
   2. General health.
   3. Educational level.
   4. Heredity.
   5. Environment.
B. Drastic personality change is rare.
   1. More often honest expression of how one feels.
   2. "Rigidity" may be due to other factors such as diseases.
C. Memory.
   1. Old memory unchanged.
   2. Long term memory.
      a. Hours to days ago.
      b. Some change.
   3. Short term or recent memory.
      a. 0–10 minutes.
      b. Poor.
D. IQ.
   1. Unchanged with information, mathematics and verbal expressions.
   2. Reduced performance on spatial perceptions and psychomotor skills.
      a. Changes in vision.
      b. Pressures of time factor.

Psychosocial Changes/Adjustments

A. Retirement.
   1. Worth often judged by productivity.
   2. Identity tied up with job role.
B. Sense or awareness of mortality.
C. Alteration in living style, i.e., nursing home, moving in with children.
D. Economic deprivation.
   1. Increased cost of living on a fixed income.
   2. Increased need for costly medical care.
E. Chronic disease and disability.
F. Social isolation loneliness.
G. Sensory deprivation (blindness and deafness).
H. Nutritional deprivation.
I. Series of losses, i.e., relationships, friends, family.
J. Loss of physical strength and agility.
   1. Body image altered.
   2. Self-concept altered.

Nursing Process

Assessment

A. Purpose.
   1. Determine patient's self-care capacities/limitations.
   2. Provide basis for individualized nursing care plan.
   3. Aid in avoiding stereotyping and labeling patient.
   4. Give patient time to answer.
B. Baseline assessment.
   1. Temperature.
      a. May be as low as 95°F.
      b. Sublingual most accurate.
   2. Pulse.
      a. Rate, rhythm, volume.
      b. Apical, radial, pedal, other sites as indicated by disorder.
   3. Respirations.
      a. Rate, rhythm, depth.
      b. Irregularity common.
   4. Arterial blood pressure.
      a. Lying, sitting, standing.
      b. Postural hypotension common.
   5. Weight—gradual loss in late years.
   6. Orientation level.
   7. Memory.
   8. Sleep pattern.
   9. Psychosocial adjustment.
C. Nervous system.
   1. Facial symmetry.

2. Level of alertness—presence of organic brain changes.
   a. Not all persons become senile.
   b. Most people have memory impairment.
   c. The change is gradual.
3. Eyes: movement, clarity, presence of cataracts.
4. Pupils: equality, dilation, construction.
5. Visual acuity—decreases with age.
   a. Do not test facing window.
   b. Use hand-held chart.
   c. Cheek condition of glasses.
6. Sensory deprivation.
7. Hearing acuity.
   a. Hearing aid.
   b. Tinnitus.
   c. Cerumen in outer ear—do not clean.
8. Presence of pain.

D. Cardiovascular system.
   1. Peripheral circulation, color, warmth.
   2. Auscultate apical pulse.
   3. Cheek for jugular vein distention.
   4. Dizziness.
   5. Fainting.
   6. Edema.

E. Respiratory system.
   1. Chest excursion.
   2. Auscultate chest/lung/breath sounds.
   3. Describe cough, if present; describe sputum.
   4. Rib cage deformity.

F. Gastrointestinal system.
   1. Nutritional status.
   2. Dietary intake.
   3. Anorexia, indigestion, nausea, vomiting.
   4. Chewing, swallowing.
   5. Condition of teeth, gums, buccal cavity.
   6. Auscultate bowel sounds.
   7. Palpate for distention, dilated colon.
   8. Constipation, diarrhea.

G. Genitourinary system.
   1. Urine: appearance, color, odor.
   2. Bladder distention, incontinence.
   3. Frequency, urgency, hesitancy.
   4. Fluid intake, output.
   5. Dysuria.
   6. Sexuality.
      a. Lack of opportunities for expression.
      b. Social stigma toward activity.

H. Integumentary system.
   1. Skin.
      a. Temperature, degree of moisture.
      b. Intactness, open lesions, tears.
      c. Turgor.
      d. Pigmentation alterations.
   2. Bruises, scars.
   3. Condition of nails.
   4. Condition of hair.
   5. Infestations.

I. Musculoskeletal system.
   1. Contractures.
      a. Muscle atrophy.
      b. Tendon shortening.
      c. Lack of adequate joint motion.
   2. Mobility level.
      a. Ambulate with or without assistance or devices.
      b. Limitations to movement.
      c. Muscle strength.
      d. Gait.
   3. Range of motion of joints.
   4. Paralysis.
   5. Kyphosis.

J. Psychosocial.
   1. Exhibits increasing dependency.
   2. Concerns focus increasingly on self.
   3. Displays narrower interests.
   4. Needs tangible evidence of affection.

K. Life story.

L. Immunization history.

Planning

A. Involve the patient and his family in planning.

B. Enlist cooperation of other health care professionals.

C. Set priorities.
   1. Patient may be content with situation as is.
   2. Encourage change, but do not force it.
   3. Safety is a major concern.

D. Prevent problems.

E. Afford patient adequate time for input.

F. Write out all plans and schedules.

Implementation

A. Provide adequate lighting.
  1. Natural lighting best.
  2. Avoid glare.
  3. Night light at all times in bathrooms, halls.
B. Encourage sensory stimulation.
  1. Large print books.
  2. Changes in environment.
  3. Colors patient can see.
C. Maintain reality orientation.
  1. Calendars.
  2. Clocks.
  3. One-to-one visits.
D. Provide circulatory care.
  1. Avoid tight/restrictive clothing.
  2. Change position, especially from horizontal to vertical.
  3. Provide warmth by applying blankets and clothing.
  4. Encourage activity to increase circulatory stimulation.
  5. Provide support and use safety measures during transfer.
  6. Use gentle friction during bath.
E. Provide respiratory care.
  1. Clean nares if nasal passages are clogged.
  2. Protect from draughts.
  3. Promote respiratory activity with exercises.
    a. Deep breathing.
    b. Forced expiration.
    c. Coughing.
    d. Inflatable toys.
  4. Oxygen therapy caution: check for carbon dioxide narcosis.
    a. Confusion.
    b. Profuse perspiration.
    c. Visual disturbance.
    d. Muscle twitching.
    e. Hypotension.
    f. Cerebral dysfunction.
F. Provide gastrointestinal care.
  1. Stimulate appetite.
    a. Small, frequent feedings of high quality.
    b. Attractive meals.
    c. Wine if allowed.
    d. Female, 1600 calories; male, 2200.
    e. Hot foods hot; cold foods cold.
    f. Preferred foods if possible; ethnic choices.
  2. Lessen/prevent indigestion.
    a. Fowler's position for meals.
    b. Antacids contraindicated.
    c. Smaller meals without gas formers.
    d. Adequate fluids.
  3. Prevent constipation.
    a. Ensure adequate bulk and fluid in diet.
    b. Encourage activity.
    c. Ensure regular and adequate time for bowel movement.
    d. Provide privacy and normal positioning.
    e. Administer laxative or suppository if above not effective.
G. Provide genitourinary care.
  1. Adequate fluid intake: 2000–3000 ml daily.
  2. Incontinence prevention.
    a. Offer opportunity to void every two hours.
    b. Keep night light in bathroom to prevent falls.
    c. Schedule diuretics for maximum effect during daylight hours.
    d. Limit fluids near and at bedtime.
  3. Sexuality.
    a. Provide counseling if desired.
    b. Provide opportunity for desired sexual expression.
    c. Encourage touching and companionship, important for older people.
H. Provide integumentary care.
  1. Bathing.
    a. Have patient take complete bath only twice a week due to dryness of skin.
    b. Use superfatted soap or lotions to aid in moisturizing.
  2. Clip facial hairs for female patients if desired.
  3. Handle gently to prevent skin tears.
  4. Cut toenails unless contraindicated.
    a. Mycosis of nails.
    b. Medical/surgical disorder.
I. Provide musculoskeletal care.
  1. Ambulate within limitations.
  2. Alter position every two hours; align correctly.

3. Prevent osteoporosis of long bones by providing exercises against resistance.
4. Provide active and passive exercises.
   a. Rest periods necessary.
   b. Paced throughout the day.
5. Provide range-of-motion exercises to all joints three times a day.
6. Educate family that allowing the patient to be sedentary is not helpful.
7. Encourage walking, which is best single exercise for the elderly.

J. Provide psychosocial care.
   1. Encourage psychological activity to aid sense of normality.
   2. Encourage life review.
   3. Assist in selecting and attending activities.
   4. Foster touching, which is a very useful tool in establishing trust.
   5. Provide dignity and the feeling of worth.
   6. Foster the wellness approach to life.

K. Maintain safety.
   1. Siderails when in bed.
      a. Often awaken disoriented for various reasons.
      b. Fall easily due to weakened muscles.
      c. Orthostatic hypotension.
   2. Bed in low position when not giving direct patient care.
   3. Handrails in bathrooms and halls.
   4. Uncluttered rooms and floors.
   5. Adequate, nonglare lighting.
   6. Restraints when necessary.

DELIRIUM, DEPRESSION AND DEMENTIA

Delirium

Definition: Acute brain syndrome that interferes cerebral functioning.

Etiology

A. Metabolic, circulatory, endocrine disorders.
B. Drugs, systemic intoxication.
C. Infection.
D. Sensory changes.

Characteristics

A. Abrupt onset, usually reversible.
B. Course can fluctuate hourly.
C. Vivid hallucinations, delusions.
D. When oriented denies confusion, tries to make "what happened" make sense.
E. Tries to answer mental status examination questions.
F. Severe, bizarre behaviors.

Implementation

A. Supportive.
B. Identify etiology and remove or treat.
   1. First step is often to discontinue all medications.
   2. Provide nutritional and fluid intake.

Depression

Definition: State of mind where person loses interest in life and finds no pleasure in activities; feels hopeless and sad.

Etiology

A. Reaction to life event.
B. Reaction to environment.

Characteristics

A. Course usually two weeks to six months, varies day to day.
B. Often aware of event and date that triggered depression.
C. Mental status examination.
   1. Often can answer correctly.
   2. Can spell "world" backward.
   3. May not try to answer.
D. Symptoms.

1. Difficulty remembering and concentrating.
2. Poor task performance.
3. Alterations in appetite and weight, sleep patterns.
4. Feels worthless, self-reproach.
5. Loss of motivation, lethargic.

Implementation

A. Supportive.
B. Antidepressants.
   1. Check cautions regarding drug use in the elderly.
   2. Few manufacturers have included geriatric dose in literature; start small.

Dementia

Definition: Acquired impairment of memory and other intellectual abilities secondary to structural brain damage; this damage may be microscopic.

Characteristics

A. Diagnostic criteria—must meet one criteria numbered 1 through 5.
   1. Sufficiently severe loss of intellectual abilities to interfere with social or occupational functioning.
   2. Memory impairment, usually short-term memory.
   3. Impairment of abstract thinking or impaired judgement or disturbance of higher cortical function or personality change.
   4. Cloudy state of consciousness.
   5. Presence of a specific organic etiology or presumed presence.
B. Onset slow, insidious, unrelated to specific situation.
C. Gradual degeneration.
D. Mental status examination.
   1. Early in the disease will attempt to find the right answer.
   2. Later will not understand question.

3. The more severe the dementia, the more errors.
E. Symptoms.
   1. Paranoid accusations.
   2. Personality changes, withdrawn.
   3. Confusion noted by others but not by the patient.
   4. Unaware of memory loss.
      a. Begins with recent memory loss.
      b. Later problem with coding and retrieving information.
   5. Oblivious to failures.

Alzheimer's Disease

Definition: Degeneration of all layers of the cortex and atrophy of the cerebrum.

A. Etiology is unknown.
B. Most common dementia in the elderly (50%).
C. Incidence in U.S. is 1.2 million over 65.
D. Diagnosis by exclusion.
   1. No other diagnosis applicable.
   2. Specific data from brain autopsy.
      a. Neurofibrillary tangles.
      b. Neuritic plaques.
      c. Amyloid clusters.
E. Possible predisposing factors.
   1. Genetic.
   2. Familial history of Down's Syndrome.
   3. Enzyme deficiency.
   4. Immune system deficiency.
   5. Slow growing virus.
   6. Aluminum toxicity.
   7. Head trauma.
   8. Acetylcholine (a neurotransmitter) deficiency.
F. Symptoms.
   1. Physically health appears good.
   2. Onset slow, progressive decline.
   3. Restless, irritable.
   4. Aphasia, can produce words but not sentences.
   5. Intellectual impairment.
   6. Disoriented to person, place and time.
   7. Motor ability declines.
   8. Incontinent.

9. Doesn't recognize staff or family.

Implementation

A. Supportive.
B. Verbal communication
1. Short words, simple sentences, verbs and nouns.
2. Call patient by name and identify yourself.
3. Speak slowly, clearly; wait for response.
4. Ask only one question, give one direction at a time.
5. Repeat, do not rephrase.
C. Nonverbal communication.
1. Use gestures, move slowly.
2. Stand directly in front of patient, maintain eye contact.
3. Move or walk with patient.
4. Listen actively; show interest.
5. Chart all phrases and nonverbal techniques used and use those that "work."
6. Maintain the patient's physical activity within limits of safety.
   a. Walk outside if grounds are fenced, alarmed or if accompanied.
   b. Exercises with simple commands.
   c. Active games.
   d. Balance activities, dance.
   e. Activities of daily living.
7. Mental stimulation.
   a. Simple hobbies.
   b. One-to-one contact.
   c. Reality orientation.
   d. Play word, number games.
8. Encourage self-care, give cues. Pantomime brushing teeth instead of brushing patient's teeth.
9. Put families in touch with support groups such as Alzheimer's Disease and Related Disorders Assoc., Inc. chapters. (ADRDA).

Associated Degenerative Diseases

A. Multi-infarct Dementia.
1. Second most common dementia in the elderly.
2. Focal neurological signs and symptoms.

3. History of significant cerebrovascular disease.
B. Korsakoffs syndrome.
1. Varied symptoms associated with chronic alcoholism.
2. Often associated with Wernicke's encephalopathy.
C. Pick's disease.
1. Rare heredogenerative process not associated with the normal aging process.
2. Similar to Alzheimer's but involvement does not include parietal lobes.
D. Huntington's chorea—genetically transmitted disorder.
1. Characterized by onset of symptoms after the age of 30.
2. Progressive mental and physical deterioration is inevitable.
E. Arteriosclerosis—a generic term referring to localized degeneration caused by vascular changes.
1. Sudden onset.
2. Occurs in 40 to 50 age group.
F. Paresis—central nervous system degeneration caused by invasion of brain cells from *Treponema pallidum* (syphilis).
1. Infection may have occurred much earlier but remained untreated by penicillin.
2. Symptoms reflect general brain disorder deterioration.

Psychological Reactions to OBS Disorders

A. Changes in self-concept.
B. Anger and frustration as reactions to forced changes in various life roles.
C. Denial used as a defense.
D. Depression.
E. Limitations accepted.
F. "Sick" role assumed.
1. Becomes dependent.
2. Lacks motivation.

Implementation

A. Meet both physical and psychological needs.

B. Help patient maintain contact with reality.
1. Give feedback.
2. Avoid small chatter.
3. Personalize interaction.
4. Supply stimulation to motivate patient.
5. Keep patient from becoming bored and distracted.
C. Assist patient in accepting the diagnosis.
1. Be supportive.
2. Maintain good communication.
3. During denial phase, listen and accept; do not argue.
4. Assist development of awareness.
5. Help patient develop the ability to cope with his or her altered identity.
D. Focus of interactions with patient.
1. Conduct short, frequent contacts with patient.
2. Use concrete ideas in communicating with the patient.
3. Maintain a reality orientation by allowing the patient to talk about his or her past and to confabulate.
4. Acknowledge the patient as an individual.
E. Provide a safe, stable, consistent environment.
F. Assess the patient's disabilities, and help to develop a nursing plan to deal with them.
G. Become a member of the rehabilitation team.

COMMON PROBLEMS FROM IMMOBILITY

Pressure Ulcers

Definition: Localized areas of necrosis of skin and subcutaneous tissue due to pressure.

Characteristics

A. Cause—pressure exerted on skin and subcutaneous tissue by bony prominences and the object on which body rests.
B. Predisposing factors.

1. Malnutrition.
2. Anemia.
3. Hypoproteinemia.
4. Vitamin deficiency.
5. Edema.
C. Common sites: bony prominences of body such as sacrum, greater trochanter, heels, elbows, etc.

Assessment

A. Stage of ulcer.
B. Identify if infection is associated with decubitus ulcer.
C. Effectiveness of ulcer treatment.
D. Healing process of the ulcer.
E. Other bony prominences for potential formation of decubiti.
F. Presence of conditions that inhibit wound healing.

Implementation

A. Prevention.
1. Relieve or remove pressure.
2. Stimulate circulation.
3. Keep skin dry.
B. Positioning.
1. Encourage patient to remain active.
2. Change position frequently.
C. Maintain good skin hygiene; inspect skin frequently.
D. Provide for active and/or passive exercises.
E. Use alternating air pressure mattress, etc.
F. Use sheepskin padding.
G. Provide for adequate nutritional intake.

External Rotation of Hip

Definition: Outward rotation of hip joint.

Characteristics

A. Cause—lying for long periods of time on back without support to hips.

B. Incorrect positioning in bed.

Implementation

A. Trochanter roll extending from crest of ilium to midthigh when positioned on back.
B. Frequent change of position.
C. Proper positioning.

Footdrop

Definition: Tendency for foot to plantar flex.

Characteristics

A. Causes.
   1. Prolonged bed rest.
   2. Lack of exercise.
   3. Weight of bed clothing forcing toes into plantar flexion.
B. Complications.
   1. Individual will walk on his toes without touching heel on ground.
   2. Unable to walk.

Implementation

A. Prevention.
   1. Position feet against footboard.
   2. Use footcradle to keep weight of top linen off toes.
   3. Provide range of motion exercises.
B. Check that soles of feet are against footboard to prevent permanent footdrop.

Contractures

Definition: Abnormal shortening of muscle, tendon, or ligament so joint cannot function properly.

Characteristics

A. Cause—improper alignment, lack of movement.
B. Result is decrease in mobility and joint movement.

Implementation

A. Proper alignment at all times.
   1. Use pillows.
   2. Provide supportive splints.
B. Provide for range of motion exercises.

Bladder Dysfunction

Definition: When an individiual is unable to void and the reflex act of micturition (urination) cannot occur.

Characteristics

A. Causes.
   1. Disease process.
   2. Lack of innervation.
   3. Lack of motivation.
B. Treatment will involve bladder retraining, surgery, drugs.

Implementation

A. Bladder training—purpose.
   1. Prevent urinary tract infection and preserve renal function.
   2. Keep individual dry and odor free.
   3. Help individual maintain social acceptance.
B. Procedure.
   1. Set up specific time to empty bladder.
   2. Give measured amounts of fluids.
   3. Position in normal voiding position.
   4. Instruct how to Credé bladder.
   5. Keep record of amount and time of intake and output.
   6. Encourage patient to wear own clothing, particularly underwear.

Bowel Dysfunction

Definition: Normal elimination does not occur due to a structural problem or disease state.

Characteristics

A. Cause.
   1. Disease process.
   2. Inadequate intake.
   3. Poor prior habits.
B. Treatment involves surgery, dietary modifications, or drugs.

Implementation

A. Identify purpose of bowel training.
   1. Develop regular bowel habits.
   2. Prevent fecal incontinence, impaction, and/or irregularity.
B. Implement nursing procedure.
   1. Establish specific time.
   2. Provide for adequate roughage and fluid intake.
   3. Use normal posture.
   4. Instruct to bear down and contract abdominal muscles.
   5. Provide privacy and time.
   6. Provide exercise.

Hypostatic Pneumonia

Definition: Inflammatory process in the lungs in which alveoli fill with exudate.

Characteristics

A. Incidence.
   1. Very young, very old.
   2. Debilitated.
   3. Immobile.
B. Cause—stasis of secretions in lungs.

Implementation

A. Prevention.
   1. Assess lung function.
   2. Encourage deep breathing, coughing.
   3. Turn every two hours.
   4. Ensure adequate hydration.
B. Provide for postural drainage, if indicated.
C. Administer oxygen, as ordered.

D. Monitor antibiotic therapy.

PROBLEM AREAS FOR ELDERLY PATIENTS

Sensory Impairment

A. Elderly experience loss of function in the senses.
   1. Ability to taste declines after age 40; taste buds are fewer in number and there is less saliva flow.
   2. Ability to smell declines.
   3. Hearing fades, especially in high frequency ranges.
   4. Regulation of body temperature in less efficient.
B. Major diseases or degeneration of organs occurs.
   1. Vision loss—see section on page 148 for Nursing Implications.
      a. Glaucoma—increased pressure causes damage to optic nerve, leading to blindness.
      b. Cataracts—clouding of the lens leading to blurred vision.
      c. Retinal detachment.
   2. Hearing loss—see section on page 151 for Nursing Implications.
      a. Otosclerosis requiring a stapedectomy.
      b. Hearing loss due to accumulation of ear wax—requires periodic irrigation of auditory canal.

Nutrition

A. Physiological requirements do change (decrease) with age.
   1. Nutrition intake must meet two major demands.
      a. Normal structural repair.
      b. Energy production for functional needs.

2. Met by protein and amino acids and adequate calorie intake.
B. Many elderly are deficient in nutrients, especially protein, B vitamins, vitamins A and C, iron, and calcium.
 1. Change in diet often responsible.
  a. Sense of taste and smell decreases, thus less conscious of hunger.
  b. Teeth in poor condition or dentures don't work properly.
  c. Physical disabilities or lack of mobility, unable to buy groceries.
  d. Loss of interest in eating.
  e. Limited income affects buying nutritious food.
 2. System cannot assimilate nutrients as well as when younger.
  a. Reduced hydrochloric acid, reduced stomach activity.
  b. Decreased salivary flow.
C. Health status affects nutritional state.
 1. Chronic diseases: heart disease, cancer, diabetes, gastro-intestinal problems, etc.
 2. Drugs: antacids, antidepressants, anticonvulsants, cathartics, diuretics, antimicrobials, etc.
D. Decreased physical activity and metabolic changes reduce caloric needs.
E. Financial resources, emotional, and physical state affect nutritional status.

Assessment

A. Hydration status, body weight, edema.
B. Anemia.
C. Appetite.
D. Ability to feed self—physical and mental.
 1. Dentition.
 2. Mastication.
 3. Swallowing.
 4. Desire to eat.
E. Fatigue, energy reserve.
F. Constipation.
G. Compliance to special diets.
H. Effects of drugs on nutrition.
 1. Gastrointestinal irritation.
 2. Food-drug interactions.
 3. Some drug side effects are nausea and vomiting.
I. Skin and mucous membrane condition.

Implementation

A. Offer/give oral fluids in small amounts every hour.
B. Plan diet to be high in nutrients.
 1. Give foods with high fiber.
 2. Balance of vitamins and minerals.
 3. Use lemon, vinegar, herbs on foods (rather than salt) to stimulate appetite.
C. Devise tools and plates which assist self-feeding.
D. Serve meals with others present to reduce isolation.

Medications

A. 25 percent of all prescriptive drugs are used by the elderly, and this does not include over-the-counter drugs.
B. 80 percent of people age 65 and over have at least one chronic medical problem that requires medications (one-third have three or more chronic problems).
C. Typical elderly American takes between four and seven prescription drugs each day in addition to over-the-counter drugs.
D. Elderly (13 percent of the population) suffer 50 percent of all drug side effects (estimated 17 per 100,000 population).
 1. Increased risk for drug toxicity.
  a. Renal excretion altered—kidneys cannot process drugs as well.
  b. Liver enzymes altered.
  c. Diminished blood circulation to liver.
  d. Receiving multiple drugs that compete for binding and interact.
  e. CNS more sensitive to drugs.
   (1) Drugs interfere with neurotransmitters (chemicals) that regulate brain function.

(2) Side effects result in confusion in elderly.
  f. Altered body mass and ratio of fat to muscle.
2. Iatrogenic illness can be caused by drug therapy.
3. Most commonly abused drugs.
  a. Tranquilizers most frequently abused.
  b. Sleeping pills.
  c. Medications to control pain.
  d. Laxatives.
E. Major problems with prescriptive drugs in the elderly.
  1. Drug interactions—people who use multiple physicians and pharmacies run risk of taking drugs that interact to cause adverse reactions.
  2. Medication errors—the more medications a person takes, the greater the risk of medication error (people over age 75 take an average of 17 prescriptions annually).
  3. Noncompliance—not taking right dose at right time or discontinuing drug without consultation; common due to lack of understanding about reason to take drug and general knowledge base of drug action.
  4. Unpredictable drug action—physiological changes in the elderly associated with age and disease may alter effects of the drugs.
  5. Drug side effects not recognized—elderly not aware or do not understand potential dangerous side effects of drugs.
  6. Inadequate monitoring—elderly often alone or not monitored consistently so drug problems are not identified.
  7. Cost of drugs—multiple medications are costly for many elderly, so they stop taking drugs.

Administration of Medications

A. Oral route.
  1. Check for mouth dryness.
    a. Drug may stick and dissolve in mouth.
    b. Drug may irritate mucous membrane.
  2. Place patient in sitting position.
  3. Crush tablets if they are very large.
  4. Do not open capsules.
  5. Do not crush enteric-coated tablets.
  6. Check with pharmacy for liquid preparations if patient has difficulty swallowing tablets.
B. Suppository.
  1. Position for comfort.
  2. May take longer to dissolve due to decreased body core temperature.
  3. Do not insert suppository immediately after removing from refrigerator.
C. Parenteral.
  1. Site may ooze medication or bleed due to decreased tissue elasticity.
  2. Do not use immobile limb.
  3. Danger of overhydration with IV.
D. Self-administration.
  1. Check compliance with amounts and times.
  2. Color code to facilitate proper administration.

Assessment

A. Changes in mental status.
B. Vital signs.
  1. Orthostatic blood pressure.
  2. Apical pulse.
C. Urine production, retention.
D. Hydration and appetite.
E. Visual disturbances.
F. Swallowing ability.
G. Evaluate effects of drug.
  1. Laboratory studies.
  2. Signs and symptoms for toxic/interaction effects of drugs.
H. Bowel function.
I. Effects of nutrition and foods on drug response.

Implementation

A. No alcohol or alcohol based elixirs when receiving benzodiazepines or antihistamines.
B. Method of administering drugs.
  1. Deep breathing and relaxation to reduce use of analgesic drugs.

2. Position patient sitting with head slightly flexed to reduce chance of aspiration.
C. Administering tablets.
1. Do not crush time-released or enteric-coated tablets.
2. Crush large tablets if not contraindicated.
3. Give with textured foods (nectar, applesauce) if not contraindicated.
D. Stroke victim—give drug on functional side of mouth.

Drug-Food Interactions for Elderly

A. Foods and vitamin-minerals can interfere with therapeutic effects of drugs.
1. Reduce absorption of drug.
2. Interfere with cellular action.
B. Medication regimen affected by nutrition may put patient at risk.
1. Important to assess patient's diet.
2. Monitor potential vitamin/drug interactions.
C. Review patient's prescriptive and over-the-counter drugs.
1. Review in relation to normal dietary intake.
2. Consider vitamin-mineral intake and supplements in terms of decreasing effect of medications.
3. Check lab values for problems.
D. Document findings so health-care team is informed of diet-drug plan.
E. Food sources of vitamins and minerals.
1. Folic acid sources: liver, kidney, fresh vegetables.
2. Niacin sources: yeast, meat, fish, milk, eggs, green vegetables, and cereal grains.
3. Pantothenic acid sources: meat, vegetables, cereal grains, legumes, eggs, milk, fish, and fruit.
4. Pyridoxine hydrochloride (vitamin B_6) sources: cereal grains, legumes, vegetables, liver, meat, and eggs.
5. Cyanocobalamin (vitamin B_{12}) sources: animal foods, liver kidney, fish, shellfish, meat, and dairy foods.

6. Ascorbic acid (vitamin C) sources: fresh fruits and vegetables.
7. Vitamin A sources: eggs, milk, cream, butter, organ meats, fish.
8. Vitamin D source: activated in body by sunlight.
9. Vitamin E sources: vegetable oils, whole grains, animal fats, eggs, and green vegetables.
10. Vitamin K sources: green leafy vegetables, spinach, broccoli, cabbage, and liver.

Lab Values in the Elderly

Urinalysis

A. Protein.
1. Normal 0–5 mg/100 ml—rises slightly.
2. May reflect changes in kidney or subclinical urinary tract infection.
B. Glucose.
1. Normal 0–15 mg/100 ml—declines slightly.
2. May reflect changes in kidney.
C. Specific gravity.
1. 1.032—decline to 1.024 by age 80.
2. 30–50 percent decline in number of nephrons affects ability to concentrate urine.

Hematology

A. Hemoglobin.
1. Men 13–18 g/100 ml—drops to 10–17 g/100 ml.
2. Women 12–16 g/100 ml—no change.
B. Hematocrit.
1. Men 45–52 percent—no change.
2. Women 37–48 percent—no change.
C. Leukocytes.
1. 4,300—10,800/cu mm—drops to 3,100–9,000/cu mm.
2. As bone marrow diminishes, hematopoiesis declines.
D. Lymphocytes.
1. 500–2,400/cu mm—T-lymphocytes fall.

2. 50–200/cu mm—B-lymphocytes fall.

E. Platelets, prothrombin time (PT) and partial thromboplastin time (PTT) no change.

Blood Chemistry Tests that Change with Age

A. Blood urea nitrogen (BUN).
1. Men 10–25 mg/100 ml—increases, may be as high as 69 mg/100 ml.
2. Women 8–20 mg/100 ml—increases.
3. Renal function decreased due to decline in cardiac output, renal blood flow, and glomerular filtration rate.

B. Creatinine.
1. 0.6–1.5 mg/100 ml—increases as high as 1.9 mg/100 ml in men and women.
2. Endogenous creatinine production as lean body mass shrinks.

3. Drugs excreted by urinary system may cause toxicity if creatinine level too high.

C. Creatinine clearance.
1. 104–125 ml/min.
2. Referenced interval: men's formula for age: 140 minus age × Kg body weight divided by 72 × serum creatinine.

D. Glucose tolerance.
1. One hour: 160–170 mg/100 ml.
Two hours: 115–125 mg/100 ml.
Three hours: 70–110 mg/100 ml.
2. With age, results rise more quickly in first two hours, then drop to baseline more slowly.
3. Alcohol, MAO inhibitors, and beta blockers can all cause a rapid fall in glucose.

E. Thyroxine (T_4) 4.5–13.5 mcg/100 ml and tri-iodothyronine (T_3) 90–220 mg/100 ml both decrease by 25 percent.

11

MATERNITY AND GYNECOLOGICAL NURSING

Anatomy and Physiology of Female Reproductive System

ANATOMY

External Genitalia

A. Collectively called the vulva.

B. Visible structures.
1. Mons veneris (mons pubis).
2. Labia majora.
3. Labia minora.
4. Clitoris.
5. Vestibule.
6. Urethral meatus.
7. Skene's and Bartholin's glands.
8. Hymen.
9. Perineum.

Internal Organs

A. Located in pelvic cavity.

B. Reproductive structures.
1. Uterus—a muscular organ with a central cavity.
   a. Functions.
      (1) Structure of fetal development.
      (2) Site of menstrual shedding.
   b. Sections.
      (1) Corpus (body)—lies below tubal insertion and composed of three layers.
         (a) Perimetrium—external layer.
         (b) Myometrium—middle layer.
         (c) Endometrium—internal layer.
      (2) Fundus—lies above tubal insertion.
2. Cervix—canal located between internal and external os.
   a. Internal os opens into body of uterine cavity.
   b. External os opens into vagina.
3. Fallopian tubes.
   a. Two slender muscular tubes extending laterally from the cornu of uterine cavity to ovaries.
   b. Passageways through which ova reach uterus.
4. Ovaries.
   a. Flat, oval-shaped organs.
   b. One ovary located on each side of uterus.
   c. Functions.
      (1) Develop and expel ova.
      (2) Secrete certain hormones.
5. Vagina.
   a. Canal extending from lower part of vulva to cervix.
   b. Functions.
      (1) Allows for passage of menstrual blood.
      (2) Allows for passage of fetus.
      (3) Provides site for copulation.

Support Structure (Pelvis)

A. Important in obstetrics.
1. Passage through which baby passes at birth.
2. Disproportions between fetus and size of pelvis make vaginal delivery difficult or impossible.

B. Bone formations.
1. Two innominate bones.
2. Sacrum.
3. Coccyx.

C. Pelvic cavities.
1. False pelvis—shallow extended portion above brim that supports abdominal viscera.
2. True pelvis—portion that lies below pelvic brim; divided into three sections.
   a. Pelvic outlet.
   b. Mid-pelvis.
   c. Pelvic inlet.

D. Pelvic types.

1. Gynecoid—nearly round or blunt; typical of normal female.
2. Android—wedge-shaped; typical of male.
3. Anthropoid—oval-shaped.
4. Platypelloid—oval-shaped, transversely.

E. Measurements of the pelvis.
   1. Diagonal conjugate (CD)—distance between sacral promontory and lower margin of symphysis pubis. Measurement greater than 11.5 cm adequate.
   2. True conjugate, or conjugate vera (CV) distance from upper margin of symphysis to sacral promontory. Measurement greater than 11 cm adequate.
   3. Tuberischial diameter (TI)—transverse diameter of outlet. Measurement greater than 8 cm adequate.
   4. Size determination.
      a. X-ray pelvimetry is most accurate means of determining size of pelvis.
      b. X-ray pelvimetry is contraindicated to avoid undue exposure of mother and infant unless pelvic contraction is suspected.

PHYSIOLOGY

Menstruation and the Menstrual Cycle

A. Menstruation.
   1. Culmination of menstrual cycle.
   2. Discharge of blood, mucus, and epithelial cells from the uterus.

B. Menstrual cycle.
   1. Occurrence—usually between ages of 12 and 45.
   2. Duration—about 28 days but varies from 21 to 35 days; ovulation occurs about 14 days before beginning of menstruation.

C. Menstrual cycle regulated primarily through phasic hormonal control of pituitary, ovaries, and uterus.
   1. Proliferative phase.
      a. Follicle stimulating hormone (FSH), released by anterior pituitary, stimulates the development of the graafian follicle.
      b. As graafian follicle develops, it produces increasing amounts of follicular fluid containing a hormone called estrogen.
      c. Estrogen stimulates build-up or thickening of the endometrium.
      d. As estrogen increases in the bloodstream, it suppresses secretion of FSH and favors the secretion of the luteinizing hormone (LH).
      e. LH stimulates ovulation and initiates development of the corpus luteum.
   2. Secretory phase.
      a. Follows ovulation, which is the release of mature ovum from the graafian follicle.
      b. Rapid changes take place in the ruptured follicle under the influence of LH.
      c. Cavity of the graafian follicle is replaced by the corpus luteum (mass of yellow-colored tissue).
      d. Main function of the corpus luteum is to secrete progesterone and some estrogen.
      e. Progesterone acts upon the endometrium to bring about secretory changes that prepare it for pregnancy. Also, progesterone maintains the endometrium during the early phase of pregnancy, should a fertilized ovum be implanted.
   3. Menstrual phase.
      a. Corpus luteum degenerates in about eight days unless the ovum is fertilized.
      b. There is a cessation of progesterone and estrogen produced by corpus luteum and blood levels drop.
      c. Endometrium degenerates and menstruation occurs.
      d. The drop in blood levels of estrogen and progesterone stimulate production of FSH and a new cycle begins.

D. Discomforts associated with menstruation.
   1. Breast tenderness and feeling of fullness.
   2. Tendency toward fatigue.

3. Temperament and mood changes—because of hormonal influence and decreased levels of estrogen and progesterone.
4. Discomfort in pelvic area, lower back, and legs.
5. Retained fluids and weight gain.

E. Abnormalities of menstruation.
1. Dysmenorrhea (painful menstruation).
   a. May be caused by psychological factors: tension, anxiety, preconditioning (menstruation is a "curse" or should be painful).
   b. Physical examination is usually done to rule out organic causes.
2. Treatment.
   a. Oral contraceptives—produce anovulatory cycle.
   b. Mild analgesics such as aspirin.
   c. Urge patient to carry on normal activities to occupy her mind.
   d. Dysmenorrhea may subside after childbearing.
3. Amenorrhea (absence of menstrual flow).
   a. Primary—over the age of 17 and menstruation has not begun.
      (1) Complete physical necessary to rule out abnormalities.
      (2) Treatment aimed at correction of underlying condition.
   b. Secondary—occurs after menarche—does not include pregnancy and lactation.
      (1) Causes include psychological upsets or endocrine conditions.
      (2) Evaluation and treatment by physician is necessary.
4. Menorrhagia (excessive menstrual bleeding)—may be due to endocrine disturbance, tumors, or inflammatory conditions of the uterus.
5. Metrorrhagia (bleeding between periods)—symptom of disease process, benign tumors, or cancer.

F. Counseling guidelines.
1. Assist with providing education about the physiology of normal menstruation and correct misinformation.
2. Assist with providing education about abnormal conditions associated with menstruation—absence of menstruation, bleeding between menstrual periods, etc.
3. Assist with providing education related to normal hygiene during menstruation.
   a. Importance of cleanliness.
   b. Use of perineal pads and tampons.
   c. Continuance of normal activities.

Development of the Fetus

Fertilization

Definition: A gamete is a matured sex cell (ovum or spermatozoon) that has undergone maturation and is ready for fertilization.

A. Fertilization takes place when two essential cells (sperm and ovum) unite; usually occurs in outer third of fallopian tube.
B. Each reproductive cell (one gamete) carries 23 chromosomes.
C. Each sperm carries two types of sex chromosomes, X and Y; when united with female, X chromosome determines the sex of the child (XY—male; XX—female).
D. After fertilization the fertilized egg descends to the uterus within three days.

Fetal Development

A. Embryo is the fertilized ovum during the first two months of development.
B. Fetus is product of conception from two months to time of birth.
C. Implantation occurs about the seventh day after fertilization.
D. During embryonic development, cells arrange themselves into three layers.
E. Fetal membranes and amniotic fluid.
   1. Fetal membranes (those which surround the fetus) are composed of two layers.
      a. Amnion (glistening inner membrane) forms early, about the second week of

Table A. Multiple Pregnancies

Double Ovum	Single Ovum
Dizygotic or fraternal twins	Monozygotic or identical twins
Ova from same or different ovaries	Union of a single ovum and a single sperm
Same or different sex	Same sex
Brother or sister resemblance	Identical genetic pattern
Two placentas but may be fused	One placenta
Two chorions and two amnions	One chorion and two amnions

embryonic development; encloses the amniotic cavity.

    b. Chorion is the outer membrane.

2. Amniotic fluid forms within the amniotic cavity and surrounds the embryo. Usually consists of 500 to 1000 ml of fluid at the end of pregnancy.

    a. Amniotic fluid contains fetal urine, lanugo from fetal skin, epithelial cells, and subaqueous materials.

    b. Function of the fluid is to provide an optimum temperature and environment for fetus and provide a cushion against injury; fetus also drinks the fluid, probably as much as 450 ml a day near term.

    c. Source is uncertain; replaced continuously at a rapid rate.

F. Placenta and fetal circulation.

1. Placenta—organ that provides for the exchange of nutrients and waste products between mother and fetus and acts as an endocrine organ. The placenta provides oxygen and removes carbon dioxide from the fetal system because its respiratory system is not yet functioning.

    a. Placenta develops by the third month.

        (1) Formed by union of chorionic villi and decidua basalis.

        (2) Fetal surface smooth and glistening.

        (3) Maternal surface red and fleshlike.

        (4) Exchange takes place between mother and fetus through diffusion.

        (5) Materials passed through placenta in addition to nutrients are drugs, antibodies to some diseases, and certain viruses. Large particles such as bacteria cannot pass through barrier.

        (6) Hormones produced by the placenta.

            (a) Chorionic gonadotropin can be detected in the urine about 15 days after implantation. This hormone stimulates the corpus luteum to maintain endometrium.

            (b) Estrogen and progesterone.

    b. Umbilical cord extends from fetus to center of fetal surface of placenta.

        (1) Main vessels in the umbilical cord are two arteries and one vein.

        (2) The umbilical cord is protected by mucoid connective tissue termed Wharton's jelly.

        (3) Length is 20 inches; width is 1 inch.

2. Circulation.

    a. Vein carries oxygenated blood.

    b. Arteries carry venous blood.

    c. There are three bypasses in fetal circulation.

        (1) Two bypasses exist because the lungs are not functioning.

            (a) Ductus arteriosus, between pulmonary artery and aorta.

            (b) Foramen ovale, between right and left atrium.

        (2) Ductus venosus bypass exists because the fetal liver is not used for exchange of waste.

    d. Bypasses must close following birth to allow blood to flow through the lungs for respiration and through the liver for waste exchange.

G. A multiple pregnancy is one in which two or more embryos are contained in the amniotic sac. May be the result of fertilization of a single ovum or two separate ova.

Table B. Fetal Growth

Age	Development
End of 1 month or 4 weeks	Form of embryonic disc No clearly defined features Body systems rudimentary form Cardiovascular system functioning
End of 2 months or 8 weeks	Head greatly enlarged, about the size of rest of body Some fetal movement as a result of beginning neuromuscular development Facial features becoming distinct Body covered with thin skin
End of 3 months or 12 weeks	Teeth forming under gums Center ossification appearing in most bones Fingers and toes are differentiated and bear nails Kidneys able to secrete Eyes have lids which are fused shut until six months Fetus swallows Sex distinguishable Fetal heart heard with ultrasonic equipment
End of 4 months or 16 weeks	Lanugo appears over body Meconium in intestines Face has human appearance Size about 6 inches long; weight about 3.5 oz
End of 5 months or 20 weeks	Skeleton begins to harden Buds of permanent teeth develop Vernix caseosa makes appearance Fetal movements stronger and felt by mother Fetal heart rate heard with fetoscope Size about 10 inches long; weight about 11 oz
End of 6 months or 24 weeks	Fat beginning to deposit beneath skin Body and head better proportioned Eyebrows and eyelashes appear Size about 12 inches long; weight about 1½ lbs
End of 7 months or 28 weeks	Skin reddish and covered with vernix Size about 14 inches long; weight about 2½ lbs May be viable if born at this time, though still immature
End of 8 months or 32 weeks	Nails are firm and extend to end of digits Lanugo begins to disappear Size about 16 inches long; weight about 4 lbs Increased chance for survival if born at this time
End of 9 months or 36 weeks	Increased fat deposits under skin Increased development Size about 18 inches long; weight about 5 lbs Chances for survival are good
End of 10 months or 40 weeks	Full term Little lanugo Smooth skin Size about 20 inches long; weight 7–7½ lbs Optimum time for survival

H. Calculation of expected date of delivery or confinement (EDC).
   1. Nägele's rule—count back three months from first day of last menstrual period (LMP) and add seven days.
      Example: LMP July 18, 1994.
      EDC April 25, 1995.
   2. Pregnancy usually does not terminate on the exact EDC. It may vary from one week before to two weeks after the expected date.

MATERNAL CHANGES DURING PREGNANCY

Physiological Changes

Reproductive Organs

A. Uterus increases in weight from two ounces to about two pounds at the end of gestation and increases in size five to six times.
   1. Changes in tissue.
      a. Hypertrophy of muscle cells and development of new muscles.
      b. Development of connective and elastic tissue, which increases contractility.
      c. Increase in the size and number of blood vessels.
      d. Hypertrophy of the lymphatic system.
      e. Growth of the uterus is brought about by the influences of estrogen during the early months and the pressure of the fetus.
   2. Other changes.
      a. Contractions occur throughout pregnancy, starting from very mild to increased strength.
      b. As the uterus grows, it rises out of the pelvis displacing intestines and may be palpated above the symphysis pubis.
B. Ligaments.
   1. Broad ligaments located in the pelvis.
      2. They become elongated and hypertrophied to help support and stabilize uterus during pregnancy.
C. Cervix.
   1. Becomes shorter, more elastic, and larger in diameter.
   2. Marked thickening of mucous lining and increased blood supply.
   3. Edema and hyperplasia of the cervical glands and increased glandular secretions.
   4. Mucous plug expelled from cervix as cervix begins to dilate at onset of labor.
D. Vagina.
   1. Increased vascularity, deepening of color to dark red or purple (Chadwick's sign).
   2. Hypertrophy and thickening of muscle.
   3. Loosening of connective tissue.
   4. Increased vaginal discharge.
   5. Secretions have high pH.
E. Perineum.
   1. Increased vascularity.
   2. Hypertrophy of muscles.
   3. Loosening of connective tissue.
F. Ovaries and tubes.
   1. Usually one large corpus luteum present in one ovary.
   2. Ovulation does not take place.

Breasts

A. Changes in tissue.
   1. Extensive growth of alveolar tissue, necessary for lactation.
   2. Montgomery's glands enlarge.
B. Other changes.
   1. Increase in size and firmness; become nodular.
   2. Nipples become more prominent, and areolae deepen in color.
   3. Superficial veins grow more prominent.
   4. At the end of third month, colostrum appears.
   5. After delivery, anterior pituitary stimulates production and secretion of milk.

Abdomen

A. Contour changes as the enlarging uterus extends into the abdominal cavity.
B. Striae gravidarum usually appear on the abdomen as pregnancy progresses.

Skin

A. Pigmentation increases in certain areas of the body.
   1. Breasts—primary areolae deepen in color.
   2. Abdomen—linea nigra, dark streak down the midline of the abdomen, especially prominent in brunettes.
   3. Face—chloasma, the "mask of pregnancy" pigmentation, distributed over the face; usually disappears after pregnancy.
   4. Face and upper trunk—occasionally spider nevi or palmar erythema develops with the increase in estrogen.
B. Pigmented areas on abdomen and breast usually do not completely disappear after delivery.

Circulatory System

A. Considerable increase (about 50 percent) in volume of blood as a result of:
   1. Increased metabolic demands of new tissue.
   2. Expansion of vascular system, especially in the reproductive organs.
   3. Increased steroid hormones which cause retention of sodium and water.
B. Increase in plasma volume is greater than increase in red blood cells and hemoglobin, although dilution is not sufficient to cause anemia (low hemoglobin in pregnancy usually caused by iron-deficiency anemia).
C. Heart increases in size and cardiac output is increased 25 to 50 percent.
D. Blood pressure *should not* rise during pregnancy.
E. Fibrinogen concentration increases until term.
F. Iron requirements are increased to meet demands of increased blood supply and growing fetus (need cannot be met by diet alone; supplement usually given).
G. Palpitations may be experienced during pregnancy due to sympathetic nervous disturbance and intra-abdominal pressure caused by enlarging uterus.

Respiratory System

A. Thoracic cage is pushed upward and the diaphragm is elevated as the uterus enlarges.
B. Thoracic cage widens to compensate so that vital capacity remains the same or is increased.
C. Oxygen consumption is increased 15 percent to support fetus and tissue.
D. Shortness of breath may be experienced in latter part of pregnancy due to pressure upon diaphragm caused by enlarging uterus.

Digestive System

A. Nausea, vomiting, and poor appetite are present in early pregnancy because of a decreased gastric motility.
B. Constipation is due to a decrease in gastrointestinal motility, reduced peristaltic activity, and the pressure of the uterus; it may be present in latter half of pregnancy.
C. Flatulence and heartburn may be present as a result of decreased gastric acidity and decreased motility of the gastrointestinal tract.

Urinary System

A. Kidneys.
   1. Kidney and renal function is increased.
   2. Renal blood flow and glomerular filtration is increased.
B. Bladder and ureters.
   1. Blood supply to the bladder and pelvic organs is increased.
   2. Pressure of uterus on bladder causes frequent urination during early pregnancy.
   3. Atonia of smooth muscles during pregnancy leads to dilatation of ureters and renal pelvis; may cause urine stasis.

4. A decrease in bladder tone is caused by hormonal influences; a decrease in bladder capacity occurs because of crowding. Such decrease may lead to complications during pregnancy and in the postpartum period.

Joints, Bones, Teeth and Gums

A. Softening of pelvic cartilages occurs, probably due to the relaxin hormone.

B. Postural changes occur as upper spine is thrown forward to compensate for increased abdominal size.

C. Demineralization of teeth does not occur as a result of normal pregnancy but may be related to poor dental hygiene.

D. Increased vascularity of gums due to hormonal changes with tendency to bleed easily.

Endocrine System

A. Placenta produces the hormones human chorionic gonadotropin (HCG) and placental lactogen (HPL).
   1. Production of estrogen and progesterone is taken over from the ovaries by the placenta/fetal unit after the second month.
   2. Normal cycle of production of estrogen and progesterone is suspended until after delivery.

B. Anterior lobe of pituitary gland enlarges slightly during pregnancy.

C. Adrenal cortex enlarges slightly.

D. Thyroid enlarges slightly and thyroid activity increases.

E. Aldosterone levels gradually increase beginning about the 15 week.

Metabolism

A. Increase in body weight (a 25-pound weight gain is usually recommended).

B. Some of the weight gain is caused by retention of fluid and by deposits of fatty tissue.

C. Water metabolism.
   1. Tendency to retain fluid in body tissues, especially in the last trimester.

   2. Reversal of fluid retention usually takes place in the form of diuresis in the first 24 hours postpartum.

D. Basal metabolic rate increases.

Emotional Changes

Altered Emotional Characteristics

A. Quick mood changes and a certain amount of emotional lability is common.

B. Emotional reactions may change during pregnancy; may range from early rejection of pregnancy to that of elation.

C. Pregnant women may become more passive and introverted in second trimester.

D. A woman may be puzzled by changes in her feelings and needs reassurance from the nurse that these are normal reactions about which one need not feel guilty.

E. Father of the baby needs to be informed that the woman's emotional lability, attitudes, and feelings toward sex are emotional reactions of pregnancy and will pass.

F. The woman may have fears and worries about the baby and herself and needs to be able to express her feelings to the nurse.

Taking on the Parental Role

A. Pregnant woman may fantasize or daydream to "experience" the role of mother before the actual birth occurs.

B. Takes on adaptive behaviors that are best suited to her own personality and situation.

C. Experiences a "letting go" of her former role (e.g., as a career woman).
   1. May experience ambivalence about letting go of her old role to take on the new one.
   2. Desire to have a baby influences adjustment and acceptance of the maternal role.

D. Father may also experience ambivalence about taking on new role and sharing wife's attention with new baby.

Childbirth Preparation

Theories of Childbirth

A. Factors that influence pain in labor.
1. Preconditioning by "old wives' tales," fantasies, and fears. Accurate information about the childbirth process can often alleviate effects of preconditioning.
2. Pain produces stress, which in turn affects the body's functioning. Interpretations of and reactions to pain can be altered by a refocusing of attention and by conditioning.
3. Feelings of isolation. Social expectations and tension may also increase feelings of pain.

B. Childbirth education classes.
1. Read method (original natural childbirth movement).
   a. Its purpose is to eradicate negative attitudes of mother through education.
   b. A basic principle establishes that childbirth is a natural occurrence and should not be painful.
   c. Presents a thorough understanding of anatomy, physiology of pregnancy, labor, and delivery.
   d. Encourages exercise to foster relaxation and prepare woman for physical work of labor; breathing (diaphragmatic, abdominal) and panting.
2. Lamaze method (psychoprophylactic method).
   a. Basic thrust is education and training.
   b. Instruction in anatomy, the physiology of the reproductive system; an extensive study of labor and delivery; replacement of misinformation and superstition with facts.
   c. Training that consists of controlled breathing and neuromuscular exercises.
   d. Husband, family member, or a friend is included in the class and serves as coach.
3. LeBoyer technique (used in delivery room to reduce stress of birth upon infant).
   a. Room temperature is increased to a comfortable level for infant, lights are dimmed, noise is controlled.
   b. Infant is placed in skin-to-skin contact on mother's abdomen and gently stroked; cord clamping is delayed until pulsation stops.
   c. Infant is submerged up to head in a bath of warm water until it appears relaxed, then is dried and wrapped snugly in a warm blanket.

Nutritional Guidelines for Pregnancy

A. Influences upon dietary habits and nutrition.
1. Food—many emotional connotations originating in infancy.
2. Eating habits influenced by:
   a. Emotional factors.
   b. Cultural factors.
   c. Religious beliefs.
   d. Nutritional information.
   e. Age—especially adolescent and aged.
   f. Physical health.
   g. Personal preferences.

B. Nutritional needs in pregnancy.
1. Influenced by above factors.
2. Must supply caloric and nutritional needs of mother as well as promote optimum fetal growth.
3. May be complicated by:
   a. Poor maternal nutrition before pregnancy.
   b. Medical complications prior to pregnancy (diabetes, anemia).
   c. Complications resulting from pregnancy (toxemia, anemia).
   d. Pica (cravings).

C. Weight gain in pregnancy.
1. Average weight gain recommended (even for obese patients)—24 pounds.
   a. 1st trimester—3 to 4 pounds.
   b. 2nd trimester—10 pounds.
   c. 3rd trimester—10 pounds.
2. Weight gain accounted by:

a. Product of conception.

Fetus—average size	7.5 pounds
Placenta	1.5
Amniotic fluid	2
Uterus	2.5
Breasts	1
Extracellular fluid	3
Blood volume	3
	20.5 pounds

b. Rest of weight gain deposited as fat stores or fluid representing energy stored for lactation.

D. Revised daily food guide.
1. Iron and folacin—cannot be ingested in sufficient quantities by dietary means. Must be supplemented during pregnancy.
2. 300 additional calories needed to meet recommended allowances.
3. Protein intake includes both animal and vegetable protein.
   a. Vegetable protein may be omitted in those whose income will allow by increasing animal servings to three 3-oz servings.
   b. One serving at least should be red meats.
4. Whole grain items are better choices than enriched breads and cereals. They contain more magnesium, zinc, folacin, and vitamin B_6.
5. At least two tablespoons of fat or oils should be consumed daily for vitamin E and essential fatty acids.

E. Special diets.
1. Adolescents.
   a. Have high proportion of low-birth-weight infants.
   b. Dietary habits often poor.
   c. Plan menu to include necessary items around foods they like.
   d. Stress balanced diet—avoid empty calories.
2. Low sodium.
   a. Presently sodium restriction is not recommended.
   b. Sodium essential in maintaining increased body fluids needed for adequate placental flow, increased tissue requirements, and renal blood flow.
   c. If moderate salt intake is necessitated, avoid highly salted foods such as canned soups, potato chips, soda pop.
3. Weight control.
   a. Presently, weight loss in pregnancy is discouraged.
   b. Even obese patient should gain 24 pounds to insure adequate nutrition for fetal growth.
   c. Strict dieting may lead to ketosis which has proven harmful to fetal brain.
   d. Stress careful dietary planning to include essential nutrients and avoid empty calories.
   e. Weight reduction program should begin *after* lactation only.

SIGNS AND DISCOMFORTS OF PREGNANCY

Signs of Pregnancy

Presumptive Signs

A. Cessation of menstruation (amenorrhea).

B. Breasts increase in size with feeling of fullness; nipples more pronounced, areola darker.

C. Nausea and vomiting ("morning sickness") appear in about 50 percent of pregnant women and usually disappears at the end of the 3rd month.

D. Frequent urination (desire to void) usually occurs in the first three to four months. Pressure on the bladder from an enlarged uterus gives the sensation of a distended bladder.

E. Quickening (first perception of fetal movement) occurs between 16th and 18th week.

F. Increased pigmentation of skin, chloasma, linea nigra, and striae gravidarum.

G. Fatigue with periods of drowsiness and lassitude during first three months.

Probable Signs

A. Enlargement of the abdomen usually occurs after the third month when the fetus rises out of the pelvis into the abdominal cavity.
B. Changes in internal organs.
   1. Change in shape, size, and consistency of the uterus.
   2. Hegar's sign—softening of the isthmus of the uterus, occurs about sixth week.
   3. Goodell's sign—softening of the cervix, occurs beginning of the second month.
C. Braxton Hicks contractions—slight, irregular contractions usually not felt by the woman until seven months, but contractions begin in the early weeks of pregnancy and continue through gestation.
D. Ballottement—pressure on an organ giving a sudden push to the fetus and feeling it rebound in a few seconds to the original position; usually possible in the fourth to fifth month.
E. Outline of the fetus by abdominal palpation (a probable sign, because a tumor may simulate fetal parts).
F. Positive pregnancy test is based upon the secretion of chorionic gonadotropin in the urine of a pregnant woman; it is usually detectable ten days after the first missed menstrual period.

Positive Signs

A. Apparent after 18th to 20th week.
B. Auscultation of fetal heart rates (120–160) with stethoscope or ultrasonic equipment. (Note: With ultrasonic equipment, fetal heart rate may be heard at 12 weeks.)
C. Active fetal movements are perceptible by the physician.
D. X-ray or sonogram examination showing fetal outline. X-ray not visible until 14th week or later, when bone calcification occurs.

Pseudocyesis (Pseudopregnancies)

A. The emotional control of physiological functioning that is psychological in origin; woman believes she is pregnant when she is not.
B. Clinical manifestations.
   1. Amenorrhea, breast changes, and secretion of colostrum.
   2. Enlargement of abdomen.
   3. Reports of quickening.
   4. Appears any age, but more common in older women.
C. Treatment.
   1. Uncover underlying emotional problem.
   2. Offer continued emotional support as this is important.

Physical Examination

A. Initial examination.
   1. Complete history is recorded (past pregnancies, medical history, family history).
   2. Physical examination of pelvis, breasts, and abdomen.
   3. Blood pressure, urinalysis, blood work including Rh factor, rubella titer, pap smear, slide for gonorrhea and VDRL.
   4. Diet and health instructions are given to patient.
B. Subsequent examinations are usually done once a month until the last trimester, then more frequently.
   1. Weight and blood pressure taken; urine tests for protein and sugar content made.
   2. Palpation of abdomen.
   3. Auscultation of fetal heart tones.
   4. Observation for untoward signs and symptoms.
   5. Continuing health care and instructions.
C. See Table B for pregnancy discomfort and relief measures.

Table B. Major Discomforts and Relief Measures

Discomfort	Trimester Most Prominent	Relief Measures
Nausea and vomiting	1st	Instead of three large meals daily, have five or six small, frequent meals In between meals, have couple of crackers or a piece of toast without fluid Avoid foods high in carbohydrates, with a strong odor, or fried and greasy Plan rest period after meals If nausea occurs at regular intervals when stomach is empty, plan ahead by eating 20 to 30 minutes earlier
Urinary frequency	1st and 3rd	Wear perineal pads if there is a leakage
Heartburn	2nd and 3rd	Avoid fatty, fried, and highly spiced foods Have small frequent feedings
Abdominal distress	1st, 2nd, and 3rd	Eat slowly, chew food thoroughly, take smaller helpings of food
Flatulence	2nd and 3rd	Maintain daily bowel movement Avoid gas-forming foods
Constipation	2nd and 3rd	Drink sufficient fluids Eat fruit and foods high in roughage Exercise moderately
Hemorrhoids	3rd	Apply ointments, suppositories, warm compresses Avoid constipation Rest
Insomnia	3rd	Exercise moderately to promote relaxation and fatigue Change position while sleeping
Backaches	3rd	Rest Improve posture Use a good abdominal support and wear comfortable shoes Do exercises such as squatting, sitting, and pelvic rock
Varicosities, legs and vulva	3rd	Avoid long periods of standing or sitting with legs crossed Sit or lie with feet and hips elevated Move about while standing to improve circulation Wear support hose
Edema of legs and feet	3rd	Elevate feet while sitting or lying down Avoid standing or sitting in one position for long periods
Cramps in legs	3rd	Extend cramped leg and flex ankles, pushing foot upward with toes pointed toward knee Increase calcium intake
Pain in thighs or aching of perineum	3rd	Alternate periods of sitting and standing Rest
Shortness of breath	3rd	Sit up Lie on back with arms extended above bed
Supine hypotensive syndrome	3rd	Change position to left side to relieve pressure of uterus on inferior vena cava
Vaginal discharge	3rd	Practice proper cleansing and hygiene Avoid douche unless recommended by physician Observe for signs of vaginal infection common in pregnancy

COMPLICATIONS OF PREGNANCY

Danger Signals

A. Bleeding from vagina.

B. Escape of amniotic fluid denoting premature rupture of membranes.

C. Abdominal pain.

D. Dizziness or blurring of vision.

E. Persistent headache.

F. Edema of face and fingers.

G. Persistent and severe vomiting.

H. Chills and elevated temperature.

Abortion

Definition: Abortion is the expulsion of the fetus before it is viable; abortion may be spontaneous or induced.

Categories of Abortion

A. Threatened—some loss of blood and pain without loss of products of conception.

B. Imminent—bleeding profuse, contractions severe, bearing down sensation; without intervention, products of conception will be lost.

C. Inevitable—bleeding, contractions, ruptured membranes, and cervical dilatation.

D. Incomplete—portion of products of conception remain in uterine cavity.

E. Complete—all products of conception expelled.

F. Habitual—abortion in three or more succeeding pregnancies.

G. Therapeutic—medically terminated for woman's physical or emotional health.

H. Criminal—termination of pregnancy outside medical or approved facilities.

Etiology

A. Abnormalities of fetus.

B. Abnormalities of reproductive tract.

C. Injuries—physical and emotional shocks.

D. Endocrine disturbances.

E. Acute infectious diseases.

F. Maternal diseases.

G. Psychogenic problems.

Assessment

A. Vaginal bleeding.

B. Intermittent contractions and pain which usually begin in the small of the back; abdominal cramping.

Treatment

A. Notification of physician immediately.

B. Endocrine therapy (usually progesterone if deficiency).

C. Correction of abnormalities or disturbances of reproductive tract.

D. Avoidance of stress and exertion during early pregnancy.

E. Bed rest and sedation; avoid climbing stairs and coitus until at least two weeks after bleeding stops.

F. Oxytocic drug may be given to hasten process of abortion, if it is inevitable, and to promote contraction of uterus after abortion.

G. Medication for pain if necessary.

H. Blood available for transfusion.

I. Dilatation and curettage may be necessary in an incomplete abortion.

J. Administration of RhoGAM in Rh-negative women.

K. Maintain sterile technique in all examinations and treatments.

Implementation

A. Offer emotional support and comfort; do not say, "Everything will be all right," if there is loss of the fetus.

B. Save all perineal pads and expelled tissue for examination.

C. Observe for and report signs of shock.

D. In criminal abortions, observe for serious complications such as septic shock, thrombophlebitis, and renal failure.

Habitual Abortion

Definition: Habitual abortion is the condition in which the patient has spontaneously aborted three or more consecutive times.

Etiology

A. Endocrine disturbances.
B. Blood incompatibilities.
C. Incompetent cervical os.
D. Chromosomal abnormalities.
E. Abnormalities of reproductive tract.
F. Fibromas of uterus.
G. Psychological.

Treatments

A. Hormone therapy (estrogen and progesterone) and thyroid therapy for endocrine disturbances.
B. Shirodkar procedure (internal os constricted by encircling suture which is removed when labor begins) for incompetent cervical os.
C. Surgical correction of abnormalities, if possible, and removal of fibromas.
D. Psychotherapy for psychological cause.

Hydatidiform Mole

Definition: Benign neoplasm of the chorion in which chorionic villi degenerate, become filled with a clear viscid fluid, and assume the appearance of grapelike clusters involving all or parts of the decidual lining of the uterus.

Incidence

A. Rare, occurs once in every 2000 pregnancies except in the Orient, where it is far less rare—may be due to protein deficiency in Orient.

B. Usually there is no fetus found.
C. May be a pathological ova.

Etiology

A. May be pathological ova.
B. High incidence in the Orient may be due to a protein deficiency in diet.

Assessment

A. Pregnancy appears normal at first.
B. Bleeding varies from spotting to profuse.
C. Rapid enlargement of the uterus.
D. Nausea and vomiting appear earlier; usually are more severe and last longer.
E. Severe preeclampsia may develop in the early part of the second trimester.
F. Hypertension may occur with the rapid expansion of the uterus.
G. Characteristic vesicles may be passed.

Diagnosis

A. Test for increased titer of chorionic gonadotropin. It is best to collect a 24-hour specimen for the total daily output.
B. Sonography which will give positive diagnosis in the first trimester.
C. Amniography—x-ray following injection with contrast dye.

Treatment and Implementation

A. Evacuation of uterus as soon as positive diagnosis is made (by dilatation and curettage or vacuum curettage suction).
B. Follow-up visits to physician for examination, because hydatidiform mole may lead to choriocarcinoma of uterus.
C. Observe for hemorrhage.
D. Provide emotional support for there may be fear of malignancy or patient may feel the loss of the baby.

Extrauterine (Ectopic) Pregnancy

Definition: A pregnancy that develops outside the uterus.

Process of Pregnancy

A. Although the fertilized ovum usually attaches to the uterine lining, it may become implanted at any point between the graafian follicle and the uterus.
B. Tubal pregnancy is the most common form (95 percent) but the ovum may attach to an ovary, the abdomen, or interligaments.
C. Implantation.
   1. Ovum attaches to tube and erodes into mucosa wall, as it would to the endometrial lining of the uterus.
   2. Tube increases in size and stretches.
   3. Pregnancy usually terminates during the first three months by:
     a. Spontaneous tubal abortion.
     b. Tubal rupture.
     c. Death and disintegration of products of conception within the tube.

Etiology

A. Progress of ovum through tube is delayed for some reason.
B. Tubal deformities that are either congenital or due to disease such as gonorrhea.
C. Tumors pressing against the tube.
D. Adhesions from previous surgery.
E. Tubal spasms.
F. Migration of ovum to opposite tube.

Assessment

A. Woman may or may not know she is pregnant.
B. May have history of missed periods and "spotting."
C. May have slight abdominal pain.
D. Early signs of pregnancy may be present.
E. Uterus enlarges and decidua develops due to hormonal influence.
F. Often first symptom is a sudden excruciating pain in lower abdomen.
G. May feel faint and have signs of shock as a result of hemorrhage into the peritoneal cavity.
H. May have little external bleeding.

Treatment and Implementation

A. Immediate removal of the affected tube.
B. Blood transfusions may be necessary.
C. Observe for signs of shock and give treatment for shock as necessary.
D. Provide emotional support; patient may be frightened and feel the loss of the pregnancy.

Placenta Previa

Definition: A placenta develops so that it partially or completely covers the internal os when ovum implants low in the uterus towards the cervix. Occurs once in every 150 deliveries.

Types

A. Complete—os entirely covered.
B. Partial—only part of os covered.
C. Marginal—margin overlaps os.

Etiology

A. Occurs more often in multiparas.
B. Occurs more often with increased age of woman.

Assessment

A. Painless vaginal bleeding after the seventh month without precipitating cause.
B. Bleeding may be intermittent.
C. As internal os begins to dilate, the part of placenta that overlies the os separates and leaves gaping vessels so that bleeding occurs.
D. Uterus usually remains soft and flaccid.

Diagnosis

A. History of painless bleeding begins late in pregnancy.

B. Localization of placenta by ultrasound.

C. Sterile vaginal or pelvic examinations are usually not done as part of diagnosis until adequate preparation has been made.

Treatment and Implementation

A. Immediate hospitalization.

B. Usually placed on bed rest.

C. Blood is typed and cross-matched for possible transfusion.

D. Treatment depends upon type of placenta previa, condition of woman, and viability of baby.
   1. Mechanical pressure applied to placental site by bringing down baby's head and occluding blood vessels; usually accomplished by the rupture of membranes.
   2. Delivery by cesarean section.

E. If baby is small and bleeding stops, delivery is usually postponed.

F. Count perineal pads.

G. Observe for hemorrhage.

H. Give emotional support, explain procedures, and help allay fears.

I. Carefully monitor fetal heart tones.

Abruptio Placentae

Definition: A separation of the placenta from the normal implantation site in upper segment of uterus before birth of baby. Occurs once in 500 deliveries.

Types

A. Complete separation—placenta becomes completely detached from uterine wall.

B. Partial separation—portion of placenta adheres to uterine wall.

C. External—blood escapes from the vagina.

D. Concealed—blood is retained in uterine cavity.

Etiology

A. Trauma.

B. Chronic vascular renal disease.

C. High parity.

D. Cocaine use.

E. Hypertensive disease.

Assessment

A. Vaginal bleeding accompanied by abdominal pain is chief external sign.

B. Concealed signs.
   1. Intense, cramplike uterine pain.
   2. Uterine tenderness and rigidity.
   3. Lack of alternate contraction—relaxation of uterus.
   4. Fetal heart tones indicate bradycardia or are absent.

Treatment and Implementation

A. Depends upon severity and extent of labor.

B. Treatment for blood loss and shock.
   1. Moderate bleeding—rupture membranes to hasten delivery and help control bleeding.
   2. Severe—immediate cesarean section.

C. Keep patient on bed rest.

D. Observe for signs of shock.

E. Carefully monitor contractions, fetal heart tones, and vital signs.

F. Maintain record of intake and output.

G. Nursing actions after delivery.
   1. Observe closely for hemorrhage.
   2. Carefully record intake and output; observe for anuria or oliguria. Anuria may develop as a result of acute tubular necrosis.

Hyperemesis Gravidarum

Definition: Pernicious vomiting during pregnancy.

Assessment

A. Usually develops during the first three months of pregnancy.
B. Persistent nausea and vomiting.
C. May have abdominal pain and hiccups.
D. Considerable weight loss.
E. May become severely dehydrated.
F. May have depletion of essential electrolytes because of unreplaced loss of sodium chloride and potassium.
G. Metabolic acidosis may develop.
H. Blood urea nitrogen increases.

Causes

A. May be caused by the addition of new substances to the body system such as a toxicity or maladjustment of the maternal metabolism.
B. Psychological disturbances may be the underlying cause, or it may be a combination of psychological and toxic factors.

Treatment and Implementation

A. Aimed at reducing the severity of symptoms.
B. Give frequent small feedings in small amounts every two hours; dry foods preferred.
C. Avoid giving spicy or fried foods.
D. Give antiemetics as prescribed along with a tranquilizer or a sedative.
E. If vomiting is persistent:
   1. Patient is usually hospitalized.
   2. Dehydration and starvation is treated by administration of parenteral fluids.
   3. Rest and sedatives are prescribed.
F. Use tact and understanding of the patient's problem.
G. Carefully record intake and output; maintain IVs.
H. Observe for acetone odor on breath.
I. Reduce stimuli and restrict visitors if necessary.
J. Monitor fetal heart tones.

Pregnancy Induced Hypertension

Definition: A group of conditions (formerly called toxemias) that usually appear after the 20th week. The major symptoms, hypertension, proteinuria, and edema, most frequently occur in young or elderly primigravidas, women with deficient diets, multiple pregnancies, polyhydramnios, and in long-standing diabetes.

Preeclampsia

Definition: An acute, hypertensive disease peculiar to pregnancy that may be mild or severe.

Assessment

A. Usually appears after the 24th week.
B. Major symptoms are hypertension, proteinuria, and edema, which may appear separately or together. Two of the three symptoms are usually needed for diagnosis.
C. Mild.
   1. Blood pressure above 140/90 or systolic 30 mmHg and diastolic 15 mmHg above normal.
   2. Edema.
   3. Proteinuria (1 gm in 24 hours).
D. Severe.
   1. Blood pressure 160/110 or above, or systolic 50 mmHg above normal.
   2. Massive edema with excessive weight gain.
   3. Proteinuria (5 gm or more in 24 hours).
   4. Oliguria (400 ml or less in 24 hours).
   5. Visual disturbances.
   6. Headache.

Treatment and Implementation

A. Mild.
   1. Patient usually remains at home.
   2. Extra rest is prescribed.
   3. Adequate fluid intake is maintained.
   4. Highly salted food is avoided.
   5. Weight is checked daily.
   6. Physician should be notified if further symptoms occur.

7. Treatment aimed at preventing further increase in disease.
B. Severe.
1. Antihypertensive, sedative drugs.
2. Increased protein diet; sodium intake is usually not restricted, but patient should avoid use of highly salted foods. (Note: This is a recent trend. The use of low-sodium diet may still be included on NCLEX.)
3. Efforts to increase diuresis (diuretics not given).
4. Maintain bed rest.
5. Administer sedatives if ordered.
6. Observe for signs of central nervous system irritability and hyperactivity.
7. Take and record vital signs.
8. Measure and record intake and output.
9. Check weight at same time each day.
10. Test urine for protein; record.
11. Limit visitors.
12. Maintain seizure precautions.
13. Provide diversional activities.

Eclampsia

Definition: A more severe form of toxemia usually accompanied by convulsions and even coma.

Assessment

A. Severe edema with tremendous weight gain.
B. Scanty urine.
C. Urine may contain red blood cells, varied casts, and protein.
D. Blood pressure may rise to 200/110.
E. There may be visual disturbances, blurring, or even blindness caused by edema of the retina.
F. Severe epigastric pain.
G. Convulsions (both tonic and clonic).
H. Labor may begin; fetus may be born prematurely or die.

Treatment and Implementation

A. Prevent and/or control convulsions.

1. Quiet, dark room.
2. Have mouth gag available.
3. Have suction available.
4. Use padded side-rails.
B. Promote diuresis; measure and record intake and output.
C. Take and record vital signs.
D. Provide oxygen as necessary.
E. Maintain IV; give fluid if ordered.
F. Monitor fetal heart tones.
G. Observe carefully for anuria and convulsions after delivery.
H. See Appendix 1 for drugs normally used during toxemia.

Polyhydramnios

Definition: An excessive amount of amniotic fluid. Usual normal amount is 500–1000 ml. In polyhydramnios there is over 2000 ml, which is excessive.

Etiology

A. Actual cause is unknown. Occurs frequently in:
1. Fetal malformations.
2. Diabetes.
3. Erythroblastosis.
4. Multiple pregnancies.
5. Toxemias.
B. Diagnosis usually made through clinical observation of the greatly enlarged uterus.

Assessment

A. Related to pressure of the enlarged uterus or adjacent organs.
B. Edema of the lower extremities.
C. General abdominal discomfort.
D. Occasional shortness of breath.

Treatment

A. Amniocentesis offers only temporary relief.
B. Delivery.

Fetal Demise (Death)

Assessment

A. Cessation of fetal movement.

B. Absence of fetal heart tones.

C. Failure of uterine growth.

D. Low urinary estriol.

E. Negative pregnancy test that may remain positive for a few weeks due to elevated human chorionic gonadotropin.

F. X-ray (overlapping of skull bones).

G. Uterus feels smaller.

Treatment and Implementation

A. Labor usually begins spontaneously a few weeks after death of fetus.

B. Labor may be induced if it does not occur spontaneously.

C. Watch patient closely for signs of disseminated intravascular disease from prolonged retention of the dead fetus.

D. Provide emotional support to parents.

E. Guide parents in planning future pregnancies.

F. Observe for hemorrhage.

G. Observe for psychological disturbances; refer for psychological counseling.

High Risk Pregnancy

Definition: A pregnancy that refers to any condition that may interfere with the normal development or delivery of the fetus; or, to any preexisting maternal disease that may increase the risk of pregnancy.

Predisposing Factors

A. Age of under 17, of over 35, or unmarried.

B. Parity (having borne five or more pregnancies).

C. Previous conditions.
   1. Previous infant death, premature birth, or congenital malformations.
   2. History of cardiac disease, diabetes, renal disease, or other maternal conditions.
   3. Difficulty in conceiving.
   4. Narcotic or alcohol addiction.
   5. Less than a year since last pregnancy.
   6. Rh incompatibility and sensitization.

Conditions Leading to High Risk

A. During pregnancy.
   1. Infection.
   2. Bleeding.
   3. Pregnancy induced hypertension.

B. Intrapartum conditions.
   1. Premature labor.
   2. Abnormal fetal positions.
   3. Premature rupture membranes.

Cardiovascular Disease

Characteristics

A. Classification.
   1. Class I—no alteration of activity.
   2. Class II—slight limitation of activity.
   3. Class III—marked limitations of activity.
   4. Class IV—symptoms present at rest.

B. Pregnancy expands plasma volume, increasing cardiac output and load on heart.

C. Most deaths are caused by cardiac failure, when blood volume is at a maximum in the last weeks of the second trimester.

D. Heart failure occurs infrequently in labor.

E. Over age 35, there is an increase in the incidence of heart failure and death.

Management During Pregnancy

A. With proper management, mortality is minimal.

B. Patient should avoid acute infections, especially respiratory infections.

C. Patient should rest frequently.

D. Strenuous activities such as rigorous excercise, stair climbing, heavy cleaning, and straining should be avoided.

E. Patients in Class III and over may be hospitalized before labor for controlled rest and diet.

F. If patient decompensates or has distress symptoms with exertion, she should remain on bed rest or in a chair.

G. Salt intake may or may not be restricted. Diuretics may be prescribed if signs of heart failure occur. The use of highly salted foods is discouraged.

H. Iron supplement is important.

I. Digitalis treatment when indicated.

J. Emotional stress should be avoided.

Management During Labor

A. Observe for signs that cardiac function is deteriorating such as pulse rate over 110 or respiratory rate over 24.

B. Relieve pain and anxiety.

C. Vaginal delivery usually preferred.

D. Patient may decompensate in early postpartum phase.

Implementation

A. Educate about special needs and danger signals during pregnancy and postpartum.

B. Be alert for signs of decompensation during pregnancy, especially in the second trimester.

C. During labor:
1. Check vital signs every 15 minutes or more often as needed.
2. Keep patient in bed and preferably lying on one side or in semirecumbent position.
3. Administer oxygen as necessary.
4. Provide calm atmosphere and emotional support to alleviate fears.
5. Administer pain medications as ordered to reduce discomfort during labor.
6. Be alert for signs of impending heart failure.
7. Monitor fetal heart tones.

D. Careful observation during postpartum period.

E. Counsel during postpartum to have help at home and planned rest periods.

Diabetes

Definition: A chronic metabolic disease caused by a disturbance in normal insulin production.

Characteristics

A. White's Classifications.
1. Class A—abnormal glucose tolerance test, indicative of latent or gestational diabetes.
2. Class B—diabetes beginning after age 20.
3. Class C—diabetes at ages 10 to 19 years, or beginning in adolescence after age 10.
4. Class D—diabetes of long duration, or onset in childhood before the age of ten.
5. Class E—evidence of pelvic vascular disease.
6. Class F—nephropathy, including capillary glomerulosclerosis.
7. Class R—malignant retinopathy.

B. Implications of diabetes in pregnancy
1. Diabetes is more difficult to control.
2. There is a tendency to develop acidosis.
3. Patient is prone to infection.
4. Toxemia, hemorrhage, and polyhydramnios are more likely to develop.
5. Latent diabetes may develop into full-blown diabetes.
6. Insulin requirements are increased.
7. Premature delivery is more frequent.
8. Infant may be overgrown but have functions related to gestational age rather than size.
9. Infant is subject to hypoglycemia, hyperbilirubinemia, respiratory distress syndrome, and congenital anomalies.
10. Stillborn and neonatal mortality rates are high, but may be reduced by proper management and control of diabetes.

Implementation

A. Reinforce teaching the effects of diabetes on the mother and fetus during pregnancy and the reasons for frequent testing of blood sugar and urine for sugar and acetone.

B. Emphasize good nutrition and health practices.

C. If hospitalized:
1. Maintain insulin on regular schedule.
2. Test urine for sugar and acetone as ordered.
3. Provide adequate diabetic diet as prescribed by physician.
4. Provide for diversion.
5. Monitor fetal heart tone.
6. Check vital signs, especially blood pressure qid and prn.
7. Weigh daily at the same time.
8. Keep accurate records of intake and output.
9. Provide support and explanations to help allay fears and reduce anxiety.
10. Watch for symptoms of hyperglycemia or hypoglycemia.

D. In labor:
1. Same as above.
2. Carefully regulate insulin and provide IV glucose as labor depletes glycogen.

E. Postpartum.
1. Close observation for insulin reaction—precipitous drop in insulin requirements usual—hypoglycemic shock may occur.
2. Close observation for early signs of infection.
3. Close observation for postpartum hemorrhage.

Anemia

A. Caused by caused by iron deficiency.
B. Symptoms.
1. Patient tires easily and looks pale.
2. Hemoglobin values are usually checked routinely in antepartum care.
3. Usually treated by diet and an iron supplement.

Urinary Tract Infection

A. Usually occurs after the fourth month or in early postpartum—affects 10 percent of maternity patients.

B. Causes.
1. Pressure on ureters and bladder.
2. Hormonal effects on tone of ureters and bladder.
3. Displacement of bladder.
C. Kidneys as well as ureters may be involved.
D. Symptoms.
1. Frequent micturition.
2. Paroxysms—pain in kidney.
3. Fever and chills.
4. Catheterized urine specimen contains bacteria and pus.
E. Treatment.
1. Bed rest.
2. High fluid intake.
3. Antibiotic treatments.
4. Urinary antispasmodics and analgesics.

Infectious Diseases

Rubella

A. In the first trimester rubella may cause congenital anomalies.
B. Vaccine is available and should be given to children from age one to puberty or to the mother in early postpartum, while she is still hospitalized. (Vaccine should not be given if pregnancy is suspected.)
C. Titer should be checked before pregnancy or on first prenatal visit.

Acute Infectious Diseases

A. Diseases such as influenza, scarlet fever, toxoplasmosis, and cytomegalovirus may be transmitted to the fetus.
B. Diseases may cause abortions or malformations in early pregnancy, premature labor or infant death in later pregnancy.

Sexually Transmitted Diseases

Syphilis

A. May cause abortion or premature labor.

B. Infection is passed to the fetus after the fourth month of pregnancy as congenital syphilis.

C. VDRL test for syphilis on first prenatal visit. (May repeat at a later date, as disease may be acquired after initial visit.)

D. Treatment—during pregnancy, procaine penicillin G with 2% aluminum monostearate, IM, normally in divided doses.

E. All cases of syphilis must be reported to health authorities for treatment of contacts.

Gonorrhea

A. Common contagious bacterial disease.

B. Incidence has been steadily rising as a result of increase in premarital sex.

C. May be mildly symptomatic in women and may persist unsuspected.

D. May cause salpingitis after third month if left untreated.

E. Slide for gonorrhea usually done on first prenatal visit.

F. Important to treat sexual partner, as patient may become reinfected.

G. Infection may be transmitted to baby's eyes during delivery, causing blindness.

H. Soon after birth all newborns have prophylactic treatment of one percent silver nitrate or an antibiotic preparation, usually erythromycin.

I. Treatment—same as for syphilis. Other antibiotics may be used for sensitivity to penicillin.

Herpes simplex type 2—genital herpes

A. Involves external genitalia, vagina, cervix.

B. Development and draining of painful vesicles.

C. Treatment—symptomatic—no specific cure identified. Safe use of Acyclovir has not been established for pregnant women.

D. Virus is lethal to fetus if inoculated during vaginal delivery. Usual mode of delivery is C-section.

For more information on Sexually Transmitted Dieseases, see Chapter 2, Nursing Through the Life Cycle.

Adolescent Pregnancy

A. Risk to mother and fetus is increased.
1. Crisis of pregnancy compounds the crises of adolescence related to physical, emotional, social development.
2. Patient may be unwed, which may cause additional problems.
3. Physical development may not be complete.
4. High incidence of prematurity and toxemia.

B. Nursing care.
1. Encourage early antepartum care.
2. Provide health instruction on pregnancy, nutrition, and hygiene.
3. Observe frequently for complications.
4. Provide emotional support and counseling.

LABOR AND DELIVERY

Definition of Terms

A. Labor is the process by which the products of conception are expelled from the body.

B. Delivery refers to the actual birth.

C. Adaptive processes.
1. During latter months of pregnancy, the fetus adapts to the maternal uterus enabling it to occupy the smallest space possible.
2. The term attitude refers to the posture the fetus assumes in utero.
3. Fetal lie is the relationship of the long axis of the baby to the long axis of the mother.

Presentation

A. A term used to describe that part of the fetus which lies closest to the true pelvis.

B. Cephalic—presentation of any part of fetal head—occurs 95–97 percent of births.
1. May be vertex, face, or brow.

2. Vertex most common and most favorable for delivery. Head is sharply flexed in the pelvis with chin near chest.

C. Breech—presentation of buttocks or lower extremities.
   1. Types.
      a. Complete or full—buttocks and feet present (baby in squatting position).
      b. Frank—buttocks only present, or legs are extended against anterior trunk with feet touching face.
      c. Incomplete—one or both feet or knees presenting, footling single or double, or knee presentation.
   2. May rotate to cephalic during pregnancy but possibility lessens as gestation nears term.
   3. May be rotated by physician but usually returns to breech position.

Position

A. A term used to describe the relationship of the fetal presenting part to the maternal bony pelvis.

B. Position is determined by locating the presenting part in relationship to the pelvis.

C. Woman's pelvis is divided into four imaginary quadrants (right anterior, right posterior, left anterior, and left posterior).

D. Most common positions (abbreviations usually used).
   1. LOA (left occiput anterior)—occiput on left side of maternal pelvis and toward front, face down, favorable for delivery.
   2. LOP (left occiput posterior)—occiput on left side of maternal pelvis and toward rear or face up.
      a. Usually causes back pain during labor.
      b. May slow the progress of labor.
      c. Usually rotates before delivery to anterior position.
      d. May be rotated in delivery room by physician.
   3. ROA (right occiput anterior)—occiput on right of maternal pelvis, toward front, face down, favorable for delivery.

4. ROP (right occiput posterior)—occiput on right side of maternal pelvis, face up. Same problems as LOP.

E. Means of assessing fetal position during labor.
   1. Leopold's maneuver—method of abdominal palpation to determine information about the fetus such as presentation, engagement, and rough estimate of fetal size.
   2. Vaginal examination.
   3. Rectal examination (rarely done at this time).

Engagement—Lightening

A. Largest diameter of presenting part has passed into the inlet of the maternal pelvis. Usually takes place two weeks before labor in primiparas, but not until labor in multiparas.

B. May be assessed by Leopold's maneuver or vaginal or rectal examination.

Station

A. Degree to which presenting part has descended into pelvis is determined by the station (the relationship between the presenting part and the ischial spines).

B. Assessed by vaginal or rectal examination.

C. Measured in numerical terms.
   1. At level of spines: 0 station.
   2. Above level of spines: –1, –2, –3 cm.
   3. Below level of spines: +1, +2, +3 cm.

D. Other terms used to denote station.
   1. High—presenting part not engaged.
   2. Floating—presenting part freely movable in inlet of pelvis.
   3. Dipping—entering pelvis.
   4. Fixed—no longer movable in inlet but not engaged.
   5. Engaged—biparietal plane passed through pelvic inlet.

Premonitory Signs of Labor

Physical Signs of Impending Labor

A. Premonitory signs—physiologic changes that take place the last several weeks of pregnancy, indicating that labor is near.

B. Lightening—descent of the uterus downward and forward which takes place as the presenting part descends into the pelvis.
1. Time in which it takes place varies from a few weeks to a few days before labor. In multigravida, it may occur during labor.
2. Sensations.
a. Relief of pressure on diaphragm, and breathing is easier.
b. Increased pelvic pressure leading to leg cramps, frequent micturition, and pressure on rectum.

C. Braxton Hicks contractions.
1. May become quite regular but do not effectively dilate cervix, thus often called false labor.
2. True labor has regular, painful contractions that continue with walking.
3. Usually are more pronounced at night.
4. May play a part in ripening the cervix.

D. Decrease in weight—there is usually a decrease in water retention due to hormonal influences.

E. Cervical changes—cervix usually becomes softer, shorter, and somewhat dilated. May be dilated 1 to 2 cm by the time labor begins.

F. Bloody show.
1. Tenacious mucous vaginal discharge, usually pinkish or streaked with blood, which is expelled from the cervix as it shortens and begins to dilate.
2. Labor usually begins within 24 to 48 hours.

G. Rupture of membranes.
1. May break any time before labor or during labor. Occasionally, they remain intact and are ruptured by the physician during labor (amniotomy).
2. May gush or trickle.
3. Patient usually advised to come to the hospital as labor may begin within 24 hours.

4. If labor does not begin spontaneously, it is induced to avoid intrauterine infections.

Implementation

A. Test vaginal secretions for alkalinity with Nitrozine paper—normal vaginal pH is acidic.
B. Keep patient on bed rest if ordered.
C. Watch for signs of infection.
D. Watch for signs of labor.
E. Watch for prolapse of cord.
F. Monitor fetal heart rate regularly.
G. Observe amniotic fluid for foul odor or signs of fetal distress (meconium staining); record time, amount, color, and odor, if present.

Assessment of Fetal Maturity and Placental Function

Studies for Delivery Capability

A. Estriol excretion.
1. Estriol level increases as the fetus grows and decreases when growth ceases.
2. Provides guide to placental functioning and fetal well-being.

B. Amniocentesis.
1. Introduction of a needle through the abdominal and uterine wall and into the amniotic cavity to withdraw fluid for examination.
2. Preparation of patient.
a. Have patient empty bladder.
b. Take fetal heart rate.
c. Make patient comfortable.
d. Explain and give reassurance that the procedure will not harm the baby.
e. Prepare abdomen with antiseptic solution.
f. Have necessary equipment available.
3. Indications:
a. Sex of baby.
b. Certain congenital defects such as mongolism.

c. State of fetus affected by Rh isoimmunization.

d. Fetal maturity.

C. Creatinine level.
1. Progressive rise as fetus approaches term.
2. Excreted in fetal urine; measures increasing muscle mass.
3. Values of 2 mg/100 ml amniotic fluid correlates with gestation of about 36 weeks.

D. Bilirubin level.
1. Amount of bilirubin in amniotic fluid decreases near term of normal fetus. Usually disappears during the last month of gestation.
2. Exposure of blood sample to light for a period greater than a few seconds invalidates the test.

E. Cytological studies—percentage of lipid globules present gives indication of fetal age (sebaceous glands of fetus begin to function and shed near term).

F. Sonography.
1. Used to measure biparietal diameter of the fetal skull after 16 weeks (should be measured weekly when growth retardation is suspected).
2. Can determine position of placenta.

G. Ultrasound.
1. A diagnostic test of intermittent high frequency sound waves that reflect off tissues according to varying densities.
2. Advantages—technique is noninvasive, nondamaging and painless.
3. Purpose—to differentiate tissue mass and do serial studies. Determines fetal movements, breathing, heart valve capability.
4. Results—detects placental location (amniocentesis, placenta previa), gestational age, presence of twins, fetal growth.
5. Procedure—patient instructed to have a full bladder; test takes 20–30 minutes to complete. Near term, anticipate supine hypotension, nausea and vertigo.

H. Oxytocin challenge test—Stress test.
1. Test designed to measure the fetus reaction to uterine contractions.

2. Performed on high risk patients (postmature diabetes).
3. If placental flow is normal, fetus remains oxygenated during uterine contractions.
4. Placental insufficiency produces characteristic late deceleration pattern during contraction. Fetal bradycardia is less than 120 beats per minute.
5. Procedure. ❖ **PROCEDURE** ❖
   a. Measured dosage of oxytocin by infusion pump; piggybacked into main IV line.
   b. Dosage is increased q 15–20 minutes until patient has three uterine contractions in ten minutes.
   c. Oxytocin is then discontinued.
   d. Patient is monitored with external fetal monitor. Baseline fetal heart rate is established prior to beginning the test.
   e. Apply external monitor and obtain baseline fetal heart rates.
   f. Observe for complications.
      (1) Fetal heart rate below 120.
      (2) Sustained uterine contractions.
      (3) Supine hypotensive syndrome.

Induction of Labor

Oxytocin Infusion

A. Indications for use.
1. Patient overdue (two weeks or more); placental functions reduced.
2. Severe preeclampsia.
3. Diabetes.
4. Premature rupture of membranes (should deliver within 24 hours).
5. Uncontrolled bleeding.
6. Rh sensitization (rising titer).
7. Excessive size of fetus.

B. Prerequisites for successful induction.
1. Fetal maturity.
2. Cervix amenable to induction (at times, patient may be induced for several days consecutively with rest at night to ripen

cervix, if it is desirable to deliver fetus because of complications).
3. Normal cephalopelvic proportions.
4. Fetal head engaged.
C. Danger signals.
1. Prolonged uterine contractions (over 90 seconds with less than 30 seconds rest period between). Safety intervention is to turn off IV—check with RN.
2. Sustained uterine contractions.
3. Fetal heart tones above 160 or below 120; change in heart rhythm.
4. Hemorrhage and shock.
5. Elevated blood pressure.
6. Abruptio placentae.

Buccal Pitocin

A. Usually oxytocin placed in parabuccal space at approximately 30-minute intervals until labor is well established.
B. May be promptly removed should adverse reactions occur.

Implementation

A. Nursing procedures.
1. Maintain patient on bed rest.
2. Provide normal care of patient in labor.
3. Monitor IV fluids.
4. Auscultate fetal heart tones.
B. Emergency measures.
1. Check patient frequently.
2. *Immediately* report abnormalities in contractions or fetal heart tones.

Process of Labor and Delivery

Theories Pertaining to Cause of Labor

A. Absolute causes unknown.
B. Alterations in hormonal balance of estrogen and progesterone increases uterine contractility.
C. Degeneration of the placenta so that it no longer provides necessary elements to fetus.

D. Overdistention of uterus incites a stimulus which triggers release of oxytocin and initiates contractions.
E. High levels of prostaglandins near term may stimulate uterine contractions.
F. It may be a combination of several of these physiological occurrences that produce the type of contraction necessary for true labor.

Forces that Produce Labor

A. Muscular contractions originate primarily in muscles of uterus and secondarily in abdominal muscles.
B. Uterine muscles contract during first stages and bring about effacement and dilatation of the cervix.
C. Abdominal muscles come into play after complete cervical dilatation and help to expel the baby.

Duration of Labor

A. Varies according to individual.
B. Average.
1. Primipara—up to 18 hours; some may be shorter, others longer.
2. Multipara—up to eight hours; some may be shorter, others longer.
C. Length of labor depends on:
1. Effectiveness of contractions.
2. Amount of resistance baby must overcome to adapt to the pelvis.
3. Stretching ability of soft tissue.
4. Preparation and relaxation of mother (fear and anxiety can retard progress).

Uterine Contractions

A. Characteristics.
1. Involuntary—cannot be controlled by will of mother.
2. Intermittent—periods of relaxation between contractions. Intervals allow mother to rest and also allow adequate circulation of uterine blood vessels and oxygenation of fetus.

3. Regular—occur once true labor is established.
4. Discomfort in back (usually starts low and radiates around to abdomen).
5. Increase in discomfort from intensity, frequency, and duration of contractions as labor progresses.

B. Methods for monitoring contractions.
  1. Place finger lightly on the fundus of the uterus (the most contractile portion), and relate what you feel in your fingers to seconds and minutes on a clock. Uterus becomes firm, then hardens, and then decreases in hardness.
  2. Use electronic monitoring device; external (less accurate) or internal (catheter inserted into uterine cavity which measures internal pressures); relay information to a graph.

C. Contractions are monitored for frequency, duration, and intensity.
  1. Frequency—measure by timing contractions from the beginning of one contraction to the beginning of next.
  2. Duration—measure time at beginning of contraction to beginning of period of decreasing intensity. Cannot be measured exactly by feeling with the hand.
  3. Intensity—measure by internal fetal monitoring device; cannot be measured by feeling.
  4. Contractions may be described as mild, moderate, or intense.

D. Purpose of contractions.
  1. To propel presenting part forward.
  2. To bring about effacement and dilatation of the cervix.

Effacement and Dilatation

A. Effacement—process by which cervical canal is progressively shortened to a stage of complete obliteration. Progresses from a structure of 1 to 2 cm in length to almost complete obliteration.

B. Dilatation—process by which external os enlarges from a few millimeters to approximately 10 cm.

C. All that remains of the cervix after effacement and dilatation is a paper-thin circular opening about 10 cm in diameter.

D. Effacement and dilatation may be measured by vaginal or rectal examination.

Changes in the Uterus

A. Uterus usually becomes differentiated in two distinct portions as labor progresses.
  1. Upper portion is contractile and becomes thicker.
  2. Lower portion is passive, becomes thinner and more expanded.

B. Boundary between the two segments is termed the *physiologic retraction ring*.

False Labor

A. Signs.
  1. Irregular contractions.
  2. Contractions that may cause discomfort.
  3. Discomfort is usually located in abdomen.
  4. Labor usually does not intensify.
  5. Discomfort may be relieved by walking.
  6. Contractions do not bring about appreciable changes in cervix.

B. Sometimes difficult to differentiate false labor from true labor until woman is observed for several hours in the hospital.

Signs of Imminent Delivery

A. Increase in bloody show.
B. Nausea, vomiting, and shaking.
C. Pressure on rectum, and woman feels the urge to push (involuntary bearing down).
D. Deep grunting sound from woman.
E. Woman states she is ready to deliver.
F. Bulging of the perineum.

Four Stages of Labor

Stage One

A. Stage one begins with first true labor contraction and ends with complete cervical dilatation.

B. Latent (effacement) phase.
1. Begins with onset of regular contraction pattern.
2. Dilatation 0 to 1 to 4 cm; membranes usually intact.
3. Contractions are mild and become well established.
4. Contractions are 5 to 15 minutes apart and last about 30 to 45 seconds.
5. Cervix thins.
6. Usually some bloody show.
7. Station is anywhere from –2 cm to +1 cm in multipara; at 0 in primigravida.
8. Woman may be quite comfortable, talkative, alert, and cheerful.
9. Woman has lots of energy and feels she can cope with labor.

C. Active (dilatation) phase.
1. Dilatation 4 to 8 cm.
2. Dilatation is more rapid.
3. Contractions are 3 to 5 minutes apart, last 30 to 45 seconds.
4. Increase in bloody show.
5. Station varies from –1 to 0 cm.
6. Woman becomes tired and less talkative and shows lack of energy.
7. Woman may need coaching on breathing techniques, or analgesia (anesthesia).

D. Transitional phase.
1. Dilatation 8 to 10 cm.
2. Contractions are intense and close (2 to 3 minutes apart, lasting 50 to 90 seconds).
3. Station +3 or +4 cm.
4. Copious bloody show.
5. Desire to bear down or defecate.
6. Membranes may rupture spontaneously if they have not done so previously; physician may rupture them artificially.

7. Woman's attention and feelings are inner-directed; she feels exhausted and no longer able to cope.
8. Signs of restlessness, shaking, nausea, vomiting, trembling, burping, or crying may be present.

Stage Two

A. Stage two begins with complete dilatation and ends with birth of baby.

B. Mechanism of labor and delivery.
1. Sequence of movements of presenting part through birth canal. Head usually enters transverse and must rotate LOA or ROA for birth.
2. Engagement—head enters pelvis.
3. Descent—movement which occurs simultaneously with passage of head through pelvis.
4. Flexion—occurs as head descends and meets with resistance. In extreme flexion the smallest diameter of the head presents.
5. Internal rotation—head usually enters with long diameter conforming to long diameter of inlet (usually transverse position) and must be rotated before it can emerge from outlet (head rotates so that smallest diameter presents to conform to pelvis).
6. Extension—follows internal rotation. The head, which is flexed as it passes through birth canal, must extend for birth.
7. External rotation or restitution—soon after birth, the head rotates to either mother's right or left side (fetal position before birth).
8. Expulsion—with delivery of shoulders, rest of body is expelled spontaneously.

C. Stage of expulsion.
1. Expulsion brought about by contractions of uterine and abdominal muscles.
2. Contractions are every 2 to 3 minutes, last 60 to 90 seconds.

Stage Three

A. Stage three, or placental stage, begins with birth and ends with delivery of placenta.
B. Phase of placental separation.
   1. Usually takes place with next few contractions after birth.
   2. Usually begins at center but may begin at edges.
   3. Some bleeding usually accompanies separation of placenta.
C. Phase of expulsion.
   1. May be expulsed spontaneously by mother, but is usually expressed manually by the physician after separation is complete.
   2. Mechanisms.
      a. Schultze (most common)—placenta is inverted on itself, and the shiny fetal surface appears; 80 percent separate in center.
      b. Duncan—descends sideways and the maternal surface appears.

Stage Four

A. Stage four begins with delivery of placenta and ends when postpartum condition of the mother is stabilized.
B. First hour after birth is critical.

NURSING CARE IN LABOR AND DELIVERY

Phase One: Latent Phase (Dilatation to 3–4 cm)

Admission

A. Details of care vary from hospital to hospital.
B. Check vital signs—temperature, pulse, respirations, and blood pressure.
C. Check fetal heart tones (FHT).
D. Determine intactness of membranes.

E. Give prep (perineal shave) and enema (if ordered by physician).
F. See that appropriate forms are completed.
G. Encourage woman to void; check urine for sugar and acetone.
H. Determine frequency, intensity (mild, moderate, severe), and duration of contractions.
I. Determine amount and character of bloody show.
J. Determine amount of cervical dilatation and effacement.
K. Keep bell cord within easy reach.

After Admission

A. Maintain bed rest if membranes have ruptured. (In some hospitals the patient may be allowed out of bed with ruptured membranes if the baby's head is well engaged and the patient is otherwise alright.)
B. Note frequency, duration, and strength of contraction every 30 minutes or prn.
C. Auscultate FHT every 15 minutes or prn.
D. Check blood pressure every 30 minutes or prn.
E. Check vital signs once per shift or more often if needed.
F. Periodic vaginal examination as indicated.
G. Observe for ruptured membranes and take FHT immediately if membranes rupture.
H. Reinforce breathing techniques or teach breathing techniques if woman has had no classes.
I. Keep family informed of progress.
J. Encourage the presence of patient's husband or a significant other person.
K. Provide support based upon woman's knowledge of the labor process.
L. Reduce stimuli if woman wants to rest.
M. Start IV if ordered; usually NPO.

Phase Two: Active Phase (Dilatation 3–4 to 8 cm)

A. Encourage breathing techniques.

B. Maintain IV fluids.

C. Encourage voiding.

D. Auscultate FHT every 15 minutes or prn.

E. Monitor contractions.

F. Take blood pressure every 30 minutes or prn.

G. Periodic vaginal examination to determine progress.

H. Observe amount and character of show.

I. Urge mother to stay off back, avoid supine hypotensive syndrome, and to lie on side.

J. Administer medications as ordered. Tranquilizing drugs may be given in early labor, but analgesics are not usually given until labor is well established.

K. Assist with anesthesia, if given, and monitor blood pressure and FHT.

L. Continue giving patient support and information.

Transitional Phase (Dilatation 8 to 10 cm)

A. Continue with care listed above.

B. Explain progress to patient and encourage her to continue with breathing and relaxing techniques.

C. Discourage bearing down efforts until dilatation is complete.

D. Encourage deep ventilation prior to and after each contraction.

E. Monitor contractions lightly with fingers as abdomen is sensitive.

F. Accept irritable behavior and aggression; continue supportive care.

G. Help patient to push when ready.

H. Observe for signs of imminent delivery, and transfer patient to delivery room when ready.

Fetal Assessment

Fetal Distress

A. Signs.

1. FHT above 160 or below 120 beats per minute.

2. Meconium-stained fluid (during hypoxia, bowel peristalsis increases, and meconium is likely to be passed).

3. Fetal hyperactivity.

B. Immediate nursing interventions.

1. Turn patient to left side; if no improvement, turn to right side. This procedure relieves pressure on umbilical cord during contractions and pressure of uterus on the inferior vena cava.

2. Report findings immediately.

Vena Caval Syndrome (Supine Hypotensive Syndrome)

Assessment

A. Assess for shocklike symptoms that occur when venous return to the heart is impaired by weight of gravid uterus causing partial occlusion of the vena cava.

B. Check for risk factors—multiple pregnancies, obesity, polyhydramnios.

C. Shocklike symptoms caused by reduced cardiac output.

1. Hypotension.

2. Tachycardia.

3. Sweating.

4. Nausea and vomiting.

5. Air hunger.

D. Fetal distress; caused by reduced flow of blood to placenta from reduced cardiac output.

Implementation

A. Assist mother to turn to left side (using a wedge pillow) to shift weight of fetus off inferior vena cava.

B. Provide oxygen with tight mask if recovery is not immediate after positioning.

C. Monitor fetal heart rate to determine fetal status.

Signs of Complications of Labor

A. Fetal distress.

B. Fetal tachycardia—persistent fetal heart rate above 160 or an increase in the basal rate, 20 to 30 beats/minute.

C. Fetal bradycardia—below 120 beats/minute.

D. Absent, minimal, or irregular FHT.

E. Foul smelling or meconium-stained amniotic fluid.

F. Fetal hyperactivity.

G. Elevated temperature in woman.

H. Dehydration.

I. Hemorrhage.

J. Inadequate uterine relaxation between contractions—over 90 seconds and less than 30 seconds between contractions.

K. Anxiety in woman.

L. Distended bladder.

Fetal Monitoring

Characteristics

A. Two types of electronic fetal monitoring.
  1. External (EFM) and internal (IFM)
  2. Continuous data readout of fetal heart rate and uterine contraction pattern.

B. Ultrasound transducer picks up motion of the fetal heart valves—provides external recording.

C. Pressure sensitive button placed over the uterine fundus—external monitoring of uterine contraction.

D. Heart rate sounds and uterine contractions are translated into electrical impulses reproduced on a printout strip on the fetal monitor.

E. Types of external fetal monitors.
  1. Abdominal electrodes—elicits fetal and maternal heart rates.
  2. Phonotransducer—picks up fetal heart tones.
  3. Ultrasonic transducer—picks up fetal heart tones.
  4. Tocotransducer—monitors uterine activity.

Implementation ❖ Procedure ❖

A. Preparation.
  1. Explain procedure to patient.
  2. Plug tocotransducer into monitor inlet.
  3. Turn monitor on and press printout button.
  4. Move stylus to zero. The printout is divided into two parts. The uterine activity waveform is found on the right side.

B. Placement of fetal monitor.
  1. Place tocotransducer over uterine fundus. (Locate fundus using Leopold's maneuvers.)
  2. Position the tocotransducer in place with belt. (Powder belt first to avoid irritating skin.)
  3. When patient is free of contractions, tighten belt until stylus on monitor moves to the 50 mmHg mark on the right side of the printout.
  4. Turn control knob until stylus moves back to the 10 mmHg mark.
  5. Test tocotransducer by pressing down on transducer. If the baseline recorder moves, tocotransducer is functioning properly.
  6. Record frequency and duration of contractions as required by hospital policy.

C. Monitoring uterine activity.
  1. *Normal fetal heart rate*: 120 to 160 beats/minute; determine baseline.
  2. *Early deceleration*: 10 to 20 beat drop in rate usually within normal range of 120 to 160 beats/minute.
  3. *Late deceleration*: decrease in fetal heart rate of 10 to 20 beats/minute—usually indicates fetal distress.
  4. *Variable deceleration*: no uniformity in pattern—may indicate cord compression.
  5. *Loss of beat-to-beat variation*: baseline is smooth—may be serious sign of fetal anoxia.
  6. *Bradycardia:* any persistent drop of 20 beats below baseline or under 120 beats/minute—may be indicative of fetal distress.

7. *Tachycardia:* increase of 10 percent over baseline or over 160 beats/minute—an ominous sign—requires intervention stat due to fetal hypoxia.

Nursing Responsibilities

Delivery Room Care

A. Transfer woman carefully from bed to delivery table; place in lithotomy position.

B. Pad stirrups to avoid pressure to popliteal veins and pressure areas. Gently raise both legs simultaneously into stirrups to avoid ligament strain. Adjust stirrups and drape patient.

C. Provide patient with handles to pull on as she pushes.

D. Cleanse vulva and perineum using sterile technique, commonly referred to as perineal "wash down."

E. Auscultate FHT every five minutes or after each push—transient fetal bradycardia not unusual due to head compression.

F. Check blood pressure and pulse every 15 minutes prn.

G. Allow baby's father in room, and position him at the head of the delivery table.

H. Encourage patient and keep her informed of advancement of baby.

I. Encourage patient to take a deep breath before beginning to push with each contraction and to sustain push as long as possible (long pushes are preferable to frequent short pushes).

Postpartum Care

A. Palpate fundus every 15 minutes and prn for first hour.

B. Massage fundus gently if it is not firm.

C. Check TPR and blood pressure upon admission; check blood pressure every 15 minutes and prn for first hour.

D. Encourage voiding and measure amount.

E. Check lochia for color, consistency, and amount.

F. Inspect perineum and episiotomy for signs of bleeding, unusual redness, or swelling.

G. Weigh pads if unusual bleeding noted.

H. Allow mother and baby's father the privacy to talk.

I. Encourage mother to rest.

J. Provide medications for pain as ordered and needed.

K. Chart all pertinent data.

L. Maintain intake and output the first 24 hours or until patient is voiding a sufficient quantity.

OPERATIVE OBSTETRICS

Obstetrical Procedures

Episiotomy

A. An incision made into the perineum during delivery to facilitate the birth process.

B. Types.
   1. Midline—incision from the posterior margin of the vaginal opening directly back to the anal sphincter.
      a. Healing is less painful.
      b. Incision is easy to repair.
   2. Mediolateral—incision made at 45-degree angle to either side of the vaginal opening.
      a. Healing process is quite painful.
      b. Incision is harder to repair.

C. Purpose.
   1. To spare the muscles of perineal floor from undue stretching and tearing (lacerations).
   2. To prevent the prolonged pressure of the baby's head on perineum.

D. Method.
   1. Generally done during contraction when the baby's head pushes against perineum and stretches it.
   2. Blunt scissors are used.

3. Mother is usually given an anesthetic (regional, local, or inhalation).

Forceps Delivery

A. Baby is extracted from the birth canal by the physician with the use of a specially designed instrument; cervix must be fully dilated.
B. Types.
   1. Low forceps—presenting part on perineal floor.
   2. Mid forceps—presenting part below or at the level of the ischial spine.
   3. High forceps—presenting part not engaged (rarely if ever used today).
C. Indications.
   1. Fetal distress.
   2. Poor progress of fetus through the birth canal.
   3. Failure of the head to rotate.
   4. Maternal disease or exhaustion.
   5. Woman unable to push (as with regional anesthesia, caudal or epidural).
D. Complications.
   1. Lacerations of the vagina or the cervix; there may be oozing or hemorrhage.
   2. Rupture of the uterus.
   3. Intracranial hemorrhage and brain damage to the fetus.
   4. Facial paralysis of the fetus.

Cesarean Delivery

A. Incision into abdominal wall and uterus to enable the delivery of an infant.
B. Types.
   1. Classical—vertical incision through the abdominal wall and into the anterior wall of the uterus.
   2. Low segment transverse—transverse incision made into lower uterine segment after abdomen has been opened.
      a. Incision made into part of uterus where there is less uterine activity and blood loss is minimal.
      b. Less incidence of adhesions and intestinal obstruction.

3. Cesarean hysterectomy—abdomen and uterus are opened, baby and placenta are removed, and then the hysterectomy is performed. Conditions indicating hysterectomy.
      a. Presence of diseased tissue or fibroids.
      b. An abnormal pap smear.
      c. Ruptured uterus.
      d. Uncontrolled hemorrhage, abruptio placentae, uterine atony, or other disorders.
C. Indications.
   1. Fetal distress unrelieved by other measures.
   2. Uterine dysfunction.
   3. Certain cases of placenta previa and premature separation of placenta.
   4. Prolapsed cord.
   5. Diabetes or certain cases of toxemia.
   6. Cephalopelvic disproportion.
   7. Malpresentations such as transverse lie.

Nursing Management

Postoperative Care

A. Take vital signs (blood pressure, pulse and respiration) every 15 minutes for 2 to 3 hours.
B. Observe site of incision for bleeding every 15 minutes for 2 to 3 hours.
C. Palpate fundus for location and tone every 15 minutes for 2 to 3 hours.
D. Check lochia for amount and color every 15 minutes for 2 to 3 hours.
E. Reinforce abdominal dressing as necessary.
F. Observe drainage from Foley catheter (amount, color, pressure of blood, and other aspects).
G. Check level of consciousness.
H. Measure intake and output.
I. Assist patient to deep breathe, cough, and turn.
J. Change perineal pad as needed.
K. Reassure the patient that the delivery is over, and give her information regarding the condi-

tion of the baby. (If something is wrong with the baby, usually the physician will first discuss this with parents.)

L. Help ambulate patient (usually the first post-partum day).

M. Give stool softener as ordered and needed.

N. Encourage patient to talk about delivery and baby.

O. Reinforce physician's teaching about care at home.
1. Planned rest periods.
2. Avoidance of heavy lifting for four to six weeks.
3. Signs of infection.
4. Care of the breasts.
5. Avoidance of constipation.
6. Nutritive diet.
7. Arrangements for postpartum checkup in four to six weeks.

COMPLICATIONS OF LABOR AND DELIVERY

Dystocia

Definition: Prolonged and difficult labor and delivery, i.e., it extends for 24 hours or more after the onset of regular contractions.

Classification

A. Dystocia may be classified in several ways; although the divisions are artificial, they are useful in looking at the processes involved.
1. Dysfunctions of powers or forces with respect to the uterus and abdominal muscles.
2. Abnormalities of the passengers (the fetus and placenta).
3. Abnormalities of the passages (bony and soft tissue).
4. May be a combination of two or more dysfunctions and abnormalities.

B. Characteristics.
1. True labor begins but fails to progress.
2. Dystocia may occur during latent or active phase of labor.
3. It is important to look at the rate of progress as well as the overall length of labor, i.e., is the patient slowly progressing or is she arrested at one spot?

Dysfunctional Labor

A. Prolonged latent phase—time required to dilate cervix to 4 cm is prolonged; primipara over 20 hours, multipara 14 hours.
1. Causes or contributing condition.
   a. Oversedation.
   b. "Unripe" cervix.
   c. False labor.
   d. Uterine dysfunction or abnormalities.
2. Treatment and nursing care.
   a. Encourage rest as woman is usually exhausted.
   b. Narcotic agent is given to stop labor and promote rest.
   c. Vaginal examination is made to determine fetal position and station.
   d. X-ray pelvimetry is made to determine the disorder.
   e. Performance of amniotomy (artificial rupture of membranes) if conditions are favorable for vaginal delivery.
   f. Oxytocin is given as a stimulant.
   g. Labor usually progresses normally after rest and stimulation by oxytocin.

B. Prolonged active phase—dilatation slower than 1.2 cm per hour for primigravida; dilatation slower than 1.5 cm per hour for multigravida.
1. Causes.
   a. Cephalopelvic disproportion (CPD).
   b. Malpositions.
   c. Excessive sedation or anesthesia.
   d. Unknown causes.
2. Treatment and nursing care.
   a. Usually no active treatment is given if dilatation is regular unless labor will be

prolonged over 24 hours; then give supportive therapy.

    b. Cesarean section may be indicated in CPD or for labor over 24 hours.

C. Arrested phase—lack of progress.

  1. Causes.

    a. CPD.

    b. Malposition of the fetus.

    c. Excessive sedation and anesthesia.

    d. Uterine abnormalities.

  2. Medical treatment and nursing care.

    a. Vaginal examination to determine position and station of fetus.

    b. X-ray pelvimetry to determine CPD.

    c. Provide rest for exhausted patient.

    d. Cautious use of oxytocic stimulation if malposition, CPD, and other abnormalities are ruled out.

    e. Cesarean section if appropriate.

D. Complications of prolonged labor (see Tables C and D).

Other Causes of Dysfunctional Labor

A. Tetanic uterine contractions—contraction lasting over 90 seconds. May lead to fetal asphyxia or uterine rupture.

B. Precipitate delivery—labor of three hours or less duration. May lead to injury of mother and fetus due to trauma.

C. Rupture of the uterus—splitting of the uterine wall accompanied by extrusion of all or part of uterine contents into the abdominal cavity. Baby usually dies and mortality rate in mothers is high due to blood loss.

  1. Signs of rupture.

    a. Acute abdominal pain and tenderness.

    b. Presenting part no longer felt through cervix.

    c. Feeling in patient that something has happened inside her.

    d. Cessation of labor pains (no contractions).

    e. Bleeding usually internal; may be some external bleeding.

    f. Signs of shock (pale appearance, pulse weak and rapid, air hunger, and exhaustion).

  2. Treatment.

    a. Laparotomy to remove fetus.

    b. Hysterectomy, although uterus may be sutured and left in.

    c. Blood transfusions.

    d. Antibiotics to prevent infection from traumatized tissues.

Implementation

A. Promote rest (darken room, reduce noise level).

B. Position patient for comfort.

C. Give patient a back rub.

D. Provide clean linen and gown; allow patient to bathe or shower if permissible.

E. Promote oral hygiene.

F. Give patient reassurance and support.

G. Explain procedures to the patient.

H. Let mother express feelings and emotions freely.

I. Watch for signs of exhaustion, dehydration, and acidosis.

J. Monitor vital signs.

K. Monitor FHT.

L. Monitor contractions for frequency, intensity, and duration.

M. Watch for signs of excessive bleeding and fetal distress.

N. Administer medications as ordered.

Abnormalities of the Passengers

Abnormal Presentations and Positions

A. Occiput posterior position.

  1. Usually prolongs labor because baby must rotate a longer distance (35 degrees or more) to reach symphysis pubis.

  2. Possible results.

    a. Persistent occiput posterior (head does not rotate).

    b. Deep transverse arrest (head arrested in transverse position).

3. Treatment.
   a. Head usually rotates itself with contraction.
   b. Rotation may be done by physician manually or with forceps.
B. Breech prolongs labor because soft tissue does not aid cervical dilatation as well as the fetal skull.
C. Face presentation is rare; results in increased prenatal mortality.
   1. Chin must rotate so it lies under symphysis pubis for delivery.
   2. If baby is delivered vaginally, the face is usually edematous and bruised, with marked molding.
   3. Cesarean section is indicated if face does not rotate.
D. Transverse lie.
   1. Long axis of fetus at right angles to long axis of mother.
   2. Spontaneous version may occur. Cesarean section is the usual method of delivery.

Excessive Size of Fetus

A. Disproportion between the size of the fetus and the size of the pelvis when fetus is ten pounds or over.
B. Head is usually large and less moldable.
C. Size of shoulders may also complicate delivery.
D. Causes.
   1. Multiparity—birth weight may progress with each pregnancy.
   2. Maternal diabetes.
E. Size of fetus may be determined by sonography and x-ray.
F. Treatment.
   1. Vaginal delivery if disproportion is not too great. Usually there are fetal injuries—brachial plexus, dislocated shoulder.
   2. Cesarean section indicated if proportion too great.
G. Fetal abnormalities.
   1. Hydrocephalus.
   2. Tumors.

Abnormalities of Passage

Cephalopelvic Disproportion

A. Disproportion may be in inlet, mid-pelvis, or outlet.
B. Pelvis is considered contracted if it is reduced enough in size to interfere with normal delivery.
C. Trial labor may be done in borderline cases.
D. Determined by x-ray of pelvis (pelvimetry).
E. Cesarean delivery is the usual method of treatment.

Other Complications of Labor

Premature Labor and Delivery

A. Occurs when pregnancy terminates after the period of viability but usually before the end of the 36th week.
B. Betamethasone or some other drug is administered to the mother to hasten fetal maturity by stimulating development of lecithin when membranes are ruptured and premature labor cannot be arrested.

Prolonged Pregnancy

A. Pregnancy of over 42 weeks gestation.
B. Complications.
   1. Amniotic fluid decreases and vernix caseosa disappears; infant's skin appears dry and cracked.
   2. Infant may weigh less.
   3. Chronic hypoxia due to placental dysfunction.
   4. Infant may pass meconium due to hypoxia.
C. Determination of gestational age usually made to ascertain actual duration of pregnancy by means of estriol studies, sonography.
D. Oxytocin challenge test to determine fetus's ability to tolerate labor.
E. Labor stimulated with oxytocin.
F. Cesarean section if induction contraindicated.

Table C. Complications and Signs of Distress in the Mother

Complication	Signs of Distress	Possible Nursing Care
Infection	Elevated temperature and pulse	Maintain sterile technique while doing vaginals Keep vaginals to a minimum Administer antibiotics as ordered
Exhaustion	Loss of emotional stability Lack of cooperation	Provide supportive therapy and comfort measures to promote relaxation and relieve tension Encourage rest Administer sedation as ordered
Dehydration	Dry tongue and skin Concentrated urine Acetonuria	Monitor IV fluids Place a wet cloth to the patient's mouth Make a frequent check of bladder elimination

Table D. Complications and Signs of Distress in the Fetus

Complication	Signs of Distress	Possible Nursing Care
Asphyxia	Irregular heart rate Heart rate above 160 or below 120 Passage of meconium in the vertex position	Administer oxygen to the mother Constantly observe and monitor FHT Check for prolapse of the cord Prepare delivery room equipment for possible resuscitation of the baby at birth
Generalized infection	Irregular heart rate Heart rate above 160 or below 120	Administer antibiotics to the mother Keep vaginals to a minimum Follow same care (except cord check) as asphyxia

Prolapsed Umbilical Cord

A. Descent of prolapsed cord through cervical canal along side of the presenting part; may even protrude from the vagina.

B. Causes.
1. Ruptured membranes before engagement.
2. Abnormal presentations.
3. Premature infant—presenting part does not fill the birth canal and allow for more space.
4. Polyhydramnios.

C. Symptoms.
1. Abnormal fetal heart pattern.
2. Cord may be palpated or seen on vaginal examination.

D. Complications—cord is compressed between presenting part and pelvis resulting in fetal asphyxia.

E. Immediate treatment and nursing care.

1. Presenting part elevated off umbilical cord.
2. Place patient in knee-chest position or exaggerated Trendelenburg's position.
3. Maintain patient on absolute bed rest.
4. Cover exposed cord with sterile dressing if available.
5. Auscultate FHT every two minutes.
6. Stay with patient and offer support.
7. Cesarean section is prescribed if cervix is not dilated enough to allow the baby to pass. Haste is important.

Emergency Delivery

Definition: Rapid or sudden labor of less than three hours duration, from onset of cervical changes to delivery of infant.

Implementation

ASSISTING WITH DELIVERY

A. Never leave mother unattended during this time and never hold baby back. Have another employee notify the physician and bring the emergency delivery pack to room.

B. Reassure mother that you will remain with her and provide care until the physician arrives.

C. Put on sterile gloves if they are available and if there is time.

D. Break membranes immediately if they have not done so spontaneously.

E. Have mother pant rather than push to avoid rapid delivery of the head.

F. With a clean or sterile towel (if available), support baby's head with one hand applying gentle pressure to the head to prevent sudden expulsion and undue stretching of the perineum or brain damage to the infant.

G. If cord is draped around baby's neck, with free hand gently slip it over head.

H. If bulb syringe is available, gently suction baby's mouth and wipe blood and mucus from mouth and nose with towel, if available.

I. Shoulders are usually born spontaneously after external rotation. If shoulders do not deliver spontaneously, ask mother to bear down to deliver them.

J. Support the baby's body as it is delivered.

K. All manipulation should be gentle to avoid injury to mother and baby.

CARE AFTER DELIVERY

A. After delivery, hold baby securely over hand and arm with head in a dependent position to allow fluid and mucus to drain.

B. If baby does not cry spontaneously, gently rub baby's back or the soles of baby's feet.

C. Dry baby to prevent heat loss.

D. Place the baby on the mother's abdomen to provide warmth. The weight on the uterus will help it to contract.

E. Palpate mother's abdomen to make sure uterus is contracting.

F. Watch for signs of placental separation.

G. Support placenta in your hand after it is expelled.

H. Clamp the cord after it stops pulsating if clamp or ties are available. Cord need not be cut; there will be no bleeding from the placental surface.

I. Wrap the baby in a blanket.

J. Put the baby to the mother's breast. This reassures the mother that the baby is all right and helps contract the uterus.

K. Check the uterus after delivery of the placenta. Make sure the uterus is contracting.

L. Keep an accurate record of the time of birth and other pertinent data.

M. If baby is delivered unassisted, in bed, before the nurse arrives (precipitate delivery), the nurse should immediately:
   1. Check the baby to make sure breathing is established.
   2. Check the mother for excessive bleeding.

N. Comfort mother.

OBSTETRIC ANESTHESIA AND ANALGESIA

Anesthesia During Labor

General Characteristics

A. No optimum anesthesia exists.

B. Ranks fourth as the cause of maternal death; other three include hemorrhage, infection, and toxemia.

C. History and physical should be obtained before administering anesthesia.

D. Should be NPO before use.

E. Should be administered by trained personnel.

F. Choice of the type of anesthesia in obstetrics is determined by the specific patient situation and condition.

General Inhalation Anesthetics

A. Advantages.
1. May anesthetize patient rapidly.
2. Depth and duration can be controlled.
3. Effects are rapidly dissipated in both infant and mother.
4. These anesthetics cause uterine relaxation when necessary for manipulation.
5. Inhalation anesthetics are preferred in hypovolemic patient and in patient whose condition prohibits the use of regional anesthetics.

B. Disadvantages.
1. Woman is not awake for delivery.
2. Brings about respiratory depression of the infant.
3. May cause emesis and aspiration in the patient.
4. May be flammable.

C. Common types.
1. Ether—seldom used.
2. Halothane—used in selected cases only.
3. Penthrane—analgesia and light anesthesia; it may be used as a self-administered analgesic.
4. Thiopental (Pentothal)—IV anesthesia usually used as an adjunct in induction of anesthesia.
5. Trichloroethylene (Trilene) is often used in self-administration by mask during labor and delivery. Never leave patient alone when she is using self-administered anesthesia.

Regional Analgesia and Anesthesia

A. Drugs given to block the nerves carrying sensation from the uterus to the pelvic region.

B. Some common agents used.
1. Novocaine.
2. Xylocaine.
3. Pontocaine.
4. Carbocaine.

C. Vasoconstrictor agents (e.g., epinephrine) are commonly used in conjunction with regional anesthetics.

1. Slow absorption and prolong the effect of the anesthetic.
2. Prevent secondary hypotension.

D. Two principle types of regional anesthesia are nerve root block and peripheral nerve block.

E. Nerve root block.
1. General considerations.
   a. Usually relieves pain completely if administered properly.
   b. Provides vasodilation below the anesthetic level which may be responsible for a decrease in blood pressure.
   c. Does not depress the respiratory center, and therefore does not harm the patient unless hypotension in the patient is severe enough to interfere with uterine flow.
   d. May cause postspinal headache.
   e. Contraindicated in a hypovolemic patient or in the case of central nervous system disease.
   f. Drug may impede labor if given too early (before 5 to 6 cm dilatation).
   g. Special skill of anesthesiologist required to administer drug.
   h. Infant may need forceps delivery because the mother usually cannot push effectively due to level of anesthesia.
2. Types.
   a. Caudal.
   b. Lumbar epidural.
   c. Saddle block.
   d. Spinal.
3. Nursing Care.
   a. Assist patient to a knee-chest position over a bolster or on her left side with head flexed and knees drawn up.
   b. Monitor blood pressure every 3 to 5 minutes until stabilized; then every 30 minutes or prn.
   c. Auscultate FHT.
   d. If hypotension does occur:
      (1) Turn mother to one side, off the inferior vena cava.
      (2) Give oxygen by mask.
      (3) Notify physician.
   e. Watch for signs of dizziness, nausea, faintness, and palpitations.

F. Peripheral nerve block.
   1. General considerations.
      a. May be done by attending physician (does not require an anesthesiologist).
      b. Local injection of anesthetic to block peripheral nerve endings.
      c. Less effective in relieving pain than nerve root block.
      d. May cause transient bradycardia in fetus, possibly due to rapid absorption of the drug into fetal circulation.
      e. Usually there are no maternal side effects.
      f. Needle guide such as Iowa trumpet usually used.
   2. Types.
      a. Paracervical.
      b. Pudendal block.
   3. Nursing management.
      a. Measure vital signs.
      b. Auscultate FHT.
      c. Assist patient to a dorsal recumbent position.
      d. Offer reassurance and support during procedure.
      e. Auscultate FHT every 5 minutes for 15 to 30 minutes and every 30 minutes thereafter.

POSTPARTUM PERIOD

Physiology of the Puerperium

Definition: Period of four to six weeks following delivery in which the reproductive organs return to the normal, nonpregnant state.

Uterus

A. Involution—rapid diminution in the size of the uterus as it returns to the nonpregnant state.
B. Lochia—discharge from the uterus, consisting of blood from vessels of the placental site and debris from the decidua.
C. Placental site—blood vessels of the placenta become thrombosed or compressed.

Cervix and Vagina

A. Cervix—remains soft and flabby the first few days, and the internal os closes.
B. Vagina—usually smooth walled after delivery. Rugae begin to appear when ovarian function returns and estrogen is produced.

Ovarian Function and Menstruation

A. Ovarian function depends upon the rapidity in which the pituitary function is restored.
B. Menstruation—usually returns in four to six weeks in a nonlactating mother.

Urinary Tract

A. May be edematous and contain areas of submucosal hemorrhage due to trauma.
B. May have urine retention due to loss of elasticity and tone and loss of sensation from trauma.
C. Diuresis—mechanism by which excess body fluid is excreted after delivery. Usually begins within the first 12 hours after delivery.

Breasts

A. Proliferation of glandular tissue during pregnancy due to hormonal stimulation.
B. Usually secrete colostrum the first two to three days postpartum.
C. Pituitary stimulates secretion of prolactin after placental hormones inhibiting the pituitary are no longer present.
D. In three to four days breasts become firm, distended, tender, and warm (engorged), indicating production of milk.
E. Milk usually produced in response to sucking of infant.

Blood

A. White blood cells increase during labor and early postpartum period and then return to normal in a few days.

B. Decrease in hemoglobin, red blood cells, and hematocrit usually return to normal in one week.

C. Elevated fibrinogen levels usually return to normal within one week.

Nursing Care of the Postpartum Patient

Assessment

A. Check vital signs every 8 hours and prn—decreased blood pressure, increased pulse, or temperature over 100.4°F.

B. Check fundus for consistency and level. Massage fundus lightly with fingers if it is relaxed.

C. Check lochia for amount, color, consistency, and odor. Watch for hemorrhage.

D. Check perineum for redness, discoloration, or swelling.

E. Check episiotomy for healing; check for drainage.

F. Check breasts for engorgement and cracking of nipples.

G. Check emotional status of new mother for depression or withdrawal.

H. Check for problems with flatus or elimination and bladder or bowel retention.

Other Nursing Considerations

A. Administer drug to inhibit lactation (if ordered and if it has not been given immediately postpartum).

B. Apply breast binder or bra after 24 hours for 7 days.

C. Administer RhoGAM as ordered within 72 hours postpartum to Rh-negative mother who is not sensitized.

D. Maintain intake and output until patient is voiding a sufficient quantity without difficulty; usually the first two voids are measured.

E. Teach mother perineal care and give perineal care until mother is able to do so.

F. Encourage ambulation as soon as ordered and as patient is able to tolerate it, giving assistance the first time.

G. Encourage verbalization of mother's feelings about labor, delivery, and baby.

H. Give perineal light as ordered.

I. Give warm sitz baths as ordered.

Emotional Aspects of Postpartum Care

The Maternal Role as Outlined by Rubin

A. Taking-in phase (the first two to three days).
   1. Mother's primary needs are her own; she needs sleep and food.
   2. Mother usually is quite talkative. She wants to discuss labor and delivery. She is assimilating and appropriating experience.
   3. Nurse can listen and help the patient interpret events to make them more meaningful.
   4. Important for nurse to interpret future mother-child relationship at this important time.

B. Taking-hold phase (from the third postpartum day to about two weeks); the phase varies with each individual.
   1. Emphasis is on present.
   2. Mother is impatient and wants to get on with reorganization of her life.
   3. Less passive and more in control of situation.
   4. Begins to take hold of "mothering" task, which takes priority over all else.
   5. May be unsure of herself. It is important for nurse to reassure mother and not make her feel awkward.
   6. Success at this time is important for the future mother-child relationship.
   7. Important time for nurse to share information without making mother feel inadequate.

C. Letting-go phase—usually occurs after discharge from hospital.

1. Mother may feel a deep loss over the separation of the baby from part of her body; she may grieve over this loss.
2. Mother may be caught in dependent-independent role; she wants to feel safe and secure yet wants to make decisions. Teenage mother needs special consideration because of the conflicts taking place within her as part of adolescence.
3. Mother may feel resentful and guilty about the baby causing so much work.
4. May have difficulty adjusting to the mothering role.
5. May feel conflict between the roles of mother and wife.
6. May feel upset and depressed at times (postpartum blues).
7. May be concerned about her other children.
8. Important for nurse to encourage vocalization of these feelings and give positive reassurance.

Role of the Baby's Father

A. Encourage the father to hold and care for the baby.
B. Encourage parents to take turns caring for the baby at night so that the mother can rest once she is home.
C. Explain the feelings that are normal to the mother at this time, e.g., tension, fatigue, insecurity in the mothering role, and her need to be dependent and independent.

Breast Feeding

Nursing Management

A. Conditions of breast when breast feeding should be postponed.
   1. Tenderness and hardness.
   2. Pain and redness.
   3. Cracking of nipples.
B. Feeding procedure.

1. Put baby to breast as soon as mother's and baby's conditions are stable (on the delivery table in some hospitals, or within 6 to 12 hours in others).
2. Have mother assume comfortable position sitting or lying down.
3. Guide baby to breast.
4. Gently press breast away from baby's nose.
5. Usually the baby is nursed two to three minutes at each breast the first time, gradually building to ten minutes or so on each side in later feedings.
6. Release suction by inserting a finger into the baby's mouth (the breast will become sore if baby is pulled off it).
7. Burp baby after feeding at each breast.
8. Stay with mother each time she nurses until she feels secure or confident with the baby and feedings.
9. Baby should not nurse more than every two hours.

C. Instruction.
   1. Explain to the mother that the baby's stool will be yellow and watery; that it is not uncommon for nursing infants to have three to four stools each day or even one for each feeding.
   2. Dry the breast after feeding and allow it to air occasionally, especially if it is sore.
   3. Use general hygiene and wash the breast once daily.
   4. Encourage the mother to eat a well-balanced diet and drink 3000 ml of fluid daily.
   5. Explain to the mother that she may offer sterile water but not formula to the baby between feedings. (The baby will not be hungry if given formula then and will not nurse well later.)
   6. Formula may be given at feeding time, or the mother may express milk manually and put it in a bottle if she plans to be away during feeding time.
   7. Breasts may leak between feedings or during coitus. Place a washcloth or pad in brassiere.
   8. Uterine cramping may occur the first few days after delivery while nursing as oxy-

tocin stimulation causes the uterus to contract.

9. Medications or drugs should be avoided unless specified by the physician (drugs are passed to infant through breast milk).
10. Some foods such as cabbage or onions may alter the taste of milk or cause gas in the infant.
11. Birth control pills are usually avoided while nursing as they decrease milk production and are passed to the infant in the milk.

CLINICAL PROBLEMS IN PUERPERIUM

Postpartum Hemorrhage

Definition: A blood loss of 500 ml or more during or after delivery.

Causes

A. Lacerations of the cervix or of the high vaginal walls, with oozing from blood vessels.
B. Retained placental tissue or incomplete separation of the placenta. This is the most frequent cause of late postpartum hemorrhage. (May occur from 12 to 21 days after delivery.)

Assessment

A. Uterine atony.
   1. Boggy, relaxed uterus.
   2. Dark bleeding.
   3. Passage of clots.
B. Lacerations.
   1. Firm fundus.
   2. Oozing of bright red blood.
C. Retained placental tissue.
   1. Boggy, relaxed uterus.
   2. Dark bleeding.
D. Shock.
   1. Air hunger (difficulty in breathing).

2. Restlessness.
3. Weak rapid pulse.
4. Rapid respirations.
5. Decrease in blood pressure.

Treatment and Implementation

A. Recognize abnormal bleeding and determine source.
B. Monitor intravenous solutions, blood, or volume expanders.
C. Administer oxytocin if uterus is boggy.
D. Assist with laceration repair.
E. Assist with removal of retained placental tissue.
F. Prevent infection.
G. Hysterectomy may be indicated if bleeding cannot be controlled.
H. Check for clotting defect.
I. Monitor vital signs every 15 minutes or until stable.
J. Palpate fundus every 15 minutes or prn while bleeding continues; then every 2 to 4 hours.
K. Gently massage fundus until firm. Be careful not to overmassage.
L. Weigh pads and linen.
M. Provide for warmth.
N. Measure intake and output.

Puerperal Infection

Definition: An infection in genitalia as a consequence of abortion or labor and delivery.

Causes

A. Organisms that were introduced during labor and delivery.
B. Bacteria normally present in vaginal tract.

Predisposing factors

A. Weakened resistance due to prolonged labor and dehydration.

B. Traumatic delivery.

C. Excessive vaginal examinations during labor.

D. Premature rupture of membranes.

E. Excessive blood loss.

F. Anemia.

G. Intrauterine manipulation.

H. Retained placental fragments.

Assessment

A. Elevated temperature of 100.4°F or more.

B. Discomfort in the abdomen and tenderness.

C. Burning on urination.

D. Foul-smelling lochia or discharge; decreased amount.

E. Pelvic pain.

F. Chills.

G. Rapid pulse.

H. Malaise.

Endometritis

Definition: An inflammation of the lining of the uterus.

General Considerations

A. Most frequent site of infection.

B. Uterus may be boggy, relaxed, and tender.

C. If untreated, may spread through lymphatic system to whole body causing septicemia.

Treatment and Implementation

A. Antibiotics.

B. May have pelvic examination.

C. Establish adequate drainage of uterus.

D. Monitor IV fluids if ordered.

E. Encourage fluid intake (3000–4000 ml) if not contraindicated.

F. Administer medications as ordered.

G. Provide high-calorie nutritive diet.

H. Place patient in Fowler's or semi-Fowler's position as ordered. Position of patient may impede extension of infection from moving upward in pelvis.

I. Provide emotional support to mother, who is usually in isolation and unable to see baby.

Thrombophlebitis

Definition: Development of a thrombi at placental site which becomes infected, causing inflammation of the deep pelvic veins. Thrombophlebitis may be confined to blood vessels in uterine wall, or it may extend to ovarian, hypogastric, or femoral veins. Femoral thrombophlebitis, commonly called "milk leg," may originate in a leg vein.

Assessment

A. Discomfort in abdomen and pelvis.

B. Tenderness localized on one side of the pelvis.

C. Femoral symptoms usually do not appear until the second week or later.
1. Edema and pain in affected leg.
2. Chills and fever.

Treatment and Implementation

A. Administer antibiotics until temperature stable.

B. Give anticoagulants.

C. Provide bed rest and diversion.

D. Apply warm compresses as ordered (for 15 to 20 minutes). Now considered controversial.

E. Bed cradle—keep bed clothes off leg.

F. Antiembolic stockings.

G. Elevate affected leg.

H. Never massage leg and teach patient not to do so.

I. Teach patient to watch for signs of excessive bleeding.

J. Allow patient to express fears and concerns.

K. Watch for signs of pulmonary embolism.

Cystitis and Pyelitis

Definition: Cystitis is an inflammation of the bladder; pyelitis is an inflammation of the renal pelvis.

Assessment

A. Usually begin several days into the postpartum.
B. Suprapubic or perineal discomfort.
C. Frequent urination.
D. Burning sensation on urination.
E. Elevated temperature.
F. Urine contains pus, bacteria, and red blood cells on microscopic examination.
G. Pain in flank area.

Treatment and Implementation

A. Observe patient closely postpartum for full bladder or residual urine.
   1. Palpate bladder for distention.
   2. Palpate fundus (full bladder displaces fundus upward and to the sides).
B. Institute measures to help patient void.
C. Insert catheter as ordered, using sterile technique.
D. Force fluids.
E. Administer drugs as ordered: antibacterials, antispasmodics.
F. Obtain urine specimens for microscopic examination.
G. Provide emotional support to patient, and allow her to express feelings about her illness and the baby.

Mastitis

Definition: An infection in breast tissue due to invading organisms, usually staphylococcus.

Causes

A. Infected hands of mother or attendants.
B. Bacteria normally present in lactiferous glands.
C. Fissure in nipples.
D. Bruising of breast tissue.
E. Stasis of milk or overdistention may injure tissue, but does not cause infection in itself
F. Infected baby.

Assessment

A. Chills.
B. Fever 103°F or above.
C. Elevated pulse rate.
D. Lobe may become hard to the touch, red, and painful.
E. May progress to abscess if untreated.

Treatment and Implementation

A. Administer medications as ordered.
B. Apply ice pack as ordered.
C. Make sure mother is wearing snug-fitting, supportive brassiere.
D. Teach mother to empty breast if nursing is to be continued.
E. Wash hands before touching patient's breast.
F. Teach mother careful handwashing and care of the breast.
G. May require incision and drainage if abscess develops.
H. Some physicians recommend breast feeding be stopped; others favor discontinuance with artificial removal of milk for a few days.

NEWBORN

Immediate Care of the Newborn

Principles of Maintenance

A. Always handle newborn with sterile gloves until after the first bath (CDC guidelines). Universal precautions essential to observe as newborn may have HIV positive mother.

Table E. Apgar Scoring

Sign	0	1	2
Heart tone	Absent	Slow (less than 100)	Over 100
Respiratory effort	Absent	Slow, irregular	Good, crying
Muscle tone	Flaccid	Some flexion of extremities	Active motion
Reflex irritability	No response	Cry	Vigorous cry
Color	Blue, pale	Body pink, extremities blue	Completely pink

B. Maintain body temperature.
  1. Place infant in heated incubator or crib with radiant heat.
  2. Wipe off fluid, mucus, and excessive vernix.
  3. Avoid excessive exposure.
  4. Wrap infant in warm blankets.
  5. Transfer to the nursery as soon as possible, after parents have seen and held infant.

C. Maintain respiration.
  1. Place infant on side, in modified Trendelenburg's position, to facilitate drainage of mucus.
  2. Suction mucus as needed with bulb or suction catheter attached to mucus trap.
  3. Provide oxygen as needed.

D. Prevent infection.
  1. Eye care—apply two drops of one percent silver nitrate in conjunctival sacs. Flush eyes with water in about two minutes; or, apply antibiotic ointment to prevent eye infection in the infant. Mother may be infected with gonorrhea or chlamydia.
  2. Cord care—use sterile gauze to cover.
  3. Carry out proper hand washing before receiving baby or wear sterile gloves.

General Observations

A. Apgar scoring, one and five minutes (see Table E); based on the scoring method developed by Virginia Apgar.
B. Congenital malformations.
C. Umbilical cord—two arteries and one vein.
D. Meconium staining—skin, nails.

E. Abnormal cry or no cry.
F. Injuries caused by birth trauma—dislocated shoulder, edema of scalp, lacerations.
G. Respiratory—nasal flaring, retractions, expiratory grunt.
H. Neurological status—reflexes, tremors, and twitching.

Implementation

A. Clamp the cord if so requested by the physician; should be clamped one inch from the base or left longer if the mother is Rh negative (in case of possible blood exchange).
B. Identify the baby with bands.
C. Show the baby to the parents and allow them to hold the infant with help (if not contraindicated).
D. Observe the mother's reactions to baby.
E. Transfer the baby to the admitting nursery with appropriate data.

Care in the Nursery

A. Care at admission and during the first 12 hours.
  1. Check rectal temperature.
  2. Weigh and measure—total length and head circumference.
  3. Place in heated crib.
  4. Check respiratory rates every hour for four to five hours and prn.
  5. Check for nasal flaring, retractions, expiratory grunt, breath sounds.

6. Check apical pulse every hour for two to three hours; watch for above 180 or below 100.
7. Keep bulb syringe available and suction as needed.
8. Administer vitamin K as ordered.
9. Bathe and dress baby when his or her temperature is stable.
10. Place in an open crib when baby's temperature is stable.
11. Administer feeding as ordered; usually water is given every four to six hours.
12. Assess baby for congenital defects.

B. Routine nursing care.
 1. Assessment.
    a. Observe for jaundice—check general skin color, blanching, sclera of the eyes.
    b. Check for respiratory difficulty—mucus, flaring of nostrils, grunting, and other signs.
    c. Note tremors, twitching, muscle tone, and reflexes.
    d. Take baby's temperature each shift.
    e. Check baby's weight daily.
    f. Note amount voided and number of stools.
    g. Check for signs of infection on the skin and cord.
 2. Apply alcohol to cord daily prn.
 3. Circumcision care.
    a. Observe for bleeding.
    b. Change petroleum gauze as necessary.
    c. Keep area clean to prevent infection.
 4. Check to see if the test for phenylketonuria has been done.
 5. Provide for nutrition and hydration.
 6. Teach mother how to hold and burp the baby.
 7. Use proper hand-washing between babies to prevent spreading infection.
 8. Isolate babies with known or suspected infections.
 9. Be sure that the mother understands the doctor's orders regarding care of the infant before she goes home and plans follow-up visits to the physician.

Physical Characteristics

Respiratory Status

A. Infant's respiratory system must function immediately after loss of placental function; adequate maturation at birth is necessary.
B. Normal respiration is about 30–40; over 60 or below 30 may indicate a problem. Respiration may be slightly elevated during crying episodes or shortly afterwards.

Circulatory Status

A. Ductus arteriosus, ductus venosus, and foramen ovale should close (may not be complete for one or two days).
B. Peripheral circulation may be sluggish (there may be mottling, acrocyanosis).
C. Pulse may be variable—normal 120–160; it may be as high as 170 with crying or below 120 when resting.
D. Anemia is common in early months because of the decrease in erythropoiesis and breakdown of red blood cells. Baby may need an iron-supplemented formula.
E. Physiologic jaundice—normal level less than 1 mg/100 ml blood.
 1. Jaundice visible in the skin, sclera.
 2. Does not become visible until the second or third day after birth.
 3. Caused by impairment in the removal of bilirubin-deficiency in the production of glucuronide transferase, which is needed to convert indirect insoluble bilirubin to direct water soluble bilirubin and then excreted.
 4. Jaundice begins to decrease by the sixth or seventh day.
 5. It may require treatment, although it usually does not if watched carefully. If needed, usual treatment is phototherapy.
F. Transitory deficiency in the ability of the blood to clot. Bacteria in the intestines are necessary for the production of vitamin K. Bacteria are not present in the intestines during the first

few days after birth. Vitamin K IM usually given after birth to aid in blood coagulation.

Ability to Maintain Body Heat

A. The baby suffers a large loss of heat because he is wet at birth and because of the coolness of the delivery room. The infant should be placed immediately in a warmer and dried off.

B. Temperature may be taken by rectum or axilla (usually taken by rectum the first time to check for patent anus).

Weight

A. Infants usually lose between 5 to 10 percent of their body weight the first few days because of low fluid intake and loss of excess fluid from tissue.

B. They usually regain weight lost within 7 to 14 days.

Head

A. Head or face may be asymmetrical due to birth trauma.

B. Molding of head may be present (elongation of head as it passes through birth canal to accommodate pelvis); usually disappears in about a week.

C. Caput succedaneum—diffuse swelling of soft tissues of scalp caused by an arrest in circulation in those tissues present over the cervix as it dilates.

D. Cephalohematoma—extravasation of blood beneath periosteum of one of the cranial bones because of a ruptured blood vessel during the trauma of labor and delivery.

E. Anterior and posterior fontanel.
1. Should be open.
2. Should neither bulge (may indicate intracranial pressure) nor be depressed (may indicate dehydration).

F. Ears well formed and cartilage present.

Gastrointestinal System

A. Salivary glands immature.

B. May have Epstein's pearls (white raised areas on palate caused by an accumulation of epithelial cells).

C. May have transient circumoral cyanosis.

D. Infant stools.
1. Meconium plug—thick gray-white mucus passed before meconium.
2. Meconium—sticky, black, tarry looking stools, consisting of mucus, digestive secretions, vernix caseosa, and lanugo; usually passed during the first 24 hours after birth.
3. Transitional stool passed second to fifth day; greenish, yellow color, and loose (partly meconium and partly milk).
4. Number of stools varies. Breast-fed infants usually have more bowel movements.
5. Stools should be observed for color, frequency, and consistency.

E. Regurgitation following feeding is common. It may be reduced by frequent burping during feedings.

Genitourinary System

A. Check presence of voiding.

B. Uric acid crystals (pink or reddish spots) may appear on diaper due to high uric acid secretion.

C. Genitalia.
1. Female.
   a. May have heavy coating of vernix between labia.
   b. Usually has mucus discharge. Mucus may be blood-tinged due to elevated hormonal levels in mother (pseudomenstruation).
2. Male.
   a. Size of penis and scrotum vary.
   b. Testicles should be descended or in inguinal canal.
   c. Circumcision—surgical removal of the foreskin of penis by physician.
      (1) Usually performed by the second or third day.

(2) Observe for bleeding from postoperative site.

(3) Observe for postoperative voiding.

Skin

A. Should be pinkish color.

B. Acrocyanosis (cyanosis of extremities) may be present for the first hour or two after birth. Persistent blueness may indicate complications such as heart disease.

C. Lanugo and vernix caseosa may be present.

D. Petechiae may be present because of the trauma of birth.

E. Milia—secretions of sebaceous materials in obstructed sebaceous glands (may be present and will disappear).

F. Hemangiomas may be present on nape of neck or upper eyelids.

G. Skin may appear dry or cracked.

H. Mongolian spots—bluish pigmented areas present on the buttocks of babies of Oriental, Negro, or Mediterranean heritage.

Effects of Maternal Hormones

A. Maternal hormones may cause enlargement of breast in both male and female infants, and "witches" milk, a milklike substance, may be excreted from the breasts.

B. Vaginal bleeding in female infant.

C. Hypertrophy of vulva or prostate.

Neurological System

A. Muscle tone.
1. Fist usually kept clenched.
2. Baby should offer resistance when change in position is attempted.
3. Head should be supported when baby is lifted.
4. Muscles should not be limp.

B. Cry.
1. Cry should be loud and vigorous.
2. Baby should cry when hungry or uncomfortable.

C. Hunger.
1. Usually becomes fretful and restless at three- to four-hour intervals.
2. May suck fingers or anything placed near mouth.

D. Sleep.
1. Sleeps about 20 out of 24 hours.
2. Often stirs and stretches while sleeping.

E. Senses.
1. Eyes.
a. Eyelids may be edematous or have purulent discharge from the chemical irritation of silver nitrate.
b. Light perception is present.
c. Eye movement is uncoordinated.
d. Usual color of eyes is blue-gray.
e. May have subconjunctival hemorrhages, which disappear in a week or two.
2. Nose.
a. Newborn breathes through nose.
b. Sense of smell is present.
3. Ears—hearing is present at birth.
4. Taste is present at birth.
5. Touch is present at birth. Responds to stimuli and discomfort.

F. Immunity.
1. May receive from the mother some passive immunity to infectious diseases, such as measles, mumps, and diphtheria.
2. Capacity to develop own antibodies is slow during first few months.
3. Has little resistance to infection.

Feeding the Newborn

Schedules of Feeding

A. First feeding. ❖ PROCEDURE ❖
1. May be breast fed on the delivery table.
2. First feeding is usually within 4 to 12 hours after birth.
3. Usually a test feeding of 5 to 10 drops of sterile water is made to determine baby's ability to swallow. Glucose is no longer given to prevent aspiration pneumonia.

B. Subsequent feeding.
   1. Routine schedule—three to four hour feedings.
   2. Self-demand—baby is fed according to his or her needs (when hungry) usually every three to six hours.

Calories and Fluid Needs

A. Fluid 150–200 ml/kg of body weight in 24 hours. More fluids should be given in hot weather or when the baby has an elevated temperature.
B. Caloric needs—approximately 110 C/kg of body weight or 50 C/lb of body weight.

HIGH RISK INFANTS

Premature Infant

Definition: An infant born before a 37 week gestation period, weighing less than 2500 gm and measuring less than 18½ inches (47 cm) long with a head circumference less than 13 inches (33 cm).

Characteristics

A. Skin is thin and capillaries are easily seen.
B. Lanugo is prominent; hair on the head is fine and fuzzy.
C. Little subcutaneous fat.
D. Body temperature is unstable and may be below normal.
E. Head is large in comparison to the rest of the body.
F. Poor muscle tone—muscles appear limp; baby assumes froglike position when placed on abdomen.
G. Feeble cry.
H. Gagging and sucking reflexes may be weak.
I. Jaundice appears later than in the normal newborn, and it may be more severe and last longer (two weeks).
J. Heightened capillary fragility and increased tendency towards hemorrhage.
K. Lack of immunity and lack of resistance to infection.
L. Poor ability to tolerate fats because of immaturity of digestive system.
M. Tendency towards periods of apnea because of immaturity of nervous system.
N. Tendency to develop respiratory distress, hypoglycemia, anemia, hypocalcemia.
O. High proportion of body surface to weight; leads to an increase in the loss of body fluids.
P. Immaturity of retina—leads to development of retrolental fibroplasia with increased levels of oxygen consumption.
Q. Immaturity of liver—difficulty detoxifying medications.
R. Renal function immature.
S. Reflexes—Moro's reflex is developed; grasp is feeble; rooting is present; sucking varies, although it is usually present at 32 weeks; poor coughing ability, gagging, and swallowing.

Implementation

A. Provide for family's needs to be met.
   1. Allow parents to visit baby frequently; as soon as possible, involve parents in infant care to promote parent-to-infant attachment.
   2. Answer questions openly, provide up-to-date information on baby's progress.
   3. Allow parents to talk freely about infant, give support as needed, and help parents to accept reality of situation.
   4. Explain specialized care to parents. Have them report to pediatrician any of the following symptoms: diarrhea, vomiting, lack of appetite, or elevated temperature.
   5. Allow mother to feel confident in caring for infant before discharge. Explain to mother infant's special needs.
B. Provide immediate care to infant.
   1. Give immediate attention in delivery room and transport to nursery to maintain heat.

    a. Maintain skin temperature at about 36°C or 97.6°F in isolette or heated crib.

    b. Gradually wean infant from heated environment and watch temperature closely until stable.

    c. Warming infant too quickly may cause apneic spells.

  2. Administer humidity (distilled water) usually between 40 to 70 percent as ordered.

C. Evaluate respiratory status.

  1. Check respiratory rate—every hour and prn.

  2. Observe for the following signs of respiratory distress:

    a. Color of skin.

    b. Flaring of nares.

    c. Grunting retractions.

  3. Auscultate breath sounds with stethoscope.

  4. Analyze oxygen concentration one to two hours or as necessary to prevent retrolental fibroplasia and to ensure adequate oxygenation.

  5. Observe for periods of apnea and stimulate by gently rubbing chest or tapping foot.

  6. Percuss, vibrate and suction as ordered to remove mucus.

D. Reposition every two hours to promote aeration lobes of lung and facilitate drainage.

E. Monitor blood gases and electrolytes frequently; IV regulated by infusion pump to prevent circulatory overload.

F. Initiate feedings as ordered (usually begin with sterile water or breast milk); progress to dilute formula or breast milk to fall strength as tolerated.

G. Give gavage feeding if respirations are about 60 breaths per minute.

  1. Use premie nipple if bottle feeding.

  2. Infants often require alternate feedings of gavage and bottle feeding.

H. Maintain intake and output including stool and weigh daily.

I. Organize care to conserve energy with rest periods after each feeding.

J. Measure head circumference and length at least once a week.

K. Maintain aseptic technique and strict isolation techniques with infected babies.

L. Prevent skin breakdown: change position, careful cleansing and handling.

M. Observe for signs of infection: vomiting, jaundice, lack of appetite and lethargy.

N. Check heart rate by apical pulse for a full minute every one to two hours.

O. Frequently check for bleeding from umbilical catheter.

  1. Apply pressure to puncture site as necessary to prevent bleeding.

  2. Administer vitamin K as ordered after birth to prevent hemorrhage.

  3. Frequently check monitors if monitored electronically.

P. Gently stroke and talk to baby when giving care.

Q. Hang colorful mobiles or other nonharmful objects in crib.

R. Hold baby during feeding as soon as condition permits.

S. Encourage parents to hold, cuddle, feed, and diaper baby as soon as baby's condition permits.

Small for Gestational Age

Definition: Refers to infants who are significantly undersize for gestational age. Also called intrauterine growth retardation (IUGR).

Characteristics

A. Postmature infants.

B. Defective embryonic development.

C. Placental insufficiency.

D. Associated factors: diabetes, toxemia, maternal infection, maternal malnutrition, cigarette smoking, multiple gestation.

E. Infant appearance.

  1. Little subcutaneous tissue.

  2. Loose, dry, scaling skin.

  3. Appears thin and wasted; old for size.

  4. May be meconium staining of skin, nails.

5. Sparse hair on head.
6. Active, alert, seems hungry.
7. Cord dries more rapidly than normal infants.

Assessment

A. Hypoglycemia: nervousness, cyanosis, apnea, temperature instability, weak cry.

B. Hypothermia: lethargy, poor feeding pattern, cold to touch, slow respiration.

C. Asphyxia: may have been deprived while in utero or aspirated amniotic fluid. Infant may require resuscitation at birth.

D. Polycythemia: usually asymptomatic but may have tachypnea, retractions.

Implementation

A. Provide care similar to premature infant until the infant is stabilized.

B. Protect from cold stress: keep warm, usually in isolette.

C. Perform tests for glucose levels.

D. Weigh daily and maintain intake and output.

Newborn with AIDS

A. Don gloves and gown to protect self from contamination.

B. Wait until newborn's temperature is stable in the nursery to provide care.

C. Wash infant carefully with Neutrogena soap.

D. Administer cord care with alcohol.

E. Wrap infant in clean blanket.

F. Dispose of gloves and gown in plastic bag.

G. Principles of care for mother of HIV baby.
1. Breast feeding is discouraged when mother tests positive for HIV.
2. Circumcisions are not done on infants with HIV positive mothers until infant's status is determined.
3. Immunizations with live vaccine (oral polio, MMR) should not be done until child's status confirmed. If child infected, live vaccine will not be given. Inactivated Polio Vaccine (IPV) will be administered.
4. Excellent hygiene procedures should be carried out in the home.
5. Inform the care giver exposed to infant's body fluids of the potential for infection transmission.
6. Teach the importance of good handwashing techniques.

DISEASES AFFECTING THE NEWBORN

Respiratory Distress Syndrome

Definition: A group of clinical symptoms signifying that the infant is experiencing problems with the respiratory system.

Etiology

A. Symptoms are the result of a decrease in the amount of surfactant in the infant's lungs as a result of one of the following conditions.
1. Prematurity—immaturity of lungs and inability to produce surfactant.
2. Hypoxia and acidosis.
3. Hypothermia.
4. High concentration of oxygen.

B. Respiratory distress syndrome is the most common cause of death in infants.

Assessment

A. Increased respirations—60/min.

B. Retractions—subcostal followed by intercostal.

C. Cyanosis.

D. Expiratory grunting.

E. Lack of activity.

F. Inability to take in sufficient oxygen leading to low oxygen and hypoxemia.

G. Respiratory acidosis due to retention of carbon dioxide as a result of inadequate pulmonary ventilation.

H. Metabolic acidosis due to increased production of lactic acid.

I. Result of x-ray examination.
1. Atelectasis—collapsed portions of lung.
2. Fibrinous membrane that lines alveolar ducts and terminal bronchioles; membrane is formed by transudation of fluid from pulmonary tissue.

Implementation

A. Primarily supportive.

B. Maintain warmth—infant usually placed in isolette or open crib with overhead warmer. Skin temperature is maintained at 97.6°F.

C. Provide for nutrition and hydration—usually give IV glucose fluids during acute periods, then gradually increase feedings as tolerated.

D. Administer oxygen, warmed and humidified, in lowest concentration possible, via hood, nasal prongs, endotracheal tubes, or bag and mask. Oxygen may be given at atmospheric or increased airway pressure.

E. Apply continuous positive pressure to lungs during spontaneous breathing.

F. Apply positive pressure to lungs during expiratory cycle when using the mechanical ventilator.

G. Check and change nasal prongs frequently if used.

H. Loosely tape and check endotracheal tube frequently for correct placement and connection at adaptor site.

I. Procedure for suctioning infant with endotracheal tube. ❖ PROCEDURE ❖
1. Disconnect from respirator at site of adaptor.
2. Instill few minims to 0.5 ml of sterile normal saline into tube to loosen secretions.
3. Suction no longer than five seconds using sterile catheter.
4. Ventilate infant as needed during procedure.
5. Reconnect tube to respirator; be certain it is in place and adaptor is secure.
6. Auscultate chest for breath sounds.

J. Provide postural drainage and percussion and suction as ordered.

K. Analyze oxygen concentration.

L. Keep parents informed of infant's progress.

M. Allow parents to visit child as much as possible and express their feelings about child's illness.

N. Gently stroke and talk with child while giving care.

Hyperbilirubinemia

Definition: An abnormal elevation of bilirubin in the newborn (above 13–15 mg/100 ml).

Etiology

A. Functional immaturity of the liver—usually appears after 24 hours and disappears after 10 days.

B. Bacterial infections.

C. ABO and Rh incompatibilities—usually show up in the first 24 hours and may be severe.

D. Enclosed bleeding, such as hematoma, from trauma of delivery.

Assessment

A. Jaundice, progressing from head to extremities.

B. Pallor.

C. Infant is lethargic and feeds poorly.

D. Urine is concentrated and stools are light in color.

E. If untreated, infant may progress to muscular rigidity or flaccidity, increased lethargy, high-pitched cry, respiratory distress, decreased Moro's reflex, and spasms.

Treatment and Implementation

A. Observe infant carefully for signs of increased jaundice.

B. Observe for and prevent acidosis/hypoxia and hypoglycemia, which decrease binding of bilirubin to albumin and contribute to jaundice.

C. Maintain adequate hydration and offer fluids between feedings as ordered.

D. Maintain temperature at 97.6°F to avoid cold stress.

E. Take measures to avoid infection.

F. Treatment with phototherapy—fluorescent light breaks down bilirubin into water soluble products. ❖ **PROCEDURE** ❖
   1. Do not clothe infant.
   2. Cover infant's eyes to prevent retinal damage.
   3. Change baby's position every two hours to ensure adequate exposure.
   4. Remove infant from light and remove eye patches during feedings.
   5. Carefully examine eyes for signs of irritation from eye patches.
   6. Keep an accurate record of hours spent under fluorescent lights.

G. Meet emotional needs of infant.

H. Reinforce physician's instruction to parents and allow parents to express concerns and feelings.

I. Exchange transfusion may be done; considered only when bilirubin reaches extremely high levels (20 mg/ml in full term infant and 16 mg/ml in premature infant).

Hemolytic Disease of the Newborn

Definition: Alteration, dissolution, or destruction of red blood cells.

Etiology

A. Rh incompatibility—Rh antigens from the baby's blood enter the maternal bloodstream. The mother's blood does not contain Rh factor, so she produces anti-Rh antibodies. These antibodies are harmless to the mother but attach to the erythrocytes in the fetus and cause hemolysis. Exchange of fetal and maternal blood takes place primarily when the placenta separates at birth.
   1. Problem may begin in early pregnancy; it may be mild to severe and can cause the death of the fetus.
   2. Sensitization usually does not occur with the first pregnancy.
   3. Diagnosis of Rh incompatibility.
      a. Begins in pregnancy, with discoveries of antibodies in an Rh negative mother's blood by means of indirect Coombs' test.
      b. Titration is used to determine the extent to which antibodies are present.
      c. Analysis of amniotic fluid for bilirubin determines the severity of the disease (the higher the bilirubin content, the more severe the disease).
      d. Testing of cord blood (direct Coombs' test) determines the presence of maternal antibodies attached to baby's cells.

B. ABO incompatibility—usually less severe.

Assessment

A. Anemia—caused by destruction of red blood cells.

B. Jaundice—develops rapidly after birth.

C. Edema—usually seen in stillborn infants or those who die shortly after birth, most likely due to cardiac failure.

Treatment

A. Immunization against hemolytic disease with RhoGAM as ordered (now given at 28 weeks and postpartum).

B. For mild forms, treat as for hyperbilirubinemia.

C. For severe, give exchange transfusion after birth or intrauterine.

Infants of Diabetic Mothers

General Considerations

A. May be delivered early to prevent intrauterine death (after 36 weeks).
B. Often delivered by cesarean section.
C. Children with diabetic mothers have a higher incidence of congenital anomalies than the general population.
D. High incidence of hypoglycemia, respiratory distress, hypocalcemia, and hyperbilirubinemia.

Assessment

A. Baby is usually excessively large in size and weight due to excess fat and glycogen in tissues.
   1. High blood sugar levels in mother cross the placenta and enter the baby's bloodstream, elevating blood sugar levels.
   2. High blood sugar stimulates infant's metabolic system to store glycogen and fat and increase the production of insulin.
B. May have puffy appearance of face and cheeks.
C. Enlarged heart, liver, and spleen.
D. Lethargy.
E. Irregular respiration.

Implementation

A. Observe for signs of hypoglycemia—twitching, difficulty in feeding, lethargy, apnea, seizures, and cyanosis.
B. Observe for signs of respiratory distress—tachypnea, cyanosis, retractions, grunting, nasal flaring.
C. Care is the same as for a premature infant.
D. Initiate feedings with sterile water, then glucose water within two to four hours after birth, as ordered by physician.

Infant Born to Mother with Drug Addiction

General Considerations

A. There is a direct relationship between the duration of the maternal addiction and dosage and the severity of symptoms in the infant.
B. Heroin addicted mother: infant may appear normal at birth with a low birth weight.
   1. Withdrawal within 12–24 hours—may last 5–7 days.
   2. Infant appears less ill than when mother is taking methadone.
   3. Heroin causes early maturity of the liver.
C. Mother on methadone.
   1. Withdrawal 1–2 days to 1 week or more; most evident 48–72 hours and may last 6 days to 8 weeks.
   2. Infant may appear to be very ill.
   3. May develop jaundice due to prematurity.
D. Mother addicted to cocaine, a stimulant.
   1. Infant evidences decreased interactive behavior, feeding problems, irregular sleep patterns, diarrhea.
   2. Seven out of 1000 mothers will have infants with major deformities—especially of the kidneys.

Assessment

A. Irritability and tremors.
B. Vomiting.
C. High-pitched cry.
D. Sneezing, nasal stuffiness.
E. Respiratory distress.
F. Fever.
G. Diarrhea.
H. Excess sweating.
I. Increased muscle tone.
J. Poor feeding.
K. Sucking of fist.
L. Convulsions (rare).

Implementation

A. Monitor respiratory and cardiac rates every 30 minutes and prn.
B. Take temperature every four to eight hours and prn.
C. Maintain warmth and swaddle infant in blanket.
D. Reduce external stimuli and handle infant infrequently.
E. Hold firmly and close to body during feedings and when giving care.
F. Pad sides of crib to protect infant from injury.
G. Administer small, frequent feedings as ordered.
H. Suction if necessary.
I. Cleanse buttocks and anal area carefully.
J. Measure intake and output.
K. Keep mother informed of infant's progress.
L. Promote mother's interest in infant.

Fetal Alcohol Syndrome

Characteristics

A. Maternal alcohol abuse throughout pregnancy results in fetal alcohol syndrome.
   1. Most serious cause of teratogenesis.
   2. In affected infants, growth is retarded; they are microcephalic with severe mental retardation.
B. Lesser amount of alcohol ingested throughout pregnancy results in less severe symptoms.
   1. Prenatal and/or postnatal growth retardation.
   2. Developmental delay.
   3. May not be diagnosed until early childhood.

Assessment

A. Respiratory distress and apnea.
B. Cyanosis.
C. Seizures.

D. Major brain dysfunction symptoms.

Implementation

A. Position on side to facilitate drainage of secretions.
   1. Keep resuscitation equipment at bedside.
   2. Have suction available, especially following feeding.
B. Administer small feedings and burp well.
C. Support family and assist to accept anomalies.

GYNECOLOGY

Examination

A. Pelvic exam.
   1. Inspection of external genitalia for signs of inflammation, bleeding, discharge, and epithelial cell changes.
   2. Speculum may be inserted for visualization of vagina and cervix.
   3. Bimanual examination is done—gloved fingers of one hand inserted into vagina while abdomen palpated with other hand.
   4. Rectal exam.
B. Breast exam may also be done when woman comes in for pelvic.
C. Papanicolaou smear.
   1. Diagnosis for cervical cancer.
   2. Vaginal secretions and secretions from posterior fornix are swabbed and smeared on a glass slide.

Conditions of the Vulva

Vulvitis

A. An inflammation of the vulva which usually occurs in conjunction with other conditions such as vaginal infections and venereal disease.
B. Signs and symptoms.

1. Burning pain during urination.
2. Itching.
3. Red and inflamed genitalia.
4. Discharge.

C. Treatment and nursing care.
   1. Apply soothing compresses and give colloidal baths.
   2. Administer medicated creams.
   3. Administer sedatives (antihistamines).

Cancer of the Vulva

A. Signs and symptoms.
   1. Long-standing pruritus (itching).
   2. Foul-smelling discharge.
   3. Bleeding.
   4. Pain.

B. Treatment and nursing care.
   1. Vulvectomy is the preferred treatment.
   2. Immediate postoperative care.
      a. Observe dressings for signs of hemorrhage.
      b. Check vital signs until stable.
      c. Assist patient to turn, cough, and deep breathe every two hours.
      d. Give pain medications as ordered.
      e. Observe drainage, and empty Hemovac as necessary.
      f. Record intake and output.
      g. Maintain IV.
      h. Maintain catheter care to reduce incidence of infection.
      i. Position for comfort.
   3. Convalescent care.
      a. Encourage patient to verbalize feelings related to change in body image.
      b. Irrigate wound as ordered, using solution as prescribed (usual solution is sterile saline hydrogen peroxide), which cleans area and improves circulation.

Conditions of the Vagina

Vaginal Infections

A. Vagina normally protected from infection by acidic environment.

B. Leukorrhea (whitish vaginal discharge) normal in small amounts at ovulation and prior to menstruation.

C. Trichomoniasis vaginalis—overgrowth of protozoan normally present in vaginal tract due to normal pH alteration.

D. Moniliasis—fungal infection caused by Candida albicans.
   1. Thrives in carbohydrate-rich environment; common in poorly controlled diabetes.
   2. Antibiotic or steroid therapy reduces protective organisms normally present.

E. Treatment—medications and vaginal inserts as prescribed.

Conditions of Ovaries and Pelvic Cavity

Endometriosis

A. Abnormal growth of endometrial tissue outside the uterine cavity.

B. This condition is a common cause of infertility.

C. Etiological theories.
   1. Embryonic tissue that remains dormant until ovarian stimulation after menarche.
   2. Endometrial tissue transported from the uterine cavity through the fallopian tubes during menstruation.
   3. Endometrial tissue transported by lymphatic tissue during menstruation.
   4. Accidental transfer of endometrial tissue to pelvic cavity during surgery.

D. Signs and symptoms.
   1. Lower abdominal and pelvic pain during menstruation due to distention of involved tissue and surrounding area by blood (symptoms are acute during menstruation).
   2. Dysmenorrhea—usually steady and severe.
   3. Abnormal uterine bleeding.
   4. Pain during intercourse.
   5. Back and rectal pain.

E. Treatment and nursing care
   1. Pregnancy may delay growth of lesions but symptoms usually recur after pregnancy.

2. Hormone therapy with oral contraceptives usually eliminates menstrual pain and controls endometrial growth.
3. Surgical intervention; total hysterectomy may be indicated.
4. Provide emotional support.

Pelvic Inflammatory Disease (PID)

A. An inflammatory condition of the pelvic cavity that may involve ovaries, fallopian tubes, vascular system, or pelvic peritoneum.
B. Etiology.
   1. Staphylococcus or streptococcus.
   2. Venereal disease.
   3. Tubercle bacilli.
C. Signs and symptoms.
   1. Elevated temperature.
   2. Nausea and vomiting.
   3. Abdominal and low-back pain.
   4. Purulent, foul-smelling vaginal discharge.
   5. Leukocytosis.
D. Treatment and nursing care.
   1. Take measures to control the spread of infection.
   2. Place patient in semi-Fowler's position for dependent drainage.
   3. Take and record vital signs every four hours.
   4. Administer antibiotics, douches, and abdominal heat as ordered.
   5. Note nature and amount of vaginal discharge.
   6. Avoid use of tampons and urinary catheterization to prevent the spread of infection.
   7. Promote good nutrition and fluid intake.
   8. Explain rationale for treatment.

Conditions of the Uterus

Displacements

A. Retroversion and retroflexion—backward displacement of the uterus.
   1. May cause difficulty in getting pregnant.

2. Treatment consists of moving the uterus to the normal position by shortening its ligaments.
B. Prolapse (usually occurs in multiparas).
   1. Weakening of uterine supports causes the uterus to slip down into the vaginal canal; the uterus may even appear outside the vaginal orifice.
   2. Prolapse may cause urinary incontinence or retention.
   3. Treatment.
      a. Pessary—instrument that keeps the uterus in place by exerting pressure on ligaments and usually used in patients of advanced age.
      B. Surgery to reposition uterus and shorten ligaments; or hysterectomy.

Tumors

A. Benign fibroid tumors.
   1. Occur in 20 to 30 percent of all women between the ages of 25 to 40.
   2. Symptoms include menorrhagia, back pain, urinary difficulty, and constipation.
   3. Fibroid tumors may cause sterility.
   4. Treatment.
      a. Removal of tumors, if they are small.
      b. Hysterectomy is performed when there are large tumors.
B. Malignant tumors of the reproductive system (second highest cause of death in the female).
   1. Cancer of the cervix—most common type of cancer in the reproductive system.
      a. Usually appears in females between the ages of 30 to 50.
      b. Signs and symptoms include bleeding between periods—may be noted especially after intercourse or douching; leukorrhea.
      c. May become invasive and include tissue outside the cervix, fundus of the uterus, and the lymph glands.
      d. Treatment depends upon extent of the disease.
         (1) Hysterectomy.
         (2) Radiation.

(3) Radical pelvic surgery in advanced cases.
2. Cancer of the endometrium (fundus or corpus of uterus).
   a. Usually not diagnosed until symptoms appear; Pap smear inadequate for diagnosis.
   b. Progresses slowly; metastasis occurs late.
   c. Treatment.
      (1) Early—hysterectomy.
      (2) Late—radium and x-ray therapy.

Hysterectomy

Types

A. Total—removal of the entire uterus but retention of fallopian tubes and ovaries.
B. Panhysterectomy—removal of the entire uterus, ovaries, and fallopian tubes.
C. Radical hysterectomy—wide removal of vaginal, cervical, uterosacral and other tissue along with the uterus.
D. Cervical.
E. Abdominal.
F. Vaginal.

Postoperative Implementation

A. Immediate care.
   1. Observe incisional site for bleeding and reinforce dressings as needed.
   2. Monitor vital signs frequently.
   3. If patient has nasogastric tube to suction, maintain NPO and observe amount, color, and consistency of drainage.
   4. Administer pain medications as ordered.
   5. Monitor IV fluids as ordered.
   6. Provide for hygienic care.
   7. Catheter care to prevent infection (observe amount and color of drainage).
   8. Assist patient to cough, turn, and deep breathe.
   9. Promote methods for decreasing pelvic congestion.
      a. Apply antiembolic stocking.
      b. Avoid high-Fowler's position.
   10. Measure intake and output.
   11. Apply range-of-motion exercises.
B. Common complications.
   1. Hemorrhage.
   2. Infection.
   3. Pneumonia.
   4. Paralytic ileus.
   5. Thrombophlebitis.
   6. Changes in body image.

Anterior and Posterior Colporrhaphy

A. Purpose.
   1. Repair of cystocele—downward displacement of the bladder towards the vaginal entrance caused by tissue weakness, injuries in childbirth, and atrophy associated with aging.
   2. Repair of rectocele—anterior sagging of rectum and posterior vaginal wall caused by injuries to the muscles and tissue of the pelvic floor during childbirth.
B. General postoperative care of the patient with cystocele and rectocele repair.
   1. Observe for foul-smelling discharge from vaginal area or operative site.
   2. Two methods of caring for perineal sutures.
      a. Sutures left alone until healing begins; thereafter, daily vaginal irrigations with sterile saline.
      b. Sterile saline douches twice daily beginning with the first postoperative day.
   3. Observe for urinary retention and catheterize as necessary.
   4. Prepare patient for discharge with instruction in perineal hygiene (no douching or coitus until advised by physician), and in detection of signs of infection.

Pelvic Exenteration

A. A surgical procedure that is performed for widespread cancer that cannot be controlled by other means.
B. Three types of pelvic exenteration.

1. Anterior pelvic—the removal of the reproductive organs, pelvic lymph nodes, adnexa, pelvic peritoneum, bladder, and lower ureter. Ureters are implanted in the small intestines or the colon.
2. Posterior pelvic—removal of the reproductive organs, vagina, adnexa, colon, and rectum. Pelvic lymph nodes may also be removed.
3. Total pelvic—removal of the reproductive organs, pelvic floor, pelvic lymph nodes, perineum, bladder, rectum, and distal portion of sigmoid colon. A substitute bladder is made from a segment of the ileum. Patient will have a permanent colostomy.

C. Care of the patient undergoing pelvic exenteration.
  1. Exercise general postoperative procedures.
  2. Observe surgical site for drainage and reinforce dressings as necessary; patient may have drainage tubes connected to suction from incision area.
  3. Apply antiembolic stockings.
  4. Encourage patient to express feelings.

Patient Receiving Radiation Therapy

A. Radiation therapy is treatment with radioactive substance given to break down cancerous tissue.
B. Therapy procedure.
  1. Radioactive cobalt, radium, or iridium inserted into endocervical canal by radiotherapist.
  2. Supplemented by external radiation.
C. Nursing care.
  1. Provide low-residue diet to prevent bowel movement and dislodging of radium.
  2. Inspect catheter to make sure it is draining (distended bladder will be in the path of radiation).
  3. Observe for unusual or profuse vaginal discharge.
  4. Instruct patient to lie on side or on back with head slightly elevated on pillow.
  5. Administer skin care to prevent tissue breakdown.

6. While giving nursing care, encourage patient to talk and express anxieties.
7. Measure intake and output.
8. Observe patient for side effects, e.g., nausea, vomiting, anorexia, and redness or blistering of skin in pelvic area.
9. Check vital signs and observe for elevated temperature.

Tumors of the Breast

Clinical Findings

A. Nontender lump in breast, usually in upper outer quadrant.
B. Dimpling of breast tissue surrounding nipple.
C. Asymmetry with affected breast being higher.
D. Nipple bleeding or retraction.

Types of Surgery

A. Simple mastectomy—removal of breast with no lymph nodes removed.
B. Radical mastectomy—removal of the breast, muscle layers down to chest wall, and lymph nodes in axillary region.
C. Lumpectomy—removal of tumor and small amount of normal tissue.

Implementation

A. Continue giving emotional support begun preoperatively during postoperative period.
  1. Patient will have altered body image.
  2. Patient may be extremely depressed.
B. Position in semi-Fowler's position with the affected arm elevated to prevent edema.
C. Turn, cough, and hyperventilate to prevent respiratory complications.
D. Turn only to back and unaffected side.
E. Hemovac placed frequently.
  1. Maintain suction.
  2. Record amount of drainage.
  3. Record drainage characteristics.

F. Prevent complications of contractures and lymph-edema by encouraging range-of-motion exercises early in postoperative period.

G. IV fluids should not be administered in affected arm.

H. Monitor vital signs for prevention of complications such as infection and hemorrhage. Take blood pressure on unaffected arm only.

I. Pressure dressings should be reinforced. Observe for signs of restriction from dressing.
   1. Impaired sensation.
   2. Color changes of skin.

J. If skin grafts were applied, treat as for any other graft.

K. Encourage visit from Reach for Recovery Group.

THERAPEUTIC ABORTION

General Considerations

A. Legality.
   1. Abortion is now legal in all states as the result of a Supreme Court decision in January 1973.
   2. It is regulated in the following manner.
      a. First trimester—decision between patient and physician.
      b. Second trimester—decision between patient and physician (state may regulate who performs the abortion and where it can be done).
      c. Third trimester—states may regulate and prohibit abortion except to preserve the health or life of the mother.

B. Indications for abortion.
   1. Medical—psychiatric condition such as chronic hypertension or disease in the mother (e.g., nephritis, severe diabetes, cancer, or acute infection such as rubella); possible genetic defects in the infant or severe erythroblastosis fetalis.
   2. Nonmedical—socio-economic reasons, unmarried, financial burden, too young to care for infant.

C. Preparation of the individual.
   1. Advise patient of available sources of abortion.
   2. Inform patient as to what to expect from the abortion procedure.
   3. Provide emotional support during decision-making period.
   4. Maintain an open, nonjudgmental atmosphere in which the individual may express concerns or guilt.
   5. Encourage and support the individual after the decision is made and after surgery.
   6. Give information about contraceptives.

D. Complications and effects.
   1. Abortion should be performed before the twelfth week, if possible, because complications and risks are lower during this time.
   2. Complications.
      a. Infection.
      b. Bleeding.
      c. Sterility.
      d. Uterine perforation.

Techniques

A. First trimester.
   1. Dilatation and curettage (D & C).
      a. Cervical canal is dilated with instruments of increasingly large diameter.
      b. Fetus and accessory structure is removed with forceps.
      c. Endometrium is scraped with curette to assure that all products of conception are removed.
      d. Process usually takes 15 to 20 minutes.
   2. Vacuum aspirator.
      a. Hose-linked curette is inserted into dilated cervix.
      b. Hose is attached to suction.
      c. The vacuum aspirator lessens the chance of uterine perforation, reduces blood loss, and reduces the time of the procedure.

B. Second trimester abortion.
   1. Intra-amniotic injection or amniocentesis abortion.
      a. Performed after the 14th to 16th week of pregnancy.
      b. From 50 to 200 ml of amniotic fluid are removed from the amniotic cavity and replaced with hypertonic of 20 to 50 percent saline that is installed through gravity drip over a period of 45 to 60 minutes.
      c. Increased osmotic pressure of the amniotic fluid causes the death of the fetus.
      d. Uterine contractions usually begin in about 12 hours, and the products of conception are expelled in 24 to 30 hours.
      e. Oxytocic drugs may be given if contractions do not begin.
      f. Complications.
         (1) Infusion of hypertonic saline solution into uterus.
         (2) Infection.
         (3) Disseminated intravascular coagulation disease may develop during procedure.
         (4) Hemorrhage.
   2. Hysterotomy.
      a. Incision is made through abdominal wall into uterus.
      b. Procedure is usually performed between the 14th and 16th week in pregnancy.
      c. Products of conception are removed with forceps.
      d. Uterine cavity is curetted.
      e. Tubal ligation may be done at same time.
      f. Patient usually requires several days of hospitalization.
      g. Operation requires general or spinal anesthesia.
   3. Prostaglandins.
      a. These hormonelike acids cause abortion by stimulating the uterus to contract.
      b. They may be administered IV into the uterine cavity through the cervical canal, into the posterior fornix of the vagina, or after 12 weeks into the amniotic cavity. The IV method is least effective and has many possible side effects.

C. Nursing care.
   1. Administer preoperative medications.
   2. Ensure that patient understands the procedure.
   3. Offer emotional support and let patient express feelings.
   4. Monitor IV.
   5. Check vital signs postoperatively.
   6. Check for excessive bleeding.
   7. Administer pain medications as ordered.
   8. Instruct patient to watch for signs of excessive bleeding (more than a normal menstrual period) and infection (elevated temperature), foul-smelling discharge, persistent abdominal pain).
   9. Administer oxytocic drug as ordered.
   10. Administer RhoGAM as ordered for an unsensitized Rh-negative patient.
   11. Offer fluids as tolerated after vital signs are stable and patient is alert and responsive.

PARENTHOOD

Influences on Parenthood

A. Tendency toward smaller families.
B. Career-oriented women who limit family size or who do not want children.
C. Early sexual experimentation necessitating sexual education and contraceptive information.
D. Reasons for tendency toward postponement of children.
   1. Completion of education.
   2. Economic factors.
E. High divorce rates.
F. Alternate family designs.

1. Single parenthood.
2. Communal family.

Methods of Birth Control

Chemical—96 to 98 percent effective

A. Foam, cream, jelly agents.
   1. Agent acts by killing or paralyzing the sperm.
   2. Combined with a compound which coats the vagina so that agent acts as a vehicle for spermicide as well as a mechanical barrier through which sperm cannot swim.
B. Oral contraceptives.
   1. Biologic mechanism.
      a. The pill artificially raises the blood levels of both estrogen and progesterone, thereby preventing the release of FSH from the anterior pituitary. Without FSH the follicle does not mature and ovulation fails to take place.
      b. Endometrial changes.
      c. Alteration in cervical mucus making it hostile to sperm.
      d. Altered tubal function.
   2. Types of birth-control pills.
      a. Combined—contain both estrogen and progesterone.
      b. Sequential (mimics normal hormonal cycle)—estrogen given alone 15–16 days, followed by combination of estrogen and progestin for the next five days.
   3. Minor side effects (usually diminish within a few months).
      a. Breast fullness and tenderness.
      b. Edema, weight gain.
      c. Nausea and vomiting.
      d. Chloasma.
      e. Breakthrough bleeding.
   4. More serious side effects.
      a. Thrombophlebitis.
      b. Pulmonary embolism.
      c. Hypertension.

Mechanical—95 to 98 percent effective

A. Diaphragm.
   1. Mechanical barrier that functions by blocking external os and closing access to cervical canal by sperm.
   2. Must be used in conjunction with vaginal cream or jelly to be effective.
B. Condom.
   1. Acts as a mechanical barrier by collecting sperm which then are not allowed contact with vaginal area.
   2. It is relatively inexpensive and may be readily purchased in a drugstore.
C. Intrauterine devices (IUD).
   1. Methods of action (not completely clear).
      a. More rapid transport of ovum through tube reaching endometrium before it is "ready" for implantation.
      b. IUD may cause substances to accumulate in uterus and interfere with implantation.
      c. IUD may stimulate production of cellular exudate which interferes with the ability of sperm to migrate to fallopian tubes.
   2. Usually made of soft plastic or nickel-chromium alloy.
   3. There are many types of devices available on market such as Lippes' loop and Saf-T-Coil.
   4. Complications.
      a. Perforation of uterus.
      b. Infection.
      c. Spotting between periods.
      d. Heavy menstrual flow or prolonged flow.
      e. Cramping during menstruation.

Biologic—60 to 75 percent effective

A. Rhythm.
   1. Based upon three principles.
      a. Ovulation usually occurs 14 days before period begins.
      b. An ovum may be fertilized 12 to 24 hours after release from ovary.

c. Sperm usually survives no longer than 24 hours in the uterine environment.
2. On these bases, if coitus is avoided during the fertile period, pregnancy should not occur.

B. Coitus interruptus.
1. Early form of contraception.
2. Requires withdrawal of penis before ejaculation.

Sterilization Procedures

A. Vasectomy.
1. Surgical procedure with local anesthesia on out-patient basis.
   a. Incision made over ductus deferens on each side of scrotum; sperm ducts isolated and severed.
   b. Ends ligated, lumen coagulated, clipped or polyethylene tubing used with a stopcock for potential reversal.
   c. Absorbable sutures used to close the skin.
2. Patient instruction for care.
   a. Apply ice for pain or swelling.
   b. Use scrotal support for one week.
   c. Inform patient that it takes 4–6 weeks and 3–36 ejaculations to clear sperm from ductus.
   d. Sperm samples (two or three) should be checked for sperm count.
   e. Patient rechecked at 6 and 12 months to insure fertility has not been restored by recanalization.
3. Possible side effects of procedure.
   a. Hematoma, sperm granulomas, and spontaneous reanastomosis.
   b. For those who wish to reverse process, 65 percent are successful.

B. Tubal ligation most common method (removal of uterus and ovaries is permanent method of sterilization).
1. Accomplished by abdominal or vaginal procedures; most common method is transection of fallopian tubes.
   a. Tubes are isolated, then crushed, ligated, or plugged (newer reversible procedure).
   b. The postpartal and mini-laparotomy procedures require hospitalization.
   c. A newer procedure, laparoscopic sterilization requires an incision at the umbilicus, the tube coagulated, and may be transected.
2. Complications of procedure include bowel perforation, infection, hemorrhage, and adverse anesthesia effects.
   a. Reversal of tubal ligations results in overall pregnancy rate of 15 percent.
   b. Three-quarters of these pregnancies result in live births and 10 percent are tubal pregnancies.

APPENDIX 1. COMMON DRUGS IN OBSTETRICS AND GYNECOLOGY

Name of Drug, Action, Dosage	Uses and Side Effects	Nursing Implications
Oxytocin, Syntocinon/Pitocin Classification: oxytocic Produces rhythmic contractions of uterine musculature Dosage: varies with method and purpose of administration. IV 5–10 USP units in 500 or 1,000 ml 5 percent dextrose in NS infused at rate 0.5–0.75 ml/min with rate gradually increased until patient has three to four good quality contractions in 10 minutes	Used to induce labor, constrict uterus, and decrease hemorrhage after delivery and postabortion Stimulates contractile tissue in lactating breast to eject milk Side effects: water intoxication; allergic reactions; death due to uterine rupture; pelvic hematomas; bradycardia	Observe for signs of sensitivity and overdose Monitor strength and duration of uterine contractions Check FHT every 15 minutes and prn Take P and BP every hour
Methergine Classification: oxytocic Produces constrictive effects on smooth muscle of uterus (more prolonged constrictive effects as compared to rhythmic effects of oxytocin or Ergotrate); also has generalized vasoconstrictive effect Usual IM dose 0.2 mg (may be repeated in 2–4 h); usual oral dose 0.2 mg 3–4 × a day for 2 days	Used primarily after delivery to produce firm uterine contractions and decrease uterine bleeding May be used to prevent postabortal hemorrhage Side effects include nausea, vomiting, dizziness, increased BP, dyspnea, and chest pain	Check BP and pulse before administration of medication and check vital signs frequently after administration Injectable form deteriorates rapidly when exposed to lights and heat-do not use if discoloration occurs
Vasodilan (isoxsuprine) Classification: vasodilator Relaxing effects on circulatory and uterine smooth muscle Usual oral dose 10–20 mg tablets 3–4 times daily Usual IM dose 10–20 mg q 2–3 hrs.	Treatment of premature labor or during labor when contractions are unusually frequent and not coordinated. Most effective when given in early latent phase of labor; rarely stops active labor. Side effects include nausea, vomiting, dizziness, transient hypotension and tachycardia	Take BP and P frequently Observe for signs of tachycardia and hypotension
Ritodrine (improved analog of isoxsuprine)	Hydrate woman prior to infusion with IV solution of 1000 cc normal saline Continuous monitoring (Swan-Ganz) of mother and infant important as mother-infant deaths have occurred	Same as above
Terbutaline B2, receptor stimulant; sympathomimetic	Treatment of premature labor and requires hospitalization Side effects: tachycardia, palpitations, sweating, tremors, restlessness lethargy, drowsiness, headache, nausea, vomiting	Same as above

APPENDIX 1. COMMON DRUGS IN OBSTETRICS AND GYNECOLOGY (*Continued*)

Name of Drug, Action, Dosage	Uses and Side Effects	Nursing Implications
Magnesium sulfate Depressive effects on central nervous system, and smooth, skeletal, and cardiac muscle Produces peripheral vasodilation Given IV in preeclampsia and eclampsia; dosage varies Usual dosage: initial dosage 4 gm in 250 ml 5% D/W at 5 ml/30 sec (approximately 20 min) or in continuous infusion	Used to prevent convulsions in preeclampsia and eclampsia. Also counteracts uterine tetany after large doses of oxytocin Side effects: *Maternal:* extreme thirst, hypotension, flaccidity, circulatory collapse, depression of CNS and cardiac system. *Fetal:* crosses placenta, lethargy, hypotonia Antidote: Calcium Gluconate. Keep available at bedside	Observe carefully for signs of magnesium toxicity: extreme thirst, feeling hot all over; loss of patellar reflex Monitor respirations (greater than 12/min), BP (hypotension), and P closely in order to assess effect of drug. Never leave patient alone Patellar reflex should be checked continuously Check urine output continuously (greater than 30 ml/hr)
Apresoline (hydralazine hydrochloride) Classification: antihypertensive Usual dosage: PO 12.5 mg bid, increased incrementally to maximum 100 mg bid Decreases peripheral resistance and peripheral vasodilatation	Side effects: flushing, headache, nausea, vomiting, tachycardia, palpitations, lupus syndrome and leukopenia	Monitor blood pressure and pulse rate Observe for orthostatic hypotension, tachycardia, palpitations, headache, dizziness, nausea, vomiting Give drug with meals to increase absorption
Estrogen preparations Classification: hormones Development and maintenance of sexual characteristics throughout adult life Common preparations Estradiol, TACE, Premarin Dosage varies, depends upon purpose for giving	Given to replace deficiencies, to control conception, relieve breast engorgement when lactation is to be suppressed Side effects include nausea, vomiting, diarrhea, skin rash, edema Diethylstilbestrol no longer used as it causes incidence of cancer in female offspring	Encourage follow-up visits to physician
Progesterone preparations Classification: hormones Normal functions—preparation and maintenance of endometrium for pregnancy. Suppresses ovulation and pregnancy and decreases uterine irritability Dosage varies	Given to control conception amenorrhea, abnormal uterine bleeding, threatened abortion Side effects include GI symptoms, dizziness, headache, allergic reactions	Encourage follow-up visits to physician

APPENDIX 1. COMMON DRUGS IN OBSTETRICS AND GYNECOLOGY (*Continued*)

Name of Drug, Action, Dosage	Uses and Side Effects	Nursing Implications
Demerol Classification: synthetic narcotic analgesic Onset of action 15 min, peaks 1 h, depresses CNS probably at both cortical and subcortical levels Dosage: 25–50 mg IM every 3–4 h prn relief of postsurgical pain	Produces analgesia in labor, postoperative relief of pain Side effects include dizziness, nausea, vomiting, dry mouth, sweating, decrease in BP	Evaluate progress of labor carefully; if given too late in labor, infant may be depressed Check for level of consciousness before administration Observe for nausea and vomiting
Morphine Classification: analgesic Combination of depressive and stimulative effects on CNS and smooth muscles of gut Raises pain threshold and produces euphoria and sedation Usual dose: 3–10 mg IM during labor; postoperative—10 mg	Produces analgesia during labor, relief of postoperative pain Side effects include nausea, vomiting, constipation, depression of respiratory center and cough, allergic reactions such as urticaria	Check level of consciousness and respiratory rate before administration Careful evaluation of progress of labor; if given too late, infant may be depressed
Nisentil Classification: synthetic analgesic Action similar to Demerol and morphine, but acts more quickly than Demerol and over a shorter period of time Dosage: 20–40–60 mg subcutaneous or IM every 2–4 h	Analgesia during labor; relief of pain after abortion Side effects include nausea, vomiting, depression of respiratory center	Monitor progress of labor carefully; if given too late in labor, infant may be depressed Check respiratory rate before administration
Nalline Hydrochloride, Narcan, Lorfan Classification: narcotic antagonists Acts as an antagonist to morphine, Demerol, and related analgesics	Treatment of respiratory depression in newborn when narcotic effect has not worn off in the mother prior to delivery Nalline may be given to the mother shortly before delivery to prevent respiratory depression due to analgesic side effects Side effects include drowsiness, lethargy, sweating	Check respiratory rate and color and cardiac rate of infant to see if medication is having desired effect

APPENDIX 2. DRUGS ADVERSELY AFFECTING THE HUMAN FETUS

Drugs	Adverse Effect	Comments
Analgesic		
Heroin and morphine	Respiratory depression; neonatal death; addiction	Near term Fairly well documented
Salicylates	Neonatal bleeding; coagulation defects	Near term
Anesthetics		
Mepivacaine	Fetal bradycardia; neonatal depression	Near term More studies needed
Antibacterials		
Chloramphenicol	"Gray syndrome" and death	Near term Fairly well documented
Nitrofurantoin	Hemolysis	Near term More studies needed
Novobiocin	Hyperbilirubinemia	Near term More studies needed
Streptomycin	8th nerve damage; hearing loss; multiple skeletal anomalies	Throughout pregnancy Debatable, more studies needed
Sulfonamides (long acting)	Hyperbilirubinemia and kernicterus	Near term Fairly well documented
Tetracyclines	Inhibition of bone growth; discoloration of teeth	2nd and 3rd trimesters Fairly well documented
Anticarcinogens		
Amethopterin	Cleft palate; abortion	1st trimester Fairly well documented
Aminopterin	Cleft palate; abortion	1st trimester Known teratogen
Cyclophosphamide	Severe stunting; fetal death; extremity defects	1st trimester More studies needed
Anticoagulants		
Warfarin	Fetal death; hemorrhage	Throughout pregnancy More studies needed
Antidiabetics		
Chlorpropamide	Prolonged neonatal hypoglycemia	Throughout pregnancy More evidence needed before implication
Tolbutamide	Congenital anomalies	Throughout pregnancy One reported case only; evidence lacking
Antimalarials		
Quinine	Deafness	More studies needed

APPENDIX 2. DRUGS ADVERSELY AFFECTING THE HUMAN FETUS (*Continued*)

Drugs	Adverse Effect	Comments
Antimitotic agents		
Podophyllum	Fetal absorption; multiple deformities	More studies needed
Antithyroid agents		
Methimazole	Goiter and mental retardation	From 14th week on Fairly well documented
Potassium iodide	Goiter and mental retardation	From 14th week on Fairly well documented
Propylthiouracil	Goiter and mental retardation	From 14th week on Fairly well documented
Radioactive iodine	Congenital hypothyroidism	From 14th week on Fairly well documented
Depressants		
Phenobarbital	Neonatal bleeding; increased rate of neonatal drug metabolism	In excessive amounts
Reserpine	Nasal block	Near term One report only More studies needed
Thalidomide	Phocomelia; hearing defect	28th–42nd day Known teratogen
Diuretics		
Ammonium chloride	Acidosis	
Thiazides (Hydrochlorothiazide) (Chlorothiazide) (Methyclothiazide)	Thrombocytopenia; neonatal death	Latter part of pregnancy One report only; evidence lacking
Stimulants		
Dextroamphetamine	Transposition of great vessels	One report only More evidence needed
Phenmetrazine	Skeletal and visceral anomalies	4th–12th week One report only More evidence needed
Sex Steroids		
Androgens, estrogens and oral progestins	Masculinization and labial fusion (early in pregnancy); clitoris enlargement (later in pregnancy)	Fairly well documented

APPENDIX 2. DRUGS ADVERSELY AFFECTING THE HUMAN FETUS (*Continued*)

Drugs	Adverse Effect	Comments
Miscellaneous		
Acetophenetidin	Methemoglobinemia	More studies needed
Cholinesterase inhibitors	Transient muscular weakness	Throughout pregnancy More studies needed
Hexamethonium bromide	Neonatal ileus and death	Throughout pregnancy More studies needed
Iophenoxic acid	Elevation of serum protein-bound iodine	
Isonicotinic acid hydrazide (INH)	Retarded psychomotor activity	More studies needed
Lysergic acid diethylamide (LSD)	Chromosomal damage; stunted offspring	1st trimester More studies needed
Nicotine and smoking	Small babies	Throughout pregnancy More studies needed
Vitamin A—large doses only	Congenital anomalies; cleft palate; eye damage, syndactyly	Throughout pregnancy
Vitamin D—large doses only	Excessive blood calcium; mental retardation	Throughout pregnancy
Vitamin K analogues	Hyperbilirubinemia; kernicterus	Near term In large doses
Cocaine	Decreased interactive behavior; feeding problems; possible deformities	Addiction throughout pregnancy

Excerpted from "Drugs Adversely Affecting the Human Fetus," 1971, Ross Laboratories, Columbus, Ohio.

APPENDIX 3. THE PREMATURE INFANT

Need	Nursing Implementation
Needs of Family	
Keep separation to a minimum	Allow parents to visit baby frequently; as soon as possible, allow parents to help care for infant.
Provide data on baby's progress	Answer questions openly, provide up-to-date information on baby's progress.
Express feelings and concerns	Allow parents to talk freely about infant, give support as needed and help parents to accept reality of situation.
Provide information	Explain specialized care to parents. Have them report to pediatrician any of following symptoms: diarrhea, vomiting, lack of appetite, or elevated temperature.
	Help mother to feel confident in care of infant before discharge.
Needs of Infant	
Warmth	Immediate attention in delivery room and transporting to nursery to maintain heat. Maintain temp at about 36°C or 97.6°F in isolette or heated crib.
	Gradually wean infant from heated environment and watch temperature closely until stable.
Oxygen and humidity	Administer oxygen (should be warmed and humidified. Administer humidity (distilled water) usually between 40–70 percent as ordered.
	Check respiratory rate—1 × h and prn.
	Observe for signs of respiratory distress, color, flaring, grunting retractions, skin color, auscultate breath sounds with stethoscope. Analyze oxygen concentration 2–4 h or as necessary to prevent retrolental fibroplasia and to ensure adequate oxygenation. Observe for periods of apnea and stimulate by gently rubbing chest or tapping foot; percuss, vibrate and suction as ordered to remove mucus.
	Reposition q 2 h to promote aeration of all lobes of lung and facilitate drainage.
	Monitor blood gases and electrolytes frequently. (Oxygen administration is determined by blood gases.)
Nutrition and hydration	May require IV feedings through umbilical catheter until stabilized. IV regulated by infusion pump to prevent circulatory overload. Initiate feedings as ordered (usually begin with sterile water or glucose water). Progress to dilute formula or breast milk to full strength formula as tolerated.
	Usually gavage feeding if respirations are about 60 breaths per minute. Use premie nipple if bottle feeding. Infants often require alternate feedings of gavage and bottle feeding.
	Maintain intake and output including stool; weigh daily and organize care to conserve energy with rest periods after each feeding. Measure head circumference and length at least once a week.
Prevention from infection	Maintain aseptic technique.
	Strict isolation techniques with infected babies.
	Prevent skin breakdown—change position, careful cleansing and handling.
	Observe for signs of infection—vomiting, jaundice, lack of appetite, lethargy, cover IV sites.

APPENDIX 3. THE PREMATURE INFANT (*Continued*)

Need	Nursing Implementation
Maintenance of circulatory functioning	Check heart rate by apical pulse for a full minute q 1–2 h.
	Frequently check for bleeding from umbilical catheter. Apply pressure to puncture site as necessary to prevent bleeding. Administer vitamin K as ordered after birth to prevent hemorrhage.
Mothering and physical stimulation	Gently stroke and talk to baby when giving care.
	Hang colorful mobiles or other nonharmful objects in crib.
	Hold baby during feeding as soon as condition permits.
	Encourage parents to hold, cuddle, feed and diaper baby as soon as baby's condition permits.

APPENDIX 4. RECOMMENDED DAILY DIETARY ALLOWANCES FOR PREGNANCY AND LACTATION

	Pregnancy		Lactation		Function	Sources
	14 to 18	Adult	14 to 18	Adult		
Calories	2400	2300	2600	2500	Meet increased nutritional needs as well as body maintenance	All foods Important to emphasize food values of foods and avoid empty calories
Protein	78	76	68	66	Augment maternal issues—bust, uterus, blood Growth and development of placenta and fetal tissue Constant repair and maintenance of maternal tissue	All essential amino acids may be found in milk, meat, eggs, and cheeses Other sources, though not complete protein by themselves: tofu, whole grains, legumes, nuts, peanut butter
Iron	+ 30 mg	+ 30 mg	18 mg	18 mg	Essential constituent of hemoglobin Part of various enzymes Fetal development and storage, especially later part of pregnancy	Good sources: liver, kidney, heart, cooked dry beans, lean pork and beef, dried fruits such as apricots, peaches, prunes, and raisins Fair sources: spinach, mustard greens, eggs
Calcium	1200 mg	1200 mg	1200 mg	1200 mg	Skeletal tissue Bones; teeth Blood coagulation Neuromuscular irritability Myocardial function Fetal stores, especially last months	Good sources: milk, cheese, ice cream, yogurt. Fair sources: broccoli, canned salmon with bones, dried beans, dark leafy vegetables
Phosphorus	1200 mg	1200 mg	1200 mg	1200 mg	90 percent compounded with calcium. Rest distributed throughout cells—involved in energy production, building and repairing tissue, buffering	Whole grain items: cereals, whole wheat bread, brown rice, milk
Sodium	0.5 g	0.5 g	0.5 g	0.5 g	Metabolic activities Fluid balance and acid-base balance Cell permeability Muscle irritability	Table salt, meat, eggs, carrots, celery, beets, spinach, salted nuts, carbonated beverages
Iodine	125 mcg	125 mcg	125 mcg	125 mcg	Necessary for health: mother and fetus; prevents goiter in mother; decreases chance of cretinism in infants	Iodized table salt, cod liver oil

	Pregnancy		Lactation		Function	Sources
	14 to 18	Adult	14 to 18	Adult		
Vitamin A	5000 IU	5000 IU	6000 IU	6000 IU	Tooth formation and skeletal growth Cell growth and development Integrity of epithelial tissue Vision—light/dark adaptation Fat metabolism	Good sources: butter, egg yolk, fortified margarine, whole milk, cream, kidney and liver Fair sources: dark green and yellow vegetables such as sweet potatoes, pumpkins, mustard greens, collards, kale, bok choy, carrots, cantaloupe, apricots
Riboflavin	1.7 mg	1.5 mg	1.9 mg	1.7 mg	Enzyme systems Tissue functioning Tissue oxygenation and respiration Energy metabolism Excreted in breast milk	Good sources: kidney, liver, heart, milk Fair sources: cheese, ice cream, dark leafy vegetables, lean meat, poultry
Thiamine	1.4 mg	1.3 mg	1.4 mg	1.3 mg	Carbohydrate metabolism Normal appetite and digestion Health of nervous system	Good sources: enriched and whole grain products—bread and cereals, dried peas, beans, liver, heart, kidney, nuts, potatoes, lean pork. Fair sources: eggs, milk, poultry, fish, vegetables
Niacin	16 mg	15 mg	18 mg	17 mg	Cell metabolism	Good sources: fish, lean meat, poultry, liver, heart, peanuts, peanut butter Fair sources: enriched and bread, whole grain cereals and milk, potatoes
Folic acid B_{12}	4.0 mg	4.0 mg	4.0 mg	4.0 mg	Cell growth Reproduction and formation of heme Enzyme activities in production of protein Deficiency results in megloblastic anemia	Dark green and leafy vegetables
Pyridoxine B_6	2.5 mg	2.5 mg	2.5 mg	2.5 mg	Essential coenzyme with amino acids Deficiency may lead to hypochromic microcytic anemia	Animal and vegetable protein such as meat, fish, beans, nuts and seeds, milk and milk products

APPENDIX 4. RECOMMENDED DAILY DIETARY ALLOWANCES FOR PREGNANCY AND LACTATION (*Continued*)

	Pregnancy 14 to 18	Adult	Lactation 14 to 18	Adult	Function	Sources
Vitamin D	400 IU	400 IU	400 IU	400 IU	Influences absorption, retention and utilization of calcium and phosphorus	Formation of bones, teeth and other tissue Good sources:fortified milk, butter, egg yolks, liver, fish oils
Vitamin C Ascorbic acid	60 mg	60 mg	80 mg	80 mg	Production of intracellular substances necessary for development and maintenance of normal connective tissue in bones, cartilage and muscles Role in metabolic processes involving protein and tissues Increases absorption of iron	Good sources: citrus fruits and juice, broccoli, cantaloupe, collards, mustard and turnip greens, peppers Fair sources: asparagus, raw cabbage, other melons, spinach, prunes, tomatoes, canned or fresh chilis

APPENDIX 5. PRENATAL INSTRUCTIONS

Nutrition

A. It is important that adequate nutrition is maintained.

B. See Appendix 4 for specific guidelines.

Use of Drugs

A. All drugs can be expected to cross the placenta and affect the fetus.

B. Greatest danger occurs in first trimester, especially when organs are developing (organogenesis).

C. Many other effects of drugs on the fetus are unknown and may not be evident for years.

D. Pregnant women should refrain from taking drugs during pregnancy; even commonly used drugs such as aspirin should only be taken by physician's order.

E. Nicotine in cigarettes may retard the growth of fetus.
1. Causes vasoconstriction of woman's vessels resulting in decreased placental flow.
2. Increases carbon dioxide levels in blood and reduces oxygen-carrying capacity.

F. See Appendix 2 for an outline on drugs that adversely affect fetus.

Exercise, Relaxation, and Rest

A. Exercise in moderation is beneficial but should never be carried on past the point of fatigue.

B. Sports may be participated in if they are part of the woman's usual activity and there are no complications present.

C. Fatigue is common in early pregnancy.

D. Frequent rest periods, at 10- to 15-minute intervals, are helpful in avoiding needless fatigue.

E. Relaxation and stress reduction important to maintain emotional stability during pregnancy.

12

PEDIATRIC NURSING

GROWTH AND DEVELOPMENT

PRINCIPLES OF GROWTH AND DEVELOPMENT†

Maturation

A. The process of maturation.
   1. Process of attaining maximum growth and development.
   2. Process of the unfolding of inherited tendencies, independent of any special practice or training.
B. Major principles of growth and development.
   1. Occurs in an orderly sequence.
   2. Continuous, but continuity may be interrupted by spurts of growth and periods of no growth.
   3. Progresses at individualized rates.
   4. Different ages vary for specific body structures.
   5. Each individual has an inherent growth pattern.
   6. Increases in structure (growth) are accompanied by increases in function (development).
C. Major influences on growth and development.
   1. Genetic factors.
   2. Environmental variations.

Profiles of Growth and Development

A. Physical development.
   1. Growth rate.
      a. Rapid during infancy.
      b. Slow and steady during childhood.
      c. Spurt during puberty.
      d. Decrease; maximum height attained during adolescence.
   2. Height.
      a. Average length is 20 inches at birth.
      b. Increases ten inches in the first year.
      c. Increases five inches in the second year.
      d. Increases three inches per year from the third to the sixth year.
      e. Increases by about two inches per year after sixth year.
      f. Peak reached by boys at about 14 years of age.
      g. Peak reached by girls at about 13 years of age.
   3. Weight.
      a. Average weight is seven and a half pounds at birth.
      b. Doubles by the end of the fifth month, and triples by the end of first year.
      c. Increases by about five pounds per year until puberty, and then increases rapidly.
      d. Levels off with only little gain after puberty.
   4. Body proportions.
      a. Striking changes from birth to maturity.
      b. At birth, head is one-fourth of the total body length; the adult head is only about one-eighth of the total body length.
   5. Bone formation.
      a. What will later be bone begins as connective tissue, which gradually becomes cartilage, and finally, through the process of ossification, becomes bone.
      b. Bone formation complete in girls at about 17 years of age.
      c. Bone formation is complete in boys at about 19 years of age.
   6. Teeth formation.
      a. First two lower central incisors appear between the fifth and seventh month followed by about one new tooth per month.
      b. The set of 20 deciduous teeth should be complete by the age of two and a half years. (For chart of dental development, see Appendix 7.)

† For Growth and Development Milestones by age group, see Chapter One.

B. Motor Development.
1. Includes learning, controlling, and integrating muscular responses.
2. Occurs in an orderly sequence, and is related to the maturation of the nervous system.
3. Begins at the head, moves downward, and proceeds from the center of the body toward the extremities.
4. Effective use of the hands for seizing and grasping objects (prehension) begins between the second and third month.
5. Ability to walk alone (locomotion) is attained gradually and begins with holding up the head; most infants have learned to walk alone between the ages of 12 and 14 months.
C. Intellectual development.
1. Intelligence is the ability to think, to reason, to remember, and to imagine.
2. Intelligence develops gradually and continuously.
D. Emotional development.
1. Emotions begin to develop early.
2. Few individuals react to the same emotion in the same way.
3. Emotions of fear, excitement, anger, and joy are recognizable at one year of age.
4. Emotions are expressed by facial expressions, vocalization, and body movements.

HOSPITALIZATION

Stages of Separation Anxiety

A. Protest.
1. Characteristics: cries loudly, throws tantrums.
2. Nursing behaviors: stay close to the child to provide warmth and support.
B. Despair.
1. Characteristics: withdraws, shows no interest in eating, playing, or interacting; typical during extended hospitalization.
2. Nursing behaviors: recognize the anxiety and establish a relationship with the child; attempt to engage and involve the child in an activity.
C. Denial.
1. Characteristics: exhibits behavior that is often mistaken for happy adjustment; ignores mother and may regress.
2. Nursing behaviors: reassure the mother, develop a relationship with the child, and provide warmth and support to the child during long hospitalization.

Hospitalization of the Infant

Psychological Implications

A. Separation from the parent is threatening.
B. Decrease in sensory stimuli.
C. Causes of breakdown in mother-infant relationship.
1. Maternal guilt.
2. Hostile, cold hospital environment.
3. Lessened opportunity for mothering role; mother may feel inadequate.
4. Subordination of the parents by the staff.

Implementation

A. Take positive nursing action to prevent the detrimental effects of hospitalization.
B. Provide a prehospitalization nursing interview with the parents and give a tour of the pediatric unit.
1. Explain procedures, regulations, and the rationale behind the rules; arrange for parents to meet the staff.
2. Encourage parents to visit frequently and/or to possibly room in.
C. Counsel the parents regarding the infant's illness.
1. Elicit their understanding of the disease as well as its likely progressive course.
2. Correct any misconceptions and, if appropriate, reassure them that they are not the cause of the illness.

D. Encourage the parents to participate in the infant's care if they show an interest in doing so.
   1. Teach the parents procedures they are capable of doing.
   2. Show respect for superior knowledge of their infant in respect to likes, dislikes, and habits.
E. Assume role of the absent mother.
   1. Limit, initially, the number of people handling the infant; allow one person to become familiar with the infant and gradually introduce others.
   2. Provide closeness and warmth by cuddling.
   3. Avoid isolating the infant from sensory stimulation.
   a. Provide stimulation during feeding.
   b. Hang brightly colored mobiles within the infant's sight.
   4. Play with the infant.

Hospitalization of the Toddler and Preschool Child

Psychological Implications

A. Hospitalization is a very threatening experience for a child.
   1. Unfamiliar situations and procedures are experienced.
   2. Growing sense of identity and independence may be disrupted.
B. Experiences separation anxiety; child mourns the absence of the mother through protest, despair and denial.
C. The loss of "body integrity" is feared.
   1. Does not realistically perceive how the body functions.
   2. May overreact to a simple procedure; some toddlers believe that drawing blood will leave a hole and that the rest of their blood will leak out.
D. Disruption of normal rituals and routines are resented; toddlers are often very rigid about those procedures that allow them a sense of security and control over otherwise frightening circumstances.
E. Loss of mobility is frustrating to a child.
F. Most recent acquired behaviors are frequently abandoned, and toddler reverts to safer, less mature patterns (regression).

Implementation

A. Introduce the child to hospital surroundings, preferably prior to hospitalization.
B. Explain all the procedures in simple terms and allow for further discussion, if desired.
C. Encourage parents to room in or to visit frequently once the child is hospitalized.
D. Suggest that the mother leave an object that the child associates with her for the child to "care for" until she can return. This procedure assures the child that his mother will return.
E. Encourage the parents to be honest about when they are going and coming. Do not tell the child they will stay all night and then leave when the child is asleep.
F. Paste family pictures to the crib.
G. Use puppet play to explain procedures and to gain an understanding of the child's perception of his hospitalization. Use puppets to work out anxiety, anger, and frustration.
H. When recording developmental history elicit exact routines and rituals that the child uses; attempt to modify hospital routine to continue these rituals.
I. Provide stretchers, wheelchairs, and carts for immobilized children.
J. Do not punish the child for reverting to less mature behavior patterns; explain the reasons for its occurrence to the parents.

Hospitalization of the School-Age Child

Psychological Implications

A. The school-age child needs to understand why things are happening as they are.

B. Child has heightened concern for privacy and needs to protect body-image.

C. Child is modest and fears disgrace.

D. Hospitalization interrupts busy school life, and child fears he or she will be replaced or forgotten by peer group.

E. Absence from peer group means a disruption of close friendships.

Implementation

A. Inform the child about his or her illness; take the opportunity to explain how the body functions.

B. Explain all procedures completely; allow the child to see special rooms (i.e., intensive care, cardiac catheter lab) prior to being sent to them for treatments.

C. Provide opportunities for the child to socialize with his or her peer group at meals and through team tournaments of cards, chess, and checkers.

D. Allow telephone privileges for calls to his or her home and friends.

E. Provide outlets (e.g., dart board and a boxing bag) for anger and frustration.

F. Give the child opportunity to make choices and exert independence.

G. Protect the child's privacy.

H. Provide tutors to prevent disruption of education.

I. Provide the opportunity to master developmental tasks of age group.

Hospitalization of the Adolescent

Psychological Implications

A. Concern with disruption of social system and peer group.

B. Fear of alteration of body image.

C. Fear of loss of independence.

D. Fear of change in future plans.

E. Concern with interruption in development of heterosexual relationships.

F. Resentment of loss of privacy.

G. The degree to which the young adult is affected depends on several factors.
1. Whether the illness is chronic or acute.
2. Whether the final prognosis necessitates a change in the young adult's future aspirations.
3. The number of changes which he or she must accept.

Implementation

A. Adolescents should be placed in rooms with their peers.

B. Allow telephone privileges with some limitations of time.

C. Enhance the adolescent's feeling of self-worth, and encourage as much independence as possible.

D. Allow reasonable heterosexual relationships to develop.

E. Provide for privacy.

F. Assist adolescent in role model identification.

G. Realistically discuss problems of the illness with the adolescent.

H. Always provide honest information.

I. Encourage the adolescent, if able, to accept reasonable responsibility for unit decorum.

General Assessment—Infant to Adolescent

General Principles

A. Maturational ability of the child to cooperate with the examiner is of major importance to adequate physical assessment.

B. When planning physical assessment of the child, the following points should be considered:
1. Establish a relationship with the child prior to the examination.
    a. Determine child's maturational level.

b. Allow the child an opportunity to become more accustomed to the examiner.
2. Explain in terms appropriate to the child's level of understanding the extent and purpose of the examination.
3. Realize that the physical examination may be a stressful experience for the child, who is helpless and depends on others for protection.
4. Limit the physical examination to what is essential in determining an adequate nursing diagnosis.
5. Proceed from the least to the most intrusive procedures.
6. Allow active participation of the child whenever possible.

Special Considerations for Each Age Group

The Infant

A. Accomplish as much of the examination as possible while the infant is sleeping or resting undisturbed.
B. Assess general condition.
1. Symmetry and location of body parts.
2. Color and condition of the skin.
3. State of restlessness and sleeplessness.
4. Adjustment to feeding regimen.
5. Quality of cry.
C. Congenital anomaly appraisal.
1. Neurological system.
a. Reflexes: absent or asymmetrical (see Appendix 2).
b. Head circumference: microcephaly, hydrocephaly.
(1) 35 cm at birth.
(2) 40 cm at 3 months.
(3) 45 cm at 9 months.
(4) At birth, the head size is 2 cm larger than the chest. Equals or exceeds chest until two years of age.
c. Fontanels: closed, bulging.

(1) Anterior measures 3.5 cm by 3.5 cm and closes by 18 months.
(2) Posterior measures 1 cm by 1 cm and closes at two months.
d. Eyes: cataracts, lid folds, spots on iris.
2. Respiratory system.
a. Breath sounds: signs of aspiration, asymmetry of lung expansion, retractions, grunting.
b. Apnea.
3. Cardiovascular system.
a. Color: cyanosis.
b. Rate and rhythm: murmurs, tachycardia, bradycardia.
c. Energy level: cannot suck for 15 minutes without exhaustion or cyanosis.
4. Gastrointestinal tract.
a. History of polyhydramnios.
b. Patency: mucus, spitting, cyanosis, cannot pass nasogastric tube to stomach.
c. Mouth: palate or lip not intact.
d. Anus: not patent.
5. Genitourinary.
a. Umbilical vessels: missing normal two arteries and one vein.
b. Urine: abnormal stream.
c. Masses: abdominal (Wilms' tumor).
d. Boys: undescended testicles, hernia, urethra not opening at the end of the penis.
e. Girls: labial adhesions.
6. Skeletal system.
a. Fractured clavicle.
b. Dislocated hip: asymmetric major gluteal folds, hip click.
c. Legs and feet: clubbing, without straight tibial line.
d. Spine: curved, inflexible, open.
D. Common problems.
1. Ear infections.
a. Increased temperature, irritability.
b. Rubbing or pulling ear.
c. Change in eating habits.
2. Upper respiratory infections.
a. Duration of symptoms, severity.
b. Wheezing, barking cough, anxiety, restlessness, use of accessory muscles.

c. If throat is sore, check white patches on tonsils.
3. Rashes.
   a. Onset, duration, description, location.
   b. Any event such as new food, exposure to animals.
4. Contact dermatitis.
   a. Allergic problems.
   b. Diaper area rash: use of soap, lotions, powders; method of cleaning cloth diapers.
5. Hernias.
   a. Inguinal: lump in groin, with or without pain.
   b. Umbilical: can it be pushed back without difficulty or pain.
6. Scalp—cradle cap.
   a. Scalp scaling, crusted; method of washing hair.
   b. Application of any lotions or balms to hair.
7. Birth marks.
   a. Change in size, color, shape.
   b. Any bleeding or irritation.
8. Eye symmetry.
   a. Frequency of a problem with eye alignment: (time of day eyes wander).
   b. Light reflex symmetrical in both eyes.

E. Screening procedures.
1. Developmental landmarks—DDST (Denver Developmental Screening Test).
2. Vision.
3. Hearing.
4. Growth charts: head circumference, weight, length.

F. Nursing guidance areas.
1. Growth and development changes.
2. Stranger anxiety.
3. Separation anxiety.
4. Transitional objects.
5. Accident prevention.

Toddler and the Preschool Child

A. General considerations.
1. Remember that separation anxiety is most acute at toddler age and body integrity fears most acute at preschool age.

2. Involve the parent in examination as much as possible.
3. Restrain child as much as necessary to protect the child from injury.
4. Give careful explanation of each portion of the exam.
5. Allow the child to handle the equipment and try out on doll.

B. Common Problems.
1. Feeding and eating.
   a. Review food ingested in last 48 hours.
   b. Types of foods, adequate source of vitamins, minerals.
2. Temper tantrums.
   a. Frequency, duration, precipitating event.
   b. Response of caretaker.
3. Toilet training.
   a. Check ability to ambulate (indicating neuromuscular maturity).
   b. Bothered by wet diapers. Interested in toileting.
4. Respiratory infections: see Infant section.
5. Communicable diseases.
   a. Onset of symptoms, progression of disease, treatment of symptoms.
   b. Observation of complications.
6. Gastrointestinal.
   a. Onset, duration, intake and output.
   b. Signs of dehydration.

C. Screening procedures (same as Infant).

School Age Child

A. General considerations.
1. Modesty important.
2. Explain all procedures.
3. Direct questions to child.

B. Common problems.
1. School.
   a. Signs of school phobias, vomits before school, delays going.
   b. Increase in physical complaints.
2. Nervous habits (stuttering, twitching, etc.).
   a. Onset, duration, precipitating event.
   b. Anxiety of child and parent over problem.

3. Accidental trauma.
   a. Understanding of accident.
   b. Prevention, physical limitations.
4. Respiratory infections: see Infant section.
5. Gastrointestinal infections: see Preschooler section.

C. Screening procedures.
   1. Snellen vision testing.
   2. Sweep check audiometry.
   3. Height and weight measurement.
   4. Inspection of skin and teeth.

D. Nursing guidance areas.
   1. Need for autonomy.
   2. Toilet training.
   3. Imaginary friends.
   4. Fear of dark.
   5. Rituals and routines.

Adolescent

A. General considerations.
   1. Examine child alone if he wishes (privacy important).
   2. Note signs of puberty.
   3. Ascertain feelings about body image.

B. Common Problems.
   1. Acne.
      a. Existing skin care program.
      b. Personal hygiene.
   2. Dysmenorrhea.
      a. Degree of pain, missed school.
      b. Use of analgesics.
      c. Amount of exercise.
   3. Obesity.
      a. Eating patterns.
      b. Family concern.
      c. Amount of exercise.

C. Screening procedures (same as School Age).

D. Nursing guidance areas.
   1. Hazards of cigarette smoking and alcohol.
   2. Transmission and symptoms of venereal disease.
   3. Review sex education.
   4. Accident prevention—particularly automobile.
   5. Principles of nutrition.

THE NEWBORN AND INFANT

CONGENITAL ANOMALIES

Cleft Lip

Definition: Fissure or split in the upper lip resulting from failure of the two sides of the face to unite properly.

Treatment and Implementation

A. Preoperative care.
   1. Use a large holed, soft nipple for feedings.
   2. Prevent infections.
   3. Place nipple on side opposite defect.
   4. Bubble frequently.

B. Surgical procedure.
   1. Closure of lip.
   2. Performed at about three months of age or when infant is ten pounds.

C. Postoperative care.
   1. Observe for respiratory distress and swelling of tongue, nostrils, and mouth.
   2. Avoid circumstances that will cause crying.
   3. Watch for hemorrhage.
   4. Use elbow restraints and provide supervised rest periods to exercise arms.
   5. Feed with rubber-tipped medicine dropper on the side opposite the repaired cleft for three weeks.
   6. After feeding, clean suture line with half-strength hydrogen peroxide.
   7. Prevent crust formation on suture line by frequent cleansing and application of ointment.
   8. Lay infant on side or back with support to prevent rolling over on the abdomen.
   9. Prevent infections.

Cleft Palate

Definition: Fissure or split in the roof of mouth (palate) resulting from failure of two sides of face to unite. There may be involvement of both the hard and soft palate.

Assessment

A. Poor sucking reflex so infant unable to form a vacuum in the mouth.

B. If able to talk, there may be a speech impediment.

C. Increased incidence of upper respiratory infections.

Treatment and Implementation

A. Preoperative care.
   1. Prevent infections.
   2. Give nothing by mouth.
B. Surgical procedure.
   1. May be performed in stages if the defect is bilateral.
   2. The repair is usually made after 18 months of age.
C. Postoperative care.
   1. Apply hand restraints to prevent damage to the mouth.
   2. Provide good oral hygiene.
   3. Prevent infections.
   4. Provide safe toys with no small parts.
   5. Sedate and attempt to keep infant content.
   6. Feed liquids using a cup or spoon.

Esophageal Atresia

Definition: Closure of the esophagus during embryonic development; usually ends in a blind pouch.

Assessment

A. Excessive amounts of saliva.

B. Drooling.

C. Respiratory distress with each feeding.

Treatment and Implementation

A. Preoperative care.
   1. Observe carefully.
   2. Clear airway.
   3. Elevate head of bed 30 degrees.
   4. Give nothing by mouth.
   5. Maintain sucking reflex.
B. Surgical procedure.
   1. Repair the esophagus.
   2. Gastrostomy for feeding access.
C. Postoperative care.
   1. Provide rest with infrequent handling.
   2. Keep gastrostomy tube open.
   3. Feed through gastrostomy tube.
   4. Maintain patent airway.
   5. Elevate head of bed 30 degrees.
   6. Maintain sucking reflex.

Hydrocephalus

Definition: Abnormal accumulation of spinal fluid within the brain causing an increase in intracranial pressure. Accumulation may be due either to blockage of the flow of spinal fluid or to the lack of proper absorption of the spinal fluid.

Assessment

A. Increase in size and shape of head.

B. Suture lines separated with bulging fontanels.

C. Dilated scalp veins.

D. Strabismus and nystagmus.

E. "Sunset" eyes (sclera visible above the iris).

F. Projectile vomiting and anorexia.

G. Irritability and lethargy.

H. Poor neck control.

Treatment and Implementation

A. Preoperative care.
   1. Feed small amounts with care to prevent vomiting.
   2. Change position frequently to prevent pneumonia and pressure sores on the head.

3. Support the infant's head when turning or moving.
4. Prevent infection.
5. Carefully observe vital signs.
6. Observe for signs of increased intracranial pressure.
7. Provide emotional support for both parents and infant.

B. Surgical procedure: ventriculovenous shunt performed to reduce the volume of spinal fluid within the ventricles.

C. Postoperative care.
1. Maintain open airway.
2. Carefully observe vital signs.
3. Look for signs of increased intracranial pressure.
4. Give nothing by mouth for four to six hours after surgery.
5. Carefully begin to feed clear fluids.
6. Meet the needs of the normal newborn.
7. Measure head circumference.
8. Position the head opposite the side of the shunt.
9. Support the head when turning or changing the position.
10. Prevent infection.
11. Give emotional support to infant and parents.

Spina Bifida

Definition: Defect in the spinal column caused either by failure of the posterior part of the laminae of the vertebrae to fuse or by absence of part of the laminae. The defect usually occurs in the lumbosacral area, but it may occur at any level of the spine.

Types of Spina Bifida

A. *Spina bifida occulta:* Bony defect in the spine that may have a visible dimple or a small tuft of hair in the area.

B. *Meningocele:* Protrusion of meninges and cerebral spinal fluid through the opening in the spine which may be covered only by a thin membranous sac.

C. *Myelomeningocele:* Protrusion of meninges, cerebral spinal fluid, spinal cord, and nerves through the defect in the spine; there may be paralysis below the level of the defect.

Treatment and Implementation

A. Preoperative care.
1. Prevent infection.
2. Observe movement of the extremities.
3. Observe bowel and bladder function.
4. Provide normal newborn care.

B. Surgical procedure.
1. Removal of the protrusion.
2. Closure of the defect.

C. Postoperative care.
1. Prevent infection.
2. Use Credé method on the bladder.
3. Provide range of motion exercises to lower extremities.
4. Provide good skin care.
5. Give emotional support to infant and parents.

Down's Syndrome

Definition: Physical malformation and degree of mental retardation resulting from a chromosomal defect, usually number 21.

Assessment

A. Face characterized by rounded shape, flattened nose, thickened tongue, almond-shaped eyes, and flattened occiput.

B. Muscles flaccid; motor development will be slow.

C. Extremities characterized by short, fat hands with simian crease on the palms and little finger curved inward.

D. Mental capacity varies from mild to severe retardation. These children are usually very happy.

Implementation

A. Individualize according to needs of the infant and the family.

B. Give assistance in contacting community agencies that can assist the family with the infant's needs.

C. Encourage developmental activities initiated at the proper time.

D. Observe for other anomalies in the infant.

E. Alert the family of the necessity to take precautions against infection.

F. Refer the family to a geneticist.

Phenylketonuria (PKU)

Definition: Failure of the body to normally metabolize the amino acid phenylalanine. High levels of this amino acid in the blood can cause mental retardation. The condition is genetically transmitted; most state health departments mandate PKU testing before the infant's discharge from the hospital.

Assessment

A. Brain development arrested by four months of age if left untreated.

B. Moderate to severe retardation by one year of age if left untreated. Retardation level correlates with high PKU levels and this condition is irreversible.

Treatment and Implementation

A. Restrict phenylalanine in the diet until about five years of age.

B. Eliminate foods high in protein, e.g., meat, poultry, fish, eggs, nuts, legumes, and milk products.

C. Observe for signs of phenylalanine deficiency, e.g., lethargy, anorexia, anemia, skin rashes, and diarrhea.

D. Suggest genetic counseling to the parents.

E. Gently remind parents to have all future children born to them screened for PKU.

Failure to Thrive

Definition: A syndrome characterized by an infant's failure to grow and develop with or without characteristic posturing or "body language." Etiology is nonspecific. May be organic or nonorganic.

Assessment

A. History of infant includes feeding problems, vomiting, sleep disturbance, irritability, sucking ability, aversion to formula, and irregularity in daily activities.

B. Abnormal nutritional intake cause may be related to deficient intake, malabsorption, or poor assimilation.
  1. Number of calories, quality of calories, and feeding patterns.
  2. Weigh daily and observe reaction to nutritional program.

C. Nature of mother-child relationship.
  1. Relationship patterns.
  2. Ability of mother to perceive infant's needs.

Implementation

A. Priority—provide sufficient nutrients so that infant will grow.
  1. Develop a structured feeding routine.
  2. Weigh daily to assess weight gain.

B. Provide nurturing to infant.
  1. Ensure a warm, loving environment through holding, cuddling, and physical contact.
  2. Spend time talking to infant and building a trusting relationship.
  3. Maintain as much eye-to-eye contact as possible.

C. Provide a positive, quiet, nonstimulating environment to promote psychosocial growth.

D. Assist mother to develop a positive relationship with infant.

E. Document feeding behaviors and monitor infant progress.

Sudden Infant Death Syndrome (SIDS)

Definition: The sudden, unexplained death of an infant during sleep.

Characteristics

A. Largest single cause of death after neonatal period.

B. Peak incidence two to four months; rare after six months.

C. Higher incidence in winter months, in low income groups, and in low birth weight infants.

D. Most deaths are unobserved and occur during sleep.

E. On autopsy, inflammation of upper respiratory tract is found.

F. Etiology unknown and controversial. Many theories involving CO_2 sensitivity, poor response to stimulus, vitamin or mineral dificiency.

Treatment

A. Support of parents—help work through feelings of guilt and loss.

B. Refer to National Foundation for Sudden Infant Death.

CONGENITAL HEART DEFECTS

Definition: A structural defect of heart or great vessels. The defects are present at birth. *Cyanotic* (with cyanosis) defects allow unoxygenated blood to circulate throughout the body. *Acyanotic* (without cyanosis) defects shunt blood previously oxygenated back to the lungs and allow oxygenated blood to go to the body.

Fetal Circulation

A. Major structures of fetal circulation.
   1. Ductus venosus—a structure that shunts blood past the portal circulation.
   2. Foramen ovale—an opening between the right and left atria of the heart that shunts blood past the lungs.
   3. Ductus arteriosus—a structure between the aorta and the pulmonary artery that shunts blood past the lungs.

B. Changes in circulation at birth.
   1. The umbilical arteries and vein and the ductus venosus become nonfunctional.
   2. The lungs expand, reducing resistance, and greater amounts of blood enter the pulmonary circulation.
   3. More blood in the pulmonary circulation increases the return of blood to the left atrium, which initiates the closure of the flap of tissue covering the foramen ovale.
   4. The ductus arteriosus contracts and the blood flow decreases; eventually, the duct closes.

C. Two major clues to presence of heart disease.
   1. Congestive heart failure.
      a. Begins before one year of age in majority of infants.
      b. Most infants are less than six months old.
   2. Cyanosis.

Coarctation of Aorta

Definition: Stenosis or narrowing of the aorta.

Assessment

A. Increased blood pressure in the arms.

B. Decreased blood pressure in the thighs; may have no femoral pulses that are palpable.

C. Headache and nose bleeds.

D. May have no audible murmurs.

Treatment and Implementation

A. Resection of the aorta or insertion of a graft.

B. Surgery delayed as long as possible, depending on the condition of the vessel.

Patent Ductus Arteriosus

Definition: Failure of the ductus arteriosus to close after birth.

Assessment

A. Dyspnea on exertion.
B. Growth failure.
C. Loud murmur.

Treatment and Implementation

A. Closing of ductus.
B. Surgery usually performed between two and five years of age.

Atrial Septal and Ventricular Septal Defects

Definition: Failure of the septum in either the atrium or the ventricle to completely develop. The extent of severity of the defect is dependent on the size and location of the opening.

Assessment

A. Frequent upper respiratory infections.
B. Cyanosis on exertion.
C. Loud murmurs.

Treatment and Implementation

A. Surgical closure to repair defect.
B. Surgery delayed as long as possible to allow child to grow.

Tetralogy of Fallot

Definition: Combination of four heart defects—ventricular septal defect, pulmonary stenosis, overriding of aorta, and hypertrophy of the right ventricle.

Assessment

A. Cyanosis.
B. Growth failure.
C. Polycythemia.
D. Black-out spells.
E. Convulsions.
F. The child normally assumes a squatting position to facilitate breathing.

Treatment and Implementation

A. Surgical closure.
B. Surgery delayed as long as possible.

Transposition of the Great Vessels

Definition: Reversal of the position of the aorta and the pulmonary artery.

Assessment

A. Cyanosis.
B. Dyspnea.
C. Tachycardia.
D. Increased respirations.

Treatment and Implementation

A. Preoperative care.
   1. Prevent infection.
   2. Encourage rest.
   3. Observe vital signs with care.
   4. Provide emotional support for the child and family.
   5. Prepare for surgery with the usual preoperative teaching of breathing exercises (e.g., cough and deep breathing; blow bottles).
B. Surgical procedure.
   1. Mustard procedure (delayed as long as possible).
   2. In infancy a shunt is usually necessary to get more oxygenated blood to the body.
C. Postoperative care.

1. Maintain pulmonary function with suctioning, oxygen, deep-breathing, and/or care of the chest tubes.
2. Observe vital signs, intake and output, and color.
3. Provide good skin care.
4. Provide adequate rest periods.
5. Maintain patient comfort with medications and necessary positioning.
6. Provide emotional support for the child and the family.

DISORDERS OF THE INFANT

Otitis Media

Definition: Inflammation of the middle ear resulting from an infection-producing organism.

Assessment

A. Pain in the ears.
B. Fever.
C. Irritability.
D. Headache.
E. Convulsions.

Treatment and Implementation

A. Antibiotics.
B. Myringotomy—incision that opens up the tympanic membrane.
C. Observe vital signs.
D. Take measures to reduce fever if present.
E. Provide good skin care; maintain cleanliness of the ear canal.
F. Irrigate ear if ordered.
G. Apply local heat to the ears if ordered.

Bronchiolitis

Definition: Inflammation of the bronchioles caused by thick mucus that traps air in the alveoli which leads to poor air exchange. Bronchiolitis usually occurs before 18 months of age.

Assessment

A. Dry, nonproductive cough.
B. Nasal discharge.
C. Dyspnea.
D. Cyanosis.
E. Dehydration.
F. Irritability.

Treatment and Implementation

A. Maintain patent airway.
B. Give nothing by mouth until dyspnea is improved.
C. Maintain intravenous feedings as ordered.
D. Provide humidity and oxygen as necessary.
E. Elevate head of bed.

Pyloric Stenosis

Definition: Obstruction in the opening between the stomach and the intestine resulting from enlargement (hypertrophy) of the pyloric muscle. The condition is more common in the male infant and usually is diagnosed between four and six weeks of age.

Assessment

A. Projectile vomiting soon after or during a feeding.
   1. Vomitus contains no bile.
   2. Formula appears to be almost the same as when ingested.
B. Weight loss and dehydration; crying and fussy.
C. Peristaltic waves during or after feeding.

Treatment and Implementation

A. Preoperative care.
   1. Elevate head of bed 30 degrees.
   2. Give nothing by mouth.
   3. Maintain intravenous feedings as ordered.
   4. Adjust nasogastric tube to low suction.
B. Surgical procedure.
   1. Pyloromyotomy—the incision of pylorus muscles.
   2. Fredet-Ramstedt procedure.
C. Postoperative care.
   1. Adjust nasogastric tube to low suction for a few hours.
   2. Maintain intravenous fluids.
   3. Feed small amounts of clear liquids frequently, and increase them as tolerated.
   4. Elevate head of bed 30 degrees.
   5. Check dressing for bleeding.

Intussusception

Definition: Invagination or telescoping of one part of the bowel into another part below it. The condition occurs most frequently in boys between the ages of four and ten months.

Assessment

A. Severe coliclike pain in the abdomen.
B. Progressive vomiting.
C. Bloody stools (like currant jelly).
D. Shock.

Treatment and Implementation

A. Barium enema, which may be effective in reducing invagination.
B. Preoperative care.
   1. Adjust nasogastric tube to low suction.
   2. Give nothing by mouth.
   3. Maintain intravenous liquids.
   4. Provide emotional support.
C. Surgical procedure.
   1. May only need to manipulate the bowel back to its normal position.

2. A resection may be required, depending on when the diagnosis was made.
3. Excision of involved area with end-to-end anastomosis.
D. Postoperative care.
   1. Maintain intravenous fluids.
   2. Adjust nasogastric tube to low suction.
   3. Begin oral feeding of clear fluids.
   4. Observe vital signs.
   5. Check dressing for bleeding.

Hirschsprung's Disease (Congenital Megacolon)

Definition: Lack of normal nerve ganglia in the distal end of the colon. Length of colon involved varies with each individual. Condition is more common in males.

Assessment

A. Newborn may or may not pass meconium.
B. Constipation is progressive as diet increases.
C. Progressive abdominal distention.
D. Anorexia.
E. Occasional vomiting.

Treatment and Implementation

A. Provide daily enemas, stool softeners, and a low residue diet.
B. Surgical procedure.
   1. Swenson's pull-through or variation of the procedure.
   2. Temporary colostomy above narrowed section.

Diarrhea

Definition: Frequent, watery bowel movements that result from an increased wavelike movement in the intestines.

Types of Diarrhea

A. Infectious—caused by either bacterial or viral organism.
B. Noninfectious—caused by an irritant in the intestinal tract, e.g., foods, drugs, laxatives, or other irritants.

Assessment

A. May be mild to severe.
B. Frequent stools, usually foul smelling, greenish in color, watery, and expelled with force.
C. Abdominal distention.
D. Irritability.
E. Weight loss and dehydration.
F. Increased rate of peristalsis.

Treatment and Implementation

A. Replace electrolytes.
B. Give antibiotics if caused by an organism and/or to prevent secondary infection.
C. Give nothing by mouth. Desire for food will increase as stools decrease.
D. Isolate infant to prevent spread of diarrhea throughout the nursery.
E. Measure intake and output.
F. Weigh infant daily.
G. Maintain intravenous feedings if ordered.
H. Give good skin care.

Sickle Cell Anemia

Definition: Tendency of red blood cells to be crescent shaped when under low oxygen tension. The disorder results from the presence of abnormal type of hemoglobin and is transmitted as a recessive dominant trait, particularly among blacks.

Assessment

A. In noncrisis state the infant experiences the following symptoms.
  1. Severe chronic anemia.

  2. Periodic crises with abdominal and joint pain.
  3. Enlarged spleen from increased activity.
  4. Jaundice from excessive red blood cell destruction.
  5. Widening of the marrow spaces of the bones.
  6. Gallstones.
B. In crisis state the infant experiences episodes with the following characteristics.
  1. Thrombotic crisis is the most frequent type and is caused by occlusion of the small blood vessels, which produces distal ischemia and infarction.
    a. Swelling of hands and feet.
    b. Large joints and surrounding areas may become painful and swollen.
    c. Severe abdominal pains.
  2. Sequestration crisis is less frequent and occurs only in young children; it is caused by pooling of blood in spleen.
    a. Enlargement of the spleen.
    b. Circulatory collapse.

Treatment and Implementation

A. Alleviate pain with analgesics.
B. Prevent dehydration with intravenous infusion if necessary and increased fluid intake.
C. Offer parents genetic counseling.
D. Counsel the family on physiology and prognosis of disease.

Thalassemias

Definition: An inherited group of hemolytic anemias caused by too few hemoglobin polypeptide chains. A chronic condition.

Assessment

A. Assess for skin breakdown, especially leg ulcers.
B. Observe for jaundice and elevated serum bilirubin.

C. Check for intolerance of fatty foods and abdominal discomfort.

D. Check blood studies, fetal hemoglobin as high as 90%.

Implementation

A. Supportive: rest, decreased activity, heat lamp to open wounds, excellent skin care.

B. Monitor packed red cells or chelating agents (Desferal) as ordered.

C. Prepare for splenectomy if transfused cells are rapidly destroyed by spleen.

Hemophilia

Definition: A sex-linked disorder in which certain factors necessary for coagulation of the blood are missing. Transmission of sex-linked traits are passed from unaffected carrier females to affected males.

Characteristics

A. Hemophilia A—Factor VIII deficiency: treated with cryoprecipitate or fresh-frozen plasma.

B. Hemophilia B—Factor IX deficiency (Christmas disease): treated with cryoprecipitate or fresh-frozen plasma.

C. Hemophilia C—Factor XI deficiency: treated with fresh-frozen plasma.

Assessment

A. Type A or B—symptoms.
   1. Possible bleeding tendency in neonatal period because factors are not passed through the placenta.
   2. Excessive bruising.
   3. Large hematomas from minor trauma.
   4. Persistent bleeding from minor injuries.
   5. Hemarthrosis with joint pain, swelling, and limited movement.
   6. Possible progressive degenerative changes with osteoporosis, muscle atrophy, and fixed joints.

B. Type C—symptoms.
   1. Usually appears as a mild bleeding disorder.
   2. Autosomal dominant trait with both sexes affected.

Implementation

A. Protect child from environment by padding crib and playpen.

B. Supervise child carefully when child is learning to walk.

C. Observe for signs of blood transfusion reaction.

D. Treatment if bleeding occurs.
   1. Apply cold compresses and pressure.
   2. Hemarthrosis (effusion of blood into joint).
      a. Immobilize joint initially.
      b. Initiate passive range of motion within 48 hours to prevent stiffness.
   3. Immobilize site of bleeding.

Anemia

Definition: A deficit of red blood cells or hemoglobin caused by impairment of red blood cell production or increased erythrocyte destruction.

Assessment

A. Assess for early changes in behavior: listlessness, fatigue, sluggishness, and anorexia.

B. Assess for late symptoms: pallor, weakness, tachycardia.

C. Check with RN to determine if nutritional deficiency is present: iron, folic acid, vitamin B_6 or B_{12}.

Implementation

A. Prevent infection by maintaining nutritious diet with vitamin supplements, excellent hygiene, adequate rest, and avoidance of exposure to infections.

B. Monitor blood transfusions and observe for signs of transfusion reactions.

C. Administer iron injections as ordered by special method (Z-track) and take special precautions.

Cystic Fibrosis

Definition: Generalized dysfunction of the exocrine glands which produce excessive mucus and abnormal secretion of sweat. The changes in secretions eventually cause dysfunction of the pancreas and the lungs. The disorder is hereditary and is inherited as a recessive trait.

Assessment

A. Pancreas involvement consists of copious, foul-smelling stools with large amount of fat but no trypsin. The infant has a good appetite but fails to gain weight.

B. Lung involvement consists of chronic cough and recurrent upper respiratory infections.

C. Sweat gland involvement consists of an increased sweat chloride test of over 60 mEq/liter.

D. An associated problem is the poor absorption of fat-soluble vitamin D; this may lead to osteoporosis.

Implementation

A. Provide special nutritive foods.
   1. Pancreatic enzymes with meals and snacks.
   2. Water soluble vitamins.
   3. A moderately low fat and high protein diet; additional salt during summer.
B. Prevent respiratory infection.
   1. Keep the lungs clear of mucus.
   2. Provide mist tent at night to liquefy secretions.
   3. Provide aerosol therapy and postural drainage.
   4. Promote breathing exercises.
C. Provide good skin care to prevent irritation.

D. Educate the parents or interested others in proper care.
   1. Teach at least two people the special procedures that are necessary for the infant's care.
   2. Teach the proper care of the equipment, especially the cleaning process.
   3. Encourage the responsible persons to participate in the infant's care while still hospitalized.
   4. Refer the parents to the Cystic Fibrosis Foundation for additional help.
   5. Refer parents to other community agencies if requested.
E. Give emotional support to child and family.

Celiac Disease (Gluten-induced Enteropathy)

Definition: A chronic disease of intestinal malabsorption precipitated by ingestion of gluten or protein portions of wheat or rye flour.

Characteristics

A. A major cause of malabsorption in children, second only to cystic fibrosis.

B. Highest incidence occurs in Caucasians.

C. Major problem is an intolerance to gluten, a protein found in most grains.

D. Basic defect is believed to be an inborn error of metabolism or an autoimmune response.

E. Inadequate fat absorption; as disease progresses it affects absorption of all ingested elements.

F. Long-term effects can be anemia, poor blood coagulation and osteoporosis.

G. Usually occurs when child begins to ingest grains. It may begin as early as six months and continue until fifth year.

Assessment

A. Diarrhea or loose stools: bulky, foul smelling, pale, and frothy.

B. Failure to gain weight after a bout of diarrhea.

C. Abdominal distention.

D. Anorexia.

E. Irritability and restlessness.

F. Celiac crisis.
1. Vomiting and diarrhea.
2. Acidosis and dehydration.
3. May be precipitated by respiratory infection.
4. Excessive perspiration.
5. Cold extremities.

Implementation

A. Monitor appropriate diet.
1. Wheat and rye gluten as well as barley and oats are eliminated.
2. Low fat.
3. Slow feedings, small amounts at a time.
4. Strict intake and output.
5. Strict calorie control.
6. Supplemental vitamins and iron.

B. Give parental support.

Wilms's Tumor (Nephroblastoma)

Definition: Rapidly developing, malignant solid tumor of the kidneys containing embryonal elements. The incidence is 1 in 10,000 and occurrence is most common in children four to eight years of age.

Assessment

A. Presence of a mass on either side of the abdomen with possible pain. (The mass itself should initiate a diagnostic work-up.)

B. Fever and hypertension.

C. Possible weight loss and anemia.

Treatment and Implementation

A. Preoperative care.
1. Avoid palpation of the tumor to prevent spreading.

2. Provide emotional support for the family.
3. Observe intake and output with care.

B. Surgical procedure.
1. Tumor can be shrunk with chemotherapy before surgery.
2. Nephrectomy if the nonaffected kidney is functioning.

C. Postoperative care.
1. Observe for toxic reactions to chemotherapy, such as mouth lesions.
2. If radiation therapy is given, provide good skin care.

Cretinism (Congenital Hypothyroidism)

Definition: Deficiency in secretions of thyroid hormones resulting from a rudimentary thyroid gland which is either hypoactive or absent. The condition is recognizable when the child is two to three months old.

Assessment

A. Body growth is retarded.

B. Eyes are puffy.

C. Tongue protrudes and is thick and large.

D. Hands and feet are short and square.

E. Skin is very dry, pale, and coarse.

F. Hair is very dry and coarse.

G. Frequently, there is an umbilical hernia.

H. Feeding difficulties include choking, lack of interest in food, and sluggishness.

I. Respiratory difficulties include apneic episodes, noisy respirations, and nasal obstructions.

Treatment and Implementation

A. Infants given thyroid hormone—Synthroid is drug of choice.

B. Cytomel is used when rapid response needed.

C. Prognosis implies that 50 percent of the children treated before the age of 6 months will achieve an IQ of 90 or more.

Epilepsy

Definition: A series of seizures that result from focal or diffuse discharges in cortical neurons—symptoms of abnormal brain function.

Etiology

A. Seizure disorders are idiopathic—cause unknown or acquired—result of brain injury caused by trauma, hypoxia, infection, toxins, or other factors.

B. Seizures more common during first two years than any other period.

C. Most common cause by age group.
   1. Young infants—birth injury, hemorrhage, anoxia, and congenital defects of the brain.
   2. Late infancy and early childhood—infections frequent cause; infrequent in middle childhood.
   3. Children older than three years—idiopathic epilepsy most common.

Assessment

A. Simple partial seizure.
   1. Localized (confined to a specific area) motor symptoms, accompanied by autonomic or somatosensory symptoms.
   2. Manifestations.
      a. Aversive seizure—most common motor seizure in children. Eye(s) turn away from focus side.
      b. Sylvan seizures—most common during sleep. Tonic-clonic movements involving face.
      c. Jacksonian march—rare in children. Sequential clonic movements.
   3. Complex partial (psychomotor) seizure.
      a. Area of brain most involved is temporal lobe (thus, this type of seizure is called psychomotor).
      b. Most common in children from three years to adolescence.
      c. Characterized by complex sensory phenomena, a period of altered behavior and amnesia (child is not aware of behavior).
      d. May perform such mannerisms as lip smacking, chewing, picking at clothes, etc.
      e. May appear dazed, but only loses consciousness for a few seconds.

B. Generalized seizures.
   1. Tonic-clonic seizures, traditionally known as "grand mal."
      a. May begin with an aura, then a tonic phase (lasting 10–20 seconds)—stiffening or rigidity of muscles, particularly arms and legs; eyes roll up; followed by loss of consciousness; may be apneic and become cyanotic.
      b. Clonic phase follows (lasts about 30 seconds, but may last as long as 30 minutes)—hyperventilation with rhythmic jerking of all extremities; may foam at the mouth and become incontinent; full recovery may take several hours.
      c. Status epilepticus—a series of seizures that run together and do not allow the child to regain consciousness between attacks.
         (1) A neurological emergency with generalized tonic-clonic seizures.
         (2) State can lead to exhaustion and death.
   2. Absence seizures, formerly "petit mal."
      a. Brief duration, often just 5–10 seconds; brief loss of consciousness; almost no change in muscle tone.
      b. May occur 20–30 times/day.
      c. Common in children; may appear to be "day dreaming," or inattentive.
   3. Myoclonic seizure.
      a. Characterized by a brief, generalized jerking or stiffening of the extremities.
      b. Seizure may throw person to the floor; no loss of consciousness.
   4. Atonic or akinetic seizures, also called "drop attacks."
      a. Onset between two and five years of age.
      b. Characterized by sudden, brief loss of muscle tone.
      c. Person may fall to ground, momentary loss of consciousness.

5. Infantile spasms.
   a. Most common between 3–12 months of age; more common in males; usually low intelligence.
   b. Characterized by sudden, brief, symmetrical contractions; head flexed, legs drawn up, arms extended.
   c. May experience numerous attacks during the day without postictal drowsiness.

Implementation

A. Prevent injury during seizure.
   1. Remove any objects that may cause harm.
   2. Remain with child during seizure and provide privacy if possible.
   3. Do not force jaws open during seizure.
   4. Tongue depressor used only with physician's orders and only prior to seizure beginning.
   5. Do not restrict limbs or restrain.
   6. Loosen restrictive clothing.
   7. Check that airway is open. Do not initiate artificial ventilation during a tonic-clonic seizure.
   8. Following seizure, turn head to side to prevent aspiration and allow secretions to drain.
B. Observe and document seizure pattern.
   1. Note time, level of consciousness, and presence of aura before seizure.
   2. Record type, character, progression of movements.
   3. Note duration of seizure and child's condition throughout.
   4. Observe and record postictal state.
C. Administer and monitor medications—complete control achieved 50–70 percent of epileptic children.
   1. Drugs prescribed for partial or generalized seizures—carbamazepine (Tegretol), phenytoin (Dilantin), and mephenytoin (Mesantoin).
   2. Drug of choice for absences is ethosuximide (Zarontin).
   3. Administer dose accurately.
   4. Keep medication out of reach of children.

D. Observe for drug side effects.
   1. Dilantin can cause hypertrophy of gums and stomatitis.
   2. Zarontin can provoke blood dyscrasia.
   3. Observe for signs of toxicity.
E. Administer postseizure procedures—will influence speed of recovery.
   1. Reduce stimuli—noise, lights, conversation.
      a. Place sources of light behind child.
      b. Keep away from fluorescent lights.
   2. Remain with child after consciousness returns.
      a. Speak and move slowly.
      b. Use simple phrases—give child time to respond.
   3. Encourage rest following a seizure (child will be exhausted) and maintain privacy.
F. Emotional factors.
   1. Assist family to understand the disease.
   2. Explain how to help child have as normal a life as possible.
   3. Prevent overprotection.

Infantile Eczema

Definition: Inflammation of the skin which can occur on any area of the body. It is most prevalent before the age of two.

Assessment

A. Local redness of the skin (erythema).
B. Papules and vesicles apparent on face, neck, and body folds.
C. Rash characterized by itching, crusting, scaling, and oozing.

Treatment and Implementation

A. Treat the symptoms.
B. Provide sedation.
C. Keep infant comfortable.
D. Prevent infections.
E, Provide emotional support.
F. Eliminate the source of allergic sensitivity if known.

THE TODDLER

DISORDERS OF THE TODDLER

Cerebral Palsy

Definition: Nonprogressive paralysis resulting from either developmental brain defects or birth trauma—effect is on motor not mental function.

Assessment

A. Poor motor development; slow at walking and in other movements.
B. Involuntary movements of extremities and head.
C. Weakness of the extremities.
D. Spasticity of the extremities.
E. One or all of the extremities may be involved.

Implementation

A. Care should be individualized to the needs of the specific child.
B. Prevention of contractures of the joints.
C. Good nutrition.
D. Good dental care.
E. Encourage activities of daily living.
F. Encourage normal growth and development.

Croup-Laryngotracheobronchitis

Definition: Group of symptoms resulting from obstruction of the larynx. The condition occurs in children under five years of age.

Assessment

A. Hoarseness and barking cough.
B. Fever may or may not be present.
C. Inspiratory stridor.

D. Asphyxia.
E. Sudden onset, but recovery usually spontaneous.

Treatment and Implementation

A. Observe vital signs with care.
B. Avoid upsetting the child.
C. Provide emotional support for the child and family.
D. Set up mist tent if severe dyspnea experienced.

Pneumonia

Definition: Inflammation of the lung tissue caused primarily by bacteria and viruses.

Assessment

A. Cough that is usually nonproductive.
B. Increased pulse and respirations.
C. Fever.
D. Vomiting and diarrhea.
E. Convulsions.
F. Increased white blood count.

Treatment and Implementation

A. Treat symptoms.
   1. Control fever.
   2. Position to aid breathing.
B. Urge fluids.
C. Observe vital signs with care.
D. Provide rest.

Bronchitis

Definition: Inflammation of the mucous membrane of bronchial tubes. No obstruction is present.

Assessment

A. Usually preceded by an upper respiratory infection.

B. Dry, nonproductive cough.

C. Irritability.

D. Fever.

Implementation

A. Provide humidified air.

B. Urge fluids.

C. Provide postural drainage.

D. Observe vital signs with care.

Lead Poisoning

Definition: Poisoning from ingestion of paint or other lead-based materials.

Incidence

A. Occurrence usually between 12 and 36 months of age.

B. Death results in 25 percent of the cases of lead encephalopathy.

C. Many neurologic residual problems in survivors.

Assessment

A. Gastrointestinal symptoms.
  1. Unexplained, repeated vomiting.
  2. Vague, chronic abdominal pain.

B. Central nervous system symptoms.
  1. Irritability.
  2. Drowsiness.
  3. Ataxia.
  4. Convulsive seizures.

Prevention and Treatment

A. Education.
  1. Inspection of buildings 25 years old or older that have lead-based paint on walls.
  2. Education of parents regarding danger of old paint or old lead pipes.

B. Treatment.
  1. IV calcium disodium edetate (EDTA) in several treatments to chelate lead from body.

2. Observe for signs of hypocalcemia or tetany from chelation treatments.

3. Provide for seizure precautions.

Poisoning

Definition: Ingestion of toxic substances which may result in death or severe illness.

A. The most common age group affected is two-year-olds because of the exploration of the environment through tasting.

B. The major cause of poisoning is improper storage of toxic agents.
  1. Legislation has mandated child-proof tops on prescription drugs, but many children can still remove the tops.
  2. Some new forms of drugs, such as transdermal patches or lozenges, are packaged so that they present a danger.

C. General principles of care for poisoning.
  1. Identify the toxic substance and retrieve the poison.
  2. Notify the local poison control center and inform them of the toxic substance.
  3. Reverse the effect of the poison.
    a. Induce vomiting with syrup of ipecac or apomorphine.
      (1) Families of small children should keep this substance in the house in case of accidental poisoning.
      (2) Dose is 15 ml for children and 30 ml for young adults; follow with tap water.
      (3) Child should vomit within 30 minutes—important to bring up the syrup of ipecac to avoid cardiac complications.
    b. Activated charcoal may be used to carry toxic substance out of the body.
  4. Vomiting is contraindicated with some substances.
    a. If child or person is in a coma, in shock, convulsing, or exhibits no gag reflex.
    b. If person has ingested low viscosity hydrocarbons or corrosive substances (acid of alkaloid).

Poliomyelitis

Definition: An acute viral infection that affects the spinal cord and brain stem; may lead to paralysis or death.

Characteristics

A. A contagious disease caused by three viruses—type 1, 2, and 3.
B. Incubation period is usually 7–14 days with range of 5–35 days.
C. Communicable—throat holds virus for about one week, feces 4–6 weeks.
D. Manifests in three forms—abortive, nonparalytic (most common), and paralytic.
E. Recent statistics indicate that parents are very susceptible to contracting polio if infants receive live vaccine when the parents have never been immunized.

Assessment

A. Assess symptoms of different types.
   1. Abortive—fever, sore throat, headache, anorexia, vomiting, abdominal pain. May last few hours to days.
   2. Nonparalytic—same as above but more severe with stiff neck, back, and legs.
   3. Paralytic (spinal and bulbar types)—similar course as nonparalytic; apparent recovery followed by paralysis.

Implementation

A. Preventive—education of public about oral trivalent polio immunization.
B. Maintain complete bedrest during acute period of infection.
C. Provide respiratory ventilation if respiratory paralysis occurs.
D. Assist with physiotherapy (most important factor in recovery) following acute stage.
E. Evaluate for potential complications.

THE PRESCHOOLER

DISORDERS OF THE PRESCHOOL CHILD

Leukemia

Definition: Unrestrained growth of abnormal, immature white blood cells which causes destruction of the red blood cells. Leukemia is the most common cancer in children.

Assessment

A. Increased number of white blood cells which are immature and do not function normally.
B. Anorexia, nausea, and vomiting.
C. Weight loss, fatigue, and weakness.
D. Abdominal pain, joint pain.
E. Fever.
F. Petechiae and bruises.
G. Enlarged liver and spleen.
H. Anemia.
I. Onset is usually rapid.

Treatment and Implementation

A. Provide supportive and symptomatic care.
B. Administer antimetabolite drugs.
C. Prevent infection.
D. Handle child gently.
E. Encourage good nutrition.
F. Provide emotional support for the child and the family during therapy.

Hemophilia

Definition: Delayed coagulation of blood due to a hereditary condition involving clot formation. Victims are frequently labeled "bleeders."

Assessment

A. Prolonged clotting time so that hemorrhage occurs with the slightest cut.
B. Bruising and swelling of affected or injured areas.

Implementation

A. Prevent injury.
B. Educate the child and family.
C. Help to rehabilitate.
D. Provide emotional support.

Acute Glomerulonephritis

Definition: Inflammation of the glomeruli which may be due to an antigen-antibody response to the beta-hemolytic streptococcus which causes changes in the glomerular filtering system.

Assessment

A. Onset usually two to three weeks following an infection in site other than kidney.
B. Edema of the face.
C. Grossly bloody urine.
D. Headache and vomiting.
E. Oliguria and anuria.
F. Fatigue.
G. Anemia and malnutrition.
H. Hypertension.
I. Encephalopathy and heart failure.

Treatment and Implementation

A. Administer antibiotics.
B. Maintain bed rest.
C. Restrict salt and fluid in diet as necessary.
D. Administer antihypertensive drugs as necessary.
E. Observe vital signs.
F. Observe intake and output.
G. Weigh daily.
H. Prevent infections.

Nephrotic Syndrome

Definition: Degenerative, noninflammatory disease of the renal tubules with an increase in permeability of the glomerular membrane and necrotic lesions of the tubules.

Assessment

A. Gradual development of generalized edema.
B. Malnutrition due to loss of appetite.
C. Anemia.
D. Susceptive to infections.
E. Nephrotic crisis indicated by abdominal pain, fever, and skin eruptions; will subside in a few days with a diuretic.
F. Abnormal laboratory tests.
  1. Urine.
     a. Increased albuminuria.
     b. Increased casts and white blood cells.
     c. Increased lipid granules.
  2. Blood.
     a. Decreased total protein to less than 4 gm/100 ml.
     b. Decreased albumin and gamma globulin.
     c. Increased blood lipids and cholesterol.
     d. Increased sedimentation rate.

Treatment and Implementation

A. Prevent infections.
B. In treatment of edema, provide good skin care, change position frequently, observe intake and output, and track weight accurately.
C. Prepare for the side effects of medications and be accurate with their dosage.
D. Provide diet high in protein, low in sodium, and high in calories.

Parasitic Worms

Roundworms

A. Life cycle.

1. Eggs are laid by the worm in the gastrointestinal tract of any host animal and passed out in feces.
2. After the worms have been ingested, egg batches are laid.
3. Larvae in the host invade lymphatics and venules of the mesentery and migrate to the liver, the lungs, and the heart.
4. Larvae from lungs reach the host's epiglottis and are swallowed; once in the gastrointestinal tract, the cycle is repeated—larvae mature and mate, and the female lays eggs.

B. Symptoms.
   1. Atypical pneumonia.
   2. Gastrointestinal symptoms—nausea, vomiting, anorexia, and weight loss.
   3. Insomnia.
   4. Irritability.
   5. Signs of intestinal obstruction.

C. Treatment—piperazine citrate.

D. Nursing management.
   1. Prevention of infection through the use of a sanitary toilet.
   2. Hygiene education of the family.
   3. Careful disposal of infected stools.

Pinworm (Oxyuriasis)

A. Life cycle.
   1. Eggs ingested.
   2. Eggs mature in cecum, then migrate to anus.
   3. Worms exit at night and lay eggs on host's skin.
   4. Itching and reingestion occur.

B. Symptoms.
   1. Acute or subacute appendicitis.
   2. Eczematous areas of skin.
   3. Irritability.
   4. Loss of weight and anorexia.
   5. Insomnia.
   6. Diagnosis by tape test—place transparent adhesive tape over anus and examine tape for evidence of worms.

C. Treatment.
   1. Piperazine hexahydrate; mebendazole.

2. All infected persons living communally must be treated simultaneously.

D. Nursing management.
   1. During treatment, maintain meticulous cleansing of the skin, particularly in the anal region, and the hands and the nails.
   2. Bed linens and clothing must be boiled.
   3. Use ointment to relieve itching.
   4. Teach careful hygiene as a preventative measure.

Hookworm

A. Life cycle.
   1. Eggs of the worm are evacuated from the human bowel in feces and left in the soil.
   2. Once the larvae are infective (in five to ten days), they invade the host when in contact with the skin—which occurs either by handling the soil or by walking barefoot.
   3. The worms live in the upper gastrointestinal tract of the host or suck blood from the intestinal wall for nourishment.

B. Characteristics.
   1. Disturbed digestion.
   2. Unformed stools containing undigested food.
   3. Tarry stool with decomposed blood.
   4. Blood loss.
      a. Pallor.
      b. Dull hair.
      c. Anemia.
      d. Increased pulse.
      e. Mental apathy.

C. Treatment.
   1. Drug—tetrachloroethylene.
   2. Possibly blood transfusions.

D. Nursing management.
   1. NPO the evening preceding the treatment.
   2. Avoid fats, oils, and alcohol for 12 hours following medication.
   3. Prevention of infection.
      a. Hygiene instruction.
      b. Use of shoes in hookworm areas.
   4. Careful disposal of stools.

Giardiasis

Definition: The most common intestinal parasite pathogen in the U.S., this condition is caused by the protozoan, *Giardia lambia*.

Characteristics

A. Very common in children in day-care centers (estimates are 9–38 percent).
B. Major mode of transmission is person-to-person, water (especially mountain lakes and streams), food, and animals.
C. Adults may be asymptomatic, but children usually manifest symptoms.

Assessment

A. Infants and young children.
 1. Diarrhea.
 2. Vomiting and anorexia.
 3. Failure to thrive.
B. Children over five years of age.
 1. Abdominal cramps.
 2. Loose stools—may be intermittent.
 3. Stools may be watery, pale and smelly.
C. Assess condition through stool specimens—may need six or more over several weeks.

Implementation

A. The most important nursing measure is to teach prevention—meticulous sanitary practices during diaper changes and cleaning of children.
 1. Inform parents of importance of handwashing.
 2. Drink water that is purified, especially when out in the open.
B. Administer drugs available for treatment: quinacrine, furazolidone (drug of choice), and metronidazole.
 1. If cost is a factor, quinacrine is usually given: administer with or after meals and crush tablets into jam or syrup.
 2. Quinacrine has most side effects: nausea and vomiting.

SCHOOL-AGE CHILD

DISORDERS OF THE SCHOOL-AGE CHILD

Rheumatic Fever

Definition: General systemic disease with damage to the connective tissue (collagen disease) caused by an antigen-antibody reaction to the beta-hemolytic streptococcus.

Assessment

A. Migratory or polyarthritis.
B. Abdominal pain.
C. Low-grade fever.
D. Weight loss and anorexia.
E. Myocarditis with a murmur.
F. Increased C-reactive protein in the blood.

Implementation

A. Maintain complete bed rest until the symptoms subside.
B. Position legs in good body alignment, and make child comfortable.
C. Provide diversional activities that do not require strenuous effort.
D. Observe vital signs, especially the pulse, with care.
E. Track weight.
F. Provide emotional support.

Nursing of Cardiac Children

General Principles

A. Encourage normal growth and development.
B. Counsel parents to avoid overprotection.

C. Deal with parents' concerns and anxieties.

D. Educate parents about conditions, tests, planned treatments, medications.

E. Assist parents in developing ability to assess child's physical status.

Congestive Heart Failure

Implementation

A. Promote rest.
   1. Provide outlets such as drawing, doll play, and reading for the child who may be frustrated by restricted activity.
   2. Organize care to limit time spent disturbing child's rest.
B. Diet supervision.
   1. Provide small frequent feedings.
   2. Make the low sodium diet more palatable through imaginative play and an attractive food arrangement.
   3. Educate parents about diet and its purpose.
C. Medication supervision.
   1. Digoxin.
      a. Monitor vital signs every hour during digitalization. If pulse under 90, notify RN.
      b. Observe for digoxin toxicity.
         (1) Nausea, vomiting, diarrhea.
         (2) Anorexia.
         (3) Dizziness and headaches.
         (4) Arrhythmias.
         (5) Muscle weakness.
      c. Always check pulse prior to giving digoxin.
   2. Diuretics.
      a. Observe for electrolyte abnormalities.
      b. Weigh the child daily.
D. Emotional support to avoid anxiety and stress.

Cardiac Surgery

Preoperative Implementation

A. Extensively prepare the child and the parents for the experience—demonstrate tubes and bandages and describe the scar that will be present after the operation.

B. Teach coughing and deep breathing to the child.

C. Conduct the child and the parents on a tour of the intensive care unit and introduce them to the staff.

D. Observe the child for signs of infection.

E. Make sure all laboratory tests are completed.

Postoperative Implementation

A. Maintain adequate pulmonary function.
   1. Keep patent airway.
   2. Patient should deep breathe and cough. Monitor use of IPPB.
   3. Suction if necessary.
   4. Oxygen.
   5. Chest suction for refilling lungs.
   6. Check rate and depth of respirations.
   7. Check water-seal chest drainage.
B. Maintain adequate circulatory functioning.
   1. Check vital signs.
   2. Replace blood where necessary.
   3. Check intake and output every hour.
C. Provide for rest through organized care.
D. Establish adequate hydration and nutrition.
E. Take measures to prevent postoperative complications.
   1. Antibiotic therapy.
   2. Turn patient frequently.
   3. Skin care.
   4. Check extremities for occlusions of major vessels with blood clots: cyanosis, paleness of extremity, or coldness to the touch.
   5. Passive range of motion.
   6. Check dressing for signs of hemorrhage.

Insulin Dependent Diabetes: Type I

Definition: A disorder characterized by metabolic conditions that interfere with the production, availability, or effectiveness of insulin. (Formerly called Juvenile Diabetes.)

Characteristics

A. Pathology.
1. Interference with the utilization of sugar.
2. Impaired transportation of glucose across cellular membranes and impaired utilization within the cell.
3. Increased glycogenesis.
4. Diuresis from hyperglycemia, resulting in glucosuria and excessive losses of electrolytes and water.
5. Increased oxidation of fats and proteins, leading to proteinuria and acidosis.

B. Prognosis: degenerative changes associated with diabetes mellitus begin in young adults who have had the disease for 10 to 20 years.
1. Arteriosclerosis with hypertension.
2. Retinal changes and cataracts.
3. Nephropathy.

Assessment

A. Rapid onset.

B. Loss of weight.

C. Increased thirst and appetite, polydipsia, polyphagia, polyuria, and nocturia.

D. Onset frequently associated with ketoacidosis—an acute, life-threatening condition.
1. Drowsiness.
2. Dryness of skin.
3. Flushed cheeks.
4. Acetone breath.
5. Hyperpnea.
6. Nausea, vomiting, and abdominal pains.

Treatment and Implementation

A. Monitor administration of insulin. (Oral hypoglycemic agents generally do not produce satisfactory results because they require some pancreatic function to be effective.)
1. Side effects: hypoglycemia with hunger, irritability, nervousness, headaches, and slurred speech.
2. Combine insulin treatment with ADA diet.

B. Monitor diet.
1. Diet should be adequate for normal growth and development and regulated according to diabetic needs.

Types	Onset (hrs.)	Peak (hrs.)	Total Duration (hrs.)
Regular	½ to 1	2 to 5	6 to 8
Semilente	1 to 2	3 to 8	10 to 16
Humulin R	½ to 1	2 to 3	5 to 7
NPH	1 to 2	6 to 12	24
Lente	1 to 3	6 to 12	18 to 24
PZI	4 to 8	10 to 20	36
Ultralente	4 to 6	8 to 24	24 to 36

2. The type of diet prescribed is influenced by the philosophy of the physician.
3. Diets vary from free diets to strict dietary control.

C. Provide family and patient education.
1. Signs and symptoms of disease, including acidosis and hypoglycemia.
2. Instruction in insulin injection, sterile technique, and urine testing.
3. Diet control as prescribed by the physician.
4. Prevention of infections through adequate skin and foot care.
5. Knowledge of the effects of increased physical activity and stress on food needs.
6. Patient's responsibility for administering insulin and managing diet.
7. Normal activity and life style appropriate.

D. Provide special counseling because of adolescent's heightened sensitivity to being different and their frequently unusual dietary habits.

Meningitis

Definition: An acute inflammation of the meninges.

Characteristics

A. May be caused by viral or bacterial agents.

B. Diagnosis based on symptoms and culture of CSF.

Assessment

A. Symptoms of nuchal-spinal rigidity: headache, irritability, nausea, vomiting, fever.

B. Positive Kernig's and Brudzinski's signs.

Implementation

A. Isolate child until the causative agent is identified.

B. Administer medications on time.

C. Manage fluids: prevent dehydration and over-hydration (causes an increase in cerebral edema).

D. Monitor neurological signs.

E. Maintain bedrest and position child comfortably; most children prefer a side-lying or flat position; sitting up increases pain.

F. Maintain patent airway; administer oxygen if ordered.

G. Provide quiet activities which are age appropriate.

Asthma

Definition: A pulmonary disorder in which physical or chemical irritants cause the release of histamine and other substances which cause edema of the bronchial walls, excess secretion of mucus by the bronchial glands, and constriction of the bronchi.

Characteristics

A. An attack may be provoked by exposure to certain foods, infections, vigorous activity, or emotional excitement.

B. Bronchiolar musculature goes into spasm.

C. Thick tenacious mucus accumulates and causes obstruction of air passages.

D. Trapping of air occurs causing obstructive emphysema.

E. Symptoms include wheezing and rales.

F. Attack may occur slowly or quickly.

G. Child usually coughs continually.

H. Neck veins may distend.

I. Cyanosis may occur.

J. Child appears anxious and upset.

K. Symptoms may become rapidly worse with acute respiratory failure with cyanosis and acidosis.

Implementation

A. Identification and removal of suspected allergen.

B. Medication supervision.
   1. Epinephrine—acts to reduce congestion and edema.
   2. Cromolyn—used prophylactically, prevents allergic responses.
   3. Aminophylline—bronchodilator.
   4. Albuterol—treatment for bronchospasm.

C. Removal and control of secretions.
   1. Large fluid intake to liquefy secretions and maintain electrolyte balance.
   2. Mist tent.
   3. Chest physical therapy and postural drainage.

D. Emotional support for parents and child to reduce anxiety.

E. Child educated to live optimally with chronic problem.

Reye's Syndrome

Definition: Acute encephalopathy with fatty degeneration resulting in marked cerebral edema and enlargement of the liver with marked fatty infiltration.

Characteristics

A. Children from 2 months to adolescence contact illness; ages 6 and 11 years most often affected.

B. Usually follows a viral infection, especially varicella and influenza B.

C. Aspirin is now contraindicated with influenza—use Tylenol. (Incidence of Reye's is down since change from aspirin to Tylenol.)

Assessment

A. Malaise, cough, rhinorrhea, sore throat.
B. Changes in level of consciousness.
C. Temperature changes.
D. Clinical stages of the syndrome.
   1. Stage 1: vomiting, lethargy and drowsiness.
   2. Stage 2: CNS changes, disorientation, delirium, aggressiveness and combativeness, central neurologic hyperventilation, hyperactive reflexes and stupor.
   3. Stage 3: comatose, hyperventilation, decorticate posturing.
   4. Stage 4: increasing comatose state, loss of ocular reflexes, fixed, dilated pupils.
   5. Stage 5: seizures, loss of deep tendon reflexes, flaccidity and respiratory arrest.

Implementation

A. Monitor for signs of increased intracranial pressure.
   1. Major effort is toward recognizing and reducing cerebral edema, as this may lead to death.
   2. Monitor IV mannitol or glycerol when administered to reduce blood osmolarity, thus reducing cerebral edema.
B. Prepare for tracheal intubation and controlled ventilation (to decrease carbon dioxide level).
C. Monitor vital signs frequently and decrease temperature as needed.
D. Monitor closely for signs of seizure activity and utilize seizure precautions.
E. Provide nursing care appropriate for semi-conscious child.
   1. Maintain head elevation at 30 degrees.
   2. Monitor reflexes as indicative of clinical stage of syndrome.
F. Provide adequate fluid balance.
   1. Ensure adequate urinary output of at least 1 ml/1 kg/hr.
   2. Provide and monitor intravenous fluids.
   3. Observe closely for cerebral edema or dehydration.
G. Provide low protein diet.
H. Provide respiratory care; suctioning, ventilation and oxygen as ordered.
I. Provide emotional and supportive care.

Brain Tumor

Definition: Benign or malignant brain mass. In children the tumor is usually located in the cerebellum or the mid-brain.

Characteristics

A. Seventy-five percent of childhood brain tumors are impossible to remove or are so situated as to cause damage if completely removed.
B. Incidence—occur most frequently in the five-to-seven age group.
C. Location—most occur in the posterior fossa.
D. Types most frequently seen in children.
   1. Astrocytoma.
      a. Located in the cerebellum.
      b. Insidious onset and slowly progressive course.
      c. Surgical removal usually possible.
   2. Medulloblastoma.
      a. Located in the cerebellum.
      b. Highly malignant.
      c. Prognosis poor.
   3. Ependymoma.
      a. Usually there is ventricular blockage, leading to signs of increased intracranial pressure.
      b. Treated with incomplete internal compression and radiation therapy.
   4. Brain stem gliomas.
      a. Seventy-five percent of childhood brain tumors.
      b. Develops slowly with initial symptoms of cranial nerve palsies.

Assessment

A. Variety of symptoms depending on location of tumor.
B. Increased intracranial pressure.

1. Vomiting without nausea; anorexia.
2. Headache.
3. Diplopia.

C. Enlargement of the head in children under four years old.

D. Mental change: lethargy, irritability, drowsiness, and stupor.

E. Unsteady gait and muscular uncoordination (ataxia).

Implementation

A. Control and relief of symptoms.

B. Seizure precautions.

C. Postoperative care for surgical removal.
1. Maintain child flat in bed on unaffected side.
2. Log roll for change of position.
3. Control fever with hypothermia mattress.
4. Frequently observe vital signs until stable.
5. Reinforce dressing, if wet, with sterile gauze.
6. Notify RN of increased wetness in dressing—possible cerebral spinal fluid leakage.

D. Provide emotional support for family and child.

Bone Tumors

Osteogenic Sarcoma

Definition: A malignant tumor originating from osteoblasts (bone-forming cells).

Characteristics

A. Tumor usually located at the end of the long bones (metaphysis).

B. Most frequently seen at the distal end of the femur or the proximal end of the tibia.

C. Primary symptoms are pain at site, swelling, and limitation of movement.

D. Lungs most common site of metastasis.

E. Occurs twice as frequently in boys as in girls.

Treatment and Implementation

A. Provide care for amputation followed by chemotherapy.

B. Administer drugs and monitor for side effects.
1. Vincristine.
2. Cytoxan.
3. Actinomycin D.

C. Provide supportive emotional care.

Ewing's Sarcoma

Definition: A malignant tumor of the bone originating from myeloblasts.

Characteristics

A. Tumor usually located on the shaft of the long bones.

B. Femur, tibia, and humerus common sites.

C. Primary symptoms.
1. Pain at site.
2. Swollen area with tenderness.
3. Fever.

D. Early metastases to lung, lymph nodes, and other bones.

E. Occurs twice as frequently in boys as in girls.

Treatment and Implementation

A. Usually radiation, sometimes followed by amputation.

B. Chemotherapy to treat tumor and prevent metastases.

C. Administer drugs and monitor for side effects.
1. Vincristine.
2. Cytoxan.
3. Actinomycin D.

D. Encourage inclusion of patient in discussions of treatment, options, risks and prognosis.

E. Listen to parents, child, and siblings as they work through denial, anger, acceptance—allow them their grieving process.

F. Promote age appropriate activities and group discussions with peers.

G. Assist parents in avoiding overprotection.

H. Treat the side effects of chemotherapy and radiation.

Pediatric Oncology

A. Signs and symptoms of pediatric malignancy may be subtle and not easily recognized.

B. Causal factors associated with cancer in children are not clearly defined.

C. Current treatment focuses on chemotherapy, radiation, a combination of the two, and surgical intervention.

Chemotherapy

Basic Principles

A. Chemotherapeutic agents work on dividing cells.

B. Tumor's location and cell type affect choice of drugs.

C. Most antineoplastic drugs are metabolized in the liver and excreted by the kidneys so these organs must be in functioning order to prevent toxicity.

Assessment

A. Assess if more than one chemotherapeutic agent is being administered.

B. Identify potential side effects of medications.
   1. G.I. disturbance.
   2. Loss of hair.

C. Assess for fluid and electrolyte imbalances associated with drug therapy.

D. Assess for adequate urine output.

E. Monitor laboratory values.

F. Assess oral cavity for irritation and bleeding gums.

Implementation

A. Establish baseline data.
   1. Nutritional status.
   2. Oral condition.
   3. Skin condition.
   4. Degree of mobility.
   5. Psychological status.
   6. Neurological condition.

B. Observe for side effects of cell breakdown.
   1. BUN on rise.
   2. Stone formation in urinary tract.

C. Observe for side effects on rapidly dividing cells.
   1. Gastrointestinal mucosa—diarrhea, nausea, vomiting.
      a. Administer antiemetics.
      b. Provide mouth care with hydrogen peroxide every four hours. No toothbrush or glycerin.
      c. Administer anesthetic spray to mouth prior to meals.
      d. Provide frequent cold, high calorie beverages.
   2. Hair follicles—loss of hair.
      a. Prepare patient for loss—suggest wig, scarf.
      b. Reassure that it will return in six weeks.
      c. Apply tourniquet around scalp during chemotherapy plus 2–3 hours following to lessen amount of hair lost.

Common Drugs

A. Prednisone.
   1. Side effects.
      a. Ravenous appetite.
      b. Change in fat distribution.
      c. Retention of fluid.
      d. Hirsutism.
      e. Occasional hypertension.
      f. Psychological disturbance.
   2. Nursing management—watch blood sugar and tapering of medication.

B. 6-Mercaptopurine.
   1. Interrupts the synthesis of purines essential to the structure and function of nucleic acids.
   2. Side effects.

a. Produces very little toxicity in children.
b. Increases amount of uric acid that the kidneys must excrete.
3. Nursing management.
a. Observe kidney function.
b. Increase fluid intake.

C. Methotrexate.
1. A folic acid antagonist that suppresses the growth of abnormal cells enough to permit regeneration of normal cells.
2. Side effects.
a. Ulceration of oral mucosa.
b. Nausea, vomiting, diarrhea, and abdominal pain.
3. Nursing management.
a. Observe for ulcerations—drug must be temporarily discontinued at the appearance of ulcers.
b. Observe renal function—primary route of drug excretion.

D. Cytoxan.
1. Alkylating agent that suppresses cellular proliferation; it has greater effect on abnormal than normal cells.
2. Side effects—hemorrhagic cystitis.
3. Nursing management—provide large quantities of fluids preceding and immediately following drug administration to prevent side effects.

E. Vincristine.
1. Alkylating agent.
2. Side effects.
a. Insomnia.
b. Severe constipation.
c. Peripheral neuritis or palsies.
3. Frequently used to induce remissions rapidly, after which the patient is maintained on another, less toxic drug.

Radiation

Basic Principles

A. Radiation affects all cells but is particularly lethal to rapidly developing cells.

B. Radiation can be utilized in conjunction with chemotherapy.
C. Radiation may be used to eradicate the tumor or to relieve pressure.

Assessment

A. Assess for fatique.
B. Assess fluid and electrolyte imbalances due to vomiting, diarrhea, and urinary frequency associated with radiation therapy.
C. Monitor hemoglobin and hematocrit.
D. Assess skin condition in radiated area.
E. Assess for dental caries and gum disease.
F. Assess condition of hair.

Implementation

A. Treatment of radiation sickness.
1. Symptoms—nausea, vomiting, malaise.
2. Offer frequent high caloric feedings (milk shakes with extra protein and vitamins).
3. Make food trays attractive, palatable.
B. Observe side effects of cell breakdown.
1. BUN on rise.
2. Accumulation of uric acid.
3. Stone formation in urinary tract.
C. Treat side effects of cell breakdown.
1. Increase fluid intake.
2. Monitor intake and output.
D. Treat skin breakdown.
1. Check patient regularly for any redness or irritation at radiation site.
2. Immediately notify physician.
3. Usual treatment—apply lotion to area, cover loosely with sterile gauze.
4. Avoid any irritation to area from clothing, soap or weather extremes.
E. Treat bone marrow depression.
1. Carefully watch lab values.
2. Isolate (low leukocytes).
3. Avoid injections (low platelets).
4. Antibiotics.

THE ADOLESCENT

DISORDERS OF THE ADOLESCENT

Obesity

Definition: Excessive accumulation of body fat which is over ten percent of that normal for a young adult with regard to age, height, and body build.

Implementation

A. Encourage adolescent to follow proper low caloric diet as prescribed by the physician.
B. Provide emotional support for the adolescent.

Ulcerative Colitis

Definition: Inflammation of the colon and the rectum in which the mucous membrane becomes hyperemic, bleeds easily, and tends to ulcerate.

Etiology

A. Unknown, although the increased incidence within families has given rise to the hypothesis that suggests a hereditary predisposition or an emotional and/or environmental causation.
B. Incidence is highest in young adults and middle-age groups.

Assessment

A. Diarrhea.
B. Weight loss.
C. Rectal bleeding.
D. Abdominal pain, nausea, and vomiting.
E. Anemia.
F. Fever and dehydration.

G. Adolescents tend to be passive, pessimistic, fearful, and strongly, though ambivalently, attached to a parent.

Implementation

A. Control infection.
   1. Supervise medication regime.
   2. Provide adequate hydration with intravenous therapy and oral fluids as indicated.
B. Provide for rest of intestinal tract.
   1. Observe for type and amount of bowel activity, symptoms of bleeding, and hyperactive peristalsis.
   2. Administer tranquilizers and observe for side effects.
C. Maintain diet therapy.
   1. Provide low residue, high fiber, bland, high protein diet and vitamin therapy.
   2. Avoid presenting cold foods because they increase gastric motility.
   3. Avoid gas-forming foods, sharp cheeses, highly spiced foods, smoked or salted meats, fried foods, raw fruits, and vegetables.
   4. Arrange for attractive environment with opportunities for socialization at mealtimes.
D. Provide counseling.
   1. Educate patient about diet, medication, and symptoms of bleeding.
   2. Observe for signs of psychological problems; initiate referral if necessary.

Infectious Mononucleosis

Definition: An infectious disease, believed to be viral in origin, that causes an increase in the mononuclear elements of the blood.

Assessment

A. Incubation period is around 11 days.
B. Symptoms.
   1. Malaise.
   2. Sore throat with pharyngitis.

3. Prolonged fever.
4. Enlargement of the lymph nodes.
5. Splenomegaly (enlargement of the spleen).
6. About 10 to 20 percent of the cases exhibit skin rashes that appear between day 4 and 10. The rash is usually the macular type, occurring primarily on the trunk.

Implementation

A. Symptomatic and supportive.
   1. Maintain bed rest initially.
   2. Increase activity gradually.
   3. Administer salicylates for fever, chills, and muscle pain as ordered.
B. No isolation procedures are required.

Hodgkin's Disease

Definition: Malignancy of the lymph system characterized by a large, primitive, reticulumlike, malignant cell. Peak occurrence is between 15 and 29 years of age.

Assessment

A. Enlarged, painless lymph nodes. Nodes are firm and movable.
B. Lessened sensitivity to specified antigens (anergy).
C. Frequent infections.
D. Prognosis is guarded (overall 5-year survival rate appears to be about 30 percent).

Stages

A. Stage I.
   1. Disease restricted to single anatomic site or localized in a group of lymph nodes.
   2. Asymptomatic.
B. Stage II.
   1. Two or three adjacent lymph nodes in the area on the same side of the diaphragm are affected.
   2. Symptoms appear.
C. Stage III.

1. Disease is widely disseminated into the lymph areas and organs.
2. Prognosis poor.

Treatment and Implementation

A. Provide for symptomatic relief for the side effects of radiation (used for Stages I, II, and III in an effort to eradicate the disease) and chemotherapy (used in combination is treatment of choice).
B. Counseling.
   1. Assist the family and the adolescent to accept the process of treatment.
   2. Encourage independence where possible.
C. Observe for pressure from enlargement of the lymph glands on vital organs, particularly for respiratory problems from the compression of the airway.

Juvenile Rheumatoid Arthritis

Definition: Systemic disease with multiple manifestations, arthritis being the most characteristic; etiology unknown.

Pathology

A. Inflammation of joints.
B. Edema and congestion of synovial tissues.
C. As the disease progresses, synovial fluid fills the joint space and causes narrowing, fibrous ankylosis, and bony fusion.
D. Growth centers adjacent to affected joints may undergo either premature closure or accelerated epiphyseal growth.

Assessment

A. Involvement of joints.
   1. Arthritis may start slowly with gradual development of joint stiffness, swelling, and loss of motion.
   2. Affects knees, ankles, feet, wrists, and fingers most frequently, although any joint may be involved.

3. Affected joints are swollen, warm, painful, and stiff.

4. Young children appear irritable and anxious, guarding their joints.

5. Weakness and atrophy of muscles appear around affected joints.

6. Chronically affected joints may become deformed, dislocated, or fused.

B. Systemic involvement.
1. Frequent occurrence.
2. Irritability, anorexia, and malaise.
3. Fever.
4. Intermittent macular rash on occasion.
5. Enlarged liver and spleen (hepatosplenomegaly) and generalized lymphadenopathy in 20 percent of the patients.
6. Anemia is common in active cases of the disease.
7. Inflammation of eyes with redness, pain, photophobia, decreased visual acuity, and nonreactive pupil.

Treatment and Implementation

A. Although there is no specific cure, care can be given to prevent joint destruction and to maintain joint mobility.
1. Exercise joints.
2. Provide night splints.
3. Educate parents in how adolescent should perform exercises, and impress upon them the adolescent's need for physical therapy and night splints.

B. Provide emotional support to the chronically ill adolescent and his family.

C. Administer medications.
1. Salicylates.
   a. Usually given in large doses.
   b. Observe for signs of toxicity and side effects.
      (1) Ringing in the ear.
      (2) Gastric irritation. (Alleviate by giving drug with milk or antacids.)
      (3) Headaches.
      (4) Disturbances of mental state.
      (5) Hyperventilation and drowsiness.

2. Gold salts.
   a. Usually given in weekly injections.
   b. Observe for side effects.
      (1) Skin rashes.
      (2) Nephritis with hematuria or albuminuria.
      (3) Thrombocytopenia.
      (4) Neurotoxicity.
   c. Weekly blood and urine tests.
3. Steroids.
   a. Observe for side effects and toxicity.
      (1) Masked infection.
      (2) Hypertension.
      (3) Vascular disorders.
      (4) Mental disturbances.
      (5) Edema with weight gain.
      (6) Increased appetite.
      (7) Peptic ulcer.
   b. Observe vital signs regularly.

D. Encourage parents to report any signs of eye problems in the adolescent immediately to the physician so eye damage may be prevented.

Scoliosis

Definition: Lateral curvature of the spine that occurs during the growth spurt at puberty.

Assessment

A. One leg shorter in length than the other.
B. One hip or one shoulder higher than the other hip or shoulder.
C. A marked curve in upper part of spine.

Treatment and Implementation

A. Preoperative care.
1. Show patient how to provide for his or her postoperative needs.
2. Provide emotional support.
B. Surgical procedure.
1. Bone graft.
2. Rod insertion.
C. Postoperative care.

1. Keenly observe for indications of pain, vital signs, and hemorrhage.
2. Change patient's position by log rolling to prevent injury to the surgical area.
3. Encourage coughing and deep breathing.
4. Encourage fluids and food; observe intake and output.
5. Use the Hemovac or similar drainage system as needed.
6. Provide emotional support.
7. Teach parents how to provide home care to adolescent who will be confined to body cast for six to nine months.

Anorexia Nervosa

Definition: A syndrome of self-starvation with underlying emotional disturbance. The psychological aversion to food results in emaciation and physical problems.

Characteristics

A. Almost exclusively female (1 in 100 are males).
B. Most common in adolescent girls and young adults.
C. Often unnoticed in early stages; female "goes on diet to lose weight."
D. Not a disturbance in appetite but distorted body image perceptions: related to disturbance in sense of self, identity, and autonomy.
E. Potentially lethal disease: mortality 15–20 percent.
F. Many anorectics have had a single episode, then recover. Factors associated with positive prognosis include: onset of problem before age 15 and weight gain within 2 years.

Assessment

A. Profound weight loss of 25 percent occurs with this disorder.
B. Delayed sexual development: amenorrhea.
C. Physical symptoms.
   1. Hypotension.
   2. Anemia.
   3. Hypoproteinemia.

4. Hypothermia.
5. Slowed heart rate.
6. Lanugo.

Implementation

A. Improve nutritional status (to stabilize medical condition).
   1. Diet.
      a. High protein, high carbohydrate.
      b. Identify foods patient prefers.
      c. Small, nutritious, attractive feedings.
      d. Maintain accurate intake records.
   2. Nasogastric feedings; if patient refuses to eat, administer tube feedings as ordered.
B. Nursing care plan.
   1. Formulate plan that all staff agree on. Do not allow manipulation. Do not engage in power struggle.
   2. Do not focus on food, taste, recipes, etc.
   3. Remain with patient when eating.
   4. Do not accept excuses to leave eating area (to vomit).
   5. Set limits on amount patient must eat. Reward when patient adheres to plan.
   6. Ensure that weight is taken same time every day with patient dressed in only a hospital gown.
   7. Work with staff on behavior therapy plan.
      a. Set limits with positive and negative reinforcement.
      b. Establish contract that specifies weight-gain privileges, restrictions, etc.
      c. Assist to correct patient's body perceptions and misconceptions about feelings, needs, self-worth, autonomy.

Bulimia

Definition: Eating disorder that involves binge eating, frequently followed by self-induced vomiting.

Characteristics

A. Etiology is unknown but this disorder is frequently accompanied by an underlying psychopathology.

B. More common in women than men.

C. Begins in adolescence or early adulthood and often follows a chronic course over many years.

D. Generally aware that eating patterns are abnormal (in contrast to anorectics).

E. Typically evidences impaired impulse control, low self-esteem, and depression.

Assessment

A. Disruption in life caused by eating disorder.

B. Depression: often due to guilt over eating binges. (New studies suggest link between bulimia and affective disorder.)

C. Weight fluctuation and potential danger of weight loss.

D. Assess potential damage to esophagus and teeth caused by vomiting.

Implementation

A. Patient is usually not hospitalized but does require therapy.

B. Behavior-modification and insight-oriented therapy used with limited success.

C. Nursing care plan is similar to anorexia nervosa with focus on interrupting binge/purge cycle and altering attitudes toward food and self.

SPECIAL PROBLEMS

The Mentally Retarded Child

Definition: Impairment of intelligence that results in a limited capacity to adapt to the environment and to achieve skills necessary for progress on the developmental continuum.

Classifications of Mental Retardation

A. Mild (educable).
1. Child can acquire simple basic learning skills.
2. IQ between 50 and 75.
3. Social and sensorimotor skills can be developed.
4. Child can learn self-support skills.

B. Moderate (trainable).
1. Child can acquire simple social skills.
a. Communication.
b. Minimal social interaction skills.
2. IQ between 35 and 50.
3. Minimal learning ability.
4. Can be independent with supervision.

C. Severe.
1. Can benefit from habit-training.
2. IQ between 20 and 35.
3. Requires supervision.
4. Poor communicative, social, and sensorimotor skills.

D. Profound.
1. Minimal capacity to function.
2. IQ below 20.
3. Requires constant supervision (custodial care).

Incidence

A. Approximately 3 percent of the general population is considered to be mentally retarded

B. Mental retardation occurs in all races and both sexes; there is no differentiation as to socioeconomic status.

C. Incidence of mental retardation according to classification.

1. Educable—75 percent.
2. Trainable—23 percent.
3. Custodial—2 percent.

Implementation

A. Treat the child according to developmental age rather than chronological age.
   1. Respond to the child on a level he or she can understand. If the developmental age is two years and chronological age is ten, respond to and deal with child as if a two year old.
   2. Assessment is often vague and inaccurate so expectations at the developmental age should not be rigid.
B. Provide the child with as much stimulation and love as a normal child.
C. Watch for infections and disease; retarded children are frequently more susceptible.
D. Challenge with behavioral modification, as it frequently works well with these children.
E. Empathize with parents' reaction to the birth of a mentally retarded child.
   1. Birth presents a threat to the parents' marital relationship and family dynamics.
   2. States of parental reaction.
      a. Denial: initial reaction of defense which protects the parents from admitting that this child, this extension of themselves, is not normal.
      b. Initial recognition: aware of difference between their child and other children.
      c. Active recognition: the parents begin to search for information on their child's problem and are ready to seek professional advice.
F. Work with staff to formulate a plan for dealing with the mentally retarded child if child is to live at home with parents.

Child Abuse

Definition: Physical maltreatment or negligence (not including accidental mishaps) of children that results from an absence of reasonable standards of protection and care by the parents or the child's caretaker.

Incidence

A. Statistics.
   1. Among 1000 newborn children, 6 become battered children.
   2. Of all injuries in children under five years of age, as seen in the hospital emergency, about ten percent are actually caused by parents or are the result of negligence.
B. Distribution.
   1. One-third of all abused victims are less than six months old.
   2. One-third of them are six months to four years old.
   3. One-third of them are over four years old.
   4. The risk of becoming a battered child is three times greater for children born prematurely than for those born full-term.
   5. Stepchildren have a higher abuse risk than do nonstepchildren.
C. Psychological factors.
   1. The abused child usually has demanding behaviors.
   2. The abuse usually occurs close in time to a crisis or stressful event.
   3. The abuse usually occurs after the parent is provoked to anger.

Clinical Indications of Abuse

A. Account of the injury/ies.
   1. The cause given for the injury is implausible.
   2. The cause given for the injury is punishment, which is inappropriate considering the age of the child.
   3. There are discrepancies in the initial account as presented by neighbors or other family members.
   4. There is a delay in seeking medical help for the child.
B. Indications for diagnosis of abuse.
   1. Physical examination.
      a. Bruises, welts, and scars in various stages of healing.
      b. Finger-mark pattern of bruises on the body.
      c. Bite, rope, or choke marks in evidence.

d. Cigarette and/or hot water burns are visible.

e. Eye damage, subdural hematoma, and/or intra-abdominal injuries.

f. Radiographic findings of multiple bone injuries at different stages of healing.

2. Other observations.

a. Child perceived as passive, noncommunicative, and/or withdrawn.

b. Child perceived as failing to thrive.

C. Characteristics of abusers—parents, caretakers, relatives.

1. Abusers usually abused as children.

2. Abusers unable to utilize outside help when angry with their children.

3. Abusers usually are isolated and lonely individuals.

4. Frequently, spouse of abuser does not know how to prevent abuse.

5. Frequently, abusive parents make unreasonable demands of their children.

6. Abusing parents often exhibit certain personality problems such as dependency, low self-esteem, immaturity, and inability to cope with feelings.

D. Legal responsibilities of health team members.

1. Both nurses and doctors have a legal responsibility to report incidences of children who are suspected of being abused to the proper authorities.

2. Designated community authorities have the responsibility to determine further placement of the abused child.

Accidents

Incidence

A. Accidents are the leading cause of childhood deaths.

B. The majority of accidents occur in or near the home.

Classification

A. Automobile accidents.

B. Aspiration of small objects.

C. Accidental falls which result in fractures and serious head injuries.

D. Accidental poisonings.

Treatment and Implementation

A. If accidental poisoning occurs, contact local poison control center for pertinent information. Keep the poison container if available.

B. Take children to the nearest emergency room for proper treatment of any type of injuries.

C. Accident prevention is very important; educate both the child and the parents.

Burns

Definition: Destruction of body tissue caused by heat. It is the most frequent accidental injury occurring to infants and children.

Degree of Burns

A. First degree—superficial—involves only the epidermis with redness, swelling, and pain.

B. Second degree—partial thickness—involves superficial skin layers with redness, blisters, and pain; scarring may occur.

C. Third degree—full thickness—involves the epidermis and some of the dermis with charring and destruction of the nerve endings, sweat glands, and hair follicles.

Treatment and Implementation

A. Exposed method (reverse isolation).

B. Pressure dressings.

C. Wet dressings (sterile).

D. Skin grafts.

E. Prevent infection.

F. Observe intake and output.

G. Align body carefully to prevent contractures.

H. Provide a well-balanced diet.

APPENDIX 1. NUTRITION

Nutrition for the Infant

A. Calories.
   1. Birth to 3 months—50 to 55 calories per pound per day.
   2. Three months to 1 year—45 calories per pound per day.
B. Fluids.
   1. First six months—two to three ounces per pound per day.
   2. Requirements increase in hot weather.
C. Number of feedings.
   1. First week—six to ten per day.
   2. One week to one month—six to eight per day.
   3. One to three months—five to six per day.
   4. Three to seven months—four to five per day.
   5. Four to nine months—three to four per day.
   6. Eight to 12 months—three per day.
D. Vitamins.
   1. Breast-fed infants—supplement with vitamins C, D, and A.
   2. Formula-fed infants—vitamin supplements depend on type of formula and which vitamins are already included in it.
E. Solid foods—recent trends indicate introduction of solid foods at three to six months of age.
   1. Cereal—infants are least allergic to rice; it can be introduced as early as four to six weeks of age.
   2. Fruits and vegetables.
      a. New foods should be introduced once a day in small amounts until the infant becomes accustomed to them.
      b. Introduce only one new food per week.
      c. Bananas and applesauce are well tolerated.
      d. Orange juice is usually not well tolerated, initially. It can be introduced, diluted with water, when the infant is two or three months old.
      e. Green and yellow vegetables can be introduced at about four months of age.
   3. Eggs.
      a. Introduce after infant is six months old.
      b. Usually yolks are well tolerated, but sometimes there are allergic reactions to egg whites.
   4. Meat.
      a. May be introduced at four months.
      b. Usually more palatable if mixed with fruits or vegetables.
   5. Starchy foods.
      a. May be introduced after the infant is six months old.
      b. Should not be substituted for green vegetables or fruit.
      c. Chief value is caloric.
      d. Zwieback and other crackers are good for the gumming infant.
F. Diarrhea (temporary).
   1. Usually caused by contaminated food.
   2. Review feeding preparation and storage of formula with caretaker.
   3. Usually corrected by withholding all solids and milk for two or three feedings and giving boiled water or balanced electrolyte solution.
G. Constipation.
   1. Increase fluid and sugar intake.
   2. In infant three months old or older, increase cereal, fruit, and vegetable intake.
   3. On occasion, prune juice (half an ounce) may be given.

Nutrition for the Second Year

A. Rate of growth is slowing down; thus there is a decreased caloric need.
B. Self-selection—children usually select a balanced diet over a period of several days.
C. Child should be feeding self, with some assistance.

Nutrition for the Preschooler

A. Child begins to imitate family's likes and dislikes.

B. Finger foods are popular.

C. Single foods are preferable to a combination of foods.

Nutrition for the School-Age Child

A. Patterns of good eating habits are established at this time.

B. Provide fruits as snacks.

Adolescent Eating Patterns

A. Adolescents often gain weight easily and then resort to fad diets.

B. Girls adapt themselves to fashionable weight goals, some of which may be unhealthy.

C. Eating of nonnutritious foods in a social setting.

Malnutrition

A. Kwashiorkor—caused by a lack of protein.

B. Rickets—caused by a lack of vitamin D.

C. Scurvy—caused by a lack of vitamin C.

APPENDIX 2. REFLEXES IN THE NEWBORN

Palmar Grasp

A. Automatic reflex of full-term newborns; elicited by placing finger in infant's palm.

B. Present at birth.

C. Disappears at four months.

Asymmetrical Tonic Neck Reflex

A. Infant assumes fencer's position—when head is turned to one side, arm on that side is extended, and opposite arm is flexed.

B. Present at birth.

C. Disappears at four months.

Moro's Reflex (Startle Reflex)

A. When infant is suddenly jarred or hears a loud noise, the body stiffens, the legs are drawn up, and the arms are brought up, out, and then in front in an embracing position.

B. Present at birth.

C. Disappears at four months.

Reciprocal Kicking

A. Movements of newborns are jerky and usually alternate in the legs.

B. Evolving at birth.

C. Disappears at nine months.

Rooting

A. When infant's cheek is brushed, the head will turn to that side.

B. Present at birth.

C. Rooting while awake disappears at three to four months.

D. Rooting while asleep disappears at seven to eight months.

Sucking

A. Infants make sucking movements when anything touches their lips.

B. Present at birth.

C. Involuntary sucking disappears at or about nine months.

Neck Righting Reflex

A. When the head is turned to one side, the opposite shoulder and trunk will follow.

B. Evolving at four months.

C. Involuntary movement disappears at 9 to 12 months.

Babinski's Sign

A. Extension of the great toe on stroking the sole of the foot.

B. Present at birth.

C. Disappears after two years.

APPENDIX 3. IMMUNIZATIONS

Age	Prevention
Birth	HBV≠
1 to 2 months	HBV
2 months	DPT°, OPV†, HbOC∞
4 months	DPT, OPV, HbOC
6 months	DPT, HbOC (HBV)
15 months	MMR±, HbOC
15 to 18 months	DPT, OPV
4 to 6 years	DPT, OPV
11 to 12 years	MMR
14 to 16 years	Td§, and thereafter every ten years

° DPT—diphtheria, pertussis and tetanus toxoids vaccine

† OPV—trivalent oral polio virus vaccine

∞ HbOC—two HbOCs are approved for children under 15 months (Haemophilus influenzae type b)

± MMR—measles, mumps and rubella vaccine; may be combined or separate

≠ HBV—hepatitis B. Infants of mothers who test seropositive must receive hepatitis B immune globulin (HBIG) at first dose, with second dose at one month and third at six months.

§ Td—combined adult tetanus toxoid and diphtheria toxoids

Immunization schedule recommended by the American Academy of Pediatrics.

APPENDIX 4. DRUG CONVERSION FOR CHILDREN

A. Clark's weight rule for pediatric dosage.

$$\frac{\text{child's weight in pounds}}{150} \times \text{adult dose}$$

= approximate dose for children

B. Intravenous microdrip usually has 60 drops/cc.

C. Conversion of administration units.

1 tsp = 5 ml
1 tbl = 15 ml
1 ml = 16 minims
1 grain = 60 mg
1 gm = 1000 mg
1 oz = 30 ml
1 dram = 4 ml

APPENDIX 5. PEDIATRIC COMMUNICABLE DISEASES

Disease	Characteristics	Transmission	Nursing Care
Chicken pox (varicella)	Acute viral disease; onset is sudden with high fever; maculopapular rash and vesicular scabs in multiple stages of healing. Incubation is 10 to 21 days.	Spread by droplet or airborne secretions; scabs not infectious.	Isolate. Treat symptoms: Tylenol, fluids for fever. Prevent scratching.

Mumps	Acute viral disease, characterized by fever, swelling, and tenderness of one or more salivary glands. Potential complications, including meningoencephalitis.	Spread by droplet and direct and indirect contact with saliva of infected person. Most infectious 48 hours prior to swelling.	Prevent by vaccination.
			Isolate.
			Treat symptoms: ice pack to neck and force fluids.
			Watch for symptoms of neurological involvement:
			    fever
			    headache
			    vomiting
			    stiff neck.

Measles (rubeola)	Acute viral disease, characterized by conjunctivitis, bronchitis Koplik's spots on buccal mucosa, dusky red and splotchy rash 3 to 4 days, and usually photophobia. Complications can be severe in respiratory tract, eye, ear, and nervous system. Incubation is 10 to 12 days.	Spread by droplet or direct contact.	Symptomatic: rest until cough and fever subside, force fluids, dim lights in room, tepid baths, lotion to relieve itching.
German measles (rubella)	Viral infection, slight fever, mild coryza, and headache. Discrete pink-red maculopapules that last about three days. Incubation 14 to 21 days. Basically a benign disease.	Spread by direct and indirect contact with droplets. Fetus may contract measles in utero if mother has the disease.	Symptomatic: bed rest until fever subsides.
Diphtheria	Local and systemic manifestations: malaise, fever, cough with stridor. Toxin has affinity for renal, nerve, and cardiac tissue. Incubation 2 to 6 days or longer.	Spread by droplets from respiratory tract or carrier.	Antitoxin and antibiotic therapy to kill toxin. Strict bed rest to prevent exertion. Liquid or soft diet. Observe for respiratory obstruction — suctioning, oxygen, and emergency tracheotomy may be necessary.
Tetanus (lockjaw)	Acute or gradual onset. Muscle rigidity and spasms, headache, fever, and convulsions. Death may result from aspiration, pneumonia, or exhaustion. Incubation 3 to 21 days.	Organisms in soil that enter body through wound. Not communicable man to man.	Toxins must be neutralized. Bed rest during illness in quiet, darkened room. Avoid stimulation that can cause spasms. Observe for complications of laryngospasm and respiratory failure.

APPENDIX 6. VITAL SIGNS FOR CHILDREN AT DIFFERENT AGES

Vital Sign Chart

Age	Range of Normal Pulse	(average)	Average Blood Pressure	Average Respiration
Newborn	70–170	120	80/45	40–90
1 year	80–160	115	96/65	20–40
2 years	80–130	110	99/65	20–30
4 years	80–120	100	99/65	20–25
6 years	75–115	100	100/56	20–25
8 years	70–110	90	105/56	15–20
10 years	70–110	90	110/58	15–20

Pulse

A. Increased rate is significant if maintained during sleep.

B. Body temperature elevation causes an increase of eight to ten pulse beats for each degree of elevation.

APPENDIX 7. DENTAL DEVELOPMENT

Deciduous

	Age at Eruption		Age at Shedding	
	Maxillary	Mandibular	Maxillary	Mandibular
Central incisors	6 to 8 months	5 to 7 months	7 to 8 years	6 to 7 years
Lateral incisors	8 to 11	7 to 10	8 to 9	7 to 8
Cuspids	16 to 20	16 to 20	11 to 12	9 to 11
First molars	10 to 16	10 to 16	10 to 11	10 to 12
Second molars	20 to 30	20 to 30	10 to 12	11 to 13

Permanent Eruption

	Maxillary	Mandibular
Central incisors	7 to 8 years	6 to 7 years
Lateral incisors	8 to 9	7 to 8
Cuspids	11 to 12	9 to 11
First molars	6 to 7	6 to 7
Second molars	12 to 13	12 to 13
First premolars	10 to 11	10 to 11
Second premolars	10 to 12	11 to 13
Third molars	17 to 22	17 to 22

13

MENTAL HEALTH NURSING

MENTAL HEALTH CONTINUUM

Mental Illness

Definition: Mental illness is the general term that is used for a variety of behavioral reactions to life stresses that range from severe personality disorganization to the milder forms of temporary inability to cope with daily stress. Mental health, according to the World Health Organization, is "the presence of physical and emotional well-being."

Characteristics

A. Mental illness is a major health problem in the United States. One out of three individuals experiences some form of mental illness during a period of his or her life.

B. There has been an ever increasing number of patients admitted to mental hospitals or special units in private hospitals.

C. The criteria of mental illness might be said to be the extent to which problems are not dealt with through rational decisions.

Community Mental Health Movement

A. National Mental Health Act placed emphasis on the quality of care hospitalized mentally ill patients received.

B. It also emphasized the level of skills necessary to deliver higher quality care and lower rate of chronic hospitalized patients.

C. Object of act was to alter the state hospital model which was linked to chronicity and severity of disease.

D. Primary objectives were stated as preventing mental illness, coping with symptoms of illness, and returning the patient to community as soon as possible.

Anxiety

Definition: Anxiety is an affective state that is subjectively experienced as a response to stress. It is experienced as painful vague uneasiness, tension, or diffuse apprehension. It is a form of energy whose presence is inferred from its effect on attention, behavior, learning, and perception.

Characteristics

A. Anxiety is subjectively perceived by the conscious portion of the personality.

B. It can occur as a result of conflicts between the personality and the environment or between different aspects within the personality.

C. It may be a reaction to threats of deprivation of something vital to the person, biologically or emotionally.

D. The individual may be unaware of the conflicts.

E. The degree of anxiety is in relation to its effect on the individual.

F. Level of anxiety is influenced by:
   1. The extent to which the self feels threatened.
   2. The extent to which behavior reduces anxiety.

G. Varying levels of anxiety are common to all individuals at one time or another.

H. Anxiety can be transmitted from individual to individual.

I. Realistic anxiety can be constructive.

J. Anxiety may be placed on a continuum of degrees.
   1. Absent (ataraxia).
      a. Uncommon.
      b. Apparent in the person who takes drugs.
      c. Indicator of a low level of motivation.
   2. Mild.
      a. Senses are alert.
      b. Attentiveness is heightened.
      c. Motivation is increased.
   3. Moderate.
      a. Selective inattention because it narrows perception.
      b. Point at which it becomes pathological depends on individual.

c. May be seen as behaviors that are complaining, arguing, teasing.

d. Can convert to physical symptoms, such as headache, low back pain, nausea, diarrhea.

4. Severe.

a. Extremely painful psychologically.

b. Nursing intervention always indicated.

c. No longer useful to patient.

d. Drains energy.

e. Defense mechanisms may be used to "solve" underlying problem.

f. Behavior becomes automatic.

g. All senses are gravely affected.

5. Panic.

a. Individual is overwhelmed.

b. Personality may disintegrate.

c. Condition is now pathological.

d. Anxiety cannot be tolerated very long.
   (1) Individual cannot control his behavior.
   (2) Individual feels helpless.
   (3) Individual is briefly psychotic.

e. Observed behavior.
   (1) Ineffective.
   (2) Wild and desperate, causing possible bodily harm to self and others.

f. Needs immediate intervention.
   (1) Physical restraint.
   (2) Constant presence of attendant.
   (3) Tranquilizers.
   (4) Nonstimulating environment.

K. Neurotic anxiety.

1. Disproportionate to the danger.

2. Involves repression and dissociation.

3. Behavior is relatively ineffective and is inflexible.

L. Anxiety is always present in emotional disorders.

M. Physiological reactions to anxiety.

1. Increased heart rate.

2. Increased or decreased appetite.

3. Increased blood supply to skeletal muscles.

4. Tendency to void.

5. Dry mouth.

6. "Butterflies" in stomach, nausea, vomiting, cramps, diarrhea.

7. "Flight" or "fight" response.

Implementation

A. Intervene when patient unable to cope with anxiety or is ineffective in reducing it.

B. Be aware of own anxiety.

C. Maintain positive attitudes toward patient.
   1. Acceptance.
   2. Matter-of-fact approach.
   3. Willingness to listen and help.
   4. Calmness and support.

D. Recognize anxiety-produced behavior.

E. Provide activities that decrease anxiety and provide an outlet for energy.

F. Establish nurse-patient relationship.
   1. Allow patient to express feelings.
   2. Proceed at patient's pace.
   3. Avoid forcing patient to express feelings.
   4. Assist patient in identifying anxiety.
   5. Assist patient in learning new ways of dealing with anxiety.

G. Provide appropriate physical environment.
   1. Nonstimulating.
   2. Structured.
   3. Arrange to prevent physical exhaustion or self-harm.

H. Administer medication as directed and, after assessment, as needed.

Crisis Intervention

Definition: Crisis intervention is the form of therapy aimed at immediate intervention into an acute episode or crisis that the individual is unable to cope with alone.

Profile of a Crisis Situation

A. The individual is typically in a state of equilibrium (homeostatic balance).
   1. State is maintained by behavioral patterns that govern interchange between the individual and the environment.
   2. The individual uses learned coping techniques to deal with simple problems as they arise.

B. A crisis situation develops when a problem (triggering event) becomes too complex to be handled by previously learned coping techniques.

    1. Functioning modes become grossly disorganized.

    2. The individual is more amenable to intervention in circumstances of inability to resolve crisis.

    3. The potential for problem resolution as a result of intervention is positive.

C. Precipitant factors of a crisis.

    1. Threat to one's sense of security.

       a. Situational crisis: may include an actual or potential loss of job, friend, or mate.

       b. Developmental crisis: may include any change in role as occurs in marriage or birth of a child.

       c. The concurrence of two or more severe problems.

    2. Precipitants typically occur within two weeks after onset of disorganization.

Characteristics

A. Crisis is self-limiting, acute, and lasts one to six weeks.

B. Crisis is initiated by a triggering event (death, loss, etc.); usual coping mechanisms are inadequate for the situation.

C. Situation is dangerous to the person; he or she may harm self or others.

D. Individual will return to a state that is better, worse, or the same as before the crisis; therefore, intervention by the therapist is important.

E. Person is totally involved—hurts all over.

F. At this time the individual is most open for intervention; therefore, major changes can take place.

Stages of Crisis Development

A. Initial perception and comprehension of scope of problem.

B. Rise in tension and anxiety which instigates the usual coping mechanisms.

C. Consultation with the usual supportive contacts.

D. Familiar methods prove unsuccessful and tension increases.

E. Seeks new problem-solving methods; if unsuccessful, the problem remains and interferes with individual's life.

    1. Functioning becomes disorganized.

    2. Extreme anxiety is likely to be experienced.

    3. Perception is narrowed.

    4. Coping ability is further impaired.

    5. Situation may cause self-harm or harm to others.

    6. Individual totally involved and hurts all over.

F. Resolution will occur within six weeks with or without intervention.

Assessment of Crisis

A. Determine period of disorganization.

    1. Extent of disorganization.

    2. Length of time situation existed.

    3. Level of functioning.

B. Evaluate precipitant event.

    1. The nature of the event that triggered the crisis.

    2. The significance of the event to the individual.

C. Examine effectiveness of coping mechanisms.

    1. History in experiencing similar situations.

    2. History in coping with similar situations.

D. Identify situational supports.

    1. Significant others.

    2. Agencies.

E. Suggest alternative coping modes.

    1. New coping alternatives.

    2. Situational supports.

Principles of Crisis Intervention

A. Goal is the return of patient to precrisis level and maintenance of functioning.

B. Intervene immediately because it is important that intervention occur within the six week time limit.

C. Assess problem accurately and keep focus on this problem with reality-oriented therapy ("here and now" focus).

D. Set limits.

E. Remain with patient or have significant person available as necessary.

F. Explore coping mechanisms available to patient.
1. Develop strengths and capitalize on them.
2. Do not focus on weakness or pathology.
3. Help explore the available situational supports.

G. Help the patient to understand the problem and to integrate the events in his or her life.

H. Determine if continuing therapy with a professional may be needed for future support.

Implementation ❖ Procedure ❖

A. Focus on immediate problem.

B. Use reality-oriented approach.

C. Stay with "here and now" focus.

D. Set limits.

E. Stay with patient or have significant persons available if necessary.

F. Explore available coping mechanisms.
1. Develop strengths and capitalize on them.
2. Do not focus on weakness or pathology.
3. Help explore the available situational supports.

G. Clarify the problem and help the individual understand the problem and integrate the events in his life.

H. When the above steps are completed, some plans for future support should be worked out by the therapist and the patient.

Defense Mechanisms

Definition: Defense mechanisms, or adjustive techniques, are methods that are assumed by an individual to relieve or decrease anxieties produced by an uncomfortable situation that threatens self-esteem.

Characteristics

A. The purpose of adjustive techniques is to attempt reduction of anxiety and reestablishment of equilibrium.

B. An individual's adjustment depends on the ability to vary responses so that anxiety is decreased.

C. Individuals use essentially the same techniques, which may vary in form.

D. The exercise of a defense mechanism may be a conscious process, but it is usually generated at the unconscious level.

E. Adjustment techniques are compromise solutions (see Appendix 1. Defense Mechanisms) that include many forms.

F. Healthy adjustment to life forces.
1. A healthy adjustment is characterized by:
   a. Infrequent need to use unconscious adjustive techniques.
   b. Ability to form new responses.
   c. Ability to change external environment.
   d. Ability to modify one's own needs.
2. Healthy adjustment mechanisms may include rationalization, sublimation, compensation, and suppression.

G. Unhealthy adjustment to life forces.
1. An unhealthy adjustment is characterized by:
   a. The inability or loss of ability to vary responses.
   b. The individual's retreat from the problem or from reality.
   c. Continual use, which may interfere with maintenance of self-image.
2. Unhealthy adjustment mechanisms may include regression, repression, denial, projection, and isolation.

Implementation

A. Be aware of your own behavior and the use of adjustive techniques.

B. Avoid criticizing the patient's behavior and use of adjustive techniques.

C. Assist the patient in learning new or alternative adjustment techniques for healthier adaptation.

D. Use techniques to help alleviate the patient's anxiety.

E. Do not attempt to arbitrarily eliminate adjustive techniques without replacement for they serve a purpose for the patient.

AFFECTIVE DISORDERS

Bipolar Disorders

Manic-Depressive Illness—Manic Episode

Definition: One manifestation of an affective disorder that involves mood swings of elation, euphoria, and grandiose behavior with or without a history of depression. Cyclothymic disorder is the second category of bipolar disorder and refers to a milder form of the same illness.

Characteristics

A. Specific etiology is unknown. May be related to a genetic predisposition to illness or to increased levels of dopamine in the brain. Attempts are now being made to discover why lithium is therapeutic in hopes of solving the mystery of manic illness.

B. Women experience this illness slightly more frequently than men. The lifetime risk of developing this illness is 1–2 percent of the population.

C. The first manic episode usually occurs before age 30 and, interestingly, is more common in the higher socio-economic group.

D. Mania refers to a pronounced, elated, high mood that is evidenced by a high level of activity and general demeanor of cheerfulness.

Assessment

A. Mood is one of euphoria which can lead to grandiose behavior and delusions.

B. Individual overresponds to stimuli.
 1. Rapid talk, with play on words and flight of ideas.
 2. Increased motor activity.
 3. Increased thought processes.

C. Individual exercises poor judgment, i.e., spends money foolishly, runs up charge accounts, erratically gives away belongings, etc.

D. Individual's attitude is narcissistic and will not tolerate guidance or criticism.

E. Individual gives little attention to physical health.
 1. Poor sleep habits with no apparent fatigue.
 2. Poor nutrition.
 3. Poor, or even bizarre, habits of grooming.

F. Behavior varies from delightful and playful to restless, irritable, sarcastic, and even antagonistic and combative.

G. If behavior is not controlled, the individual will become incoherent, overtly aggressive, and hostile.

Implementation

A. Maintain safe environment.
 1. Reduce external stimuli such as noise, people, and motion.
 2. Eliminate patient's participation in competitive activities.
 3. Redirect patient's energy into brief but useful activities.

B. Establish one-to-one relationship.
 1. Maintain an accepting and nonjudgmental attitude.
 2. Create conditions favorable to the development of mutual trust.
 3. Avoid entering into patient's playful, joking activity if it appears to be a manic reaction.
 4. Allow the patient to verbalize his or her feelings, especially hostility.

C. Set realistic limits on behavior.
 1. Set scope and limitations to behavior to provide for a sense of security.

2. Restrain destructive behavior.
3. Be firm and consistent.
D. Give attention to physical needs.
   1. Provide a diet that is high in calories, vitamins, and fluids.
   2. Ensure adequate rest and sleep.
   3. Protect patient from inadvertent self-harm.

Major Depressive Episode

Definition: A unipolar condition in which the feeling state of the individual is abnormal and manifests itself by a complex of symptoms. The symptoms may be mild and only slightly debilitating or pathological, implying overwhelming intensity and long duration.

Characteristics

A. The most common of all psychiatric illnesses, depression is a symptom probably experienced by 15 out of 100 adults in our society.
B. One cause is now thought to involve a genetic link; other possible causes are personality traits such as low self-esteem, neuro-chemical imbalances, and other biological factors.
C. Most acute depressive episodes are self-limiting and last from a few weeks (with treatment) to a few months.
D. More than half of those persons who experience a first episode go on to suffer a recurrence.
E. About 20–25 percent never return to their premorbid state of mental health.

Assessment

A. The distinguishing quality of depression is mood; affect is one of sadness or gloom.
B. Behavior is slowed down with purposeful movement nearly diminished.
C. Personal appearance is neglected.
D. Thought processes are slowed down until there is paucity of thinking.
E. Attitudes are pessimistic and self-denigrating, and focus is on the problems and uselessness of life. The individual lacks inner resources and strengths to cope effectively.
F. Physical symptoms usually reflect a preoccupation with body and poor health. Weight loss, insomnia, and general malaise are typically in evidence.
G. Social interaction is reduced and inappropriate. The depressed patient feels isolated but cannot resolve that condition because he or she cannot contribute to a relationship.
H. A common outcome of depression is possible suicide (refer to section on suicide).

Major Depressive Episode Subtypes

A. Depression with melancholia.
   1. Predisposing factors appear to be dissatisfaction with accomplishments in life and loss of pleasure in the usual activities.
   2. Emphasis is on the vegetative signs and variation in mood (often called involutional melancholia).
   3. Common symptoms that accompany this disorder are a general depressed mood that is worse in the morning, psychomotor retardation, or agitation and anorexia which may result in weight loss.
B. Depression with psychotic symptoms.
   1. This subtype of depression is accompanied by an inability to test reality: delusions, hallucinations, and confusion.
      a. May also have severe impairment of personal and social functioning.
      b. May be severely withdrawn.
   2. Approximately 10 percent of those depressed have psychotic symptoms.
   3. Psychotic depressions are considered to be biologically based.

Dysthymic Disorder (Depressive Neurosis)

A. Symptoms of depression fluctuate and are less severe than with the major depressive disorder.
   1. Mild symptoms are present for at least two years.
   2. Depression may be episodic or constant.

B. Psychosis is not present.

C. Several of the following symptoms are usually present with this diagnosis.
  1. Low energy level.
  2. Loss of interest in pleasurable activities.
  3. Pessimistic attitude toward the future; thoughts of suicide.
  4. Tearful, crying demeanor.
  5. Feelings of low self-esteem.
  6. Decreased ability to concentrate.

Implementation

A. Provide a safe milieu, and protect the patient from self-injury (prevent suicide).

B. Provide a structured environment to mobilize the patient.
  1. Encourage daily activities, and allow time for them.
  2. Provide stimulation for occupational and recreational activity.
  3. Reactivate interests outside of the patient's present concerns.
  4. Motivate patient for treatment.
  5. Encourage psychotherapy and occupational therapy activities.

C. Build trust through one-to-one relationship.
  1. Employ a supportive and unchallenging approach.
  2. Project behaviors and attitudes that are accepting and nonjudgmental.
  3. Show interest. Listen and give positive reinforcement.
  4. Redirect the patient's monologue away from painful and depressing thoughts.
  5. Focus on the patient's underlying anger, and encourage its expression.

D. Help build the self-esteem of the patient.
  1. Encourage simple tasks that invite successful experiences.
  2. Limit decision-making with the severely depressed.
  3. Support use of defenses to alleviate suffering.

E. Be attentive to the patient's physical needs: provide adequate nutrition and opportunity for sleep and exercise.

Table 1. Affective Illness

Depression Type	Distinguishing Feature
Bipolar	
Manic-depressive disorder	History of elation episodes with or without depression
Cyclothymic disorder	
Unipolar	
Major depressive disorder	History of depression without any history of elation
Depression with melancholia	
Depression with psychotic features	
Dysthymic disorder	

Suicide

Definition: The act of killing oneself intentionally.

Characteristics

A. Suicide is the seventh most common cause of death in the United States today.

B. Suicide statistics.
  1. Suicide ranks fourth as the cause of death in the 15 to 40 age group.
  2. For every successful suicide, it is believed that there are five to ten attempted suicides.
  3. Women make more suicide attempts than men.
  4. Suicide is more common in the elderly age group.
  5. Adolescent suicide is increasing.
  6. Suicides are incurred by means of auto accidents; because they are not reported as such, statistics remain low.

C. Causes of suicide attempts.
  1. Depression is the primary cause.
  2. The secondary cause is alcohol.
  3. Inability to cope with problems in living.

4. Attempts to control others.

D. Depressed individuals, when severely ill, rarely commit suicide.
   1. They do not have the drive and energy to make a plan and follow it through when severely depressed.
   2. Danger period is when depression begins to lift.

E. Eight out of ten known suicide cases give warnings or messages through direct or indirect means.

F. Danger symptoms range from depression, disorientation, and defiance to intense dependence on another.

Implementation

A. Provide safe environment to protect patient from self-destruction.

B. Observe closely at all times, especially when depression is lifting.

C. Establish supportive relationship, letting the patient know you are concerned for his welfare.

D. Encourage expression of feelings, especially anger.

E. Determine patient's capacity to entertain suicide ideas.
   1. Ask questions such as, "Are you thinking of suicide?" "Did you think you might do something about it?" "What?" "Have you taken any steps to prepare?" "What are they?"
   2. Important to recognize a continued desire to commit suicide.

F. Focus on strengths and successful experiences that can enhance self-esteem.

G. Follow a structured schedule, and involve the patient in activities with others.

H. Help structure a plan for coping when patient next experiences ideas of suicide.

I. Help the patient plan for continued professional support after discharge.

SOMATOFORM DISORDERS

Definition: Somatoform disorders (also called psychosomatic disorders) are physical diseases that may involve any organ system, and whose etiologies are in part related to emotional factors.

Characteristics

A. An individual must adapt and adjust to stresses in life.
   1. The way a person adapts depends on individual characteristics and extent of inner stability.
   2. Emotional stress may exacerbate or precipitate an illness.

B. Psychosocial stress or anxiety is an important factor in symptom formation.
   1. If stress or anxiety cannot be expressed through verbalization, it finds expression through particular organ symptoms.
   2. Exact relationship between stress and illness is unknown.
   3. It is thought that somatic symptoms occur in individuals who have never had to resolve dependent-independent struggles of childhood; dependent needs not met.
   4. Illness provides focus for individual away from original anxiety, thereby providing secondary gains of sympathy and attention from others.

C. Structural changes in body systems may occur and pose a life-threatening situation.
   1. Individual not faking illness; it is real and requires direct medical attention.
   2. Correcting physical illness may not alter the underlying cause of anxiety.

D. There can be synergistic reaction from repressed feelings and overexcited organs.

E. Psychosomatic illness provides individual with coping mechanisms.
   1. Means to handle anxiety and stress.
   2. Ways to gain socially acceptable attention.
   3. Rationalization for failures.
   4. Means for adjusting to dependency needs.
   5. Ways to handle anger and aggression.
   6. Ways to punish self and others.

F. Kinds of adjustive techniques used (see Appendix 1. Defense Mechanisms).
   1. Repression.
   2. Denial.
   3. Projection.
   4. Conversion.
G. A psychosomatic disorder may involve any body system.
   1. Gastrointestinal system.
      a. Peptic ulcer.
      b. Colic.
      c. Ulcerative colitis.
   2. Cardiovascular system.
      a. Hypertension.
      b. Tachycardia.
      c. Migraine headaches.
   3. Respiratory system.
      a. Asthma.
      b. Hay fever.
      c. Hiccoughs.
   4. Skin (most expressive organ of emotion).
      a. Blushing.
      b. Flushing, perspiring.
      c. Dermatitis.
   5. Nervous system.
      a. Chronic general fatigue.
      b. Exhaustion.
   6. Endocrine.
      a. Dysmenorrhea.
      b. Hyperthyroidism.
   7. Musculoskeletal system.
      a. Cramps.
      b. Rheumatoid arthritis.
   8. Other associated disorders.
      a. Diabetes mellitus.
      b. Obesity.
      c. Sexual dysfunctions.
      d. Hyperemesis gravidarum.
      e. Accident proneness.

Implementation

A. Observe closely and assess patient's condition.
   1. Collect data about the physical illness, psychosocial adjustment, life situations, natural stresses, strengths, etc.
   2. Report the kinds of things that aggravate or release the symptom.

B. Attend to the whole person, physically and emotionally.
C. Reduce demands on the patient.
D. Develop nurse-patient relationship.
   1. Respect the patient and acknowledge his or her problems.
   2. Assist the patient to express his or her feelings.
   3. Help the patient to release anxiety and explore new coping mechanisms.
   4. Allow the patient to meet dependency needs.
   5. Allow the patient to feel in control of his or her life.
E. Encourage the patient to work through problems and to learn new methods of responding to stress.
F. Provide safe and nonthreatening environment.
   1. Balance therapy and recreation.
   2. Decrease distracting stimuli.
   3. Provide activities that can deemphasize or help to alleviate the patient's physical symptoms.

Conversion Disorder

A. Anxiety that results from an unconscious conflict is converted into physical symptoms for which there is no organic explanation.
B. Specific nursing approaches.
   1. Understand that patient's lack of concern or indifferent attitude is at the same time a symptom of the illness.
   2. Recognize that illness is frequently used for primary gains, i.e., solving conflict by not solving it and removing the source of stress. Illness used as secondary gains provide patient with sympathy and attention to physical handicap.
   3. Do not confront the patient with his or her illness.
   4. Divert patient's attention from symptoms. Do not respond to patient's secondary gains.
   5. Reduce pressure or demands on patient.
   6. Create positive relationship.
   7. Use a matter-of-fact approach.

8. Provide patient with recreational and socializing activities.
9. Teach necessities of daily living, and give assistance as needed, i.e., if patient is blind, help and show how to feed self.

Hypochondriasis

A. A severe, morbid preoccupation with one's own body; abnormal anxiety about one's health.
B. Specific nursing approaches.
1. Accept the patient and his or her complaints.
2. Provide diversional activities in which the patient can succeed.
3. Use friendly, supportive approach.
4. Provide for patient's physical needs.
5. Assist patient to refocus interest.

ANXIETY DISORDERS

Definition: A mild to moderately severe psychological disorder that affects thought and feeling processes. The individual suppresses and represses unpleasant thoughts and/or feelings to alleviate the discomfort of the resulting anxiety. The consequent conflicts are handled by means of anxiety reaction, phobias, obsessive-compulsive reaction, dissociation, hypochondriasis, and neurasthenia.

Characteristics

A. No apparent physiologic basis for symptoms.
B. Threats to ego cause anxiety, and ego protects the person by developing defenses.
C. A neurosis is an attempt to deal with anxiety.
D. Individuals have little difficulty talking, but conversation may be vague and unrevealing.
E. Individual is generally unaware of his or her behavior patterns.
F. Individual becomes more dependent as time goes on.
G. Secondary gains from anxiety become associated problems.

1. These are the fringe benefits that patient receives from symptoms.
2. Secondary gains reinforce maladaptive behavior.
H. Common defense mechanisms include repression and projection.
I. Evidence of low self-esteem is observable.
J. No gross distortion of reality.
K. Personality is not grossly disorganized.
L. The martyr syndrome is common.
M. Individual is highly suggestible.

Implementation

A. Nurse needs to understand and recognize own feelings and attitudes in dealing with neurotics.
B. Convey an attitude of acceptance and understanding of patient's symptoms because patient relies on them to control anxiety.
C. Plan nonthreatening activities that will reduce anxiety and enhance self-esteem.
D. Do not make unreasonable demands upon the patient.
E. Remain with extremely anxious patient.
F. Avoid using labels for patient's behaviors.
G. Provide a safe, supportive environment.
H. Be alert to the specific needs of patient as demonstrated by their behavior.

Generalized Anxiety Disorder

A. Anxiety is diffuse (free-floating).
B. Anxiety cannot be controlled by means of defense mechanisms.
C. Psychological symptoms.
1. Cannot concentrate on work.
2. Feels depressed and guilty.
3. Harbors fears of sudden death or insanity.
4. Dreads being alone.
5. Confused.
6. Tense.
7. Agitated and restless.
D. Physiological symptoms.
1. Tremors.

2. Dyspnea.
3. Palpitations.
4. Tachycardia.
5. Numbness of extremities.
E. Specific nursing approaches.
1. Calm, serene approach with recognition of own anxiety.
2. Nonverbal reassurance.
3. Listen.
4. Provide physical outlet for anxiety.
5. Remain with patient.
6. Decrease environmental stimuli.

Phobic Disorders

A. By means of displacement, anxiety is transferred from the original source to a symbolic idea or situation.
B. Phobic disorders are classified into three types.
1. Agoraphobia—most common form.
   a. Marked fear of and avoidance of being alone or in public places where escape might be difficult or help not available in case of sudden incapacitation.
   b. Increasing constriction of normal activities until fear dominates the individual's life.
2. Social phobia.
   a. A persistent irrational fear and compelling desire to avoid a situation in which the individual is exposed to scrutiny by others.
   b. Fear of acting in a way that may be humiliating or embarrassing.
   c. Distress about disturbance and feelings.
3. Simple phobia.
   a. A persistent irrational fear and compelling desire to avoid an object or a situation other than agoraphobia or social.
   b. Fear of heights, closed spaces, or animals.
   c. Distress about symptoms.
C. Specific nursing approaches.
1. Slowly develop a trusting relationship with the patient.
2. Do not force patient into feared situations.
3. Divert patient's attention from the phobia.
4. Direct patient's focus to awareness of self.
5. Encourage but do not force patient to discuss fears and feelings.
6. Support patient during program of phobic desensitization.

Obsessive-Compulsive Disorder

A. Anxiety is associated with the persistence of undesired ideas or impulses; repetitive ritualistic actions alleviate anxiety.
B. Specific nursing approaches.
1. Avoid punishment or criticism for compulsive repetition of acts.
2. Set limits to protect patient from harmful acts.
3. Provide climate of acceptance and understanding.
4. Orient nursing care around patient's need to perform rituals.
5. Provide for patient's physical needs.

SCHIZOPHRENIC DISORDERS

Definition: Schizophrenia is a syndrome that carries with it varied etiology, psychodynamics, and psychopathology. The clinical course of the illness varies from patient to patient, so the nurse should view the disease as a syndrome with varying clinical entities. It is characterized by disturbances in thought, communication, relationships, behavior, and perception.

Characteristics

A. Schizophrenia may be the result of many variables: genetic constellation, individual adaptive patterns, poor family relationships, lack of ego strength, earlier traumatic experiences, or distorted cognition.
B. Regression and repression are regarded as the primary mechanisms of schizophrenia.
C. Major maladaptive disturbances: impaired interpersonal relationships, ineffective mental

and emotional processes, and disturbances in overt behavior patterns.
D. Individuals generally demonstrate personality disorganization and coping difficulty.
E. Schizophrenic reactions may become acute and/or chronic.

Primary Disturbances

A. Thoughts are confused and disorganized so that ability to communicate clearly is limited.
B. Feelings (affect) may be expressed in an inappropriate manner.
C. Behavior may be bizarre or lack purposeful direction.
D. Close and trusting interpersonal relationships are difficult to establish.

Assessment

A. The four "A's."
   1. *Affect*—feelings or subjective aspect of emotions are minimal, i.e., "flat affect"; apathetic, inappropriate expression of moods and responses.
   2. *Associative looseness*—no connection between thoughts and expressed ideas; difficulty in discerning logical from illogical thought.
   3. *Autistic thinking*—thoughts are self-serving and focus inward, i.e., patient uses neologisms or invented words and lives in a world of inner fantasy.
   4. *Ambivalence*—two equally strong feelings, such as love and hate, neutralize each other and immobilize patient.
B. Other important clinical signs.
   1. *Reality testing* difficulty—objective facts cannot be distinguished from wishes or imagination.
   2. *Delusions*—fixed misinterpretation of reality. False beliefs maintained despite evidence to the contrary.
   3. *Hallucinations*—sensory input (smell, taste, sound, touch, sight) that has no basis in the real world. One "hears" voices, "sees" visions, etc.
   4. *Withdrawal*—behavior that signifies the patient's desire to regress into more satisfying world of own making (autism).
   5. The above signs may manifest themselves in singular or combined forms.

Implementation

A. General approaches.
   1. Establish nurse-patient relationship.
      a. Develop positive and trusting relationship.
      b. Provide a safe and secure environment.
   2. Stress situational reality.
      a. Help patient to reality-test and come out of fantasy world.
      b. Involve the patient in reality-oriented activities.
      c. Help the patient to find satisfaction in the external environment.
   3. Accept the patient as he or she is.
      a. Do not invalidate disturbed thoughts or fantasies.
      b. Do not invalidate the patient's sense of self by your inappropriate responses.
   4. Use only therapeutic communication techniques.
      a. Encourage patient to express negative and/or positive emotions.
      b. Encourage patient to express thoughts, fears, and problems.
      c. Match your nonverbal with your verbal communications.
      d. Communicate clearly with the patient.
   5. Do not foster a dependency relationship.
   6. Avoid stressful situations that can increase the patient's anxiety.
B. Approaches to specific behaviors.
   1. Working with delusions.
      a. Help the patient to recognize distorted views of reality.
      b. Focus on patient's strengths.
      c. Provide a safe, nonthreatening milieu.
      d. Divert focus from delusional material to reality.
      e. Provide situations that can create successful experiences for the patient.
      f. Specific nursing responses:

(1) Avoid confirming or feeding into delusion.

(2) Stress reality by denying you believe the patient's delusion.

(3) Respond to patient's feelings, i.e., validate his or her feelings by saying, "I sense you are afraid. Is this true?"

2. Working with withdrawn behavior.

a. Assist patient in developing a satisfying relationship with you.

(1) Initiate interaction.

(2) Show sincerity for a trusting relationship by being consistent in keeping appointments, in attitudes, and in nursing practice.

(3) Be honest and direct in what you say and do.

(4) Deal with your feelings incurred by patient's hostility or rejection.

b. Help patient to modify self-perception.

(1) Structure situations in which patient will succeed.

(2) Focus on patient's assets or strengths to enhance self-esteem.

(3) Relieve patient from making choices until able to make decisions.

c. Teach patient how to restore social skills.

(1) Gradually increase opportunities for social contacts with staff and other patients.

(2) Increase opportunities for social contact with significant others (family) as appropriate.

d. Focus on reality situations.

(1) Use nonthreatening approach.

(2) Provide safe nonthreatening milieu.

e. Attend to physical needs of nutrition, sleep, exercise, occupational therapy.

Schizophrenic Subtypes

A. Catatonic type.

1. Secondary symptoms of motor involvement are present.

a. Underactivity results in bizarre posturing.

b. Overactivity leads to agitation.

2. Negativism: doing the opposite of what is asked.

a. Rigidity is the simplest form of negativism.

b. Mute behavior is another form of negativism.

B. Disorganized type.

1. Inappropriate affect: giggling and silly laughter (formerly labeled hebephrenia).

2. Disorganization of speech.

3. Regression.

4. Absence of systematized delusions.

C. Undifferentiated type.

1. This type is characterized by a combination of symptoms, none of which discriminates a specific type of disorder.

2. Flat affect and/or autism is usually present.

3. Association disorders and thought disturbance, such as delusions or hallucinations, are usually present.

4. This condition includes other behavioral maladaptations that cannot be otherwise classified.

D. Paranoid schizophrenia.

1. A type of schizophrenic reaction that manifests delusions of persecution and other maladaptive behavior.

2. Characteristics.

a. Individual is extremely suspicious and withdraws from emotional contact with others.

b. The onset is gradual and usually occurs between the ages of 30 and 40.

c. Certain stressful events in the individual's life may precipitate onset of paranoid reaction.

(1) Real or imaginary loss of a loved one.

(2) Experiences of failure with subsequent loss of self-esteem.

d. Individual expresses abnormal concern with health (hypochondriasis).

(1) Complains of insomnia and weakness.

(2) Complains of strange bodily sensations.

      (3) Complains of other somatic distur-
         bances.
  e. Individual projects common paranoic
    delusional thoughts.
      (1) Feels persecuted, i.e., individual
         fears that people are out to harm,
         injure, or destroy him or her.
      (2) Behaves as if in a state of grandeur.
      (3) Expresses jealousy.
  f. Paranoic reactions can occur in organic,
    senile, alcoholic, and other mental ill-
    nesses.
3. Clinical signs and symptoms.
  a. Extreme suspiciousness and mistrust of
    others.
  b. Hostility toward others.
  c. Delusions of persecution or grandeur.
  d. Chronic insecurity, inadequate self-con-
    cept, low self-esteem.
  e. Chronic high anxiety level.
  f. Patient denies delusional role.
  g. Hypochondriasis.
4. Nursing care.
  a. Establish a trusting relationship.
    (1) Be consistent and friendly despite
       patient's hostility.
    (2) Avoid talking and laughing when
       the patient can see but not hear
       you.
    (3) If patient is very suspicious, relate
       one-to-one and not in a group situ-
       ation.
    (4) Involve the patient in the treatment
       plan.
    (5) Give nonpunitive support.
  b. Reduce anxiety associated with inter-
    personal interactions.
    (1) Avoid power struggles, i.e., do not
       argue with the patient because it
       increases anxiety and hostility.
    (2) Proceed with nursing therapy slow-
       ly because a paranoid patient is
       suspicious and often mistrustful of
       others.
    (3) Show consistency and honesty.
  c. Help patient differentiate delusion
    from reality (refer to section on delu-
    sions).

Table 2. Profile Differentiation

Schizophrenic	Non-Schizophrenic
Major ego impairment. Includes faulty reality testing, delusions, hallucinations (especially auditory).	No grave impairment of reality testing. No hallucinations or delusions.
Serious impairment of patient's life, including social, vocational, and sexual.	Difficulty in relating, but interaction with others not prevented. Personality usually remains organized.
Little insight into problems and behavior. Patient generally does not recognize he or she is ill.	Some awareness into problems. Keenly feels subjective suffering. Often unconsciously fights any changes in status (getting well).
Severe personality disorganization, e.g., judgment, memory, and perceptions.	Less severe disorganization. Can function but with decreased efficiency.
May be caused by both physiological or psychological factors.	Always a functional disorder; not organic in origin.
Usually requires hospitalization and long-term treatment.	Usually does not require hospitalization. May require long-term treatment.
Maladaptive adjustment mechanisms used in rigid, fixed way. May be seen as severe regression.	Suppression and repression used to handle internal conflicts; defenses are largely symbolic.
No secondary gain received.	Symptoms generally exploited for secondary gain.

    (1) Do not explain away imagined
       thoughts for they are real to the
       patient.
    (2) Use reality-testing whenever possi-
       ble.
    (3) Focus on reality situations in the
       environment.

Paranoid Disorders

Definition: Diagnosis of paranoid disorder is made when paranoid features dominate the personality. Other symptoms of maladaptive behavior may be absent.

Characteristics

A. Paranoia is characterized by extreme suspiciousness and withdrawal from all emotional contact with others.
B. The onset is usually gradual.
C. The onset of paranoid reactions may be precipitated by certain stressful events in patient's life.
    1. Real or imaginary loss of a love object.
    2. Experiences of failure with subsequent loss of self-esteem.

Assessment

A. Intense focus on hypochondriasis.
B. Complaints of insomnia and weakness.
C. Complaints of strange bodily sensations.
D. The more common paranoid psychosis is manifested by delusional thoughts:
    1. The most common delusions are of persecution (people are out to harm, injure, or destroy).
    2. Other delusions may center around grandeur, somatic complaints, or delusions of jealousy.
E. Suspiciousness and mistrust of others.
F. Hostility toward others.

DISSOCIATIVE DISORDERS

Definition: This disorder is a sudden temporary alteration in the integrative functions of consciousness, identity, or motor behavior.

Characteristics

A. Patient attempts to deal with anxiety through various disturbances of by walling off certain areas of the mind from consciousness.
B. Patient remains in contact with reality.
C. Repression is used.

Assessment

A. Amnesia: circumscribed, selective, generalized and continuous.
B. Fugue or physical flight.
C. Interference in lifestyle and interpersonal relationships.
D. Accompanying symptoms such as depression, suicide ideation, etc.

Implementation

A. Support therapeutic modality as established by treatment team.
B. Reduce anxiety-producing stimuli.
C. Redirect patient's attention away from self.
D. Avoid sympathizing with patient.
E. Increase socialization activities.

PERSONALITY DISORDERS

Definition: An individual with a personality disorder adjusts to life situations with difficulty and interacts with others in an unsatisfactory manner. Behavioral problems rather than symptoms are exhibited. This individual is known as a psychopathic or sociopathic personality.

Characteristics

A. Experiences difficulty in developing warm interpersonal relationships.
    1. Affective responses are shallow.
    2. Relationships tend to be superficial.
B. Responds poorly to intellectual and emotional demands made of them.
C. Aggressive and sexual impulses are expressed overtly.
D. Tolerance for anxiety is low so that the person will go to any length to avoid situations that provoke anxiety.
    1. The attempts to gain relief from anxiety produce inappropriate behavior.

2. Individual is unaware that behavior is contrary to social expectations.

E. Exhibits poor impulse control and poor judgment; rejects all authority.

F. Social assets include intelligence and charm; skilled in manipulation.

G. Behavior often perceived as direct or indirect attack on laws and mores of society.

H. Personality profiles.
1. Antisocial (dissocial) personality.
   a. Lies, cheats, and steals (a pathologic diagnosis common in prisons).
   b. Patient shows evidence of emotional immaturity.
   c. Indicates little or no capacity for good judgment.
   d. Rationalizes behavior so that it appears justified; lacks a moral conscience.
   e. Is the typical "con artist."
2. Inadequate personality.
   a. Responds to intellectual and emotional demands ineffectively.
   b. Does not learn from experience or punishment, indicating poor judgment.
   c. Is socially unstable.
   d. Lacks ability to adapt.
3. "Social deviate" personality types.
   a. Sadist—inflicts pain on another.
   b. Masochist—inflicts pain on self.
   c. Voyeur—enjoys "peeping Tom" behavior.
   d. Exhibitionist—exposes own body for pleasure.
4. Addictive personality (see section on addiction).
5. Schizoid personality.
   a. Lacks close interpersonal relationships.
   b. Is shy and behavior is withdrawn.
   c. Projects eccentric behavior patterns.
   d. Unable to express hostility; affect is flat.
6. Paranoid personality.
   a. Suspects intentions of others.
   b. Unable to sustain interpersonal relationships because of inability to trust.
   c. Experiences jealousy and envy in relating to others.

Implementation

A. Participate in planning a therapeutic nurse-patient relationship that focuses on reinforcement of positive behavior.
1. Accept the patient for what and where he or she is (in terms of abilities).
   a. Set realistic expectations.
   b. Assess capabilities realistically so that excessive expectations will not reinforce failure.
2. Maintain control, and protect other patients from antisocial behavior.
3. Allow patient to express frustration and hostility.
4. Assist patient to tolerate frustration and postpone satisfaction.
5. Explore new alternatives for patient's living patterns that are socially acceptable.
6. Be aware of your own negative attitudes that may arise in working with these patients.

B. Set limitations firmly and with consistency.
1. Avoid falling into the patient's charming and manipulative ways.
2. Understand that the patient's anxiety will increase if manipulative behavior is ineffective.

C. Recognize that punishment does not resolve problems or change behavior.
1. Confront behavior but do not demean the patient.
2. Plan a supportive environment.
   a. Provide the patient with a sense of security.
   b. Provide opportunities for patient to learn how to cope with impulses.

D. Help patient to formulate realistic future plans.

E. Set specific guidelines for working with sociopathic and/or psychopathic behavior.
1. Attempt to develop a trusting relationship; it is difficult because the patient usually does not want help.
2. Follow the total care plan as determined by the physician. This is important because therapy is oriented toward reconstruction of personality.

3. Focus on reality, and do not allow patient to manipulate.
4. Give approval only for acceptable behavior.

Nursing Approaches to Maladaptive Behavior

Aggressive or Combative Behavior

A. Observe sharply for clues that the patient is getting out of control.
1. Note rising anger from patient's verbal and nonverbal behavior.
2. Note erratic or unpredictable responses to staff or other patients.

B. Intervene immediately when aware that patient's loss of control is imminent.

C. Approach the patient in a nonthreatening manner.

D. Set firm limits on unacceptable behavior.

E. Maintain calm demeanor, and do not show fear.

F. Avoid engaging in an argument or provoking the patient.

G. Summon assistance only when indicated: sudden involvement of many people will increase the patient's agitation.

H. Remove the patient from a threatening situation as soon as possible.

I. Use seclusion and/or restraints only if necessary.

J. Attempt to calm the patient so that control can be regained.

K. Be supportive and remain with the patient.

L. Use a problem-solving focus following outburst of aggressive or combative behavior.
1. Encourage discussion of feelings surrounding incident.
2. Attempt to discuss causal factors of the behavior.
3. Examine the patient's initial response to stimulus, and explore alternative responses.

4. Point out consequences of aggressive behavior.
5. Discuss the patient's role in taking responsibility for his aggressive behavior.

Verbally Abusive Behavior

A. Do not respond in kind to abusive comments.

B. Try not to take abuse personally.

C. Interact with the patient on a therapeutic basis.
1. Help the patient examine own feelings.
2. Do not reject the patient.
3. Give patient feedback concerning your reactions to abusive comments.
4. Teach alternative ways to express feelings.

D. Maintain a calm, accepting approach to patient.

Demanding Behavior

A. Do not ignore demands; they will only increase in intensity.

B. Attempt to determine causal factors of behavior, e.g., high anxiety level.

C. Set limits to your own response patterns when patient is demanding.

D. Control own feelings of anger and irritation.

E. Teach alternative means for getting needs met.

F. Plan nursing care to include frequent contacts that are initiated by the nurse.

G. Alert the staff to try to give patient needed reassurance.

Rape Intervention

Definition: Rape is a sexual assault on a person that is basically an act of violence; only secondarily considered a sex act.

Characteristics

A. Recognize that the assault of rape is a humiliating and violent experience and that the victim is experiencing severe psychological trauma.

B. Accept the fact that the victim was indeed raped and that the victim is to be supported, not treated as the "accused."

C. Understand that the victim's behavior might vary from hysterical crying and/or laughing to very calm and controlled.

D. Crisis response
1. Acute: shock, crying, high anxiety, hysterical, incoherent, agitated, fearful, volatile, poor problem-solving ability.
2. Beginning to cope: denial, appears calm and controlled, withdrawn, fearful, begins to talk about feelings, expresses anger, makes decisions.
3. Resolution: realistic attitudes, able to express feelings, controlled anger, acceptance of facts.

Implementation

A. Treatment focus.
1. Emotional—crisis counseling and call Women Against Rape.
   a. Degree of emotional trauma.
   b. Presence of symptoms.
2. Medical—immediate medical care: assess assault and degree of trauma.
   a. Assist with a complete physical examination.
   b. Carefully assess and document all physical damage: injuries; signs of physical entry.
3. Legal—do not bathe, douche, or change clothes; gather evidence.

B. Interventions.
1. Provide immediate privacy for examination.
2. Choose a staff member of the same sex to be with the victim.
3. Remain with the victim.
4. Administer physical care.
   a. Do not allow patient to wash genital area or void before examination; these actions will remove any existing evidence such as semen.
   b. Keep patient warm.
   c. Prepare patient for complete physical examination to be completed by physician (same sex as patient if possible).
   d. Physical exam includes:
      (1) Head-to-toe exam.
      (2) Pap smear.
      (3) Saline suspension to test for presence of sperm.
      (4) Acid-phosphatase to determine recency of attack.
   e. Physical treatment may include:
      (1) Prophylactic antibiotics.
      (2) Tranquilizers.
5. Provide emotional support.
   a. Demonstrate a nonjudgmental and supportive attitude.
   b. Express warmth, support, and empathy in relating to the victim.
   c. Listen to what the victim says and document all information.
   d. Encourage the victim to relate what happened, having her tell you in her own words if it appears that she would like to talk about the experience.
   e. Do not insist if patient chooses not to talk; allow the victim to cope in her own way.
   f. During the interview, continue to be sensitive to the victim's feelings and degree of control. If, in relating the attack, she becomes hysterical, do not continue questioning at this time.
6. Termination of crisis relationship.
   a. Counsel patient to receive repeat test for sexually transmitted diseases in three weeks or sooner if symptoms appear.
   b. Help reestablish contact with significant people.
   c. Refer to appropriate community resource for follow-up care.
   d. Keep accurate records, as they may be important in future legal proceedings

SUBSTANCE ABUSE

Definition: Substance abuse includes any process by which an individual ingests any mind-altering, nonprescribed chemical that produces physiological and/or psychological dependence. Withdrawal symptoms are usually manifest when substance is not taken.

Characteristics

A. Psychological dependence—emotional dependence, desire, or compulsion to continue taking the substance or drug.
B. Tolerance—the gradual increase of the amount required to obtain the desired effect.
C. Physical dependence—physical need for the substance manifested by appearance of withdrawal symptoms when substance is withheld.

Alcoholism

Definition: The abuse of any alcoholic substance combined with physical and psychological addiction.

Characteristics

A. Alcohol consumption is permitted by law and supported by most people in our society as a recreational activity.
B. A fine line exists between the social drinker and the addicted or problem drinker.
C. The greatest difference involves the degree of compulsion to drink and the inability to survive the trials of everyday living without the ingestion of alcohol.
D. Alcoholism, the third largest health problem in the United States (heart disease and cancer rank first and second), affects 15 million people.
E. Alcoholism is involved in about 30,000 deaths and one-half million injuries (auto accidents) every year.
F. Alcoholism decreases life span 10 to 12 years.

G. Loss to industry caused by alcoholism is estimated at 15 billion dollars a year (affecting primarily the 35 to 55 age group).
H. Major U.S. social concern is the dramatic rise in teenage alcoholism (estimated to affect 3 million adolescents).

Dynamics of Alcoholism

A. Alcoholic disease implies the consumption of alcohol to the point where it interferes with the individual's physical, emotional, and social functioning.
  1. The syndrome consists of two phases: problem drinking and alcohol addiction.
  2. Dependence on other drugs is very common.
B. No hereditary or organic basis for alcoholism has been proven to date.
C. Alcohol blocks synaptic transmission, depresses the central nervous system (CNS), and releases inhibitions. It acts initially as a stimulant but is actually a depressant.
  1. Chronic excessive use can lead to brain damage (sedative effect on CNS).
  2. High blood levels may cause malfunctions in cardiovascular and respiratory systems.
D. Blood level of 0.10% or more of alcohol is considered the level of intoxication.
E. Psychological effects of alcohol appear to be the gratification of oral impulses and the reduction of superego forces; abuse leads to shame and guilt and impaired ego function.
F. Alcohol may be said to be a defense against anxiety; therefore, the patient needs to work on problems causing his or her anxiety.
G. Illnesses associated with alcoholism.
  1. Korsakoff's syndrome.
  2. Delirium tremens.
  3. Chronic gastritis.
  4. Poor nutritional intake resulting in beriberi, pellagra, cerebellar degeneration, and anemia.
  5. Laënnec's cirrhosis and hepatitis.
  6. Peripheral neuropathy.
  7. Osteoporosis.

8. Individual is prone to infection.

Characteristics of an Alcoholic

A. Dependent personality but resents authority.

B. Sets high self-expectations but has a low tolerance for frustration.

C. Inclined toward patterns of failure.

D. Uses alcohol to gain a false sense of success, power, confidence, and self-worth.

E. Uses alcohol to ease suffering, reduce anxiety, and to help cope with life stresses.

F. Functions with less intellectual, emotional, and social ability as need for alcohol increases.

Implementation

A. Help reestablish the patient's healthy physical condition.
   1. Provide adequate nutrition with fluids and a high vitamin, high calorie, and high protein diet.
   2. Promote adequate rest and sleep.
   3. Observe patient for symptoms of impending delirium tremens.

B. Maintain a controlled and structured environment until the patient is able to manage his or her own circumstances.
   1. Set behavior limits, and confront the manipulative patient.
   2. Suggest group interaction for lonely patients.
   3. Remember that the patient needs support, firmness, and a reality-oriented approach.

C. Treatment techniques.
   1. Patient must first go through detoxification—intensive care to prevent the toxic state and then the return to a nonalcoholic state.
   2. Stress need for a change in attitudes.
      a. To accept fact that alcoholism is an illness.
      b. To accept fact that life must be managed without the support of alcohol.
   3. Promote psychotherapy techniques of group and family therapy; establish positive nurse-patient relationship therapy.

   a. Therapy goals.
      (1) Focus on the underlying emotional problems.
      (2) Offer assistance in handling anxiety.
      (3) Focus on relief of inferiority feelings and low self-esteem.
   b. Advantages of group therapy.
      (1) Patient receives support from peers.
      (2) Patient can receive negative feedback from peers without feeling threatened.
      (3) Patient can be supported in efforts to change by nonprofessional groups (AA), but change will not occur unless patient wants to be helped.
   4. Encourage rehabilitation or long-term supportive care.
      a. Continued psychotherapy on an outpatient basis.
      b. Referral to Alcoholics Anonymous.
      c. Medication such as Antabuse (alcohol sensitizing drug that causes vomiting and cardiovascular symptoms if the patient drinks after taking drug).
      d. Referral to social or vocational rehabilitation community program.

D. Nursing attitudes.
   1. Maintain a nonjudgmental attitude toward the alcoholic.
   2. Approach patient with firmness and consistency.
   3. Accept the individual but not his deviant behavior.
   4. Support patient's attempts to change life patterns.
   5. Assist patient to develop a support system—AA, church, etc.

Drug Addiction

Definition: Drug addiction is the dependency on drugs other than alcohol or tobacco that alter perception and/or mood.

Characteristics of Narcotic Addiction

A. The most common narcotics are heroin and morphine.
B. Emotional dependence on the drug (to alter mood) is followed by physical dependence on the drug.
C. Narcotics have a sedative effect on the CNS.
D. As tolerance level increases, greater amounts of the drug are necessary to produce pleasurable effects.
E. Addiction tends to be chronic; the rate of relapse is high.
F. Withdrawal symptoms.
  1. Anxiety.
  2. Nausea and vomiting.
  3. Sneezing, yawning, and watery eyes.
  4. Tremor and profuse perspiration.
  5. Stomach cramps and dehydration.
  6. Convulsions and coma.
G. Characteristics of the narcotic addict personality.
  1. Emotionally immature with feelings of inadequacy and inferiority.
  2. Difficulty in establishing interpersonal relationships; untruthful and insecure.
  3. Poor judgment and inability to tolerate frustration.

Characteristics of Barbiturate Addiction

A. The most common barbiturates are Seconal and Sodium Amytal.
B. Barbiturates have a sedative effect on the CNS.
C. Danger of death from overdose.
D. Emotional dependence on the drug is followed by physical dependence on the drug.
E. Originally may have been taken to relieve pain or sleeplessness.
F. Addicts usually have emotional problems and an anxious temperament.

Characteristics of Other Common Addictions

A. Amphetamines.
  1. The most common amphetamines are Benzedrine and Dexedrine.
  2. They are CNS stimulants so that overuse may result in brain damage.
  3. They have the effect of producing a "high."
  4. Large doses produce a hyperactive and agitated state.
  5. They produce an emotional addiction, especially for persons who feel insecure and inadequate.
  6. They reduce appetite and awareness of bodily needs so that the person's physical condition suffers.
B. LSD, or "Acid."
  1. A hallucinogenic drug that mimics hallucinations seen in psychoses.
  2. Produces changes in perception and logical thought processes.
  3. Not considered addictive per se, but individual may become emotionally dependent on the drug.
  4. Experiences following LSD ingestion range from ecstasy to terror; the consequences are unpredictable.
C. Marijuana.
  1. The abuse potential is minimal because it produces neither tolerance nor physical dependence.
  2. Produces "dreamy" state and feelings of euphoria, hilarity, and well-being.
  3. Moods vary according to environmental stimuli.
  4. Changes in perception of space and time seem to distort and extend.
  5. High dosage may produce hallucinations and delusions.
D. Cocaine.
  1. Classified as a stimulant.
  2. Usually sniffed or used intravenously.
  3. Strong psychological dependence may occur.
  4. Does not develop a physical dependence or tolerance.
E. PCP—"crystal," "elephant tranquilizer."
  1. Usually smoked with marijuana. May also be ingested or injected.

2. Reactions vary from sense of well-being to total disorientation and hallucinations.
3. Considered an extremely dangerous street drug.
4. Psychological dependence may occur.
5. Cerebral cellular destruction and atrophy may occur with even small amounts.
6. Overdoses or "bad trips" are characterized by erratic and unpredictable behavior, withdrawal, disorientation, self-mutilation, and self-destructive behaviors.
7. Overdoses are treated with sedatives, with a decrease of environmental stimuli, and with protection of the patient from self-harm and harm of others.

Implementation

A. General nursing approaches and attitudes are similar to those enumerated for alcoholism.
B. Special approaches to drug addiction.
   1. First step is withdrawal treatment; accomplished abruptly ("cold turkey") or gradually over a period of days.
   2. The substitute drug methadone is used to reduce the physical reaction to withdrawal.
   3. Extended medical and psychiatric treatment for physical and emotional deterioration must be part of convalescence.
   4. Resocialization process of patient needs supportive treatment from professional and/or community resources.
   5. Rehabilitation programs must be directed toward helping the person reenter the mainstream of society.
      a. Many organizations operated by ex-addicts offer help in rehabilitation.
      b. Therapeutic communities and group therapy programs also assist with rehabilitation.
   6. Specific guidelines.
      a. Provide a structured environment, and set consistent and strict limits.
      b. Identify patient's attempts to manipulate; maintain control.
      c. When patient distorts reality, affirm the situational facts.

d. Give equal concern to patient's physical, social, and emotional needs.

ADJUNCT THERAPIES

Psychotropic Drugs

Definition: Psychotropic drugs are those used in psychiatry in conjunction with other forms of therapy to temporarily modify behavior. They control symptoms but do not cure disorder.

Characteristics

A. Psychotropic drugs affect both the central and autonomic nervous systems.
B. These drugs affect behavior indirectly by chemically interacting with other chemicals, enzymes, or enzyme substrates.
   1. Changes in cellular, tissue, and organ functions occur.
   2. Drug effects vary from cellular activity to psychosocial interaction.

Antipsychotic Drugs

A. These drugs are also known as ataractic, neuroleptic, or major tranquilizers.
B. Introduced about 1953.
C. Most common drugs are phenothiazine derivatives (Thorazine, Stelazine, Trilafon, Vesprin, and Prolixin).
D. Antipsychotic drugs control hallucinations, delusions and bizarre behavior and can calm an excited patient without producing a marked impairment of motor function or sleep.
E. Side effects.
   1. Blood dyscrasias.
      a. Agranulocytosis occurs in first 3–5 weeks of treatment. *Symptoms:* fever, sore throat.

b. Leukopenia, preceded by altered white blood count.
2. Extrapyramidal effects occur in 30 percent of patients, affecting the voluntary movements and skeletal muscles.
   a. Parkinsonism—symptoms occur 1–4 weeks; signs are similar to classic parkinsonism: rigidity, shuffling gait, pill-rolling hand movement, tremors, dyskinesia, and masklike face.
   b. Akathisia—very common; occurs 1–6 weeks; uncontrolled motor restlessness, foot-tapping, agitation, pacing.
   c. Dystonia—occurs early, 1–2 days; limb and neck spasms; uncoordinated, jerky movements; difficulty in speaking and swallowing, and rigidity and spasms of muscles.
   d. Tardive dyskinesia—develops late in treatment; estimated to occur in up to 50 percent of chronic schizophrenics. Antiparkinson drugs are of no help in decreasing symptoms. This is a permanent side effect; symptoms are shuffling gait, drooling, and general dystonic symptoms.
3. Hypotension—orthostatic hypotension may occur. Monitor closely when patient is elderly. Keep patient supine for 1 hour and advise to change positions slowly.
4. Anticholinergic effects—dry mouth, blurred vision, tachycardia, nasal congestion and constipation. Treat symptomatically.
5. Potentiate CNS depressant, especially alcohol.
6. Antacids reduce absorption.
F. Another common antipsychotic drug is derived from butyrophenone (Haldol).
1. These drugs are less sedative than phenothiazines.
2. High incidence of severe extrapyramidal reactions.
3. Side effects include leukocytosis, blurred vision, dry mouth, urinary retention.
4. Avoid alcohol.
G. Clozapine (Clozaril) is a new drug for management of psychotic symptoms in patients who do not respond to other antipsychotics.

1. Side effects—similar to other antipsychotics: be aware of blood dyscrasias (leukopenia, neutropenia, agranulocytosis, eosinophilia).
2. Monitor monthly bilirubin, CBC, liver function studies.
H. Other classes of drugs are Thioxanthenes (Taractan and Navane) and Dibenzoxazepines (Loxitane).

Antianxiety Drugs

A. These drugs induce sedation, relax muscles, and inhibit convulsions; major use to reduce anxiety.
B. These drugs are the most frequently prescribed drugs in medicine; demand is great for relief from anxiety and they are safer than sedative-hypnotics.
C. They potentiate drug abuse. Greatest harm occurs when combined with alcohol and other CNS depressants.
D. They are prescribed in neuroses, psychosomatic disorders, or functional psychiatric disorders, but do not modify psychotic behavior.
E. Drugs from two major classes. Benzodiazepines: safer and more common (Librium, Valium, Centrax, Serax, and Xanax—being tested for use in depression and panic disorders). Nonbenzodiazepines: Vistaril, Equanil, and Miltown.
F. Side effects.
1. Drowsiness (avoid driving or working around equipment).
2. Blurred vision, constipation, dermatitis, mental confusion, anorexia, polyuria, menstrual irregularities, and edema.
3. Habituation and increased tolerance.
4. Pancytopenia, thrombocytopenia, and agranulcytopenia.

Antidepressant Drugs

A. The tricyclics, the most commonly used antidepressants, include Elavil, Norpramin, Tofranil, Aventyl, and Vivactil.

1. Anticholinergic: take 1–4 weeks to be effective. Produce antagonism of the parasympathetic system.
2. Patients with morbid fantasies do not respond well to these drugs.
3. Side effects.
   a. Anticholinergic effects: dry mouth, blurred vision, constipation, postural hypotension.
   b. CNS effects: tremor, agitation, angry states, mania.
   c. Cardiovascular effects: palpitations. Exert a quinidinelike effect on the heart so assess any patient with history of myocardial infarction.
4. If patient is switched from a tricyclic drug to an MAO inhibitor, a period of 1–4 weeks must elapse.

B. The monoamine oxidase inhibitors include Marplan, Niamid, Nardil, and Parnate.
   1. MAO inhibitors are toxic, potent, and produce many side effects.
   2. They should not be the first antidepressant drug used; effect is at best equal to a tricyclic and side effects more dangerous.
   3. Side effects.
      a. Most dangerous is hypertensive crisis.
      b. Drug interactions can cause severe hypertension, hypotension, or CNS depression.
      c. Postural hypotension, headaches, constipation, anorexia, diarrhea, and chills.
      d. Tachycardia, edema, impotence, dizziness, insomnia, and restlessness.
      e. Manic episodes and anxiety.
   4. All patients must be warned not to eat foods with high tyramine content (aged cheese, wine, beer, chicken liver, yeast), drink alcohol, or take other drugs, especially sympathomimetic drugs (amphetamines, L-Dopa, epinephrine).
   5. MAO inhibitors must not be used in combination with tricyclics.

C. Hypertensive crisis.
   1. Severe symptoms: headache, confusion, drowsiness, vomiting.
   2. Monitor for potential complications: encephalopathy, heart failure.
   3. Treatment.
      a. Drug of choice: Regitine, IV 5 mg with close monitoring; antihypertensive.
      b. Monitor vital signs, EKG and neurological signs; BP q 5 minutes.
      c. Norepinephrine is administered for severe hypotension.

D. Prozac, introduced in 1988, is chemically and pharmacologically distinct from other antidepressant drugs.
   1. A selective inhibitor of the uptake of serotonin.
      a. Studies suggest that increased serotonin in critical areas of the brain modifies certain affective behavior. Results in the increased concentration of active serotonin in critical synaptic areas in the brain.
      b. A number of neurochemical pathways can be affected by existing antidepressants—Prozac is highly selective for the serotonin pathway and exerts little or no effect on the uptake of other neurotransmitters or receptor sites.
   2. Prozac exhibits less side effects than other antidepressant drugs.
      a. Anticholinergic side effects such as dry mouth, constipation are fewer with Prozac.
      b. Side effects observed are nausea, the most common, anxiety/nervousness, insomnia, drowsiness, and headache.
      c. Co-administration of alcohol and Prozac is not recommended.
   3. Recommended starting and maintenance dose is 20 mg per day—daily dose should never exceed 80 mg.

Antimanic Drugs

A. These drugs control mood disorders, especially the manic phase.

B. Before lithium therapy is begun, baseline studies of renal, cardiac and thyroid status obtained.

C. Most common form of drug is lithium carbonate, a naturally occurring metallic salt.

D. Drug must reach certain blood level before it is effective.
   1. Stabilizing concentration occurs in 5–7 days; therapeutic effects 7–10 days.
   2. Serum level can be simply and reliably measured in mEq/liter of blood.

E. Lithium is metabolized by the kidney.
   1. Deficiency of sodium results in more lithium being reabsorbed thus increasing risk of toxicity.
   2. Excessive sodium causes more lithium to be excreted and may lower level to a nontherapeutic range.
   3. Normal dietary intake of sodium with adequate fluids to prevent dehydration.
   4. Serum levels measured 2–3 times weekly (12 hours after last dose) in beginning of therapy; for long term maintenance therapy, every 2–3 months.

F. Drug concentration and side effects.
   1. Therapeutic range of serum levels is 0.8–1.2 mEq/liter; for acute manic state, 1.2–1.5 mEq/liter.
   2. Side effects occur at upper ranges, usually about 1.5 mEq/liter.
   3. Gastrointestinal disturbances, metallic taste in mouth, muscle weakness, fatigue, thirst, polyuria, and fine hand tremors.
   4. Hypothyroidism.

G. Lithium toxicity.
   1. Appears when blood level exceeds 1.5–2.0 mEq/liter. Many appear sooner depending on individual patient.
   2. Central nervous system is the chief target.
   3. Initial symptoms include nausea, vomiting, drowsiness, tremors, slurred speech, blurred vision.
   4. If drug is continued, coma, convulsions, and death may result.
   5. Treatment for toxicity: gastric lavage, correction of fluid balance, drug (Mannitol) to increase urine excretion.

Antiparkinson Drugs

A. The term "extrapyramidal disease" refers to motor disorders often associated with pathologic dysfunction in the basal ganglia.
   1. Clinical symptoms of the disease include abnormal involuntary movement, changes in tone of the skeletal muscles, and a reduction of automatic associated movements.
   2. Reversible extrapyramidal reactions may follow the use of certain drugs.
   3. The most common drugs are the phenothiazine derivatives.

B. Antiparkinson drugs act on the extrapyramidal system to reduce disturbing symptoms.
   1. They are usually given in conjunction with antipsychotic drugs.
   2. Two of the most common drugs are Artane and Cogentin.
   3. Side effects are dizziness, gastrointestinal disturbance, headaches, urinary hesitancy, and memory impairment.

C. Benadryl, an antihistamine, is often given in place of Artane or Cogentin.
   1. Controls the extrapyramidal side effects of phenothiazines.
   2. Preferred because it does not cause as many untoward side effects as other antiparkinson drugs.

Drug Administration in a Psychiatric Setting ❖ PROCEDURE ❖

A. Give correct *drug* and *dose* at correct time to correct *patient* according to physician's orders.

B. Learn the specific actions and uses of drugs.

C. Become familiar with the side effects and precautions associated with major drug groups.

D. Observe patient carefully for side effects.

E. Be familiar with the drug groups that are not compatible.

F. Refer to psychotropic drug classification chart in Appendix 2.

Other Forms of Therapy

Electroshock Therapy

A. Passing of electric current through brain to induce seizures as treatment for depression; breaks up behavior patterns by causing temporary amnesia.

B. In several weeks, as memory returns, most of the self-depreciation and sadness will have dissipated.

C. Provide support by listening to the patient's expression of fear concerning the procedure.

D. Assure patient that she or he will not be alone during or after treatment.

E. Remove patient's dentures (if present), and give nothing by mouth prior to treatment. Assist physician during treatment.

F. Reorientate patient following procedure, and explain feelings of confusion.

G. Observe and record patient's response to treatments.

Insulin Coma Therapy

A. Used infrequently in treatment of schizophrenia.

B. Carefully observe patient for signs and symptoms of insulin shock following treatment.

Socialization or Motivational Therapy

A. Intended to motivate and get patient moving again.

B. Patient can socialize and be motivated by means of group therapy, occupational therapy, environmental therapy.

C. Encourage patient's participation in therapy.

D. Support patient's efforts to share feelings.

APPENDIX 1. DEFENSE MECHANISMS

Compensation
Covering up a lack or weakness by emphasizing a desirable trait, or making up for a frustration in one area by overemphasis in another area. Learned early in childhood and may be recognized in adult behavior, for example, the physically handicapped individual who is an outstanding scholar.

Denial
Refusal to face reality. The ego protects itself from unpleasant pain or conflict by rejecting obvious facts or truth. Example, a person not seeing a doctor because he does not want to know the truth. Individual who avoids reality by becoming ill.

Displacement
Discharging pent-up feelings from one object to a less dangerous object. Example, your supervisor yells at you and you yell at your husband.

Fantasy
Gratification by imaginary achievements and wishful thinking. Example, children's play.

Fixation
Persistence into later life of interests and behavior patterns appropriate to an earlier age.

Identification
Assumption of desirable personality attributes of one admired. Satisfaction can be derived from assuming the success or the experience of others. Example, nurse who feels sick watching a traumatic procedure on her patient.

Insulation
Passive withdrawal. Inaccessible to avoid further threatening circumstances. Sometimes the person appears cold and indifferent to his surroundings. Insulation is usually harmless, but can become very serious if it prevents interaction with others.

Isolation
Walling off of certain ideas, attitudes, or feelings. Isolation is separating the feelings from the intellect, by putting our emotions concerning a specific traumatic event into an isolated compartment. Example, the individual talks about a significant situation such as an accident or death without a display of feelings. This pattern can be positive if used temporarily to keep the ego from being overwhelmed.

Projection
Attribution of one's own undesirable traits to someone else. Example, the child who says to a parent, "You hate me," after the parent has spanked the child. In an adult, this technique may be a predominant indicator of paranoia.

Rationalization
The attempt that is almost universally employed to prove or justify behavior. It is face saving to give a reason that is acceptable rather than the real reason, as in remarks such as, "It wasn't worth it anyway" "It's all for the best." This mechanism relieves anxiety temporarily and helps the person avoid facing reality.

Reaction-Formation
Prevention of dangerous feelings and desires from being expressed by exaggerating the opposite attitude—a kind of denial. The overly neat, polite, conscientious individual may have an unconscious desire to be untidy and carefree. The behavior becomes pathological when it interferes with tasks or produces anxiety and frustration.

APPENDIX 1. DEFENSE MECHANISMS (*Continued*)

Regression | Resorting to an earlier developmental level in order to deal with reality. Regression is an immature way of responding, and is frequently seen during a physical illness. It is sometimes used to an extreme degree by the mentally ill, who may regress all the way back to infancy.

Repression | The unconscious process in which undesirable and unacceptable thoughts are kept from entering the conscious. This repressed material may be the motivation for some of our behavior. The superego is largely responsible for repression; the stronger, more punitive the superego, the more emotion will be repressed. The child who is frustrated and downtrodden by a parent may rebel in later life against authority.

Sublimation | The mechanism by which a primitive or unacceptable tendency is redirected into socially constructive channels. This adjustment pattern is at least partly responsible for many artistic and cultural achievements, such as painting and poetry.

Suppression | The act of keeping unpleasant feelings and experiences from awareness.

Symbolization | An idea or object used by the conscious mind to represent an actual event or object. Sometimes the meaning is not clear because the symbol may be representative of something unconscious. Children use symbolization in this way and have to learn to distinguish between the symbol and the thing being symbolized. Examples include obsessive thoughts or behavior (hand washing, cleansing) and the incoherent speech of the schizophrenic (by the time the painful thoughts reach the surface, they are so jumbled that they lose their painfulness).

Undoing | A specific action is performed that is considered to be the opposite of a previously unacceptable action. This action is felt to neutralize or "undo" the original action. Example, Lady MacBeth rubbing and washing her hands.

APPENDIX 2. DRUG CLASSIFICATION CHART

Common Psychotropic Drugs

Major Tranquilizers

Drug	Method of Administration	Daily Dose
Thorazine	Tablets, concentrate, syrup, IM, IV, suppositories	25–1500 mg
Sparine	Tablets, concentrate, syrup, capsules, IM, IV	50–100 mg
Mellaril	Tablets, concentrate	100–800 mg
Serentil	Tablets, concentrate, IM	30–400 mg
Trilafon	Tablets, concentrate, syrup, IM, suppositories	6–64 mg
Prolixin, Permitil	Tablets, concentrate, IM	0.5–20 mg
Stelazine	Tablets, concentrate, IM	2–50 mg
Quide	Tablets	10–180 mg
Compazine	Tablets, capsules, syrup, concentrate, IM, IV, suppositories	15–150 mg
Taractan	Tablets, concentrate, IM	30–600 mg
Navane	Capsules, concentrate, IM	6–60 mg
Haldol	Tablets, concentrate, IM	2–40 mg

Minor Tranquilizers (Antianxiety)

Drug	Method of Administration	Daily Dose
Atarax	Tablets, syrup	50–400 mg
Vistaril	Capsules, suspension,	50–400 mg
	IM only	50–100 mg
Librium, Librax	Tablets, capsules, IM, IV	10–100 mg
Valium	Tablets, IM, IV	2–40 mg
Serax	Capsules, tablets	30–120 mg
Equanil	Tablets, capsules, suspension	400–1200 mg
Miltown	Tablets	400–1200 mg

Antidepressants (Mood Elevators)

MAO Inhibitors

Drug	Method of Administration	Daily Dose
Marplan	Tablets	10–30 mg
Niamid	Tablets	125–200 mg
Nardil	Tablets	15–75 mg
Parnate	Tablets	20–30 mg

Tricyclics

Drug	Method of Administration	Daily Dose
Tofranil	Tablets, IM	75–300 mg
Elavil	Tablets, IM	50–200 mg
Norpramin	Tablets	75–150 mg
Aventyl	Capsules, liquid	20–100 mg
Vivactil	Tablets	15–60 mg
Sinequan	Capsules	25–300 mg

APPENDIX 2. DRUG CLASSIFICATION CHART (*Continued*)

Common Psychotropic Drugs

Drug	Method of Administration	Daily Dose
Antimanic		
Lithium carbonate, Lithane, Litho-Tabs, Lithonate	Tablets, capsules	600–1800 mg
Antiparkinson		
Cogentin	Tablets, IM	1–6 mg
Artane	Tablets, elixir, capsules	1–10 mg
Akineton	Tablets, IM, IV	1–8 mg
Kemadrin	Tablets	6–15 mg

APPENDIX 3. GLOSSARY

Acting out   Expression of unconscious emotional conflicts of hostility or love in actions that the person does not consciously know are related to such conflicts of feelings.

Affect   Generalized feeling, tone, or mood.

Aggression   Any verbal/nonverbal activity that may be forceful abuse of self, another person, or thing.

Ambivalence   The simultaneous existence of contradictory and contrasting emotions toward a person or object at the same time, that is, love and hate.

Amnesia   A condition where the individual experiences a loss of memory because of physical or emotional trauma.

Anxiety   A persistent feeling of tension and apprehension arising from within the individual. Response to vague, unspecific danger that may be real or imagined.

Apathy   Pathological indifference.

Autism   Detachment from reality when self-preoccupation and involvement predominate.

Compulsion   An irresistible urge to repeat an act that must be carried out to avoid anxiety.

Conflict   A struggle between two or more opposing forces.

Covert   Hidden, below the surface.

Cyclothymia   Alternations in mood from high to low.

Defense mechanism   Originally identified by Anna Freud, an activity of the ego which defends itself by not allowing unacceptable thoughts or feelings to come into awareness to cause anxiety.

Delusion   A false belief maintained in spite of facts or evidence to the contrary.

Depression   An unshakable feeling of sadness accompanied by feelings of hopefulness, worthlessness, and the feeling of a bleak future.

Disorientation   A condition where the individual manifests loss of ability to recognize or locate himself in respect to time, place, or other persons.

Echolalia   A condition where the individual constantly repeats what is heard.

Echopraxia   A condition where the individual mimics what is done.

Ego   A Freudian term denoting that aspect of the psyche which is conscious and most in touch with external reality; the "I" part of the person. Also, that part of the personality that makes decisions, is conscious, and represents the thinking-feeling part of a person.

Electroshock   A medical procedure of applying electric current to certain areas in the brain. Used in the treatment of certain psychiatric disorders (especially depression).

Etiology   The cause or causes of disease.

Euphoria   A feeling of elation or joy.

Fear   Response to an actual person or situation of external danger.

Fixation   A stage in development when there is an abnormal attachment; inability to move on to later developmental tasks.

Frustration   A feeling that may contain elements of anger, hopelessness, or defeat, which results when goals set by perceived needs are blocked.

Fugue   A condition experienced as a transient disorientation-patient is unaware that he or she has physically escaped or run to another place.

Functional   Used in psychiatry to denote mental illness existing without known physical causes or structural changes.

Hypochondriasis   A state of morbid concern about one's body or health for which there is no physical evidence.

Hysteric   Involves elements of both conscious and unconscious exaggerated reaction, often in a dramatic manner, to some stimuli situation.

Id   A Freudian term denoting a division of the psyche from which come blind, instinctual impulses that lead to immediate gratification of primitive needs, dominated by the pleasure principle.

Ideas of reference   A distortion of reality where a person believes that activities of others have a personal reference to one's self.

Illusion   Distorted perceptual experience where the individual misinterprets actual data from the environment. Examples: a mirage on the desert; seeing a lake when it is only light refraction.

Insight   An individual's understanding of the origin and mechanisms of his or her attitudes and behavior.

Interpersonal   Existing between two or more persons.

Intrapersonal   Existing within one person.

Labile   Refers to rapid shifts in emotions from high to low.

Manipulation   The process by which one individual influences another individual to function in accordance with his needs without regard to the other's needs or goals.

Mental retardation   A term for mental deficiency or lack of normal development of intelligence.

Milieu   The total environment, emotional as well as physical.

Narcissistic   Loving one's self excessively in a childish or an infantile fashion.

Negativism   A strong resistance to suggestions coming from others.

Neologism   A term that refers to the coining of a new word, as seen in schizophrenia.

Obsession   A persistent repetitive and unwanted thought.

Organic   Based on structural alterations, gross or microscopic.

Overt   Discernible; out in the open.

Parataxic   A term coined by Sullivan to mean distorted perception.

Phobia   The dread of an object, an act, or a situation that is not realistically dangerous but that has come to represent a danger.

Premorbid personality   The status of an individual's personality (conflicts, defenses, strengths, weaknesses) before the onset of clinical illness.

Psyche   A term meaning the mind or the mental and emotional "self."

Psychogenic   Originating within the psyche or mind. Sometimes used to describe physical disorders that are believed to stem from the emotions.

Rapport   A component of a relationship where one feels harmony or empathy with another.

Regression   Reverting to types of behavior characteristic of an earlier level of development.

Resistance   A mechanism an individual employs to avoid certain ideas or feelings coming into consciousness.

Schizoid   A term used to describe a form of personality disorder characterized by an unsocial, withdrawn, shy type of personality.

Seclusive   A term describing persons who are unsociable, reserved, secretive, and adverse to interacting with people.

Soma   A term meaning body.

Superego   A Freudian term referring to a system within the total psyche that is developed by incorporating parental standards such as moral values; the two components of superego are conscience and ego ideal.

Unconscious   A term coined by Freud to refer to that part of the mind where mental activity is always going on, but not on a conscious level.

Undoing   A defense mechanism aimed at the removal of a painful memory.

Waxy flexibility   A condition associated with catatonic schizophrenia, where a posture is maintained for long periods of time.

APPENDIX 4. MENTAL ASSESSMENT SUMMARY

General appearance, manner, and attitude

Assess *physical appearance*.

Note *grooming*, mode of dress, and *personal hygiene*.

Note *posture*.

Note speed, pressure, pace, quantity, volume, and diction of *speech*.

Note relevance, content, and organization of *responses*.

Expressive aspects of behavior

Note *general motor activity*.

Assess *purposeful movements* and gestures.

Assess style of *gait*.

Consciousness

Assess level of *consciousness*.

Thought processes and perception

Assess coherency, logic, and relevance of *thought processes*.

Assess *reality orientation*: time, place, and person.

Assess *perceptions* and reactions to stimuli.

Thought content and mental trend

Ask questions to determine general themes that identify *degree of anxiety*.

Assess *ideation* and *concentration*.

Mood or affect

Assess prevailing or variability in mood by observing behavior and asking questions such as "How are you feeling right now?" Check for presence of abnormal *euphoria*.

If you suspect *depression*, continue questioning to determine depth.

Memory

Assess *past and present memory* and *retention* (ability to listen).

Assess *recall* (recent and remote).

Judgment

Assess *judgment* and interpretations.

Insight

Assess *insight*, the ability to understand.

Intelligence and fund of information

Assess *intelligence*.

Assess *fund of information*.

Sensory ability

Assess the five *senses*.

Developmental level

Assess patient's *developmental level*.

Addictive patterns

Identify *addictive patterns*.

Coping devices and defense mechanisms

Identify *defense-coping mechanisms* and their effect.

14

LEGAL ISSUES IN NURSING

NURSE PRACTICE ACT

Composition

A. A series of statues enacted by each state's legislature to regulate the practice of nursing in that state.
B. Establishment of scope of nursing practice for which the registered nurse and/or the vocational/practical nurse is held legally responsible by a particular state.

Provisions

A. Definition of nursing to include functions, responsibilities, and personal qualifications.
B. Authorization to practice (licensure).
C. Educational requirements.
D. Implementation and reinforcement of act by State Board of Nursing.
E. Proceedings and penalties of professional misconduct.

Scope of LPN/LVN Functions

A. Administer nursing care, utilizing basic scientific knowledge and understanding, under the direction and supervision of a registered nurse, or licensed physician.
B. Assist the registered nurse or licensed physician with patients who require more complex medical care.

STATE BOARDS OF NURSING

Composition

A. A group invested with authority by a state to administer its Nurse Practice Act.

B. Members of a board are appointed from among the nursing profession and interested public.

Responsibilities

A. Accredits schools of nursing which meet preestablished standards.
 1. Withholds accreditation from schools which do not meet standards.
 2. Withdraws accreditation from the schools which do not conform to standards.
B. Provides guidelines and minimum standards for nursing curriculum.
C. Governs all aspects of licensing.
 1. Administers the official nursing examinations.
 2. Grants licenses to authorized applicants.
 3. Takes necessary legal action required for denial, revocation, and suspension of license.
D. Conducts investigations and hearings on violations of established standards, laws, and regulations.
E. Interprets the nurse pracice act based on practice, standards of care, and information from all states.

Licensure

A. Licensure is granted to individuals who have met predetermined standards.
 1. One main reason for licensure is protection of the public from unqualified practitioners.
 2. It is the responsibility of the LVN or LPN to be familiar with the laws of the state in which he or she will practice.
B. Requirements for practice.
 1. A license to practice is mandatory requirement in some states.
   a. Without license, titles of LVN or LPN may not be used.
   b. Without license, compensation for services as LVN or LPN cannot be received.

2. Some states have a permissive law that allows one to practice without a license.

C. Methods of obtaining a license.
   1. Application reviewed by State Board of Nursing.
   2. Attain established educational and personal standards and pass licensing examination.
   3. If licensed in another state, some states will recognize that license and grant a license by *reciprocity* or *endorsement*.

D. Basis for disciplinary action.
   1. Obtaining a license fraudulently.
   2. Practicing nursing during period of revocation or suspension of license.
   3. Permitting or aiding unlicensed person to perform those nursing activities requiring a license.
   4. Performing duties beyond scope of nursing practice.
   5. Practicing in a manner that is judged to be incompetent and/or negligent.
   6. Practicing when functional ability is impaired by drugs, alcohol, or other disability.

THE NURSE AND PATIENT

Patient's Rights

A. A violation of a patient's right, or claim to a right, may be established by a court of law.

B. A nurse should be totally familiar with all aspects of a patient's rights when those rights are associated with health care.

C. Basic rights are guaranteed by the United States Constitution.
   1. Freedom of expression.
   2. Due process of law.
   3. Freedom from cruel and inhumane treatment.
   4. Equal protection for all citizens.

D. Patients have the right to courteous, individual care without discrimination.

1. Patient's Bill of Rights is a statement of expectations from the institution.
2. The Patient's Bill of Rights is adopted by the American Hospital Association.

Consent to Receive Health Services

A. Consent is the approval by a patient, or those authorized to give consent, to have his or her body touched by health services personnel (e.g., physician, nurse, or other allied health personnel).

B. Factors in consent-giving process.
   1. Consent may be implied or expressed in either written or verbal form.
   2. Consent must be *informed consent*.
      a. Patient must be fully informed regarding the mode and extent of tests, surgery, and varieties of treatment to be administered.
      b. Patient must understand that intended results may not be accomplished.
      c. Patient must understand that unintended, potentially harmful consequences may result.
      d. Does not mean a patient can insist on having whatever he wants.
      e. The patient has the right to make choices between "acceptable options."
      f. To make decisions, the patient must have the emotional/mental/legal capacity to do so.
   3. A prior consent may be rescinded in either verbal or written form.

C. Individuals authorized to give consent for health services.
   1. Mentally competent adult patients.
   2. Parents or legal guardians of minors.
   3. Court-approved individuals responsible for the mentally incompetent patient.
   4. Holders of durable power of attorney.

D. Emergency situations requiring immediate life-preserving action require no prior consent.
   1. Serious injury and extreme body dysfunction (e.g., cardiac or respiratory arrest).
   2. Imminent deaths from other causes.

E. Liabilities of a nurse regarding consent.
   1. Nurse is liable if he or she requests signature of a patient on a consent form when he or she knows (or *should have known*) patient had not been informed by either the physician or authorized hospital staff regarding potential harmful consequences of treatment, procedures, or surgery.
   2. Nurse is liable if he or she does not respect rights of a mentally competent adult patient to refuse health care.

Medical Records

A. A medical record is a complete and accurate written account of a patient's medical history which includes past and present medical conditions, a recording of all tests, surgeries, procedures, medications, and other relevant data.
B. A medical record functions as a tool of communication within a hospital, clinic, or physician's office for allied health personnel.
   1. Provides continuity of health care given and to be given to patient.
   2. Provides data for purposes of research.
   3. Provides data necessary for assessing quality care by hospital obligations.
C. Nurse's legal and ethical obligations.
   1. Help to maintain complete and timely records.
   2. Sign or countersign only those entries which are accurate and complete.

PUBLIC LAW AND THE NURSE

The Law

A. Binding rules and standards of an extended community which are formally recognized, obeyed, and enforced by authority.
B. The purpose of the law is the preservation of order and the promotion of safety.

C. Obligations of a nurse to the law are no different from that required of other citizens.
   1. An individual is responsible for his or her own behavior unless that individual is mentally incompetent.
   2. An individual is responsible to know the law and its ramifications.
   3. Punitive action may be taken against the individual who fails to abide by the law.

Nursing Contracts

A. A contract is a binding agreement (usually in printed form) between two or more individuals that gives evidence to specified terms and conditions expected of both parties to the agreement.
B. A contract entered into by a nurse and employer may be in the form of either a written or verbal agreement.
C. Conditions of the agreement.
   1. The nurse is required to perform all nursing duties with skill and knowledge.
   2. Performance is to be in accordance with the standards of care established by the Nurse Practice Act for licensure.
   3. The employer is required to issue fair compensation for services given.
D. Breach of the agreement (contract) occurs when one or more parties to the agreement fail to fulfill the obligations stipulated within it.

Civil Torts

A. Wrongful act committed by one person against another.
B. Types of litigation (lawsuit).
   1. *Negligence* is failure to perform the extent of care a reasonable and prudent person would exercise.
      a. *Malpractice* is negligent performance by a physician, RN, LVN, LPN, or other allied health personnel.
      b. *Respondeat superior* is the legal doctrine that holds an employer responsible for negligent acts of employees in

course and scope of employment. (A nurse continues to be liable for negligent performance.)

2. *Invasion of privacy* is the interference by one individual of another individual's right to privacy. (Refers only to nonpublic individuals.)
   a. Make another individual's private affairs public.
   b. Exhibit another individual's likeness publicly.
3. *Defamation of character* is the harm of an individual's reputation or the disgrace of character by a second individual.
   a. *Libel* is a written or published defamation.
   b. *Slander* is an oral defamation.

Criminal Law

A. *Crime* is an offense against the public for which the state prosecutes and seeks punishment.
B. *Felony* is a serious crime punishable by imprisonment or death.
C. Felonious acts.
   1. *Assault* is the threat or attempt to do harm or come into physical contact with another individual without consent.
   2. *Battery* is actual use of force or contact with another individual without consent.
   3. *Euthanasia* is the act of killing a hopelessly ill or injured individual for reasons of mercy.
   4. *False imprisonment* is the intentional restraint of an individual against his or her will without legal justification.
D. *Misdemeanor* is a crime less serious than a felony.

PROFESSIONAL ORGANIZATIONS

Purpose

A. Maintain and improve nursing standards.
B. Provide a vehicle for continuing education.
   1. Workshops.
   2. Publications.
   3. National and state conventions.
C. Provide opportunity to share professional interests.
D. Enhance an individual's sense of belonging.

National Associations

A. National Association of Practical Nurse Education and Service, Inc. (NAPNES).
   1. Membership—extended to any individual with an interest in education of practical nurse and/or other aspects of practical nursing.
   2. Publication—*The Journal of Practical Nursing*.
B. National Federation of Licensed Practical Nurses (NFLPN).
   1. Membership—limited to licensed practical or vocational nurses.
   2. Publication—*Journal of Nursing Care*.
C. National League for Nurses (NLN).
   1. Membership—extended to any individual with an interest in nursing.
   2. Publication—*Nursing and Health Care*, *Nursing Research* and professional directories.
   3. Functions.
      a. Prepare and score selection and achievement tests.
      b. Conduct workshops.
      c. Nationally accredit schools of registered nursing.
D. American Nurses' Association (ANA).
   1. Membership—limited to registered nurses, students of vocational/practical nursing.
   2. Publication—the *American Journal of Nursing*.

VOCATIONAL ETHICS

A. Ethics is a study that deals with issues of good and bad, moral duty and obligation.
B. Issues are frequently translated into principles of conduct that govern individual or group behavior.

Characteristics of a Set of Principles

A. Principles are generally predetermined and set down by the same group of individuals whose conduct will be guided by them.
B. The group will abide by these principles voluntarily.
C. The moral duties and obligations governing nursing care practice are embodied in the set of guiding principles.
D. The principles clarify desirable attitudes that ought to be basic to a nurse's performance.

NAPNES Code of Ethics

A. The licensed practical/vocational nurse shall:
1. Consider a basic obligation the conservation of life and the prevention of disease.
2. Promote and protect the physical, mental, emotional, and spiritual health of the patient and his or her family.
3. Fulfill all duties faithfully and efficiently.
4. Function within established legal guidelines.
5. Accept personal responsibility (for his acts) and seek to merit the respect and confidence of all members of the health team.
6. Hold in confidence all matters coming to his knowledge, in the practice of his profession, and in no way and at no time violate this confidence.
7. Give conscientious service, and charge just remuneration.
8. Learn and respect the religious and cultural beliefs of his or her patient and of all people.
9. Meet his or her obligation to patients by keeping abreast of current trends in health care through reading and continuing education.
10. As a citizen of the United States of America, uphold the laws of the land and seek to promote legislation which shall meet the health needs of its people.
B. The code of ethics provides principles to guide the performance of licensed practical/vocational nurses.

APPENDIX 1. DIRECTORY OF BOARDS OF NURSING

Executive Officer
Board of Nursing
770 Washington Avenue, RSA Plaza
Montgomery, Alabama 36130-3900

Executive Secretary
Alaska Board of Nursing
3601 "C" Street, Suite 722
Anchorage, Alaska 99503

Secretary
Health Services Regulatory Bd.
LBJ Tropical Med. Ctr.
Pago Pago, American Samoa 96799

Executive Director
Arizona State Board of Nursing
2001 W. Camelback, Suite 350
Phoenix, Arizona 85015

Executive Director
Arkansas State Board of Nursing
1123 South University, Suite 800
Little Rock, Arkansas 72204

Executive Officer
Board of Vocational Nursing and Psychiatric
Technical Examiners
1414 K Street, Suite 103
Sacramento, California 95814

Program Administrator
Colorado State Board of Nursing
1560 Broadway, Suite 670
Denver, Colorado 80202

Executive Officer
Department of Health Services
150 Washington Street
Hartford, Connecticut 06106

Executive Director
Delaware Board of Nursing
O'Neill Building, P. O. Box 1401
Dover, Delaware 19901

Chairperson
District of Columbia Board of Nursing
614 H Street NW
Washington, DC 20013

Executive Director
Florida State Board of Nursing
111 E. Coastline Drive, East
Jacksonville, Florida 32202

Executive Director
Georgia Board of Examiners of Licensed
Practical Nurses
166 Pryor Street, SW, Suite 300
Atlanta, Georgia 30303

Administrator
Guam Board of Nurse Examiners
P. O. Box 2816
Agana, Guam 96910

Executive Secretary
Hawaii Board of Nursing
Box 3469
Honolulu, Hawaii 99503

Executive Director
Idaho State Board of Nursing
280 N. 8th Street, #210
Boise, Idaho 83720

Nursing Education Coordinator
Department of Professional Regulation
320 W. Washington Street
Springfield, Illinois 62786

Board Administration
Indiana State Board of Nursing
402 W. Washington Street
Indianapolis, Indiana 46204

Executive Director
Iowa Board of Nursing
1223 E. Court Avenue
Des Moines, Iowa 50319

Executive Administrator
Kansas State Board of Nursing
900 SW Jackson Street, Suite 551S
Topeka, Kansas 66612-1256

Executive Director
Kentucky Board of Nursing
4010 Dupont Circle, Suite 430
Louisville, Kentucky 40207

Executive Director
Louisiana State Board of PN Examiners
1440 Canal Street, Suite 1722
New Orleans, Louisiana 70112

Executive Director
Maine State Board of Nursing
35 Anthony Avenue
State House Station 158
Augusta, Maine 04333-0158

Executive Director
Maryland Board of Nursing
4201 Patterson Avenue
Baltimore, Maryland 21215

Executive Secretary
Board of Registration in Nursing
100 Cambridge Street, Room 150
Boston, Massachusetts 02202

Board Secretary
Michigan Board of Nursing
P. O. Box 30018, 611 West Ottawa
Lansing, Michigan 48909

Executive Director
Minnesota Board of Nursing
2700 University Avenue West 108
St. Paul, Minnesota 55114

Supervisor
Health Occupations Education
Divison of Vocational Education
Department of Education
P. O. Box 771
Jackson, Mississippi 39205

Executive Director
Missouri State Board of Nursing
3605 Missouri Boulevard
Jefferson City, Missouri 65102

Executive Director
Montana State Board of Nursing
111 Jackson, Arcade Building
Helena, Montana 59620-0407

Associate Director
Bureau of Examining Board
P. O. Box 95007
Lincoln, Nebraska 68509

Executive Director
Nevada State Board of Nursing
2670 Chandler #9
Las Vegas, Nevada 89210

Executive Director
State Board of Nursing
Division of Public Health
6 Hazen Drive
Concord, New Hampshire 03301

Executive Director
New Jersey Board of Nursing
P. O. Box 45010
Newark, New Jersey 07101

Executive Director
New Mexico Board of Nursing
4253 Montgomery NE, Suite 130
Albuquerque, New Mexico 87109

Executive Secretary
New York State Board of Nursing
The Cultural Center, Room 3023
Albany, New York 12230

Executive Director
NC Board of Nursing
P. O. Box 2129
Raleigh, North Carolina 27602

Executive Director
North Dakota Board of Nursing
919 S. 7th Street, Suite 504
Bismarck, North Dakota 58504-5881

Executive Director
Ohio Board of Nursing
77 S. High Street, 17th Floor
Columbus, Ohio 43266-0316

Executive Director
Oklahoma Board of Nursing
2915 N. Classen Boulevard Suite 524
Oklahoma City, Oklahoma 73106

Executive Director
Oregon State Board of Nursing
800 NE Oregon Street, #25
Portland, Oregon 97232

Executive Secretary
Pennsylvania State Board of Nurse Examiners
P. O. Box 2649
Harrisburg, Pennsylvania 17105

Director
Department of Education
Practical Nurse Accreditation
Box 759
Hato Rey, Puerto Rico 00919

Director
Board of Registration in Nursing
3 Capital Hill
Providence, Rhode Island 02908-5097

Executive Director
State Board of Nursing for South Carolina
220 Executive Center Drive, Suite 220
Columbia, South Carolina 29210

Executive Secretary
South Dakota Board of Nursing
3307 South Lincoln
Sioux Falls, South Dakota 57105

Executive Director
TN Board of Nursing
283 Plus Park Boulevard
Nashville, Tennessee 37217

Executive Director
Board of Vocational Nurse Examiners
9101 Burnet Road, Suite 105
Austin, Texas 78758

Executive Secretary
Utah State Board of Nursing
160 East 300 South, Box 45802
Salt Lake City, Utah 84145

Executive Director
Vermont Board of Nursing
Licensing and Registration Division
109 State Street
Montpelier, Vermont 05602

Executive Secretary
Virgin Islands Board of Nurse Licensure
P. O. Box 7309
St. Thomas, Virgin Islands 00801

Executive Director
Virginia State Board of Nursing
6606 Broad Street, 4th Floor
Richmond, Virginia 23230-1717

Executive Director
State Board of Practical Nursing
1300 Quince Street, Ey-27
Olympia, Washington 98504

Executive Secretary
Board of Examiners for Practical Nurses
922 Quarrier Street, Suite 506
Charleston, West Virginia 25301

Administrative Officer
Wisconsin Department of Regulation & Licensing
P. O. Box 8935
Madison, Wisconsin 57208-8935

Executive Director
State of Wyoming Board of Nursing
2301 Central Avenue, Barrett Building
Cheyenne, Wyoming 82002

Other NCLEX-PN Review Aids

by

Sandra F. Smith, RN, MS

❖ *NCLEX-PN Review Questions*

❖ *NCLEX-PN/VN Assessment Test*

For further information on current editions,
prices and delivery, telephone 1.800.950.4095 or
FAX 415.941.4354.

National Nursing Review

SIMULATED NCLEX-PN CAT TEST

1. An adult patient has come to the clinic complaining of pain in her joints. Her records show a diagnosis of osteoarthritis. Comfort measures for this patient may include

1. Applying warm, moist packs to her joints.
2. Undertaking exercises that stress her muscles.
3. Wearing a copper bracelet to lessen her pain.
4. Sleeping on a soft mattress to ease her pain.

2. Acetylsalicylic acid is helpful to people with osteoarthritis because it acts as an

1. Analgesic.
2. Antipyretic.
3. Adrenergic blocker.
4. Antispasmodic.

3. An adult patient is scheduled to undergo arthroplasty of the hip. A priority postoperative nursing intervention is to

1. Turn the patient to the operated side.
2. Maintain abduction of the affected hip.
3. Maintain acute flexion of the hip.
4. Keep the patient prone for four days.

4. On the second morning following arthroplasty of the hip, the patient is allowed out of bed. To accomplish this, the first intervention would be to assist the patient to

1. Dangle legs at the bedside.
2. Transfer from the bed to a chair.
3. Transfer from the bed to a walker.
4. Transfer from the bed to crutches for support.

5. Test results indicate that Mrs. Mary King, 30 years old, is pregnant. Her LMP began eight weeks ago (1/21/94). According to Nägele's Rule, Mrs. King's EDC would be

1. 10/28/94.
2. 10/14/94.
3. 11/21/94.
4. 10/1/94.

6. If a pregnant woman does not know her LMP date, the sign most useful to calculate her EDC would be the

1. Appearance of linea nigra.
2. Fetal size detected by ultrasound.
3. Estriol level at 12 weeks.
4. Detection of Goodell's sign.

7. Before a patient goes to surgery, an operative permit must be signed. The most appropriate sequence for having the permit signed is to

1. Have the patient sign the permit as soon as she is admitted so she knows what surgery she will be having.
2. Prepare the patient for surgery, give the preoperative narcotics, and have her sign the permit before she goes to sleep.
3. Ensure that the surgeon has explained the surgery to the patient, answer her questions, have her sign the permit, and then complete the final preparations for surgery.
4. Have the patient sign the operative permit and then call the physician to come and talk with her.

8. The charge nurse asks you to give a pregnant patient diet counseling. The patient says she does not want to gain too much weight because her husband likes her thin. Which of the following responses would be the best?

1. "It's best for the baby if you don't try to stay too thin."
2. "If you are careful about the foods you eat, especially those high in calories, you will not gain too much."
3. "Let's talk about the importance of good nutrition and weight gain in pregnancy."
4. "Why don't you have your husband come to the clinic next time, and we can all talk about nutrition."

9. A 70-year-old patient is admitted to a skilled nursing facility (SNF) with the diagnosis of organic brain syndrome. The patient is often disoriented. This is most likely to occur

1. When he first gets out of bed after breakfast.
2. After he ambulates in the hall.
3. After his family visits.
4. When he awakens, especially at night.

10. A 62-year-old patient is admitted to the hospital with congestive heart failure. She has had angina for many years, and recently her symptoms have been getting worse as a result of arteriosclerosis. In establishing a patient care plan, a primary goal of treatment is to

1. Reduce the workload of the heart.
2. Promote rest for the heart.
3. Reduce fluid retention.
4. Reduce circulating blood volume.

11. A 6-month-old infant is admitted to the pediatric unit with a diagnosis of severe diarrhea. The most important nursing objective is to

1. Make constant assessment of the infant's dehydration level.
2. Accurately record the number of the infant's stools.
3. Dispose of the infant's stools in proper containers.
4. Monitor the infant's electrolyte lab results.

12. The most effective means of controlling external bleeding of an extremity is

1. Direct pressure.
2. Pressure points.
3. Tourniquets.
4. Elevation.

13. A depressed 50-year-old patient is admitted to the hospital. You are assigned to work with the patient and orient her to the unit. One of your first goals would be to

1 Show the patient where she will be sleeping.
2 Introduce the patient to the other patients.
3 Allow the patient to do as she wishes.
4 Establish a nurse-patient relationship.

14. A 35-year-old patient is brought to the hospital by her husband. She has been hearing voices, acting bizarre, and singing her sentences instead of talking. A tentative diagnosis of schizophrenic disorder is made. The patient begins to take chlorpromazine (Thorazine) 200 mg t.i.d., and by the second day, she is having limb spasms and jerky movements. You should assess this behavior as

1 Dystonic movements.
2 Tardive dyskinesia.
3 Parkinsonism.
4 Extrapyramidal movements.

15. The physician orders a medication to counteract the adverse effects of chlorpromazine (Thorazine). You may expect that this will be

1 Haloperidol (Haldol).
2 Trifluoperazine hydrochloride (Stelazine).
3 Benztropine mesylate (Cogentin).
4 Levodopa (L-Dopa).

16. A premature infant is placed in an Isolette. The air in the Isolette will be humidified to

1 Improve respiratory capacity.
2 Prevent hyperbilirubinemia.
3 Increase the infant's temperature.
4 Prevent drying of bronchial secretions.

17. A patient gives birth to a normal, premature, female infant. The infant's physician diagnoses respiratory distress syndrome. The concentration of oxygen that the infant receives will be regulated based on her pO_2 and pCO_2 levels. You understand that this is necessary because high levels of oxygen

1 Produce kernicterus.
2 Cause retinal spasms leading to the development of retrolental fibroplasia.
3 Cause peripheral circulatory collapse.
4 May cause respiratory damage.

18. An adult patient has just returned from the recovery room following lower bowel surgery for an obstruction. She is unable to void and her physician orders a Foley catheter. You will perform the catheterization implementing

1 Surgical asepsis.
2 Clean technique using universal precautions.
3 The physician's instructions.
4 Medical asepsis.

19. A 63-year-old patient was recently diagnosed with cervical cancer and is receiving radium therapy. When working with the charge nurse to prepare the patient for discharge, you should tell her that she

1 Will suffer no adverse symptoms.
2 Will suffer from radioactive symptoms for at least six weeks.
3 Should report vaginal or rectal bleeding immediately to the physician.
4 May have persistent nausea and vomiting for awhile after discharge, but these symptoms are not significant.

20. An adult patient who sustained a head injury when he fell off a ladder is admitted to a neurological unit. He develops increased intracranial pressure. The earliest sign of intracranial pressure would be

1 Vomiting.
2 Increased blood pressure.
3 Agitation.
4 Lethargy.

21. The day before scheduled abdominal surgery, the results of a patient's laboratory tests indicate a white blood cell count of 9,800/cu mm. The most appropriate intervention is to

1 Call the operating room and cancel the surgery.
2 Notify the surgeon immediately.
3 Take no action because it is a normal value.
4 Call the laboratory and have the test repeated.

22. Nursing responsibilities for the preoperative period would include notifying the charge nurse if the patient's

1 Erythrocyte count is 6 million/cu mm.
2 Oral temperature is 99.6°F.
3 Hemoglobin is 14 gm/100 ml.
4 Urinalysis indicates ketonuria.

23. An adult patient whose diagnosis is Personality Disorder, Borderline, is committed for 14 days on the locked unit. When confronted with his inappropriate behavior of talking another patient into leaving the unit without permission, he responds, "Well, if it wasn't me, someone else would have talked her into leaving." This response is an example of

1 Denial.
2 Rationalization.
3 Suppression.
4 Reaction formation.

24. An adult patient with a diagnosis of epilepsy is being admitted to the hospital for a general work-up and medication management. As you go into the patient's room, you observe that he is just beginning to have a seizure. The first nursing action would be to

1 Push the patient's emergency help buzzer.
2 Protect the patient's head and body from damage.
3 Hold the patient down.
4 Place a tongue blade between the patient's teeth.

470

25. A hospitalized 24-year-old is constantly trying to manipulate the staff as a way of getting his needs met. Which response to the patient would indicate that the nurse understands how to therapeutically respond to manipulation?

1 "I won't allow you to manipulate me."
2 "I won't do as you ask, but I will stay with you and talk."
3 "If this behavior doesn't stop, I shall have to tell your doctor."
4 "Let's focus on your anxiety so we can deal with all this manipulation."

26. A 9-year-old boy who has been hospitalized for a week with cystic fibrosis is about to be discharged. Before he is discharged from the hospital, you teach his mother about administering pancreatic enzymes. You will know she understands the instructions when she says that the medication should be taken

1 At 8-hour intervals with a large glass of milk.
2 Following breakfast, lunch, and dinner.
3 At six- to eight-hour intervals with the timing based on whatever is most convenient for the family schedule.
4 Prior to breakfast, lunch, and dinner.

27. When establishing discharge goals for a 9-year-old with cystic fibrosis, a major goal of the child's care at home will be to

1 Avoid catching a cold.
2 Continue breathing exercises.
3 Control fat intake.
4 Continue an antibiotic regimen.

28. For patients with peptic ulcer disease, nursing assessment should include observations for possible complications including

1 Pain with defecation.
2 Mucus in the stool.
3 Bright-red bloody stools.
4 Tarry stools.

29. Cimetidine (Tagamet) is ordered for a patient with peptic ulcer disease. The drug has been effective when the patient no longer

1 Tells you she is nauseated after eating.
2 Complains of intermittent pain.
3 Complains of pain when her stomach is empty.
4 Tells you she can only eat small, bland meals.

30. A 14-year-old patient who is admitted to the hospital will most likely experience a fear of

1 Being displaced.
2 Separation.
3 Loss of independence.
4 The unknown.

31. A 14-year-old patient has been admitted to the adolescent unit with a diagnosis of juvenile diabetes mellitus. Symptoms that the patient will exhibit when her insulin injection is delayed include

1 Thirst, polyuria, and decreased appetite.
2 Flushed cheeks, acetone breath, and increased thirst.
3 Nausea, vomiting, and diarrhea.
4 Weight gain, acetone breath, and thirst.

32. When teaching a 14-year-old patient about regulating his diabetes at home, you should include information about

1 Limiting vigorous exercise.
2 Eliminating sugar from his diet.
3 Testing his blood for sugar at regular intervals.
4 Limiting carbohydrates in his diet.

33. An adult patient is admitted to the hospital with a diagnosis of acute glomerulonephritis. His symptoms have been mild, consisting of fatigue, anorexia, and mild hypertension. One of the primary goals of the patient's treatment would be to

1 Restore his fluid and electrolyte balance.
2 Encourage bed rest during the acute phase of his illness.
3 Give him a high-protein diet to restore nutritional status.
4 Treat his hypertension.

34. A nursing action that will lessen the severity of a patient's orthostatic hypotension is to

1 Turn him from side to side every two hours.
2 Limit times he will have to get in and out of bed.
3 Change his position routinely, especially from horizontal to vertical.
4 Encourage him to move very slowly.

35. When caring for a patient whose physician has ordered furosemide (Lasix), you should recognize that the medication is having the desired effect when

1 He becomes very thirsty.
2 He passes stones in the urine.
3 Infection is decreased.
4 Production of urine is increased.

36. An adult patient who was admitted to a psychiatric unit two days ago with a diagnosis of acute depression attempts suicide. The staff intervenes in time to prevent the patient from harming herself. The most important rationale for having the staff discuss the suicide attempt is that they must

1 Reenact the attempt so they can understand exactly what happened.
2 File an accident report so the hospital administration is kept informed.
3 Discuss the patient's behavior prior to the attempt to identify cues that might have warned them.
4 Prevent a second suicide attempt because there is high probability that the patient will try again in the immediate future.

37. A curarelike medication and a barbiturate that are given to patients before electroconvulsive therapy (ECT) are aimed at reducing the likelihood of

1 Cardiac arrest and loss of memory.
2 Convulsions and fractures.
3 Fractures and anxiety.
4 Anxiety and loss of memory.

38. A 4-week-old infant is brought to the hospital by her mother, who is concerned about her weight loss and frequent crying. Pyloric stenosis is the suspected diagnosis. As you are assessing the infant, you should know that the most obvious sign or symptom is

1 Constant hunger and fussiness.
2 Peristaltic waves passing left to right after a feeding.
3 Frequent diarrhea.
4 Spitting up after a feeding.

39. The most important nursing goal prior to surgery for correction of pyloric stenosis would be to

1 Prevent dehydration.
2 Educate the parents about the procedure.
3 Provide sensory stimuli for the infant.
4 Prevent development of a negative attitude toward feeding.

40. An infant is usually placed in a heated crib immediately after birth to

1 Prevent loss of body heat.
2 Increase oxygen intake.
3 Facilitate drainage of mucus.
4 Provide an environment similar to the uterus.

41. A 38-year-old patient is admitted to the hospital with right upper quadrant tenderness and jaundice. Infectious hepatitis is suspected. Before the diagnosis is confirmed, the nursing care plan should include

1 Observing enteric precautions.
2 Not using isolation techniques.
3 Using only needle precautions.
4 Using universal precautions.

42. Which of the following symptoms would indicate possible thrombophlebitis?

1 Pain along a vein.
2 Severe cramping.
3 Edema.
4 Area surrounding a vein is warm to touch.

473

43. A patient who has received a diagnosis of infectious hepatitis tells you she is a very active person and wants to get out of bed and walk around the hospital. The most appropriate response is

1 "You must remain on complete bed rest."
2 "You must remain on bed rest for a few days, but you can get up to go to the bathroom."
3 "You may walk around for short periods of time every day."
4 "You may be up as much as you wish."

44. A 72-year-old patient in a long-term care facility has a diagnosis of Alzheimer's disease. The patient shuffles up to the station, crying and screaming, "Nobody cares if I live or die! You all hate me! All hate me!" The response by the nurse that would be most therapeutic is

1 "What makes you think we hate you?"
2 "You are always saying that, and you know we all love you."
3 "Here is a cigarette. Now go in the dayroom and watch TV.'
4 "You seem very upset. Let's take a walk and talk about it."

45. A 7-year-old patient received a diagnosis of sickle cell anemia. When her parents are given genetic counseling, they will be told that if one parent has the sickle cell trait, the number of children who will get the disease is

1 None.
2 All of the children.
3 Half of the children.
4 Twenty-five percent.

46. The group of signs and symptoms that best describe a patient who is experiencing heat stroke would be

1 Pale, moist skin; rapid pulse; and slow, deep respirations.
2 Hot, dry skin; rapid pulse; and slow, deep respirations.
3 Hot, dry skin; normal pulse; and normal respirations.
4 Pale, moist skin; weak pulse; and rapid respirations.

47. In planning the daily schedule of a patient who has Alzheimer's disease, it is important for the nurse to understand that this patient

1 May have moderate to severe memory impairment and short periods of concentration.
2 Will respond to a rigid daily schedule, which will help him be more comfortable.
3 Is more likely to be able to remember current experiences than past ones.
4 Can usually be trusted to be responsible for his daily care needs.

48. When assessing an infant who was born 24 hours ago, you should know that the normal apical pulse rate on a newborn is between

1 120 and 160 beats per minute.
2 60 and 80 beats per minute.
3 80 and 100 beats per minute.
4 180 and 200 beats per minute.

49. An adult patient was admitted to the hospital with a diagnosis of carcinoma of the left lung. Following a left lobectomy, the patient is returned to the unit with a chest tube in place. The chest tube is inserted to

1 Supply oxygen to the thoracic cavity.
2 Remove fluid from the alveolar sacs.
3 Provide a means of instilling medication into the thoracic cavity.
4 Provide for removal of air and fluid from the pleural space.

50. When a chest tube is inserted, it is connected to a water-seal suction. The purpose of the water is to

1 Provide humidity for the oxygen.
2 Maintain a closed system so air cannot enter the pleural space.
3 Provide a sterile environment for drainage.
4 Provide an accurate means to measure drainage.

51. An important preoperative nursing procedure for a patient who is scheduled for a craniotomy would be a

1 Hair shampoo.
2 Cleansing enema.
3 Complete bath.
4 Shaving of the head.

52. Following a craniotomy, postoperative nursing care for the patient will include

1 Placing him in Trendelenburg's position.
2 Administering morphine sulfate for pain.
3 Placing him in a belt restraint and soft wrist restraints.
4 Recording rectal temperatures frequently.

53. A 45-year-old patient is scheduled to have an abdominal hysterectomy. While you are orienting the patient to her surroundings, she states that she is afraid of what will happen the next day. The most appropriate nursing response is to

1 Assure her that the surgery is very safe and that problems are rare.
2 Let her talk about her fears as much as she wishes.
3 Explain that she has an excellent physician and that she has nothing to worry about.
4 Explain that anxiety has been proven to prolong length of hospitalization.

54. When caring for a patient who has undergone an abdominal hysterectomy, which of the following nursing measures would best prevent atelectasis?

1 Have her turn, cough, and deep breathe every two hours.
2 Put pillows under her knees to decrease pressure on the incision, thereby increasing her willingness to take deep breaths.
3 Apply a scultetus binder as soon as she is fully awake to assist with deep breathing.
4 Closely observe her intake of fluids to liquefy secretions.

55. A 40-year-old patient is a candidate for prenatal diagnosis by amniocentesis because of her age. Amniocentesis would be primarily performed to detect

1 The presence of twins.
2 Down's syndrome.
3 Tay-Sachs disease.
4 The sex of the fetus.

56. A 35-year-old patient was admitted to the nursing unit four hours ago with a diagnosis of asthmatic reaction. When assessing the patient, you should consider that a characteristic symptom of asthma is

1 Flushed skin.
2 Wheezing type of respiration.
3 Hemoptysis.
4 Chest pain.

57. When a patient becomes dyspneic, the priority nursing action indicated is to

1 Elevate the head of the bed.
2 Keep the patient warm.
3 Administer oxygen as ordered.
4 Turn the patient onto his side.

58. A patient who is experiencing dyspnea appears anxious. The best nursing approach is to

1 Ignore the anxiety, understanding it will decrease when his breathing improves.
2 Stay with him and be supportive.
3 Tell him his breathing will soon improve.
4 Notify the physician.

59. When caring for a senile elderly patient, which of the following should be considered necessary for comfort and safety?

1 Hand rails in halls.
2 A portable walker.
3 Floors with wall-to-wall carpeting.
4 Hand rails by the toilets.

60. A pregnant mother of a 10-year-old son says that he has begun to ask questions about the pregnancy. She is afraid he's going to ask her "where the baby comes from" and asks you what to say. Which of the following responses would be best?

1 "Ignore it and gently change the subject."
2 "Ask a male family member to discuss it with the boy."
3 "Give him a simple explanation of the facts of reproduction."
4 "Redirect the question to him to find out what he specifically wants to know."

61. When caring for a patient who has renal failure, you should be concerned about a change in

1 Blood pressure.
2 Pulse.
3 Proteinuria.
4 Respirations.

62. After a normal delivery, the newborn appears jaundiced. The physician has ordered a continuous bili light and forced fluids between feedings. An important nursing action when an infant has phototherapy is to

1. Cover the eyes with eye patches to prevent retinal damage.
2. Dress the infant to prevent chilling.
3. Isolate the infant to prevent cross-contamination.
4. Avoid handling the infant so as not to interfere with the treatment.

63. When caring for a newborn infant, you should know that physiologic jaundice in a newborn usually appears

1. Within the first 24 hours and disappears after 3 days.
2. Within the first 24 hours and lasts 6 to 7 days.
3. On the second or third day and lasts 48 hours.
4. On the second or third day and begins to decrease on the sixth or seventh day.

64. Confabulation is a symptom frequently seen in dementia. Confabulation can be best defined as

1. Amnesia of recent events.
2. A defense mechanism to control anxiety.
3. The falsifying of facts to fill in memory gaps.
4. A mechanism to lower self-esteem.

65. When preparing a patient for an intravenous pyelogram (IVP), nursing care will include

1. An NPO regimen.
2. Forced fluids.
3. Enemas until clear.
4. A 24-hour urine collection.

66. A 36-year-old male patient comes to the emergency room with complaints of severe right flank pain radiating to the inguinal and testicular area. He is pale, diaphoretic, and nauseated. The physician orders an analgesic, a routine urinalysis, and admission to the hospital. The patient should be instructed to

1. Save his urine for measurement and straining.
2. Drink as much fluids as possible.
3. Notify the nursing staff of the amount of his voidings.
4. Refrain from eating and not drink until further notice.

67. The charge nurse asks you to check on any allergies a patient who is scheduled for an immediate intravenous pyelogram (IVP) may have. The reason for obtaining this data is

1. The intravenous dye contains iodine.
2. It is routine information.
3. The patient will require antibiotic therapy.
4. The patient's symptoms may suggest an allergic reaction.

68. A patient is experiencing dyspnea associated with congestive heart failure. A nursing measure that would relieve the dyspnea would be to place her in

1 Supine position.
2 High Fowler's position.
3 Reverse Trendelenburg's position.
4 Semi-Fowler's position.

69. When monitoring a patient who is receiving a blood transfusion, you should know that the signs and symptoms that are most characteristic of an allergic reaction to blood are

1 Fall in blood pressure, distention of neck veins, and rash.
2 Backache, increased temperature, and chills.
3 Wheezing, hives, and laryngeal edema.
4 Tachycardia, hives, and flushed skin.

70. If an allergic reaction to a blood transfusion occurs, your first action should be to

1 Notify the physician.
2 Call the charge nurse.
3 Slow the rate of infusion.
4 Shut off the transfusion.

71. A 41-year-old patient has been admitted with a diagnosis of severe hyperthyroidism. She complains of weight loss, nervousness, and personality changes. The goal of nursing care that you anticipate will be the most difficult to achieve for the patient is

1 Adequate rest.
2 Eye care.
3 Diet.
4 Skin care.

72. The physician has scheduled a thyroidectomy for a patient. A postoperative complication of thyroidectomy surgery that should be continually assessed for is

1 Pineal damage.
2 Facial nerve damage.
3 Hypercalcemia.
4 Respiratory distress.

73. A patient who has undergone a thyroidectomy will be maintained in semi-Fowler's position postoperatively to

1 Assist her to be more comfortable.
2 Prevent respiratory distress.
3 Avoid strain on the suture line.
4 Prevent bleeding.

74. One day, a terminally ill patient says to the nurse, "Well, I've given up all hope. I know I'm going to die soon." The most therapeutic response to this statement is

1 "One should never give up all hope. We are finding new cures every day."
2 "Would you like to talk about dying?"
3 "You've given up all hope?"
4 "You know, your physician will be here soon. Why don't you talk to him about your feelings and giving up all hope?"

75. The condition of a patient who has been on an oncology unit for two months becomes critical. Of the following tasks, the one with the highest priority is to

1 Attend to her physical needs and assess her condition for changes.
2 Support the family and give them needed encouragement.
3 Encourage her to express and talk about her fears of dying.
4 Contact her lawyer so she can tie up loose ends.

76. A patient's physician has ordered that he be fed via hyperalimentation. This procedure is a method of

1 Providing the necessary fluids and electrolytes to the body.
2 Providing complete nutrition by the intravenous route.
3 Tube feeding that provides necessary nutrients to the body.
4 Blood transfusion.

77. An important nursing goal in planning care for a patient with chronic organic brain syndrome is to

1 Encourage the patient to function dependently.
2 Continually orient the patient to reality.
3 Provide an unstructured environment with appropriate recreational activities.
4 Plan a daily schedule that is varied and interesting.

78. Regression is a defense mechanism used by psychiatric patients. The best description of this mechanism is that it

1 Is an immature way of responding.
2 Works most effectively to eliminate anxiety.
3 Fosters dependence.
4 Provides security through childlike behavior.

79. You should expect that the dietary requirements of a patient who has been admitted with jaundice will

1 Limit carbohydrates.
2 Restrict fatty foods.
3 Avoid all juices.
4 Include parenteral fluids.

80. The RN asks you to teach a patient how to care for his new colostomy. In teaching him to irrigate his colostomy, you tell him that he should irrigate

1 By gravity flow from a container placed at a height of three feet above the ostomy opening.
2 By gravity flow from a container placed at shoulder height.
3 By gravity flow several inches above the ostomy opening.
4 At any height as long as the flow is regulated by gravity.

81. Mrs. Mary Wakins, 55 years old, was brought to the hospital by ambulance after telling her husband that she had intense chest pain, anxiety, and nausea. Her admitting diagnosis is suspected myocardial infarction. When providing care for Mrs. Wakins in the emergency department, the nurse should understand that myocardial infarction results from a

1 Critical reduction in blood supply to the myocardium.
2 Marked increase in cardiac output.
3 Sudden irregularity of cardiac contraction.
4 Marked decrease in cardiac output.

82. An elderly patient develops arrhythmias while she is being admitted to the hospital. Which of the following medications should the nurse expect to be administered first?

1 Morphine sulfate, U.S.P.
2 Lidocaine hydrochloride, U.S.P.
3 Nitroglycerin (Nitrostat).
4 Meperidine hydrochloride (Demerol).

83. Christopher Sherlock, 3 days old, is admitted to the pediatric unit from the nursery. His diagnosis is esophageal atresia, type III. Mrs. Sherlock says to the nurse, "I feel as though I've done something wrong to make my baby sick." Which of the following responses would be appropriate?

1 "Your baby was born with this. You've done the best you can."
2 "It does no good to feel that way. Your baby is sick and needs you."
3 "A lot of mothers feel guilty when their babies are sick."
4 "I can understand your feelings, but remember that this is a congenital defect that you did not cause."

84. A child returns from surgery with a gastrostomy tube in place. On the second postoperative day, the nurse should

1 Return the tube to gravity drainage.
2 Secure the tube above the level of the stomach.
3 Leave the tube as it is.
4 Plug the tube.

85. Anticoagulants are prescribed for an adult patient. The nurse should understand that this type of medication will

1 Relieve pain from myocardial damage.
2 Prevent extension of a coronary thrombus.
3 Improve coronary circulation.
4 Improve cardiac output.

86. The physician prescribes a soft diet for an adult patient who has a diagnosis of congestive heart failure. She complains to the nurse about the diet. The nurse should explain that the purpose of this diet is to

1 Minimize the effort of mastication and digestion.
2 Increase elimination.
3 Prevent an increased workload on the heart.
4 Reduce the caloric intake.

87. Ms. Kaye Benson, 30 years old, comes to a clinic with symptoms that include pain and numbness in her legs. A tentative diagnosis of multiple sclerosis is made. The nurse should understand that multiple sclerosis is the

1 Formation of fluid-filled cavities in the central part of the spinal cord.
2 Formation of fibrous tissue causing pressure on nerve roots.
3 Chronic inflammation of the coverings of the central nervous system.
4 Patchy destruction of the myelin sheath.

88. When teaching a patient about multiple sclerosis, the nurse should counsel her that she should *avoid*

1 Activity.
2 Fatigue.
3 A great deal of rest.
4 A regular program of exercise.

89. Following a normal, spontaneous birth by a diabetic mother, the infant is admitted to the newborn nursery. After a first feeding of sterile water, the infant is given glucose water. The next nursing action should be to

1 Observe the infant for hyperbilirubinemia.
2 Administer formula or, preferably, breast milk to the infant.
3 Monitor the infant's respiratory status.
4 Monitor the infant's glucose levels using Dextrostix.

90. Mrs. Anne Martin, 50 years old, was admitted to a hospital for a breast biopsy. Following the biopsy, Mrs. Martin was scheduled for surgery. After her radical mastectomy, the nurse should position Mrs. Martin

1 On her operative side.
2 On her unoperative side.
3 In semi-Fowler's, with her affected arm flat on bed.
4 In semi-Fowler's, with her affected arm elevated.

91. After discharge from the hospital, a patient is being treated with chemotherapy and radiation therapy at an outpatient clinic. Before radiation therapy begins, it would be most important for the nurse to tell the patient that

1 Radiation therapy can cause pneumonitis.
2 Radiation ionizes atoms in the chemical system of the cells and causes side effects.
3 Radiodermatitis will occur in the course of therapy.
4 Radiation therapy causes cell damage that may result in gastrointestinal side effects.

92. Mrs. Beth Ramsey, a postoperative cataract extraction patient, is to be instructed in the use of eyedrops before discharge. The nurse's instructions should include

1 Looking down when instilling the eyedrops in the lower eyelid.
2 Dropping the medication in the lower eyelid near the nose.
3 Dropping the medication in the center of the lower eyelid.
4 Looking up when instilling the eyedrops on the lens.

93. To best facilitate the breathing of a child who has croup, the nurse should place her in

1 Prone position.
2 Semi-Fowler's position.
3 Supine position.
4 Low Fowler's position.

94. Immediately following a normal, spontaneous birth, the newborn infant is dried thoroughly and banded and erythromycin is placed in both eyes. The mother asks the nurse, "Why are you putting medicine in my baby's eyes?" The nurse's reply should be based on an understanding that erythromycin is administered optically to infants to prevent

1 Gonorrheal infection.
2 Retrolental fibroplasia.
3 Blindness.
4 Transferral of human immunodeficiency virus (HIV).

95. When performing a newborn assessment, the nurse should know that signs of hypoglycemia in the infant will include

1 Restlessness and a whining cry.
2 Stuporlike behavior with no cry.
3 A high-pitched cry.
4 A weak, soft cry.

96. The nurse is providing care for a patient who just learned that she has terminal cancer. She says to the nurse, "I don't know why you are all so concerned; I'm not that sick." The defense mechanism she is using is

1 Denial.
2 Rationalization.
3 Projection.
4 Regression.

97. The nurse should understand that vitamin K is administered to infants in the newborn nursery to

1 Help conjugate bilirubin in the infant.
2 Prevent Rh sensitization in the infant.
3 Reduce the possibility of hemorrhage in the infant.
4 Increase the infant's resistance to infection.

98. Oxygen therapy may be prescribed for a patient who is oxygen deprived. The nurse should know that the primary purpose of oxygen is to

1 Minimize myocardial necrosis.
2 Increase cardiac output.
3 Decrease cardiac output.
4 Dilate coronary blood vessels.

99. When providing nursing care for a patient who is receiving oxygen, the environment should be kept free of all possible sources of sparks or fire because oxygen

1 Supports combustion.
2 Will burn rapidly.
3 Is explosive.
4 Is present in higher concentrations than normal.

100. A depressed patient refuses to join group activities and sits in a corner all day. To deal with this aspect of depression, the nurse should

1 Assign the patient to clean the unit kitchen.
2 Insist that the patient join group therapy.
3 Formulate a structured schedule of daily activities for the patient.
4 Allow the patient to not participate until the medication is effective.

101. Mr. Ben Abram, 23 years old, is admitted to an emergency room with first-degree (superficial, partial thickness) burns of his entire right arm and second- (partial thickness) and third-degree (full thickness) burns of his neck, abdomen, and back. Assessing Mr. Abram's burns according to the Rule of Nines, the nurse should calculate that the burns affect

1 1 to 18 percent of his body.
2 19 to 33 percent of his body.
3 34 to 49 percent of his body.
4 Over 50 percent of his body.

102. The nurse should understand that the major loss to the body of a severely burned patient is in

1 Electrolytes.
2 Water.
3 Blood.
4 Skin.

103. A severely burned patient has an IV of lactated Ringer's solution infusing. The physician has ordered insertion of a nasogastric tube. The nurse should understand that the nasogastric tube will prevent

1 Taking fluids by mouth.
2 Paralytic ileus.
3 Overload of fluids in the body.
4 Vomiting of stomach contents.

104. After the first week of hospitalization for a severely burned patient, the nurse should expect his diet to include foods that are

1 High protein, low sodium and low carbohydrate.
2 Low fat, low sodium and high calorie.
3 High protein and high carbohydrate.
4 High protein, high vitamin B-complex and low sodium.

105. Marlise Border, 18 months old, is brought to the clinic by her parents for a checkup. Marlise is a normal, healthy toddler. Because Marlise is at the age of exploring, it would be most important for the nurse to counsel Mr. and Mrs. Border to be aware of

1 Safety hazards, such as poisons and medicine, that are within Marlise's reach.
2 The need for giving Marlise plenty of opportunity for exercise.
3 The danger of spoiling Marlise with too much love and affection.
4 The possibility that Marlise may show extreme jealousy toward others.

106. A patient who is receiving radiation therapy comes to the clinic for a scheduled treatment. The nurse notices that the patient's skin appears wet and weeping. The nurse should

1 Not give the treatment and tell the patient to avoid bathing the skin until the weeping has stopped.
2 Give the treatment and make a note on the patient's record concerning the skin condition.
3 Not give the treatment and notify the charge nurse of the patient's skin condition.
4 Give the treatment and instruct the patient to use antibiotic lotion on the lesions.

107. The nurse will know that a patient understands the specific dietary guidelines for patients receiving radiation if she says that she avoids eating

1 Cheese, fried eggs, nuts, and raw fruit.
2 Beef, pork, bread, and cooked vegetables.
3 Lunch meat, canned soups, tomatoes, and yellow vegetables.
4 Milk, eggs, canned vegetables, and fish.

108. Jamie Bell, 7 months old, has received a tentative diagnosis of mental retardation. Her parents have come to the hospital for further assessment and counseling. During the nursing assessment, an observation that will help confirm the diagnosis of mental retardation is that Jamie

1 Is unable to sit unsupported for brief periods.
2 Is able to approach a toy and grasp it.
3 Frequently rolls from back to stomach.
4 Can grasp a spoon and bring it to her mouth.

109. When working with parents of a retarded child, the nurse should formulate a nursing plan that

1 Is based on a careful family assessment, including the parents' grief reaction.
2 Will help the parents make decisions about long-term plans for the child.
3 Will interpret the parents' feelings about their child and the grief process they are experiencing.
4 Presents information about institutional placement for the child.

110. When administering intermittent positive pressure breathing (IPPB) therapy to an adult patient, the nurse should be alert for the side effects of

1 Increased venous return to the heart.
2 Increased cardiac output.
3 Reflex bradycardia secondary to increased blood pressure.
4 Decreased venous return to the heart.

111. When providing dietary teaching for a patient who is receiving intermittent positive pressure breathing (IPPB) therapy, the nurse should

1 Suggest small, frequent meals.
2 Insist on a low-salt diet.
3 Suggest a high-protein diet that includes no carbohydrates.
4 Force fluids.

112. A pregnant patient who has a history of mild diabetes that is controlled by insulin asks the nurse what will happen to her insulin requirements during her pregnancy. Which of the following responses would be best for the nurse to make?

1 "Because your case is so mild, you are not likely to need much insulin during your pregnancy."
2 "It's likely that, as the pregnancy progresses to term, you will need increased insulin."
3 "Every case is individual, so there's really no way to say."
4 "If you follow the diet well and don't gain too much weight, your insulin needs should stay about the same."

113. When reviewing the urinalysis report of a patient with the diagnosis of cystitis, the nurse should be surprised to find that it shows

1 RBCs present in the urine.
2 Negative glucose.
3 Specific gravity, 1.015.
4 No WBCs or RBCs in the urine.

114. The urinalysis report of a patient with the diagnosis of cystitis shows that neither RBCs nor WBCs are present in the urine. Based on this report, the initial nursing action would be to

1 Notify the charge nurse immediately.
2 Check to determine that an error was not made in identifying the specimen.
3 Tell the patient the test results are fine.
4 Request that the test be repeated.

115. Mr. Jim Nelson, 56 years old, is admitted to a hospital with a diagnosis of pneumonia. He is an alcoholic who has recently resumed heavy drinking. One day, when approached by the nurse, he says, "I'm really no good. I drink and don't take care of my family, and I'm a rotten father." Which of the following responses to this statement would be most therapeutic?

1 "But now you are doing something about your problem, Mr. Nelson."
2 "It sounds as though you are feeling pretty guilty about drinking."
3 "I'm sure that you are a good father, Mr. Nelson."
4 "What makes you think you are no good?"

116. When assessing the developmental level of a 3-month-old infant at a well-baby clinic, the nurse should expect the infant to

1   See objects only as shapes and shadows.
2   Focus her eyes only momentarily.
3   Distinguish between light and dark only.
4   Focus her eyes on objects and people.

117. When a 57-year-old male patient comes to a clinic for a periodic checkup, he receives a diagnosis of angina pectoris, with no subsequent cardiac involvement. His physician prescribes nitroglycerin. The nurse should know that this medication is given sublingually because

1   Superficial blood vessels promote rapid absorption of the medication.
2   Stomach acids destroy the medication.
3   Saliva helps break down the medication for absorption.
4   The medication is too rapidly absorbed in the stomach.

118. Part of the nursing care plan for a patient who is taking nitroglycerin is to instruct him to store this medication

1   In the refrigerator.
2   In a clear, tightly closed glass jar.
3   In a dark, tightly closed glass jar.
4   Not more than three months.

119. Mrs. Karen Barry, 30 years old, was brought to a hospital by her husband. Mrs. Barry's diagnosis is bipolar disorder, manic episode. She manifests an excess of energy and cannot sit still. The most useful activity that the nurse might suggest for Mrs. Barry would be to

1   Play volleyball outside.
2   Engage in group exercises.
3   Play table tennis in the day room.
4   Deliver linen to other patients' rooms.

120. Following ileostomy surgery, one of the goals is to prevent thrombus formation from venous stasis. A nursing action to achieve this goal is to

1   Help the patient to perform total range-of-motion exercises every two hours.
2   Administer acetaminophen (Tylenol) to the patient as prescribed.
3   Put antiembolic stockings on the patient.
4   Elevate the foot of the patient's bed.

121. When teaching a woman about the adequate nutrition that is essential during early pregnancy for optimal fetal development, the nurse should recommend a nutritious daily diet that is supplemented by

1   Iron and folacin.
2   Vitamin C.
3   Additional minerals.
4   Vitamin B complex.

122. Ms. Terry Learner, 45 years old, returned to the unit following exploratory abdominal surgery yesterday with a nasogastric tube in place. Understanding possible early complications of abdominal surgery, the nurse should evaluate Mrs. Learner for

1 Constipation.
2 Clay-colored stools.
3 Infection.
4 Hemorrhage.

123. Prior to administering the third dose of digoxin to a five-year-old child, the nurse observes that the child's temperature is 37.7°C (99.8°F) and her pulse rate is 100. The appropriate nursing action would be to

1 Notify the charge nurse.
2 Recognize that these are signs of digoxin toxicity and withhold the dose.
3 Administer the medication.
4 Administer the medication, but tell the charge nurse that the child's pulse rate is lower than normal.

124. After a normal labor and delivery, the infant weighs 2400 gm (5 lb) and is considered premature. Which of the following actions should the nurse consider most important for providing adequate nutrition for the infant?

1 Use a regular nipple with a large hole.
2 Offer a feeding every four to six hours.
3 Use a premie nipple for bottle feeding.
4 Use milk high in fat for the formula.

125. The mother of a premature infant visits her every day. During a visit, the nurse asks the mother if she would like to feed the infant. She says, "Oh, no; you do it so well. I want my baby to be well cared for." The most appropriate response is to say

1 "I'll feed her today. Maybe tomorrow you can try it."
2 "It's not difficult at all. She is just like a normal baby, only smaller."
3 "You can learn to feed her as well as I can; I wasn't good when I first fed a premature infant either."
4 "It's frightening sometimes to feed an infant this small, but I'll stay with you to help."

126. Which of the following signs would indicate to the nurse that a newly inserted nasogastric tube is in the appropriate place?

1 Regular intermittent bubbling when the end of the tube is submerged in water.
2 Hearing a rush of air in the stomach when 1 ml of air is injected into the tube.
3 The presence of mucus after aspiration through the tube.
4 No coughing or choking when the tube was inserted.

127. When Mrs. Jean Godfrey, 28 years old, comes to a clinic, she is experiencing suprapubic tenderness with urinary urgency and dysuria. She receives a diagnosis of cystitis. The nurse should know that Mrs. Godfrey will be instructed to take

1 Restricted fluids by mouth.
2 Unrestricted fluids by mouth.
3 NPO.
4 Only certain limited foods.

128. Considering the diagnosis of cystitis, the nurse should teach a patient the importance of

1 Restricting her physical activity.
2 Maintaining good perineal hygiene.
3 Limiting her intake of certain foods to maintain normal bladder pH.
4 Limiting her oral fluids for the duration of the problem.

129. A diabetic mother-to-be asks the nurse about breast feeding. The statement that is most accurate about breast feeding and diabetes is that it is

1 Contraindicated because insulin is passed to the infant through the milk.
2 Contraindicated because the diabetic's milk production mechanism is faulty.
3 Contraindicated because it puts too much stress on the mother's body.
4 Not contraindicated.

130. The nurse should understand that it is most difficult to control a pregnant woman's diabetes

1 Early in the pregnancy.
2 Early in the postpartum period.
3 During the delivery process.
4 During labor.

131. A 16-year-old patient and her mother have come to a clinic for counseling and contraceptive information. The nurse should know that many of the fears and fantasies of adolescents can be avoided if

1 Sex education is accurate and complete.
2 Religion is respected and valuable to them.
3 They are kept physically active.
4 All mixed gatherings are carefully chaperoned.

132. Ms. Judy Moore, 27 years old, has been ill for four days. She has just been admitted with a diagnosis of pneumococcal pneumonia. She has a temperature of 38.9°C (102°F), and she feels nauseated and lethargic. When providing care for Ms. Moore, the nurse must recall that one of the most important goals in the treatment of pneumonia is to

1 Keep the environment aseptic.
2 Administer limited fluids.
3 Conserve the patient's energy.
4 Encourage the patient to frequently turn and cough.

133. The nurse must handle nasal and bronchial secretions from a patient with pneumonia carefully because

1 Bloody sputum will be present.
2 These secretions may spread the disease.
3 The sight may be upsetting to the patient.
4 Universal precautions must be observed for all patients with pneumonia.

134. Tara Carter, 1 month old, is brought by her mother to a well-baby clinic for a check-up and to receive her first immunization. Mrs. Carter is concerned because Tara sleeps so much of the day. The nurse should tell Mrs. Carter that infants

1 Sleep all day and stay awake most of the night until they get on a regular routine.
2 Should have only one nap during the day.
3 Need at least 12 hours of sleep out of every 24 hours.
4 Usually sleep about 20 hours out of every 24 hours.

135. A patient who has a diagnosis of esophageal varices has had a Sengstaken-Blakemore tube inserted to control the bleeding. The most important nursing intervention for this patient is

1 Providing good mouth care.
2 Monitoring IV fluid intake.
3 Assessing respiratory status.
4 Deflating the balloons on a regular basis.

136. An infant weighs 2880 gm (6 lb) at birth. By 6 months of age, the infant should weigh about

1 9.6 kg (21 lb).
2 3840 gm (8 lb).
3 5760 gm (12 lb).
4 11.8 kg (26 lb).

137. Mrs. Estelle Green, 82 years old, has had an open reduction of the hip, with fixation by the use of a nail. Postoperatively, the primary nursing intervention is to

1 Keep her affected hip in acute flexion.
2 Elevate her affected leg to avoid edema.
3 Keep her affected hip in abduction.
4 Keep the head of the bed flat.

138. Following a patient's hip replacement surgery, a Hemovac is in place to assist with drainage. During the first postoperative hours, the nurse should observe the Hemovac frequently to check for

1 Infection of the incision site.
2 Hemorrhage.
3 Color of drainage.
4 Edema at the incision site.

139. A patient's disruptive behavior on the unit has been extremely annoying to the other patients. One approach the nurse may find effective is to

1 Tell the patient that she is bothering others and confine her to her room.
2 Ignore the patient's behavior, realizing that it is consistent with her illness.
3 Set consistent limits on the patient's behavior.
4 Make a definite, structured plan that the patient will have to follow.

140. Mrs. Rene Lourdes, 32 years old, is in her 37th week of pregnancy and is showing early signs of preeclampsia. When assessing Mrs. Lourdes, the nurse should observe for the most common early signs of preeclampsia, which are

1 Increased blood pressure, proteinuria, and edema.
2 Decreased blood pressure, proteinuria, and edema.
3 Increased blood pressure, glucose in the urine, and weight gain.
4 Hypertension, hyperreflexia, and edema.

141. The nursing care plan for a pregnant patient includes assessing for further signs of preeclampsia that the nurse will report to the team leader. Indications that preeclampsia is progressing to a more severe state would be

1 Severe hypertension, glycosuria, and polyuria.
2 Hyperreflexia, oliguria, and epigastric pain.
3 Hypertension, weight loss, and diuresis.
4 Hypertension, convulsions, and polyuria.

142. An adult patient who was diagnosed as having cholelithiasis has had several episodes of gallbladder attacks over the past year. Which of the following symptoms should the nurse recognize as the one that would most likely cause the patient to go to a physician?

1 Chronic pain in the lower right abdomen.
2 Chronic pain in the lower left abdomen.
3 Fatty food intolerance while eating.
4 Fatty food intolerance several hours after eating.

143. The nursing action that will provide the best source of relief for a woman in labor with back pain would be to

1 Direct her attention to the television or talk to her.
2 Help her to walk around.
3 Administer a prescribed narcotic analgesic to her.
4 Apply counterpressure to her sacrum.

144. While assessing a patient who is taking lithium carbonate, U.S.P, to treat manic-type behavior disorders, the nurse should be alert for signs and symptoms of

1 Dehydration.
2 Muscle weakness.
3 Drowsiness.
4 Anuria.

145. A teenaged girl comes to a prenatal clinic where it is determined that she is 12 weeks pregnant. When helping her select the best protein foods from the school cafeteria, the nurse should suggest that she choose

1 A slice of pizza.
2 Pasta.
3 A peanut butter sandwich.
4 Tomato soup and crackers.

146. The nurse should teach a mother-to-be that energy requirements of pregnancy increase the daily calorie requirement. The nurse will know the mother-to-be understands when she says the daily calories should be increased by

1 500 calories.
2 100 calories.
3 300 calories.
4 50 calories.

147. The most effective nursing measure to maintain optimal positioning and function for a patient who has had a cerebrovascular accident (CVA) is to

1 Place the patient in a prone position for 15 to 30 minutes, 3 times a day.
2 Change the patient's position every 4 hours.
3 Maintain the patient on the affected side as much of the time as possible.
4 Change the patient's position from the affected to the unaffected side every 2 hours.

148. Mrs. Marilyn Ferrar, 45 years old, is brought to a hospital by her husband because she refuses to get dressed or go out, cries most of the time, and says life is not worth living. A major depressive episode is the admitting diagnosis. A priority goal of Mrs. Ferrar's nursing care plan should be to

1 Provide a safe environment.
2 Build up Mrs. Ferrar's self-esteem.
3 Pay attention to Mrs. Ferrar's physical needs.
4 Establish a nurse-patient relationship.

149. The most important developmental task for the nurse to encourage a mother to teach her child prior to surgery for cleft palate repair would be

1 Drinking with a straw.
2 Using a spoon.
3 Using a soft nipple.
4 Drinking from a cup.

150. A mother is unable to breast feed her sick infant, who has a gastrostomy tube in place. An appropriate nursing action is to encourage the mother to

1 Accept the fact that the infant will need formula while in the hospital.
2 Discontinue the idea of breast feeding.
3 Pump her breasts and bring the milk to the hospital.
4 Wait until the infant leaves the hospital and then resume breast feeding.

151. Tranylcypromine sulfate (Parnate) is prescribed for a depressed patient about to be discharged. The nurse should tell the patient that

1 Parnate takes two to three weeks to become effective.
2 Drowsiness and blurred vision can be dangerous side effects of Parnate.
3 Parnate potentiates the action of other drugs.
4 Parnate should not be taken with foods that are aged or that contain tyramine.

152. Sandy Biggs, 10 years old, is admitted to a hospital with a diagnosis of congestive heart failure. She is now being digitalized. Before administering digoxin, the appropriate nursing action is to

1 Obtain an EKG.
2 Assess Sandy's blood pressure.
3 Measure Sandy's temperature.
4 Count Sandy's pulse rate.

153. When caring for a patient following abdominal surgery, the appropriate nursing intervention to prevent pulmonary complications would be to

1 Administer oxygen to the patient as prescribed.
2 Instruct the patient to turn, cough, and deep breathe every two hours.
3 Encourage the patient to hyperventilate every hour.
4 Assist the patient out of bed to a chair on the second postoperative day.

154. When discussing family planning methods with a couple, the nurse should

1 Include only the female in the discussion.
2 Ensure that the couple have a thorough understanding of the method they choose.
3 Choose the method that would best suit the couple.
4 Point out that most methods are 99.9 percent effective, so it makes no difference which method they choose.

155. When a patient returns to the unit following a cardiac catheterization, the nursing activity that should immediately follow taking vital signs is

1 Placing the patient in a warm bed and encouraging sleep.
2 Providing the patient with fluids.
3 Assessing the patient's peripheral pulses.
4 Reapplying the patient's dressing where the dye was injected.

156. An unconscious patient is brought to an emergency room. To determine if the airway is clear, the nurse should first perform

1 Forceful mouth-to-mouth ventilation.
2 Endotracheal tube insertion.
3 Head tilt-neck lift.
4 Cardiopulmonary resuscitation (CPR).

157. Ms. Jennifer Holmes, 23 years old, is admitted to a hospital at 8:00 P.M. with a diagnosis of possible appendicitis. On admission, she states that she has been experiencing pain all day. During the initial assessment of Ms. Holmes, the nurse should be especially alert for

1 High fever.
2 Nausea and vomiting.
3 Tenderness in the upper right abdominal quadrant.
4 Lethargy.

158. Following the completion of laboratory studies, a patient is scheduled for an appendectomy. Nursing interventions during the preoperative period will include keeping the patient

1 Lying flat in bed, with no heat or ice applications to the affected area.
2 In bed in semi-Fowler's position, with ice to the affected area.
3 In any position, with a heating pad on the tender area.
4 In any position, with an ice bag on the tender area.

159. The preoperative nursing care plan for a patient scheduled for an appendectomy should include

1 Increasing the patient's protein intake to help prevent post-operative protein depletion.
2 Giving the patient fluids, but no solid food, to prevent dehydration.
3 Keeping the patient NPO to decrease peristalsis.
4 Beginning IV therapy because the patient is NPO.

160. A teenaged girl comes to a clinic and tells the nurse that she is sexually active and would like some form of birth control. After discussing the various methods of contraception, she decides she would like to use an oral contraceptive. The nurse should tell her that the physician will need to know

1 The names of her sexual contacts.
2 A complete history of her sexual experiences.
3 If she has a history of thrombophlebitis or migraine headaches.
4 If her parents approve and will sign a written consent.

161. When preparing a 5-year-old child for a cardiac catheterization, the nurse should consider the fact that children at this age

1 Are beyond the stage of fearing intrusive procedures.
2 Respond poorly to verbal directions.
3 Understand simple directions.
4 Are quiet, shy, and withdrawn.

162. A 15-year-old patient with scoliosis has been admitted to an adolescent unit and will be having surgery the following day for the insertion of a Harrington rod. Following surgery, the nurse will turn the patient using

1 Adduction.
2 Abduction.
3 Log-rolling method.
4 An overhead traction device.

163. The nurse can best establish whether a patient is unconscious by observing the patient's response to

1 Verbal stimuli.
2 Pupillary reaction to light.
3 Pinching the earlobe.
4 Opening the airway.

164. Ms. Jane Manning, 24 years old, is brought into an emergency room by her roommate. She appears to be unconscious, is unresponsive, and her friend can give no information about the cause of her condition. The period of time allowed for checking Ms. Manning's level of unresponsiveness would be

1 Less than 4 seconds.
2 4 to 10 seconds.
3 5 to 8 seconds.
4 10 to 12 seconds.

165. The nurse should recognize that the most appropriate method of ordering low-sodium meals for a 6-year-old child would be to

1 Help the child fill out the menu.
2 Have one of the child's parents fill out the menus after learning about the diet.
3 Fill out the menu for the child.
4 Ask the dietitian to order the meals.

166. The best maneuver for the nurse to use when opening the airway of a patient who has a suspected neck injury is the

1 Head tilt.
2 Head tilt-chin lift.
3 Head tilt-neck lift.
4 Jaw-thrust.

167. A pregnant woman asks the nurse at a maternity clinic about snacks to increase her protein intake. The nurse should suggest

1 One-half cup of dry-roasted, unsalted peanuts.
2 Two apples.
3 A beef jerky stick.
4 One cup of low-fat milk.

168. Mrs. Sharon Klein, 60 years old, is admitted to a hospital for treatment and rehabilitation after suffering a cerebrovascular accident (CVA). Mrs. Klein has some residual expressive aphasia. The most therapeutic nursing action would be to

1 Anticipate all of her needs and requests.
2 Encourage her communication by writing or using an alphabet board.
3 Encourage every attempt to communicate without correcting words or usage.
4 Encourage Mrs. Klein to use pantomime as a way of communicating.

169. When a patient has a visual loss in the right half of each visual field, the most effective nursing approach to assist her in compensating for this loss would be to

1 Place the items that she frequently uses on her unaffected side.
2 Position her so that her unaffected side is toward the activity in the room.
3 Frequently encourage her to position and turn her head to scan the environment on her affected side.
4 Approach her on her unaffected side.

170. Mrs. Rebecca Franc, 26 years old, is admitted to a hospital at 40 weeks' gestation in active labor. Initial assessment indicates that her cervix is 4 cm dilated, and she is having strong contractions every 4 minutes, lasting 40 seconds. She complains of back discomfort and an urge to bear down. The nurse should suspect that

1 Her cervix is fully dilated.
2 The fetus is in a posterior position.
3 She requires analgesic medication.
4 She needs to get up and walk around.

171. A patient returns to the unit from the recovery room following a cholecystectomy. During surgery, a T-tube was placed in the common bile duct. Goals of nursing care following a T-tube insertion should include

1 Placing the patient in semi-Fowler's position to facilitate drainage.
2 Placing the patient in prone position to promote bile drainage.
3 Connecting the T-tube to a drainage bottle kept at the level of the bed.
4 Clamping the T-tube and only releasing it at intervals.

172. The nurse should understand that the major postoperative complication following a cholecystectomy is

1 Paralytic ileus.
2 Thrombophlebitis.
3 Pneumonia.
4 Hemorrhage.

173. The nurse should know that the most appropriate breakfast for a patient on the third postoperative day following a cholecystectomy would be

1 Cocoa, cereal with half-and-half, grapefruit, and toast and jelly.
2 Tea, boiled eggs, pork sausage, and toast and butter.
3 Coffee, oatmeal with half-and-half, scrambled egg, and toast and butter.
4 Tea, banana, boiled egg, and toast and jelly.

174. The nurse should know that the primary goal of keeping a depressed patient busy and active is formulated to

1 Refocus the patient's attention.
2 Mobilize the patient to help lift the depression.
3 Keep the patient busy until the prescribed antidepressant medication takes effect.
4 Avoid having the patient sit around the unit thinking depressing thoughts.

175. Which of the following laboratory values should the nurse recognize as the normal serum potassium level?

1 1.010 to 1.030.
2 3.5 to 5.5 mEq/L.
3 135 to 145 mg.
4 22 kg.

176. A 40-year-old patient has orders for continuous bladder irrigation following a transurethral resection (TUR). This procedure is used primarily to

1 Provide hemostasis at the incisional site.
2 Maintain adequate bladder drainage.
3 Ensure adequate hydration.
4 Promote adequate urine output.

177. Bethanechol chloride (Urecholine) is prescribed prn for a patient following a transurethral resection (TUR). The nurse will administer the medication when the patient

1 Complains of bladder spasms.
2 Complains of severe pain.
3 Is unable to void.
4 Has frequent episodes of painful urination.

178. Iodine is being administered to a patient with hyperthyroidism. Patient teaching should include telling him to take the medication

1 On an empty stomach.
2 With milk to prevent gastritis.
3 With 8 ounces of water and following a meal.
4 With the meal.

179. The nurse is concerned that a patient who is receiving mydriatic eyedrops is experiencing a systemic anticholinergic effect as a result of absorption. The nurse should assess the patient's

1 Complaints of light headedness and headache.
2 Respirations that are becoming more shallow.
3 Perspiration and complaints of blurred vision.
4 Decreased pulse and blood pressure.

180. A patient has an order to be log rolled following a lumbar laminectomy. The most appropriate method to turn the patient is to use

1 One nurse positioned at the patient's back.
2 Two nurses, one in front and one in back.
3 Three nurses, two in front and one in back.
4 Four nurses, two on each side.

ANSWERS WITH RATIONALE

1. (1) Heat increases circulation to the area. There is no scientific evidence that stressing muscles with exercise or copper bracelets helps arthritis in any way. A soft mattress would cause greater strain on joints.

2. (1) Acetylsalicylic acid relieves pain in muscles. In arthritis, much of the pain comes from muscle spasms.

3. (2) Abduction of the hip should be maintained and acute flexion avoided. She may be turned to the side affected only with physician's orders. She does not have to remain prone.

4. (3) You want to avoid flexion of the hip, so do not dangle the patient's legs or move the patient to a chair. The correct action is to use a walker to provide support for walking. Crutches will not provide enough support.

5. (1) Nägele's Rule is to subtract three months and add seven days. Using this formula, Mary's EDC would be 10/28/94.

6. (2) Fetal size is usually detected by ultrasound. Another gestational age determinant is quickening, which is first perceived between 17 and 19 weeks gestation.

7. (3) Informed consent by a patient who is mentally competent is required in order to have an operative permit signed. This means the physician must talk to the patient, and the patient must not be under the influence of narcotics. The operative permit does not have to be witnessed.

8. (3) Adequate nutrition and weight gain in pregnancy are directly related to decreased mortality and morbidity in the newborn.

Helping the patient understand the role of nutrition and weight gain will help her to explore the best way to talk with her husband about his concerns.

9. (4) Because of an elder's slowness in adapting to dim light, the patient is most likely to be disoriented if he awakens in the dark.

10. (1) Congestive heart failure results when the heart is unable to pump adequate amounts of blood. The cardiac workload and activity should be reduced to allow the heart to rest.

11. (1) While all the objectives listed in the answers are important, assessment of dehydration level and acidosis are the most crucial, for this condition can be life-threatening.

12. (1) Direct pressure is the most effective way of controlling bleeding. It can be augmented by elevating the wound above the level of the heart. Pressure points only slow bleeding, as collateral circulation is almost always present. Tourniquets are seldom needed.

13. (4) With a psychiatric patient, establishing a relationship where she can begin to trust another person is a primary goal and should begin during orientation. During this process you will also accomplish answers (1) and (2).

14. (1) Although these side effects are Parkinson-like and are extrapyramidal, the more specific answer is dystonia, the form that occurs in the first one or two days.

15. (3) The drugs of choice to counteract the extrapyramidal side effects are Cogentin or Artane. Haldol and Stelazine are used in place of Thorazine to control behavior; L-Dopa is

used in Parkinson's disease, not for Parkinson-like side effects.

16. (4)   The infant will have a weak cough and gag reflex and have difficulty removing mucus. Should the bronchial secretions become dry, they become tenacious and almost impossible for the infant to cough up, as well as difficult to remove by suctioning. Oxygen is very drying to the mucous membranes and should always be humidified while being administered, whether to an infant or adult.

17. (2)   High blood levels of oxygen cause spasms of the retinal vessels, and the destruction of these vessels can cause retrolental fibroplasia and blindness.

18. (1)   Nurses observe surgical asepsis while performing catheterizations because of the sterility of the system being entered. Physician's instructions do not include the procedure for catheterization.

19. (3)   Any sign of vaginal or rectal bleeding during a radium implant should be reported immediately to the physician, as it would indicate that complications have developed.

20. (4)   Lethargy is the earliest sign of increased intracranial pressure. It is due to compression of the brain from edema or hemorrhage (or both).

21. (3)   The normal WBC is 5000 to 10,000 per cu mm. If the results were abnormally high, the surgeon would have to be notified, and the surgery may be canceled. Tests with abnormal results are not routinely repeated unless the results are grossly abnormal.

22. (4)   All the other reports are within normal range. The ketonuria indicates a probable diabetic complication or other metabolic condition.

23. (2)   Rationalization is the most common defense mechanism used by borderline individuals. They usually do not feel guilt.

24. (2)   The primary nursing goal during a seizure is to protect the patient from physical injury and, if possible, to maintain a patent airway. After a seizure has begun, you would not use a tongue blade because it can cause damage.

25. (2)   It is important to set limits but not to reinforce low self-esteem, so staying with the patient would be therapeutic.

26. (4)   The purpose of pancreatic enzymes is to replace the enzymes in the child's system that assist with the digestion of fats; therefore, they should be taken prior to the ingestion of food.

27. (2)   The major objective is to keep lungs clear of mucus. Since these children tend to have shallow breathing, breathing exercises are an important goal.

28. (4)   A bleeding duodenal ulcer would cause tarry stools. Bright-red bloody stools indicate a bleeding problem low in the gastrointestinal tract.

29. (3)   Tagamet blocks gastric acid secretion, so the patient will no longer experience pain when her stomach is empty. Nausea is not an expected side effect of the drug.

30. (3)   Having recently achieved some measure of independence, adolescents have a fear of losing it.

31. (2)   All the other choices have one wrong answer. Decreased appetite (1), diarrhea (3), and weight gain (4), are symptoms not usually associated with this condition.

32. (3)   Regular testing for sugar via finger sticks is important as a guide to dietary and insulin control. If a patient is in good health and understands the increased glucose needs of

the body following exercise, there is no reason to restrict activities. All sugar is usually not eliminated if correct ADA exchanges are used and carbohydrates make up 60 percent of the diet.

33. (2) Bed rest would protect the poorly functioning kidneys (activity may increase urinary abnormalities), as well as facilitate diuresis. Protein is usually restricted if oliguria is present.

34. (3) Orthostatic hypotension occurs more frequently with a shift in body position and can be lessened by routinely altering the patient's position.

35. (4) Furosemide (Lasix) actually increases blood flow to the kidney, thereby increasing the production of urine. The patient may become thirsty, but answer (4) is more specific. The patient may or may not have kidney stones and Lasix is not given for this diagnosis. Answer (3) is wrong because Lasix is not antimicrobial.

36. (3) Even though all of the reasons are important and should not be ignored, the most important task is that the staff learn to assess the patient's behavior correctly and to identify cues that might indicate an impending suicide attempt.

37. (3) The curarelike drug lessens strong muscular contractions during the convulsion that can cause fractures, and the barbiturate is given to reduce anxiety by putting the patient to sleep for 5 to 10 minutes.

38. (2) Observing peristaltic waves is one of the most distinctive signs of pyloric stenosis.

39. (1) Dehydration from persistent vomiting is the most frequent complication of pyloric stenosis.

40. (1) The infant is wet and delivery rooms are usually cool, resulting in heat loss from the

infant through conduction, convection, and radiation. Placing the infant in a heated crib decreases heat loss. Trendelenburg's position is used to facilitate drainage, not the heated crib itself.

41. (1) Recognizing that these symptoms may represent infectious hepatitis which is communicable by excreta, the nurse will protect patients and personnel by observing enteric precaution isolation until the diagnosis is confirmed. After the diagnosis is confirmed, the patient will be infectious for one week. (Three weeks prior to and one week after developing jaundice.)

42. (4) The area surrounding a vein would be warm to touch and red, indicating an inflammatory response. Pain may be present, but it would not be along a vein.

43. (2) During the acute phase, the patient must remain on bed rest with bathroom privileges; reasonable activity is allowed during subsequent phases.

44. (4) The nurse acknowledges the patient and his feelings without focusing directly on them. Answer (1) asks for an analysis of feelings; (2) is making light of the patient's feelings; (3) is ignoring the problem.

45. (1) No children will get sickle cell anemia. Both parents must have the recessive gene to have a child with the disease. One parent can pass the gene on so that the children may be carriers.

46. (2) A person experiencing heat stroke will most likely have hot, dry skin; a rapid pulse; and slow, deep respirations.

47. (1) It is important to remember that these patients usually have some memory and concentration impairment. The degree depends upon the individual and is influenced by the basic personality structure and the cause of the problem. Past experiences are more likely to

be remembered. This patient cannot be responsible for his daily needs.

48. (1)   Normal cardiac rate in an infant is 120 to 160 beats per minute. It may drop down to 100 when the infant is resting and increase to 180 when he is crying. Rates above or below those parameters indicate a cardiac or circulatory problem.

49. (4)   Air enters the chest cavity when it is opened, and fluid collects during surgery. A tube is placed in the pleural space to drain this collection of fluid and to allow for the reexpansion of the lung.

50. (2)   The end of the drainage tube is kept under water; this water seals the tube so air cannot enter and be drawn back into the pleural space.

51. (1)   While a complete bath is usually given, the most important preoperative procedure is the shampoo. A cleansing enema is usually not given because of the potential increase in intracranial pressure. The physician will shave the patient's head.

52. (4)   Hyperthermia is a complication of brain surgery, and since the patient probably is not fully oriented, a rectal temperature should be taken. Trendelenburg's position increases intracranial pressure; morphine may depress respirations. Restraints are not routinely used; however, side rails are used for safety.

53. (2)   Allowing the patient to express her fears results in a decrease in anxiety and a more realistic and knowledgeable reaction to the situation.

54. (1)   Atelectasis is collapse of alveoli caused by mucus plugs in the small bronchioles due to inadequate ventilation. Turning, coughing, and deep breathing improve ventilation and help prevent the collapse. Liquefying secretions is important, but answer (1) is more critical.

55. (2)   Amniocentesis is done primarily to determine fetal trisomy 21 (Down's syndrome) in pregnant women over 35 years of age. Carrying twins (1) is not relevant to performing this test. Ashkenazic Jews (3) have a high incidence of Tay-Sachs disease, and for a person with this ethnic background, the test might be performed; it is not related to age. While this test does reveal the sex of the fetus (4), it is not the purpose.

56. (2)   Asthma is defined as recurrent paroxysms of dyspnea with a characteristic wheezing.

57. (1)   With the head of the bed elevated, the diaphragm drops down and allows the lungs to expand. This should be the first nursing action. If this does not decrease dyspnea, then giving O_2 as ordered is indicated.

58. (2)   The dyspneic patient may be very anxious and will look to the nurse for support and reassurance. The best way to provide this is to remain with him. Do not ignore the anxiety; it is a symptom of the condition. Telling him his breathing will improve is giving him false reassurance.

59. (4)   The patient should be encouraged to use toilet rails for support. Hall hand rails are useful but not as important as rails by the toilet. The patient is not yet ready for a walker. Carpeting has been found to hold unpleasant odors and is difficult to clean.

60. (4)   Always clarify with children what it is they want to know before giving them facts; then give them simple, direct answers. Ignoring the question may only postpone the answer or, worse, give the child the idea that it is an unspeakable subject.

61. (1)   While pulse and respirations may change, hypertension is the major concern. Patients in early stages of renal failure become hypertensive due to poor kidney perfusion and function, probably caused by renal ischemia.

62. (1) The infant's eyes are covered with patches during treatment because of the possibility of damage to the retina. The light is warm, so the baby will not be fully dressed. This condition is not contagious, so isolation is not indicated.

63. (4) Physiologic jaundice shows up as the bilirubin level in the blood rises. As liver function increases, bilirubin is excreted and blood levels of bilirubin go down.

64. (3) As the patient experiences memory gaps, he fills them with stories unsubstantiated by facts to preserve his self-esteem, not lower it.

65. (1) Realizing that the patient could require surgical removal of an existing stone, the nurse places him NPO as a precautionary measure.

66. (1) The patient's urine should be measured and strained for stones. If surgery is anticipated, the patient will be maintained NPO regardless of the status of his nausea.

67. (1) Anaphylactic reactions have occurred in patients with hypersensitivity to iodine derivatives from the intravenous dye used for the pyelogram. If he is allergic to shellfish, which contains iodine, he may well be allergic to the dye.

68. (2) High Fowler's position allows for good lung expansion, as well as decreasing venous return from the lower extremities.

69. (3) These are classic symptoms of an allergic reaction. Answer (2) lists symptoms of a hemolytic reaction. All other symptoms listed are a combination of allergic and transfusion reactions.

70. (4) If the nurse suspects an allergic reaction, the blood should be shut off immediately, and then the charge nurse and the physician should be notified.

71. (1) Persons with hyperthyroidism are hyperactive, nervous, and irritable; provision for adequate rest is a major nursing challenge.

72. (4) Respiratory distress may occur, so it is important to keep a tracheostomy tray at the bedside. Other common postoperative complications are laryngeal nerve damage and tetany or hypocalcemia.

73. (3) You want to avoid strain on the sutures, which could cause bleeding. This position will not prevent respiratory distress, but will help relieve it.

74. (3) This reflective response will open communication and enable the patient to express whatever concerns or feelings she has without confining her to a discussion of dying (2).

75. (1) The highest priority is observing for changes in physical status and then giving the patient emotional support. Supporting the family is part of your role as a nurse, but contacting the lawyer is not your responsibility.

76. (2) This is a method that involves infusion of a solution of protein, glucose, electrolytes, vitamins, and minerals—complete nutrition by the intravenous route.

77. (2) OBS patients require frequent orientation to reality as they forget recent events. They should be encouraged to function independently in a safe, structured environment. The daily schedule should be planned and predictable.

78. (2) Regression is a way to reduce anxiety and cope with different situations by going back to a time when the patient felt more safe, secure, and comfortable.

79. (2) Gallbladder and liver functions are stimulated by ingestion of fats, so they will be restricted. Juices and carbohydrates will be included in the diet.

80. (2)   It is important to use a Laird tip on the catheter and irrigate no higher than shoulder height to reduce the risk of perforation.

81. (1)   Critical reduction of blood supply to the myocardium for a prolonged period results in sustained oxygen deprivation. As a result, cardiac muscle is destroyed.

82. (2)   Death-producing arrhythmias must be treated immediately with lidocaine or another antiarrhythmic medication. Although a narcotic analgesic will also be given to decrease pain and a nitroglycerin IV drip will probably be started, these medications are not the priority.

83. (4)   The nurse recognizes the mother's feelings, but tries to show that they are not based on fact.

84. (1)   The gastrostomy tube is returned to gravity drainage until the infant can tolerate feedings. After the second or third day, the gastrostomy tube is pinned to the infant's shirt, above the level of the stomach. This prevents draining of stomach contents out through the tube.

85. (2)   Anticoagulants are administered to decrease the occurrence of venous thrombosis and emboli, as well as to prevent the extension of a clot that has already formed.

86. (3)   A soft diet decreases bulk and promotes elimination of solid wastes. Ease in defecation prevents straining and an increased workload for the heart.

87. (4)   Patches of sclerotic tissue and nerve degeneration occur in the area of myelin sheath destruction.

88. (2)   The patient should avoid fatigue, stress, and exposure to infection. She should have a regular program of exercise and rest, with adequate activity.

89. (4)   Dextrostix results yield data about the blood glucose level; this is essential data for monitoring hypoglycemia in the infant of a diabetic mother.

90. (4)   Semi-Fowler's position with her arm elevated will enhance lymphatic and venous drainage of fluid in the affected arm.

91. (4)   All of the information is accurate regarding radiation; however, the patient's initial symptoms usually are related to GI function. She should not be told about pneumonitis but could be told to report any unusual symptoms. Answer (2) is technical and not necessary for patient understanding of the disease process.

92. (3)   The patient is instructed to look upward while the eyedrops are placed in the center of the lower eyelid. In order to accomplish this, the patient needs to keep her eye open and be careful to not touch the lid. Contamination of the eyedropper will occur if it touches the lid.

93. (2)   Semi-Fowler's position is the most appropriate to facilitate breathing. Some children prefer being on their abdomen, which is also acceptable.

94. (3)   Every newborn receives silver nitrate 1%, or more commonly, a broad spectrum antibiotic such as erythromycin in the eyes. The purpose of this is to prevent blindness caused by the mother having a sexually transmitted disease, such as Chlamydia or gonorrhea.

95. (3)   Infants with signs and symptoms of hypoglycemia usually have a high-pitched cry.

96. (1)   The patient is simply refusing to accept her terminal illness to protect herself from the unpleasant reality of possible death. Denial is a stage of the grief process.

97. (3)   Vitamin K is necessary for blood coagulation. The newborn has a transitory deficiency in the clotting ability of the blood. Bacteria are necessary for the production of vitamin K in the intestines, and bacteria are not present in

sufficient numbers in the newborn until several days after birth.

98. (1) Myocardial infarction results from a sustained interruption in the blood flow to the myocardium. Administering oxygen helps relieve pain, prevent arrhythmias, and minimize myocardial necrosis. Caution must be used if the patient has chronic obstructive lung disease.

99. (1) Oxygen itself does not burn, but, if it is present, it will allow a small fire to spread rapidly.

100. (3) An important goal for depressed patients is to keep them busy with a structured schedule. It may be too early for the patient to join a group, and cleaning the kitchen may not increase self-esteem.

101. (3) According to the Rule of Nines, Mr. Abram's right arm would be considered as 9 percent; his abdomen, 9 percent; and his back, 18 percent, for a total of 36 percent. Burn degree is not taken into account.

102. (2) Water loss occurs from fluid moving from the vascular compartment in the burned area to interstitial tissues surrounding the burned area, causing edema.

103. (2) Paralytic ileus, a neurogenic type of obstruction of the bowel, can occur due to traumatic disturbance of the autonomic nervous system.

104. (3) A diet high in protein and carbohydrates is essential so that the protein is available for tissue-cell rebuilding and repair. Sodium is not a factor for burn diets.

105. (1) Toddlers are interested in all things within their reach, and they will explore and indiscriminately put items in their mouths. All dangerous substances and items should be made safety proof. Children at this age will

automatically get a lot of exercise (2). There is no danger of spoiling a child with love.

106. (3) During the time the reaction occurs, patients are taken off radiation therapy and instructed to use antibiotic lotion and steroid cream to prevent infection.

107. (1) These foods are difficult to digest and can be irritating to the GI tract. They can lead to additional GI symptoms.

108. (1) At six months, a child should be sitting with minimal support. Often, with retarded children, their flaccid muscles and loose joints prevent the attainment of simple developmental milestones. The ability to sit is one of the most important milestones.

109. (1) Parents cannot be expected to make decisions and long-term plans for the child while they are still experiencing grief. The focus of nursing should be on accepting parents' feelings and promoting communication.

110. (4) Intermittent positive pressure breathing raises intrathoracic pressure, compressing the heart and thoracic vessels. The sympathetic nervous system recognizes any drop in blood pressure and responds by increasing the heart rate to compensate for the deceased cardiac output and decreased venous return to the heart.

111. (4) Forcing fluids is necessary to liquefy secretions so that the IPPB therapy can be as effective as possible.

112. (2) Because of the diabetes and normal changes caused by pregnancy, there is usually an increased need for insulin in the second and third trimesters.

113. (4) White blood cells and red blood cells are usually present in urine samples from patients with cystitis. White blood cells are a response to the inflammation; the irritation of the

mucosa and irritation of the urethra cause bleeding.

114. (2) The nurse should evaluate the possibility of a nursing or laboratory identification error, then have the test repeated.

115. (2) The nurse paraphrases the patient's comments to give feedback, to show an understanding of what was said, and to encourage the patient to continue expressing feelings.

116. (4) At three months, an infant is able to focus on objects or people.

117. (1) Sublingual administration allows for rapid absorption, which is of prime importance in the treatment of angina. Sublingual administration of nitroglycerin relieves anginal pain in one to three minutes.

118. (3) Nitroglycerin should be kept in a dark, tightly closed jar. The potency is six months, not three.

119. (4) This activity would channel her energy, but would not increase external stimuli as group activities would do.

120. (3) Antiembolic stockings and leg exercises are the best means of preventing thrombus formation. Total ROM is not appropriate, as the hip must remain in abduction. ASA is given, not Tylenol, as an anticoagulant.

121. (1) Iron and folacin cannot be ingested in sufficient quantities by dietary means; thus, they must be supplemented during pregnancy. Additional vitamins, C and B complex, and minerals may be appropriate, but they are not critical daily nutrients.

122. (4) Because an incision has been made into the abdomen, hemorrhage is occasionally a complication of abdominal surgery.

123. (3) A normal pulse rate for a five-year-old child is 100; elevated temperature is not a sign of digoxin toxicity.

124. (3) A regular nipple is too hard and will make it difficult for the infant to suck, causing unnecessary fatigue. A soft premie nipple should be used.

125. (4) The nurse, while recognizing and accepting this mother's apprehension, assures her that she will have assistance.

126. (2) Hearing the rush of air in the stomach is the best indicator that proper tube placement has occurred. Though answer (4) is partially correct, it does not definitely indicate that the tube is in the correct position.

127. (2) Unrestricted fluids are usually given by mouth to help flush the bladder. The amount of output will help evaluate the function of the kidneys, and adequate fluid intake will decrease the irritation of the bladder mucosa.

128. (2) One of the most common causative organisms is Escherichia coli, which is normal bowel flora and may be the result of poor perineal hygiene. Restricting her activity and fluids may lead to calculi formation. Limiting certain foods is not likely to affect bladder pH. Drinking more juices, especially cranberry, will help to maintain normal pH.

129. (4) Insulin does not cross into the milk. The mother's calorie intake needs to be adjusted with an increase in protein intake. Insulin must be adjusted and care must be exercised during weaning.

130. (2) Early postpartum is a crucial period, for the placenta contains the hormone insulinase, which blocks the use of insulin during pregnancy.

131. (1) Adolescents need information about their bodies and what to expect.

132. (3) The patient's energy should be conserved to enable the body to use all of its resources for fighting the disease. Fluid intake should be at least 3000 ml per day.

133. (2)   Pneumonia may be caused by a virus, bacteria, or fungi, which would be present in the secretions. Universal precautions are always good nursing care, but there is no rule that they must be observed for pneumonia.

134. (4)   Most newborns are awake for eating and care only. The mother should not worry if the infant sleeps most of the time because this is normal.

135. (3)   The respiratory system can become occluded if the balloon slips and moves up the esophagus, putting pressure on the trachea. This would result in respiratory distress. Scissors should be kept at the bedside so that the tube can be cut if distress occurs.

136. (3)   Infants should double their birth weight by five to six months of age.

137. (3)   The hip should be kept in abduction to prevent flexion. The hip must not be in acute flexion. If the affected leg is elevated, flexion of the hip occurs and this could cause dislocation of the hip. Position should be changed frequently and can be done by raising or lowering head of the bed.

138. (2)   You will observe for hemorrhage during the first few hours. Later you may observe for infection. It is also important to check for patency of the Hemovac.

139. (3)   Setting limits is important to prevent the patient from being rejected by others, with subsequent lowering of self-esteem.

140. (1)   Classical manifestations of mild preeclampsia (also called pregnancy-induced hypertension or PIH) are elevated blood pressure, proteinuria, and edema.

141. (2)   Hyperreflexia occurs with increased irritation of the central nervous system. Epigastric pain is usually due to edema or bleeding into the liver capsule. Other signs include oliguria, edema, and hypertension.

142. (4)   Pain is due to contraction of the gallbladder, which has stones present. The gallbladder empties when fat is present in the stomach. The gallbladder is located in the upper right side of the abdomen along the side of the liver.

143. (4)   Counterpressure provides much pain relief by supporting the sacrum as the fetus's head is driven down by the contraction. Also try positional changes. Knee-chest position often provides pain relief. It is too early for any analgesics.

144. (2)   Muscle weakness is an expected side effect and one that the patient may have to live with. Dehydration is not a side effect, and drowsiness is a toxic side effect. A usual side effect is polyuria, not anuria.

145. (3)   A peanut butter sandwich has 12 gm of protein, more than the other foods. A teenager requires 78 gm of protein a day.

146. (3)   The increased energy and nutritional demands of pregnancy require approximately 300 additional calories a day.

147. (1)   Changing the position to prone three times a day will encourage optimal functioning. The position protocol is 2 hours on the unaffected side, 20 minutes on the affected side, and 30 minutes prone t.i.d. Prolonged pressure on the affected side contributes to contractures, deformities, and decubitus ulcers due to loss of motor tone and circulation.

148. (1)   The highest priority is to protect the patient from self-injury by providing a safe milieu to prevent suicide. The other goals are also important, but have lower priority.

149. (4)   It is imperative that the child know how to drink from a cup, since that is the only way the child can drink following this surgery.

150. (3)   While the gastrostomy tube is in place, the mother cannot breast feed. It is important,

however, to continue the flow of milk so that when the baby is ready, breast feeding can be resumed.

151. (4)   Parnate is an MAO inhibitor and cannot be taken with foods high in tyramine, such as cheese, wine, and chocolate. Answers (1) and (2) refer to tricyclic medications. MAO medications should never be taken with alcohol or other medications.

152. (4)   The nurse should always check the pulse rate prior to administering digoxin because of its slowing effect on the heart.

153. (2)   The most effective method of preventing pulmonary complications is to instruct the patient to turn, cough, and deep breathe frequently.

154. (2)   Contraceptive methods must be thoroughly understood if they are to be used properly and prevent pregnancy. Both partners should be informed.

155. (3)   You must ensure that the peripheral circulation is intact. The other activities are completed but are not considered priority.

156. (3)   Head tilt with neck lift is the first action. Forceful mouth-to-mouth ventilation should only be used as a last resort in clearing an airway obstruction. This action may blow an obstruction past the narrow point of the airway (larynx and epiglottis) and provide a partial airway. An endotracheal tube would be inserted if the airway cannot be cleared.

157. (2)   Patients will have a low-grade temperature, tenderness in the lower right quadrant, and nausea and vomiting unrelated to eating. Pain is primarily in the lower right quadrant.

158. (2)   Semi-Fowler's position relieves abdominal pain and tension. Ice is used to decrease pain. Heat is never used because it could cause the appendix to rupture, thus causing peritonitis.

159. (3)   Before surgery for appendicitis, she will be kept NPO to decrease peristalsis and avoid more pressure on the appendix.

160. (3)   Since one of the suspected side effects of the pill is thrombophlebitis, it is important to know the patient's history. If the history indicates a predisposition, the pill would not be the contraceptive method of choice. Regardless of her age, she may obtain contraceptive counseling. Names of sexual contacts are important for tracing sexually transmitted diseases.

161. (3)   A preschooler can understand simple directions. Although a five-year-old may be quiet and shy, these qualities are not applicable to this situation.

162. (3)   The log-rolling method is essential to maintain alignment of the spine. Abduction is the position for total hip replacement.

163. (1)   A patient's response (or lack thereof) to verbal stimuli is the best indicator of unconsciousness. An unconscious patient's pupils may continue to react to light. Pinching the lobe of the ear offers little in the way of pain stimuli. Opening the airway is not an appropriate stimulus.

164. (2)   You should take 4 to 10 seconds to check unresponsiveness in a patient who appears to be unconscious. Give the patient a chance to awaken and respond.

165. (1)   Ordering meals in this manner allows the child some independence and control, while providing an excellent teaching opportunity.

166. (4)   The jaw-thrust maneuver would be the best choice for opening an airway in a patient with a suspected neck injury. This can be done with the patient's neck and head in a neutral position, thus not further endangering the spine.

167. (1) One-half cup of peanuts has twice as much protein as one cup of milk or the beef jerky. Apples contain very little protein.

168. (3) Recovery of language is related to frequent attempts to communicate with a responsive listener. Allowing the patient to use her own form of communication to express needs encourages further attempts to communicate. Pantomime is useful but should not replace verbal communication.

169. (3) Homonymous hemianopsia is a common visual deficiency associated with hemiplegia. Loss of the visual field must be compensated for by the patient's increased conscious awareness of hazards to personal safety.

170. (2) A posterior fetal position often causes severe back pain and a bearing-down sensation during contractions.

171. (1) Patients are positioned in semi-Fowler's position to promote drainage. The T-tube can be clamped before meals to accumulate enough bile for digestion. The drainage bottle is positioned below the level of the bed to facilitate drainage.

172. (3) Patients with high abdominal incisions tend to splint and do not like to cough and deep breathe because of associated pain. Pneumonia can be a complication related to this surgery.

173. (4) This breakfast has the lowest total grams of fat. The egg will provide some of the daily allotment of protein necessary for tissue building. Fat in the diet should be avoided for at least several weeks postoperatively.

174. (2) The primary goal of activity is to mobilize the patient. Activity has the effect of lifting the depression through the mind-body interaction.

175. (2) Electrolytes (potassium) are measured in mEq/L, and 3.5 to 5.5 mEq/L is the normal serum potassium level.

176. (2) Maintaining adequate bladder drainage will assist with rinsing out debris, such as blood clots, following the surgery. The catheter must remain patent in order to achieve this goal. Hemostasis can also occur if bleeding should be evident; however, this is not the primary function of the irrigation.

177. (3) Bethanechol chloride (Urecholine) stimulates the parasympathetic nervous system. It increases the tone and motility of the smooth muscles of the urinary tract, thus it is used frequently following a transurethral resection (TUR) when the patient has a lack of muscle tone and is unable to void. Bladder spasms can be relieved with Belladonna or opium suppositories.

178. (3) Taking iodine following a meal and with at least 8 ounces of water will dilute the medication and minimize gastric distress.

179. (3) These are signs of a systemic anticholinergic effect. In addition to these symptoms, the patient may experience loss of sight, difficulty breathing, flushing, or eye pain. If these symptoms occur, the medication must be discontinued and the physician notified.

180. (3) The two nurses positioned in the front will receive the patient as he is turned. The nurse in back maintains the patient's alignment during the turning process.

INDEX

A antigens: testing for, 110–11
Abbreviations: for drug orders, 88
Abdominal pregnancy, 316
Abducens nerves, 121
ABO blood groups, 50; incompatibilities, 354, 355; testing, 110–11
Abortion: complications of, 344–45, 362, 363; spontaneous, 314–15; therapeutic, 28, 362–63
Abruptio placentae, 317
Abscesses: diagnosis of, 124
Absence seizures, 135, 136–37, 396, 397
Abuse behavior: nursing approaches to, 440, 453
Abused children, 28, 416–17
Accessory nerves, 121
Accidents, 432; childhood, 417
Acetazolamide, 151
Acetest, 230
Acetone breath odor, 223, 231, 233
Acetone in urine, 223, 230
Acetylcholine, 138, 139, 155, 291
Acid ash diet, 98
Acid-base balance, 46–50; imbalances in, 110, 188. See also pH
Acid-fast bacilli: gastric washings for, 114, 201
Acidifiers, 73
Acidosis: diabetic, 99, 113; metabolic, 47, 110, 318; respiratory, 48–49, 110
Acne, 384
Acoustic nerves, 121
Acquired immunodeficiency syndrome. See AIDS
Acrocyanosis: in newborn, 350
Acromegaly, 223–24
Activated charcoal, 399
Active exercise: defined, 63
Active transport, 43
Acute brain syndrome, 290
Acute closed-angle glaucoma, 149–51
Acute gastritis, 204–5
Acute glomerulonephritis, 219, 401
Acute infectious diseases: in pregnancy, 322. See also Infections
Acute lymphocytic leukemia (ALL), 174
Acute myelogenous leukemia (AML), 173, 174
Acute pancreatitis, 215
Acute pulmonary diseases, 185–87
Acute pulmonary edema, 166–67
Acute renal failure, 217–18
Adaptation, 10–11
Addiction: alcohol, 442–43; drug, 443–45
Addisonian crisis, 225, 226
Addison's disease, 116, 222, 223, 225
Adhesions, 209

Adolescents: alcoholism in, 442; assessment of, 381–82, 384; death and, 24; disorders of, 411–15; hospitalization of, 381; immunizations of, 420; nutrition for, 419; personality development, 22; physical development, 19, 378–79, 422; pregnant, 311, 323; sexual development of, 25; social development, 19–20. See also Children; Pediatric nursing
Adrenal cortex: in pregnancy, 309
Adrenal corticoid treatment: dietary therapy, 99
Adrenalectomy, 226–27
Adrenal gland: disorders of, 222, 225–27; surgical procedure, 226–27
Adrenalin. See Epinephrine
Adrenergics, 72
Adrenocorticosteroids, 58
Adulthood, 20–21; death and dying and, 24; sexuality and, 26–28. See also Parenting
Affect, 435, 453
Affective disorders, 428–31
Afferent nerves, 120, 121, 122
Ageism, 284
Aggression: defined, 453; nursing approaches to, 440
Aging: assessment of, 287–88; death concept in the aged, 24; defined, 284; developmental tasks of, 21; disorders of, 290–93; drug-food interactions and, 298; drugs and, 296–98; factors influencing, 285; fears of the aged, 284; general principles of, 284; immobility problems, 293–95; lab values in the aged, 298–99; major problems of, 22; nursing implementation, 287–90; nutrition and, 100–101, 295–96; physiological changes of, 22, 285–87, 295–96; process of, 284–87; psychological changes of, 22–23, 287; psychosocial changes of, 22–23, 287, 288; sensory impairment and, 285, 295; theories of, 284–85
Agoraphobia, 434
Agranulocytosis, 173, 445
AIDS, 175–76; HIV antibody test, 117; mothers and newborns with, 353
Airway: cardiopulmonary resuscitation and, 279–80; maintaining, 181, 188; structure and function of, 177; suctioning, 191
Akathisia, 446
Akinesia, 140
Akinetic seizures, 136–37, 396, 397
Albumin: serum, 115, 156; urine testing for, 113, 114
Albuminuria levels, 114
Albuterol, 406
Alcohol: addiction to, 442–43; cancer and, 260; central nervous system effects of, 71; cirrhosis from, 214; fetal alcohol syndrome, 357

Aldomet, 159
Aldosterone: aging process and, 286; in pregnancy, 309
Alimentary tract, 198–200. See also Gastrointestinal system
Alkaline phosphatase, 115
Alkalinizers, 73
Alkalosis: metabolic, 47–48, 110; respiratory, 49–50, 110
Alkylating agents, 266
Allergens: defined, 71
Allergies: anaphylactic shock and, 272, 274–75; asthma and, 182, 406; contact dermatitis, 237–38, 383; eczema, 238; to gluten, 394–95; hay fever, 432; in infants, 383; poison ivy, oak, and sumac, 237; stress and, 10; to transfusions, 52
Alopecia: from chemotherapy, 267
Alphachymotrypsin, 148
Alpha hydroxybutyric dehydrogenase, 10
Alveoli, 177, 178, 179; disorders of, 58, 179, 183, 186, 354, 398
Alzheimer's disease, 291–93
Amantadine, 140
Ambiguous genitalia, 26
Ambivalence, 435, 453
Ambulation: postoperative, 255–57
Amenorrhea, 304, 311
American Nurses' Association (ANA), 461
Amino acids, 90, 92; metabolism abnormalities diet, 97
Aminophylline, 197, 275, 406
Ammonia: for fainting, 71; liver function and, 115–16, 212, 213
Amnesia, 438, 453
Amniocentesis, 325–26
Amniocentesis abortion, 363
Amniography, 315
Amnion, 304–5
Amniotic fluid, 305, 319; meconium staining of, 325, 331
Amniotomy, 335
Amphetamines, 444
Amphiarthroses, 245
Amputation, 252–53, 257
Amylase, 93
Amylopsin, 93
Amyotrophic lateral sclerosis, 144
Analgesics: central nervous system effects of, 71; defined, 41; in labor, 339–41; narcotic, 56–57, 71
Anaphylactic shock, 272, 274–75. See also Bee stings
Anastomosis, 207, 391
Androgens, 225
Androgynous nature, 25
Android pelvis, 303
Anemia: alcoholism and, 442; aplastic, 172; diet for, 99; hemolytic, 355; in infants, 393–94; in newborn, 348, 351, 355; per-

516

Electrolytes. *See* Fluid and electrolytes

Electromyography (EMG), 125

Electronic monitoring: of fetus, 332–3333

Electroshock therapy, 449, 453

Electrosurgery, 262

ELISA test, 117

Elixirs, 74

Embolisms: fat, 62; preventing, 248; pulmonary, 61–62, 192

Embryo: development of, 304, 306

Emergency nursing, 187–88, 270–81; bee sting, 276; burns, 277–78; cardiopulmonary resuscitation, 279–81; chest injury assessment, 187–88; choking, 276–77; cold exposure, 277; consent requirements, 459; delivery of baby, 338–39; disasters, 270; first aid care, 270–71; fractures, 278; heat exposure, 277; poisoning, 277; shock, 272–74; snake bite, 275–76; sprains and strains, 278–79; tourniquets, 167, 276; wounds, 271–72

Emetics, 72

EMG, 125

Emotional disorders. *See* Mental health nursing

Emotions: development of, 379; postpartum, 342–43; in pregnancy, 309; regulation of, 121

Emphysema, 183

Emulsions, 74

Encephalitis, 131

Encephalopathy: acute, 406–7

Endarterectomy: carotid, 132

Endocarditis: bacterial, 168

Endocardium, 152

Endocrine glands, 222

Endocrine hormones, 222, 224

Endocrine system, 222–35

Endogenous creatinine clearance, 112

Endolymphatic system: dilatation of, 143

Endometriosis, 358–59

Endometritis, 345

Endometrium, 302, 303, 305; cancer of, 360

Endoscopy, 201

Endotracheal tube: suctioning infant with, 354

Enema: barium, 201; after hemorrhoidectomy, 211

Engagement: in labor, 324, 329

Engle, George, 23

Enteric coated tablets, 74

Enteritis: diet for, 100

Enterokinase, 93

Enteropathy: gluten-induced, 116, 394–95

Enucleation, 256

Envenomation, 275

Enzyme-linked immunosorbent assay (ELISA) test, 117

Enzymes, 58; digestive, 93, 199; from heart muscle damage, 109; kidney, 216; liver

function and, 115, 212; serum, 158

Ependymoma, 407

Ephedrine, 197

Epicardium, 152

Epidermis, 236; inflammation of, 238

Epididymitis, 22

Epidural block, 340

Epidural hematomas, 130–31

Epiglottis, 177

Epilepsy, 135–37, 396–97

Epinephrine: for anaphylactic shock, 275, 276; for asthma, 406; as cardiovascular drug, 162; as ophthalmic drug, 151; for respiration, 197–98; from sympathetic nervous system, 155

Epiphysis, 244

Episiotomy, 333–34, 342

Epithelioma: basal cell, 242–43

Epstein-Barr virus antibodies (EBV) test, 117

Epstein's pearls, 349

Equanil, 446, 452

Erepsin, 93

Erikson's stages of personality development, 22

Erythema, 236, 243

Erythematosus: lupus, 241–42

Erythrocytes (red blood cells), 156; formation of, 156, 244; in labor and postpartum, 342; testing, 106, 113; in urine, 113–14

Erythrocyte sedimentation rate (ESR), 106

Esophagogastroduodenoscopy (EGD), 201

Esophagus, 199; atresia of, 385; cancer of, 204, 260; hernia of, 204; infection of, 203; irritation of, 203; varices of, 203

Estriol level: in pregnancy, 325

Estrogen: aging and, 286; drug preparations of, 367; menstrual cycle and, 303, 304; in oral contraceptives, 364; pregnancy and, 305, 307, 309

Ethopropazine, 140

Euphoria: defined, 453

Euthanasia: defined, 461

Evisceration, 60

Ewing's sarcoma, 408–9

Exchange transfusion, 355

Exenteration: pelvic, 257, 360–61

Exercises: for the aged, 290; for amputation patients, 252; coronary artery disease and, 162; for diabetes mellitus patients, 232–33; for knee surgery patient, 251–52; for myasthenia gravis patients, 139; perineal, 221; pregnancy and, 376–77; rehabilitative, 63–64; for spinal cord injury patients, 130; for thoracic surgery patients, 192

Exertional dyspnea (DOE), 156

Exfoliative cytology, 262

Exhibitionists, 439

Exocrine cells (pancreas), 200

Exophthalmic goiter, 227, 228

Expected date of confinement (EDC), 307

Expectorants, 58, 73

Expiration (breathing), 178

Expiratory reserve volume (ERV), 178

External auditory canal: irrigation of, 152

External os, 302

External rotation of hip, 65, 293–94

Extracellular fluid volume, 42

Extrapyramidal disease, 448

Extrapyramidal structures, 121, 140

Extrauterine pregnancy, 316

Eyes: aging process and, 285, 288, 295; conditions of, 148–51, 295; fetal development of, 306; foreign body removal from, 150–51; instilling drops in, 150; neurologic control of, 121; sunset, 385; surgical positions and ambulation, 256; surgical procedures, 148, 149, 150; testing, 384; of unconscious or immobilized patients, 126–27

Face: "butterfly", 242; moon, 226; pain from trigeminal neuralgia, 142; paralysis of, 142–43; pregnancy and, 308

Face presentation: in delivery, 337

Failure to thrive, 387

Fainting, 71, 157

Fallopian tubes, 302, 304; ligation of, 365; pelvic inflammatory disease and, 359; in pregnancy, 307

False imprisonment: defined, 461

False labor, 325, 328

False pelvis, 302

False pregnancy, 312

Family planning. *See* Parenting

Fantasy: defined, 450

Fat bodies: in urine, 114

Fat embolism, 62

Father: assuming role of, 309, 343. *See also* Parenting

Fatigue: in cardiovascular disease, 156; general nursing care for, 176; in pregnancy, 312, 376; psychosomatic, 432; shock and, 61, 273

Fat necrosis, 134

Fats: cancer and, 260; diets that control, 97–98; as essential nutrient, 90, 92; metabolism of, 92–93, 115; therapeutic recommendations, 95

Fatty acids, 90; pregnancy and, 311

Fear: in the aged, 284; of the dark, 384; defined, 454. *See also* Phobic disorders

Fecal impaction, 209

Federal Food, Drug, and Cosmetic Act of 1938, 84–85

Feedback: defined, 37

Felony, 461

Female reproductive system: anatomy and

Motor nerves, 120, 121, 122, 246
Mouth, 198; cancer of, 203; inflammation of, 203; ulcerative lesions in, 176; of unconscious or immobilized patients, 127
MRI, 124
Mucokinetic agents, 198
Mucolytic agents, 58
Mucomyst, 198
Mucous gland, 199
Mucous membranes: drug absorption by, 68; of ventilation tract, 177, 178
Mucous plug: cervical, 307
Mucus discharge: in female newborn, 349
Multigravida, 325, 335
Multi-infarct dementia, 292
Multipara, 327, 329, 335
Multiple pregnancies, 305
Multiple sclerosis, 137–38
Mumps, 421; immunization against, 420
Muscles: cardiac muscle, 122, 155; contractures of, 65, 248, 294; controlling movement of, 121, 122; convulsions and, 134–35; of newborn, 350, 351; weakness of, 61, 137–40, 144, 273. See also Motor function
Muscle setting exercise: defined, 63
Musculoskeletal system, 244–55; aging process and, 286–87, 288, 289–90; anatomy and physiology of, 244–47, 378; assessment of, 288, 382; disorders of, 247–55, 413–14, 432; surgical positions and ambulation, 267; surgical procedures, 251–53; unconscious or immobilized patients and, 126. See also Motor function
Mustard procedure, 389
Mute behavior, 436
Myasthenia gravis, 138–40
Myasthenic crisis, 139, 140
Mycobacterium tuberculosis, 187
Mydriatics, 151
Myelin sheath, 120, 137, 143
Myelocytic leukemia: chronic, 173–74
Myelogenous leukemia: acute, 173, 174
Myelography, 123
Myelomas, 261
Myocardial infarction, 164–65
Myocarditis, 168
Myocardium, 152, 153
Myoclonic seizures, 135–37, 396, 397
Myometrium, 302
Myoneural junction, 246
Myringotomy, 390
Myxedema, 116, 223, 227

Nägele's rule, 307
Nails: aging process and, 286, 289; blanching of, 250; fetal development of, 306
Nalline hydrochloride, 368
Narcan, 368

Narcotic addiction, 443–45
Narcotic analgesics, 56–57, 71
Nardil, 447, 452
Nasal. See Nose
Nasogastric tube: management of, 206, 207; metabolic alkalosis and, 48; for nutrient feeding, 94–96; purpose of, 206
Nasopharynx, 177, 198
Nasotracheal suctioning, 196
National Association of Practical Nurse Education and Service, Inc. (NAPNES), 461
National Council Licensure Examination (NCLEX): overview, 2–6; review guidelines, 6–8; test-taking strategies, 7–8
National Federation of Licensed Practical Nurses (NFLPN), 461
National League for Nurses (NLN), 461
National Mental Act, 424
Natural childbirth, 310
Nausea, 202; in pregnancy, 308, 311, 312, 317–18
NCLEX. See National Council Licensure Examination (NCLEX)
Neck righting reflex, 419
Needle aspiration, 261
Negativism, 436, 454
Negligence, 460
Neisseria gonorrhoeae, 30–31
Neonate. See Newborn
Neoplasms: benign and malignant, 261. See also Cancer; Oncology nursing
Nephrectomy, 219, 257
Nephroblastoma, 395
Nephrolithotomy, 257
Nephrons, 216
Nephropathy, 231
Nephrostomy, 219, 256
Nephrotic crisis, 401
Nephrotic syndrome, 401
Nerve blocks, 340–41
Nerve fibers, 120
Nerves: cranial, 121; disorders of, 142–44; motor, 120, 121, 122, 246; spinal, 121–22
Nervous system. See Neurologic system
Neuralgia: trigeminal, 142
Neurectomy, 41
Neurogenic shock, 60, 272
Neuroglia cells, 120
Neurolemma cells, 120
Neuroleptic drugs, 445–46
Neurologic system, 120–52; aging process and, 285, 287–88; conditions of, 125–44, 432; diagnostic procedures, 123–25; of newborn, 347, 350; positions for neurological conditions, 147, 255; surgical procedures, 41, 128, 144–47. See also Autonomic nervous system; Central nervous system
Neurons: structure and function of, 120

Neuropathy, 231
Neuroses, 433, 446
Neurosurgery, 41, 128, 144–47
Neurotic anxiety, 425
Neutrophils, 156
Newborn, 346–57; with AIDS, 353; Apgar scoring, 347; caring for, 346–48; circulation of, 388; congenital anomalies, 382, 384–90; diseases affecting, 353–57; feeding, 350–51; physical characteristics of, 348–50, 378; premature, 351–52, 372–73; reflexes in, 419; small for gestational age, 352–53; universal precautions for, 346; vital signs of, 422. See also Children; Infants; Pediatric nursing
Niacin: deficiency in, 94; food sources of, 92, 298, 375. See also Vitamins
Niamid, 447, 452
Nicotine. See Smoking; Tobacco
Nifedipine, 159
Nipride, 160
Nisentil, 368
Nitroglycerin, 163–64
Nitrosoureas, 266
Norepinephrine, 155
Norpace, 162
Norpramin, 446–47, 452
Numorphan, 57
Nurse-patient relationship, 36
Nurse Practice Act, 458
Nursery: care of newborn in, 347–48
Nursing. See Breast feeding
Nursing contracts, 460
Nursing diagnosis, 35
Nursing process, 3
Nutrition, 90–104; for the aged, 100–101, 289, 295–96; alcoholism and, 442, 443; assessment of, 102; assimilation of nutrients, 91–93; basic four food groups, 93, 103–4; cancer and, 260; eating disorders, 202, 414–15; essential nutrients, 90–91, 92; hospital-based problems, 94; for infants, 418; malnutrition, 94, 100–101, 419; for newborn, 350–51, 352, 372; postoperative, 56, 100, 101; for pregnancy, 97, 99, 100–101, 310–11, 313, 374–76; for premature infants, 352, 372; preoperative, 101; recommended daily dietary allowances, 93; therapeutic, 93, 96–101; tube feeding, 94–96; for unconscious or immobilized patients, 126, 127. See also Appetite; Calories; Diets; Food; Nasogastric tube
Nutritional marasmus, 94

Obesity, 432; adolescent, 384, 411; cancer and, 260; chest wall compliance and, 180; coronary artery disease and, 162; diet for, 100; endocrine disorders and, 222, 226
Obsession: defined, 454

cle (boil), 238–39; herpes simplex, 31, 239, 323; herpes zoster, 239; impetigo, 238; radiodermatitis, 263–64; rashes, 383, 412; syphilis, 242. *See also* Burns
Skin test: tuberculin, 181, 187
Skull, 121
Skull fractures, 130–31
Skull series, 123
Slander, 461
Sleep: newborn and, 350; regulation of, 121
Small for gestational age newborn, 352–53
Small intestine, 199; diagnostic procedures, 200–201; resection of, 256; surgical procedures, 209–10
Smell sense: aging process and, 295; in newborn, 350
Smoking: cancer and, 260; coronary artery disease and, 162; fetal growth and, 376; peripheral vascular problems and, 171
Smooth muscle, 122
Snake bites, 71, 275–76
Snellen vision testing, 384
SOAP charting, 35
Social development, 12–19
Social deviate personality types, 439
Socialization therapy, 449
Social phobia, 434
Sociopathic personality, 438–40
Soda bicarbonate, 48, 72
Sodium: foods high in, 99, 374; imbalance in, 44–45, 107; pregnancy and, 311, 319, 321, 374; restriction of, 99; testing, 107, 112. *See also* Minerals
Sodium nitroprusside, 160
Soft diet, 101
Somatic neurons, 120
Somatoform disorders, 431–33
Somogyi effect, 232
Sonography, 312, 315, 326
Spasms, 123; infantile, 397
Specific gravity: in the aged, 298; testing, 112, 113
Sperm, 304
Sphincters: cardiac, 199; pyloric, 199
Spider bites, 71
Spider nevi, 308
Spina bifida, 386
Spinal block, 340
Spinal cord: diagnostic procedures, 123, 125; structure and function of, 121; surgical procedures, 253. *See also* Central nervous system (CNS)
Spinal cord injuries, 128–30; sexuality and, 28
Spinal fusion, 253, 257
Spinal nerves, 121–22
Spinal shock, 129, 130
Spine: curvature of, 413–14; fusion of, 253, 257. *See also* Musculoskeletal system
Spirits, 74

Spleen, 156; rupture of, 175; sequestration crisis, 392
Splenomegaly, 412, 413
Splinting, 278
Spontaneous abortion, 314–15
Spots: floating, in retinal detachment, 148
Sprains, 278
Sputum: bloody, 157, 181, 182; examination of, 180–81
Squamous cell carcinoma, 243
Staging, 262
Stapedectomy, 151–52, 256
Staphylococcus infections: furuncle, 238–39; impetigo, 238; mastitis, 346; meningitis, 141–42. *See also* Pneumonia
Startle reflex, 351, 419
State boards of nursing, 458–59, 462–65
Station of presenting part: in labor, 324, 329
Status epilepticus, 137, 396
Steapsin, 93
Steatorrhea, 115, 201
Steinmann pins, 248, 250
Stenosis: aortic, 168, 388; heart valve, 165; mitral, 168; pyloric, 390–91; tricuspid, 168
Sterilization (contraceptive), 365
Steroid hormones, 225
Steroids, 145, 413. *See also* Corticosteroids
Stimulants, 71
Stokes-Adams syndrome, 167
Stomach: cancer of, 208; decompressing, 206; diagnostic procedures, 114, 181, 200, 201; diet for surgery of, 100; inflammation of, 204–5; pyloric stenosis of, 390–91; structure and function of, 199; tubes, 206; ulceration of, 206
Stomatitis, 203
Stools: analysis of, 114–15, 201–2; newborn, 349. *See also* Bowel function
"Storm"/thyroid crisis, 228–29
Strains, 278–79
Streptococcus infections: glomerulonephritis, 219; impetigo, 238; meningitis, 141–42. *See also* Rheumatic fever
Stress, 10–11; cancer and, 260; regulation of stress response, 121. *See also* Anxiety; Somatoform disorders
Stress test, 157; fetoplacental status, 326
Striae gravidarum, 308, 311
Stridor, 182
Stroke, 147; drug administration to stroke victims, 298
Stroke volume (SV), 155
Stryker boots, 248
Stryker frame, 129
Stuttering, 383
Subarachnoid fluid, 121
Subarachnoid hematomas, 130–31, 147
Subarachnoid space, 121, 123, 125
Subcutaneous injections, 74–75, 79–81

Subdural hematomas, 130–31, 147
Sublimation: defined, 451
Sublingual salivary gland, 198
Submaxillary salivary gland, 198
Submucous resection (SMR), 190
Substance abuse, 442–45
Substantia nigra, 140
Sucking reflex, 419
Sucrase, 93
Suctioning: of chest, 191–92, 193–97; infant with endotracheal tube, 354; of tracheostomy, 191
Sudden infant death syndrome (SIDS), 388
Suicide, 430–31
Sulfamylon, 241
Sulfonamides, 70
Sulfonylureas, 231–32
Sunset eyes, 385
Superego: defined, 454
Supine hypotensive syndrome, 313, 331–32
Suppositories, 73; and the aged, 297
Suppression: defined, 451
Suprapubic cystostomy, 220
Suprapubic prostatectomy, 221
Supraventricular tachycardia, 161
Surfactants, 179
Surgical asepsis, 52
Surgical floor: nursing care on, 56
Suspensions, 74
Sweat glands, 236; aging process and, 286
Sweep check audiometry, 384
Swenson's pull-through, 391
Sylvan seizures, 396
Sylvan Technology Centers, 4–6
Symbolization: defined, 451
Symbols: for drug orders, 88
Sympathectomy, 41
Sympathetic nervous system: cardiovascular system control by, 153, 155–56; drug effects on, 72; function of, 122; origin of fibers of, 121
Synapses, 120
Synarthroses, 245
Syncope, 71, 157
Synergist muscles, 246
Syphilis, 29–30, 242, 292; pregnancy and, 242, 322–23; testing for, 117
Syrup of ipecac, 399
Syrups, 74
Systole, 34, 154, 285

T_3 resin uptake, 116, 223
T_4 resin uptake, 116, 223
Tablets, 73, 298
Tachyarrhythmias, 162, 167
Tachycardia, 432; drugs for, 161, 162; fetal, 332, 333; shock and, 61, 272
Tachypnea, 182; shock and, 61, 272
Talwin, 57
Tardive dyskinesia, 446